SPAS
The International Spa Guide™

5th Edition
1999-2000

**An International Passport to
Beauty, Fitness and Well-Being**

Co-editor --- Joseph H. Bain
Co-editor --- Eli Dror
Marketing --- Rafael Da Costa
Front Cover Design --- Robert Richards
Back Cover Photos ----------------------------------Chiva Som (Thailand), Grand Nirvana (Israel)

B.D.I.T., INC.
Port Washington, New York

B.D.I.T., Inc.
P. O. Box 1405
Port Washington, New York 11050
Email: bditusa@aol.com
Web: www.bdit.com

ISBN 0-890618-00-4
ISSN: 1041-2417

BDIT

ACKNOWLEDGMENT

B.D.I.T., Inc. wishes to acknowledge the assistance of the national tourist offices, the individual spas
and hotels, travel agents and tour operators, and advertisers who provided information, encouraged,
and supported the publication of the fifth edition of **Spas - The International Spa Guide**®.

CONTENTS

XIII FOREWORD
History, Classifications, Programs, Treatments,
Holistic, European Spas, Categories, Symbols

INTERNATIONAL SPAS

1 ANDORRA
Escaldes: Centre Thermal Andorra

3 ANTIGUA
St. John's: Sandals Antigua Resort & Spa

3 ARGENTINA
Buenos Aires: Tamara di Tella; Club Olympus;
Spa Marino
Mar Del Plata: Club de Mar;
Sheraton Mar del Plata Hotel
Colon: Quirinale Spa

5 ARUBA
Palm Beach: Radisson Aruba Resort, Spa & Casino;
Wyndham Aruba Beach Resort & Casino - La Spa

6 AUSTRALIA
Coolum (QLD): Hyatt-Regency Coolum & Spa
Brisbane (QLD): Clear Mountain Health Spa
Daylesford (VIC): Lake House
Kingston (TAS): Anubha Mountain Retreat
Katoomba (NSW): Lilianfels Blue Mountains
Kerrajong (NSW): Kurrajong Heights Health Farm
Surfers Paradise (QLD): Radisson Watermark
Sydney (NSW): The Observatory Hotel Day Spa,
Health & Leisure Club

9 AUSTRIA
Achenkirch: Posthotel Achenkirch
Bad Aussee: Hotel Erzherzog Johann; Villa Kristina
Bad Hall: Herzog Tassilo Kurhotel
Bad Hofgastein: Grand Park Hotel;
Kur & Sporthotel Moser; Kurhotel Germania;
Norica Kur & Sporthotel; Hotel Palace Gastein
Bad Ischl: Kurhotel Bad Ischl
Bad Kleinkirscheim: Hotel Romerbad;
Themenhotel Das Ronacher
Bad Mitterndorf: Vital Hotel Heilbrunn
Bad Tatsmannsdorf:
Steigenberger Bad Tatsmannsdorf
Bad Walternsdorf: Der Steirerhof;
Steigenberger Bad Walternsdorf Hotel
Baden bei Wien: Parkhotel Baden;
Sauerhof Grand Hotel; Hotel Schloss Weikersdorf

Badgastein: Best Western Hotel Weismayr;
Elisabethpark Hotel; Europäischer Hof;
Hoteldorf Grüner Baum; Kur & Sporthotel Miramonte;
Mozart Hotel; Slazburgerhof Hotel; Wildbad Hotel
Blumau: Rogner-Bad Blumau
Elbigenalp: Vital & Erlebnishotel Alpenrose
Ellmau: Der Baer Hotel
Gaschurn: Dr. Felbermayer
Dornbirn: Rickatsschwende
Haldensee: Hotel Liebes Rot-Flüh
Hirschegg: Ifen Hotel
Igls: Kurzentrum Parkhotel; Schlosshotel
Ischgl: Trofana Royal
Kitzbühel: Polly's Vital-Center
Leutasch: Hotel Quellenhof
Maurach: Sporthotel Alpenrose
Mieming: Wellnes Resort Schwartz
Obertauren: Kohlmayr Hotel
Pertisau: Hotel Fürstenhaus
Reuthe: Kurhotel Bad Reuthe
Saalfeden: Sporthotel Gut Brandlhof
Salzburg: Hotel Kobenzl; Hotel Schloss Fuschl
Schöcken: Hotel Widderstein
Schwaz: Natur Hotel Grafenast
Seefeld: Vital Hotel Royal
St. Leonhard: Sport & Vitalhotel Seppl
Telfs-Buchen: Interalpen-Hotel Tyrol
Warmbad-Villach: Josefinhof Hotel Im Park
Warth a. Arlberg: Wellnesshotel Warther Hof

25 BAHAMAS
Cable Beach / Nassau: Sandals Royal
Bahamian Resort & Spa

26 BELGIUM
Brussels: Metropole Hotel
Chaudfontaine: Palace Hotel
Knokke: la Reserve Hotel & Thalassa Center
Limelette: Chateau de Limelette & Centre Thalgo
Oostende: Iridia Thalassa; Thermae Palace
Spa: Hotel Alfa Balmoral; Domaines des Hautes Fagnes;
The Thermes de Spa

29 BELIZE
Maskal Village: Maruba Resort Jungle Spa

31 BERMUDA
Southampton: Sonesta Beach Hotel & Spa

32 BONAIRE
Kralendijk: Harbour Village Beach Resort

CONTENTS - THE INTERNATIONAL SPA GUIDE

33 BRAZIL
Caldas Novas: Pousada do Rio Quente
Florianoplis: The Brain Spa
São Paulo: The Maskoud Plaza

35 BULGARIA
Albena: Dobroudja Hotel & Spa; Hotel Imperial
Golden Sands: Hotel International
Kyustendil: Velbuzhd Hotel & Spa
Sandanski: Sandanski Hotel
St. Constantine: Grand Hotel Varna

40 CAMBODIA
Phenom Penn: Hotel Le Royal
Siem Reap: Grand Hotel D'Angkor

41 CANADA
Banff (BC): Banff Springs Hotel
Clinton (BC): Echo Valley Ranch Resort
Fairmont Hot Springs (BC):
Fairmont Hot Springs Resort
Harrison Hot Springs (BC):
Harrison Hot Springs Hotel
One Hundred Mile House (BC):
The Hills Health Ranch
Cambridge (ON):
Langdon Hall Country House Hotel & Spa
Chatam (ON): Best Western Wheels Inn
Grafton (ON): Ste-Anne's Country Inn & Spa
McKellar (ON): The Inn at Manitou
Zephyr (ON): High Fields Country Inn & Spa
Carleton-sur-Mer (QC): Acqua-Mer Thalassotherapie
Eastman (QC): Centre de Santé d'Estman
Magog-Orford (QC): Clinique Algothérapie;
Spa Chéribourg
Montréal (QC): Relais Santé Effi-Corp
Montpellier: Château Les Beaulne
Notre Dame de Lourdes (QC):
Station Santé - Maison d'Orient
Piedmont (QC): Relais des Monts
Pointe-au-Pic: Manoir Richelieu
Québec City (QC): Château Bonne Entente
Saint-Faustin (QC):
Centre de Santé - Sonia Blancard
Saint-Georges de Beauce (QC):
Hôtel le Georgesville
Saint-Paulin (QC): Le Baluchon
Shawinigan (QC): L'Escale Santé

52 CAYMAN ISLANDS
George Town: The Beauty Spa

52 CHILE
Maitencillo: Marbello Resort

Patagonia: Termas de Puyuhuapi Hotel & Spa
Santiago: San Cristobal Tower & Neptuno Spa

53 CHINA
Beijing: The Palace Hotel
Shanghai: Hotel Sofitel Hyland
Tianjin: Hyatt Tianjin

55 CHINA (HONG KONG)
Kowloon: Gold Coast Hotel - Balinese Spa;
The Peninsula Hotel & Spa

56 COSTA RICA
San José: Melia Comfort Carobici Hotel & Spa;
El Tucano Hotel; San José Palacio Spa & Casino;
Tara Resort Hotel

57 CROATIA
Duga Uvala: Hotel Croatia Duga Uvala
Opatija: Thalassotherapia
Sibenik: Thalassotherapy Institute & Hotel Ivan

59 CUBA
Piñar del Rio: San Diego de los Baños
Topes de Collantes: Topes de Collantes
Villa Clara: Horizontes Elguea Hotel & Spa
Viñales: Horizontes Rancho San Vicente

61 CURAÇAO
Piscadera Bay: Sonesta Beach Hotel & Casino

62 CYPRUS
Larnaca: Lordos Beach Hotel
Lefkosia: Cyprus Hilton Hotel
Lemesos: Four Seasons Hotel
Paphos: Coral Beach Hotel & Resort;
Paphos Amathus Beach Hotel

65 CZECH REPUBLIC
Frantiskovy Lazne: Imperial Hotel
Jachymov: Akademik Behounek;
Spa Sanatory Rodium Palace
Karlovy Vary: Bristol Spa Hotel; Elwa Sanatorium;
Grandhotel Pupp; Hotel Dvorak; Spa Hotel Imperial;
Spa Hotel Central; Spa Hotel Sirius; Spa Hotel Kolonáda
Lazne Beohrad: Ann'a Peat Spa
Luhacovice: Hotel Zalesi; Sanatorium Palace;
Spa House Moroava; Spa House Bedricha Smetany
Marianske Lazne: Hotel Exce;siar;
Spa Hotel Centralni Lazne; Spa Hotel Hvizda;
Spa Hotel Palace; Spa Hotel Royal
Podebrady: Hotel Bellevue Tlapak;
Spa Hotel Libensky
Trebon: Spa Sanatory Aurora

CONTENTS - THE INTERNATIONAL SPA GUIDE

72 DOMINICAN REPUBLIC
La Romana: Casa de Campo
Santo Domingo:
Renaissance Jaragua Hotel & Casino

73 EGYPT
Aswan: Hotel Aswan Oberoi Hotel & Spa
Hurghada: Dawar El Omda

75 FINLAND
Ikaalinen: Ikaalinen Spa
Kuusamo: Kuusamo Tropical Spa
Lapland: Spa Hotel Levitunturi
Naantali: Naantali Spa Hotel
Nokia: Nokia Spa Hotel Eden
Porvoo: Haikko Manor Spa
Tampere: Spa Hotel Tampere
Turku: Health Spa Ruissalo

80 FRANCE
Ajjacio: Best Western Eden Roc;
Sofitel Thalassa Portccio
Arzon: Hotel Miramar Port Crouesty
La Baule: Hotel Royal Thalasso
Biarritz: Miramar Hôtel
Capvern les Bains: Hôtel Le Laca
Contrexville: Hôtel Cosmos
Deauville: Biotherm Deauvile
Eugenie-Les-Bains: Les Pres d'Eugenie
Evian les Bains: Royal Club Evian
Paris: Royal Monceau Hôtel
Quiberon: Sofitel Diététique; Sofitel Thalassa Hôtel
Toulouse: Grand Hotel de L'Opera
Vichy: Hotel Les Celestins; Novotel Thermalia Hôtel

89 GERMANY
Bad Alexandersbad: Hotel Alexandersbad
Bad Bevensen: Grünings Landhaus Hotel
Bad Bruckenau: Dorint Hotel
Bad Duerkheim: Kurparkhotel
Bad Ems: Atlantis Kurhotel
Bad Füssing: Hotel Garni Villa Fortuna
Bad Griesbach: Gulfhotel Maxmilian; Parkhotel;
Hotel Fürstenhof
Bad Harzburg: Seela Hotel
Bad-Kissingen: Bristol Hotel;
Steigenberger Kurhaushotel
Bad Kreuznach: Hotel der Quellenhof;
Park Hotel Kurhaus
Bad-Lautenberg: Kneipp Kurhotel Heikenberg
Bad Mergentheim: Maritim Parkhotel
Bad Neuenahr-Ahrweiler:
Giffels Goldener Anker; Steigenberger Hotel
Bad-Orb: Steigenberger Bad Orb

Bad Reichenhall: Parkhotel Luisenbad;
Steigenberger Hotel Axelmanstein
Bad Saarow: Kempinsky Hotel Sporting Club Berlin
Bad Sazuflen: Maritim Staatabadhotel
Bad Urach: Hotel Graf Eberhard
Bad Wiesse: Hotel Graf Eberhard
Bad Wildbad: Sommerberg Hotel
Bad Wildungen: Maritim Badehotel
Bad Wöerishofen: Kneipp-Kurhotel;
Kurhotel Eichwald
Baden-Baden: Badhotel Zum Hirsch;
Brenner's Park Hotel & Spa; Quisisana Privathotel;
Schlosshotel Bühlerhöhe Beauty Farm & Health Spa;
Steigenberger Avance Badischer Hof
Badeweilier: Hotel Römebad
Bergisch Gladbach: Lancaster Beauty Farm
Berlin: Hotel Berlin
Freudenstadt: Schwartzwaldhof Hotel
Hindelang: Hotel Prinz-Luitpold-Bad;
Romantik Hotel Bad - Hotel Somme
Juist: Nordsee-Hotel Freese
Kassel: Parkhotel Emstaler Höhe
Rodach bei Coburg: Kurhotel am Thermalbad
Schlangebad: Parkhotel Schlangebad
Schliersee: Annabella Alpenhotel
Seesen: Hotel Seesen mit Beautyfarm
Speyer: RR Binshof Resort
Timmendorfer Strand: Maritim Seehotel
Weisbaden: Aukamm Hotel; Hotel Baeren;
Schwarzer Bock Hotel

105 GREAT BRITAIN - ENGLAND
Bath: Bath Spa Hotel;
Combe Grove Manor Hotel & Country Club
Droitwich Spa: Chateau Impney Hotel
Grayshott: Grayshott Hall
Henlow: Henlow Grange Health Farm
Hoar Cross: Hoar Cross Hall Health & Spa Resort
Ipswich: Shrubland Hall Health Clinic
Kintbury: Inglewood Health Hydro
Liphook: Forest Mere
New Milton: Chewton Glen Hotel
Packington: Springs Hydro
Ragdale: Ragdale Hall
Taplow: Cliveden
Taunton: Cedar Falls Health Farm
Torquay: Lorrens Haelath Hydro
Wigginton: Champneys

113 GREAT BRITAIN - SCOTLAND
Auchterarder: Champneys the Health Spa
East Kilbride: Stakis East Kilbride
Edinburgh: The Balmoral Edinburgh;
Dalmahoy Hotel Golf & Country Club

CONTENTS - THE INTERNATIONAL SPA GUIDE

Peebles: Peebles Hydro Hotel
St. Andrews: The Old Course Hotel Golf Resort & Spa
Troon: Marine Highland Hotel
Turnberry: Turnberry Hotel, Golf Courses & Spa

116 GREECE
Kamena Vourla Spa: Astir Hotel Galini
Loutraki (Pozar): Loutraki Spa
Loutraki Spa: Hotel Poseidon Club; Therme Loutraki
Siderokastro: Siderokastro Spa
Vravrona: Mare Hostrum Thalasso
Crete Island: Royal Mare Thalasso
Ikaria Island: Ikaria Spa
Lesvos Island: Thermi Spa

119 GRENADA
St George's: Allamanda Beach Resort & Spa;
La Source

120 HUNGARY
Budapest: Danubius Aquincum Hotel; Danubius
Grand Hotel Margitsziget; Danubius Hotel Gellerit;
Danubius Thermal Hotel Margitsziget;
Danubius Thermal Hotel Helia
Bukfurdo: Danubius Thermal & Sporthotel Bük
Eger: Hotel Flöra
Gyula: Hotel Erkel
Heviz: Danubius Thermal Hotel Aqua;
Thermal Hotel Héviz; Rogner Hotel Lotus Therme
Sarvar: DanubiusThermal Hotel Sarvar
Zalakrosi: Men Dan Thermal Aparthotel

128 ICELAND
Hvergerdi: Nature Health Association of Iceland
Ryekjanes Peninsula: The Blue Lagoon

129 INDIA
Goa: Four Seasons resort Leela Beach
Jaipur: Rajvilas Jaipur

130 INDONESIA
Bali Island
Jimbaran Bay: Four Seasons Bali Jimbaran Bay
Legian Beach: Hotel Imperial Bali;
Hotel & Residence Jaykarta Bali; The Oberoi Bali;
The Legion Bali; White Rose Hotel
Manggis: The Seai Hotel
Nusa Dua: Aston Bali Resort & Spa; Club Med Bali;
Gran Mirage Resort; Nusa Dua Beach Resort;
Nikko Bali Resort & Spa;
Padma: Bali Padma Hotel
Ubud: Banyan Tree Kamandalu;
Four Seasons Bali Sayan; The Chedi Ubud
Ungasan: Bali Cliff Resort

Java Island
Yogyakata: Hyatt Regency Yogyakarta
Lombok Island
Kelamata Pujut Praya: Novotel Lombok Coralia
Medana Beach: The Oberoi Lombok

135 IRELAND
Coolakay: Powerscourt Springs Health Farm
Cork: Thalassotherapy Centre
Galaway: Galaway Bay Health Farm
Horseleap: Temple Country House & Spa
Killaloe: Tinarana House
Mooresfort: An Tearmann Beag
Westport: Cloona Health Centre

138 ISRAEL
Dead Sea Spas: Caesar Premier Hotel Dead Sea;
Carlton Galei Zohar Hotel; Ein Gedi Resort Hotel & Spa;
Grand Nirvana on the Dead Sea Spa; Hod Hotel;
Hyatt Regency Dead Sea Resort & Spa;
Radisson Moriah Gardens Dead Sea;
Radisson Moriah Plaza Dead Sea Hotel & Spa
Eilat: Herods Sheraton Resort; Orchid Hotel & Resort
Haifa: Carmel Forest Spa Resort
Rosa Pina: Mitzpeh Ha'Yamim Hotel
Tiberias: Holiday Inn Tiberias

146 ITALY
Abano Terme: Bristol Buja Hotel; Columbia Hotel;
Due Torri Morisini; Grand Hotel Trieste & Victoria;
Metropole Terme; President Hotel, Quisisana Terme Hotel;
La Residence Hotel; Ritz Terme Hotel;
Smeraldo Terme Hotel; Terme Patria
Bellagio: Grand Hotel Villa Serbelloni
Capri Island: Europa Palace Hotel - Capri Beauty
Farm; Hotel Punta Tagara
Castrocaro Terme: Grand Hotel Terme
Chinciano Terme: Spadeus
Fiuggi: Grand Hotel Palazzo della Fonte;
Silva Hotel Splendid
Ischia Island - Ischia Porta:
Continental Terme Hotel; Grand Hotel Excelsior Belvedere;
Grand Hotel Punta Molino Terme; Jolly Hotel delle Terme
Ischia Island - Lacco Ameno:
Albergo Terme San Montano; La Reginella Terme;
Regina Isabella Hotel
Merano: Palace Hotel
Montecatini Terme: Cappelli-Croce di Savoia;
Grand Hotel Croce di Mata; Grand Hotel e la Pace;
Grand Hotel Tamerici & Principe; Grand Hotel Vittoria
Montegrotto Terme: Continental Hotel Terme;
Hotel Espalanade Tergesto; Ineternational Hotel Bertha
Rimini: Il Grand Hotel
Rome: Rome Cavalieri Hilton

CONTENTS - THE INTERNATIONAL SPA GUIDE

Salsomaggiore: Centrale Bagni Hotel; Grand Hotel Poro
Sardinia Island: Forte Village
Saturnia: Terme di Saturnia
Sirmione: Grand Hotel Terme
Stresa: Centro Benessere di Stresa

163 JAMAICA
Irishtown: Strawberry Hill - Aveda Spa
Montego Bay: Half Moon Golf Tennis & Beach Club;
Round Hill Hotel & Villas;
Royal Court Hotel & Natural Health Retreat
Negril: Sandal Negril Beach Resort & Spa; Swept Away
Ocho Rios: Charlie's Spa at Sans Souci;
Elysium Spa & Salon; Enchanted Garden;
Sandals Dunn's River Golf Resort & Spa

166 JAPAN
Atami: New Fujiyia Hotel
Beppu: Sunginoi Hotel
Fukuoka City: Grand Hyatt Fukuoka
Hakodate: Hokodate - Onuma Prince Hotel;
Hakodate Yunokawa Wakamatsu
Hakone: Fujiya Hotel; Ichinoyu
Ibusuki: Ibusuki Iwasaki Hotel;
Ibusuki Park Hotel Hakusikan
Matsuyama City: Funaya Hotel
Misasa Spa: Hotel Mansuiro
Naha City: Loisir Hotel Okinawa;
Renaissance Okinawa Resort
Naruko: Yusaya Country Inn
Noboribetsu: Daiichi Takimotokan;
Noboribetsu Grand Hotel; Kanko Hotel Takinoya
Osaka City: Imoerial Hotel Osaka;
Hotel Nikko Kansai Airport; Rits-Carlton Osaka
Sendai: Hotel Zuiho
Shima Spa: Sekizenkan
Shirabu: Nakaya Ryokan
Tochiomata: Hogando
Tokyo: Four Seasons at Chinzan-So; Hotel Nikko Tokyo
Yunohira: Shimizu Ryokan

176 JORDAN
Aman: Hotel Intercontinental Jordan
Hammamat Ma'in: Ashtue Ma'in Hotel
Salt Land Village: Dead Sea Spa Hotel

177 LATVIA
Jurmala: Baltija Hotel; Majori Spa; Rigas Licis Hotel

178 LITHUANIA
Druskininkai: Spa "Egle"

179 LUXEMBOURG
Mondorf-les-Bains: Mondorf le Domaine Thermal

180 MACAU
Taipa Island: Hyatt Regency Macau

181 MALAYSIA
Johor Bahru: Hyatt Regency
Kuala Terengganu:
Berjaya Redang Golf & Spa Resort

182 MALDIVES
Male: Banyan Tree Maldives; Kuda Huraa Reef Resort

183 MALTA
Gozo Island
San Lawrenz: Thalgo Marine Cure Center
Malta Island
St. Julians: The Apollo Club; Westin Dragonara
Resort; Spa Mediteranée Thalassotherapie
San Anton: Athenaum Spa

186 MEXICO
Cabo San Lucas: Villa Del Palmar Resort & Spa;
Casa del Mar; Melia Cabo Real Beach & Golf Resort
Cancun: Calinda Beach & Spa Cancun;
Casa Turquesa; Fiesta Americana Condesa Cancún;
Melia Cancun Resort & Spa
Cihuatlan: Hotel Bel-Air Costa Careyes
Cuautla: Hotel Hacienda Cocoyoc
Cuernavaca: Hosteria las Quintas;
Mission del Sol Resort & Spa
Guadalajara: Rio Caliente Hot Springs Spa
Isla Mujeres: Puerto Isla Mujeres Resort & Yacht Club;
Ixtapan: Hotel Spa Ixtapan
Lake Tequesquitengo:
Villa Bejar Hotel & Grand Spa
Mazatlan: El Cid Mega Resort
Mexico City: Hotel Marquis Reforma & Spa
Playa del Carmen: El Dorado Resort & Spa
Puerto Vallarta: La Jolla de Mismaloya Resort & Spa;
La Jolla de Mismaloya Resort & Spa; Paradise Village
Beach Resort & Spa; Qualton Club & Spa Vallarta;
Velas Vallarta Grand Suites Resort
Rosarito: Rosarito Beach Hotel & Spa
San Miguel de Allende:
La Puertercita Boutique'otel & Spa
Tecate: Rancho La Puerta
Valle de Bravo: Avandaro Golf & Spa Resort

197 MONACO
Monte Carlo: Les Thermes Marines

199 NETHERLANDS
Bad Valkenburg a/d Geul: Thermae 2000
Bergambacht: Hotel de Arendshoeve
Houthem/St. Gerlach: Château L'Ermitage

CONTENTS - THE INTERNATIONAL SPA GUIDE

Nieuweschans: Golden Tulip Fontana Spahotel
Ootmarsum: Hotel de Wiemsel
Schevningen: Kuur Thermen Vitalizee
Venlo: De Bovenste Molen Hotel
Zandvoort: Golden Tulip Zandvoort Hotel

203 NEW ZELAND
Hanmer Springs: Alpine Spa Lodge;
Hanmer Springs Thermal Reserve
Motueka: Kimi Ora Health Resort
Queenstown: Millbrook Resort
Rotorua: Millenium Rotorua; Moose Lodge;
Polynesian Spa; Regal Geyserland Hotel;
Sheraton Rotorua Hotel

206 PALAU (REPUBLIC OF)
Koror: Outrigger Palasia Hotel Palau

206 POLAND
Busko: Marconi
Ciechocinek: Dom Zdrojowy
Cieplice Zdroj: Dom Zdrojowy
Inowroclaw: Inowroclaw Health Resort
Kolobrzeg: Mewa V & Muszelka
Krynica: Nowy Dom Zdrojowy
Kudowa: Zameczek
Polanica: Wielka Pieniawa
Polczyn: Irena

213 PORTUGAL
Algarve: Vilalara Thalasso
Termas de Curia: Grand Hotel da Curia
Termas de Luso: Grand Hotel de Luso
Vidalgo: Vidalgo Palace Hotel

217 PUERTO RICO (U.S.A)
Dorado: Hyatt Regency Dorado Beach & Cerromar Beach
Los Croabas: El Conquistador Resort & Country Club
Rio Mar: The Westin Rio Mar Beeach Resort
San Juan: Caribe Hilton; Ritz-Carlton San Juan Hotel &
Casino; San Juan Grand Beach Resort & Casino:

218 ROMANIA
Baile Felix: Baile Felix Spa
Baile Herculane: Baile Herculane Spa
Bucharest: Flora Hotel; Otopeni Clinical Centre
Coastal Spas: Doina Cure Hotel; Eforie Nord Spa;
Europa Hotel; Mangalia Cure Hotel
Covasna: Covasna Spa
Sinaia: Mara Hotel
Sovata: Sovata Spa

225 RUSSIA
Moscow: Aerostar Hotel; Hotel Metropole Moscow

Sochi: Dagomys Tourist Complex; Kamelia Hotel

227 SINGAPORE
Singapore: Clark Hatch Life Spa; Lifestyle Spa &
Fitness Centre; Ritz Carlton Millenia Singapore;
Sheraton Towers Singapore; St. Gregory Javanna Spa

228 SLOVAKIA
Bardejov: Bardejovské Kúpele - Ozón
Piestany Spa: Balnea Esplanade; Balnea
Grand-Splendid; Minotel Magnolia; Thermia Palace
Strbske Pleso: Helios
Trencianske Teplice: Krym Hotel; Pax Hotel

234 SLOVENIA
Atomske Toplice: Atomske Toplice Health Resort
Catez: Terme Hotel
Moravske Toplice: Moravske Toplice Spa
Portoroz: Grand Hotel Palace
Radenci: Radenci Health Resort
Rogaska Slatina: Rogaska Health Resort
Smarjeske Toplice: Smarjeske Toplice Health Resort

239 SOUTH AFRICA
Badplaas: Aventura Badpas
Cape Town: The Table Bay Hotel at the Waterfront
Pretoria/Erasmia: Hoogland Health Hydro
Stellenbosch: High Rustenberg Hydro
Warmbaths: Aventura Spa

242 SPAIN
Archena: Hotel Termas
Barcelona: Princesa Sofia Inter-Continental Barcelona
Cadiz: Iberostar Royal Andalus Golf Hotel
Caldas de Malavella: Vichy Catalan
Fuengirola: Hotel Baylos Andaluz
Isla de la Toja: Gran Hotel de la Toja
Mallorca Island: Arabella Golf
Marbella: Incosol Spa & Resort
Puente Viesgo: Gran Hotel Puente Viesgo
Tarragona: Hotel Termes Montbrio
Vila de Caldes: Vila de Caldes Hotel & Spa

249 ST. LUCIA (W.I.)
Castries: Jalousie Hilton Resort & Spa;
Le Sport; Royal St. Lucian

251 ST. MAARTEN (N.A.)
Pelican Key: L'Aqualigne
Maho Bay: Peter's Health Spa

252 SWITZERLAND
Adelboden: Park Hotel Bellevue

CONTENTS - THE INTERNATIONAL SPA GUIDE

Ascona: Hotel Casa Berno; Hotel Eden Roc; Giardino Ascona
Bad Ragaz: Grand Hotel Hof Ragaz; Grandholtel Quellenhof; Hotel Tamina
Bad Schinznach: Kurhotel Im Park
Bad Vals: Kurhotes Therme Vals
Baden: Hotel Verenahof
Cademario: Kurhaus Cademario
Clarens-Montreux: Centre de Révitalisation Clinique; Clinic La Prairie
Crans / Montana: Hotel Crans Ambassador
Gstaad: Grand Hotel Park
Hüttwilen: Schloss Steinegg
Interlaken: Victoria-Jungfrau Grand Hotel & Spa
Kastanienbaum: Seehotel Kastanienbaum Luzern
Lake Geneva: Le Mirador Resort Hotel & Spa
Lausanne: Lausanne Palace
Lenk: Kurhotel Lenkerhof
Leukerbad: Badhotel Bristol; Grichting & Badnerhol Hotel; Maison Blanche Grand Bain
Montreux: Grand Hotel Excelsior / Biotonus Montreux
Morschach: Swiss Holiday Park
Rheinfelden: Park-Hotel am Rhein
St. Moritz: Badrutt's Palace Hotel; Kulm Hotel; Parkhotel Kurhaus
Vals: Hotel Therme
Yverdon-les-Bains: Grand Hotel des Bains
Zurzach: Parkhotel Golden Tulip

268 TAIWAN
Kaoksiung: Grand Hi-Lai Hotel
Taitung: Hotel Royal Chipen Spa

269 THAILAND
Bangkok: Oriental Bangkok; Sheraton Grande; Sukhumvit Grand Spa & Fitness Club; The Westin Banyan Tree & Banyan Tree Spa
Chiang Mai: The Regent Chiang Mai
Hua-Hin: Chiva-Sam International Health Resort
Phuket: Banyan Tree Phuket & Banyan Tree Spa
Ranong: Jansom Thara Hot Spa Health Resort

272 TRINDAD & TOBAGO
Black Rock: Le Grand Courlan Resort & Spa
Scarborough: Coco Reef Resort & Spa

273 TUNISIA
Sousse: Abou Nawas Diar El Andalouss Hotel
Tunis: Le Palace Tunis

274 TURKEY
Balçova-Izmir: Balçova Agamemnon Thermal Hotel; Thermal Prenses
Bursa: Celik Palas Hotel Thermal; Kervansarai Hotel

Cesme: Altinyunus Holiday Resort; Turban Cesme Hotel
Pamukkale: Club Colossea; Hierapolis Thermal
Silivri: Klassis Golf & Country Club & Thalgo Health Farm

278 TURKS & CAICOS
Providenciales Island: Beaches Resort & Spa

279 UNITED STATES OF AMERICA

279 ALASKA
Artic Crcle: Circle Hot Springs Resort
Chena Hot Springs: Chena Hot Springs Resort

280 ARIZONA
Carefree: Golden Door Spa at the Boulders
Mesa: Buckhorn Mineral Wells Spa
Phoenix/Scottsdale: The Arizona Biltmore Resort & Spa; Hyatt Regency Scottsdale; Marriott's Camelback Inn; The Mist Spa; The Phoenician; Scottsdale Hilton Resort & Villas; Scottsdale Princess Spa;
Sedona: Enchantmenrt Resort & Spa; Los Abrigados
Tucson: Canyon Ranch; Golden Door Spa/The Lodge; Loews Ventura Canyon Resort; Miraval Life in Balance; Omni Tucson National Resort & Spa; Stepping Stone Spa; The Westin La Paloma; Westward Look Resort

287 ARKANSAS
Eureka Springs: Palace Hotel & Bath House
Hot Springs: Arlington Resort Hotel & Spa; Downtowner Hotel & Spa; Hot Springs Park Hilton Hotel; Majestic Hotel & Spa

289 CALIFORNIA
Big Sur: Post Ranch Inn & Spa; Ventana Inn
Calbasas: The Ashram Health Retreat
Calistoga: Dr. Wilkinson's Hot Springs; Golden Haven Hot Springs Spa; Mount View Hotel; Silver Rose Inn; Village Inn & Spa
Carlsbad: La Costa; Olympic Resort Hotel & Spa
Carmel Valley: Carmel Country Spa
City of Industry: Industry Hills Sheraton Resort & Spa
Corona: Glen Ivy Hot Springs
Coronado: Le Meridien San Diego
Del Mar: L'Auberge Del Mar Resort & Spa
Desert Hot Springs: Desert Hot Springs Spa Hotel; Lido Palms Spa Resort; Mineral Springs Hotel & Spa; Two Bunch Palms Resort & Spa; We Care Health Retreat
Escondido: Castle Creek Inn Resort & Spa; Golden Door
Garberville: Heartwood Institute
Grass Valley: Sivananda Ashram Yoga Farm
Indian Wells: Hyatt Grand Champions Resort; Renaissance Esmeralda Resort & Spa
La Jolla: Chopra Center For Well Being

CONTENTS - THE INTERNATIONAL SPA GUIDE

La Quinta: Spa La Quinta
Los Angeles: Miyako Inn & Spa;
The New Otani Hotel & Garden
Murrieta: Murrieta Hot Springs Resort & Health Spa
Oakland: The Claremont Resort & Spa
Ojai: The Oaks at Ojai; Ojai Valley Inn & Spa
Palm Desert: Marriot's Desert Springs;
Palm Valley Country Club
Palm Springs: Merv Griffin's Resort Hotel &
Givenchy Spa; Palm Springs Hilton Resort;
The Palms at Palm Springs; Spa Hotel & Casino
Rancho Mirage: The Spa at the Ritz Carlton
Redwood City: Sandra Caron European Spa
San Diego: San Diego Hilton Resort & Spa
San Francisco: Hotel Nikko San Francisco
Santa Barbara: Radisson Hotel Sanata Barbara
Santa Monica: Pritikin Longevity Center & Spa
Sonoma: Sonoma Mission Inn & Spa
South Lake Tahoe: The Keys at Lake Tahoe
St. Helena: Inn at Southbridge's Health Spa Napa
Valley; Spa at Meadwood Resort; White Sulfur Springs
Resort & Spa
Ukiah: Vichy Hot Springs Resort Inn
Vista: Cal-A-Vie
Woodside: The Lodge at Skylonda

309 COLORADO
Beaver Creek: The Charter At Beaver Creek
& Spa Struck
Breckenridge: The Lodge at Breckenridge
Colorado Springs: The Spa at the Broadmoor
Denver: Oxford Aveda Spa & Salon
Glenwood Springs: Glenwood Hot Springs Lodge
Gunnison: Waunita Hot Springs Ranch
Idaho Springs: Indian Springs Resort
Ouray: Box Canyon Lodge & Hot Springs; Wiesbaden
Hot Springs Spa & Lodgings
Telluride: The Peaks at Telluride & Golden Door Spa
Vail: The Lodge & Spa at Cordillera;
Marriott Vail Mountain Resort & Spa Struck;
Sonnenalp Resort of Vail; Vail Athletic Club Hotel & Spa;
Vail Cascade Hotel Club & Spa
Ward: Four Seasons Spa at Gold Lake Mountain Resort

313 CONNECTICUT
Norwich: Norwich Inn & Spa
Wesrbrook: Water's Edge Inn & Resort

314 FLORIDA
Bonita Springs: Shangri-La & Spa
Clearwater: Belleview Biltmore Resort & Spa
Coral Gables: The Biltmore Hotel
Fort Lauderdale: Hyatt Regency Pier 66 & Spa;
Wyndham Resort & Spa

Fort Myers: Sonesta Sanibel Harbour Resort
Hallandale: Regency Spa
Key West: Caribbean Spa & The Pier House Resort
Lake Buena Vista: Buena Vista Palace Resort &
Spa; Grand Floridian Spa Health Club; Hilton Walt Disney
World Village; Spa at the Disney Institute
Miami / Miami Beach: Agua at the Delano
Hotel; Doral Golf Resort & Spa; Eden Roc Resort & Spa;
Fontainebleau Hilton Resort & Spa; Hotel
Inter-Continental Miami; Lido Spa Hotel; The Spa
Internazionale at Fisher Island; Turnberry Isle Health Spa
Palm Beach / West Palm Beach:
Four Seasons Palm Beach; Hippocrates Health Institute;
PGA National Resort & Spa; Ritz-Carlton Palm Beach
Pompano Beach: Spa Atlantis; The Spa at Palm-Aire
Ponte Verda Beach: Ponte Verda Inn & Club
St. Petersburg: Don CeSar Beach Resort & Spa
Sarasota: The Colony Beach & Tennis Resort
Tampa: Safety Harbor Resort & Spa;
The Spa at Saddlebrook Resort Tampa

325 GEORGIA
Atlanta: Ritz-Carlton Buckhead; Swissotel Atlanta
Braselton: Chateau Elan Winery & Resort
Sea Island: The Sea Island Spa at The Cloister

327 HAWAII
Hawaii Island
Kamuela/Kohala: Four Seasons Resort
Hualalai Spa & Sports Club; Kohala Spa at Hilton
Waikoloa Village; Kona Village Resort; The Orchid at
Mauna Lani
Kauai Island
Koloa: Hawaiian Wellness Holiday; Hyatt Regency
Kauai Resort & Spa
Lihue: Kauai Marriott Resort & Beach Club
Maui Island
Hana: Hana-Maui Wellness Center
Kapalua: Ritz Calton Kapalua
Wailea Beach: Grand Wailea Resort & Spa
Oahu Island
Kapolei: Ihilani Resort & Spa

331 IDAHO
Coeur d'Alene: Spa at Coeur d'Alene Resort

332 ILLINOIS
Chicago: Four Seasons Hotel Chicago
Gilman: The Heartland

333 INDIANA
Chesterton: Indian Oaks Resort & Spa
French Lick: French Lick Springs Resort
Maukport: Orbis Farm

X

CONTENTS - THE INTERNATIONAL SPA GUIDE

334 IOWA
Des Moines: Savery Hotel & Spa
Fairfield: The Raj Maharishi

335 LOUISIANA
New Orleans: Avenue Plaza & Spa

336 MAINE
Poland Springs: Poland Springs Health Institute
Raymond: Northern Pines Health Resort

337 MASSACHUSETTS
Boston / Cambridge: Boston Harbor Hotel;
Four Seasons Hotel Boston; The Charles Hotel
Lancaster: Maharishi Ayur-Veda
Lenox: Canyon Ranch; Kripalu Center for Yoga & Health

340 MINNESOTA
Litchfield: Birdwing Spa
Minnetonka: Spa at The Marsh

341 MISSOURI
Excelsior Springs: The Elms Resort & Spa
Osage Beach: The Lodge of Four Seasons;
Marriott's Spa at Tan Tar A Resort
Washburn: Wholistic Life Center

342 MONTANA
Anaconda: Fairmont Hot Springs Resort
Boulder: Boulder Hot Springs Hotel
Pray: Chico Hot Springs Lodge

343 NEVADA
Crystal Bay: Cal Neva Resort Hotel, Spa & Casino
Genoa: Walley's 1862 Hot Springs Resort
Las Vegas: Bellagio - The Resort Spa Bellagio;
Caesars Palace; Cenegenics Ant-Aging Center;
Desert Inn Hotel & Casino; Golden Nugget Hotel &
Casino; Luxor Las Vegas; MGM Grand Hotel Casino;
The Mirage; Treasure Island at The Mirage
Mesquite: CasBlanca Casino Resort Spa
Reno: Silver Legacy

347 NEW JERSEY
Atlantic City: The Spa at Bally's Park Place;
The Spa at Trump Plaza
Long Branch: The Spa at Ocean Place Hilton Resort
Short Hills: The Hilton at Short Hills

349 NEW MEXICO
Galisteo: Vista Clara Ranch Resort Spa
Ojo Callente: Callente Mineral Springs Spa
Santa Fe: The Thousand Waves

250 NEW YORK
Bolton Landing: The Sagamore
Hunter: Cooperhead Inn & Spa;
Vatra Mountain Valley Lodge & Spa
Lake Placid: The Spa at The Mirror Lake
Montauk: Guerney's Inn Resort & Spa
Neversink: New Age Health Spa
New York City: The Barbizon Hotel; Essex
House - Hotel Nikko; The Peninsula New York & Spa
Saratoga Springs: Gideon Putnam Hotel

353 NORTH CAROLINA
Blowing Rock: Westglow Spa
Durham: Duke University Diet & Fitness Center;
Structure House Village
Lake Toxaway: The Spa at The Greystone Inn

355 OHIO
Aurora: Mario's Int'l Spa & Hotel
Grand Rapids: The Kerr House

357 OREGON
Detroit: Breitenbush Hot Springs
Warm Springs: Kah-Nee-Ta Resort

358 PENNSYLVANIA
East Stroudsburg: Deerfield Manor
Farmington: Nemacolin Woodlands

359 SOUTH CAROLINA
Charleston: Charleston Harbor Hilton Resort;
Woodlanbds Resort Inn
Hilton Head: Hilton Head Health Institute

361 TENNESSEE
Waynesboro: Tennessee Fitness Spa

361 TEXAS
Arlington: The Greenhouse
Austin: Barton Creek Conference Resort;
Lake Austin Resort
Dallas: The Spa atThe Cooper Aeobics Center;
Wyndham Anatole Hotel; Four Seasons Resort & Spa
Houston: The Spa at The Houstonian;
The Woodlands Executive Conference Center & Resort
San Antonio: Alamo Plaza Spa The Menger Hotel

365 UTAH
Hurricane: Pah Tempe Hot Springs Resort
Ivins: Red Mountain Spa
St. George: Green Valley Spa Tennis & Fitness Resort
Park City: Stein Eriksen Lodge
Snowbird: The Cliff Lodge & Spa

CONTENTS - THE INTERNATIONAL SPA GUIDE

368 VERMONT
Killington Ski Area: Killington at The Woods;
New Life Hiking Spa; Green Maountain at Fox Run
Manchester Village: The Equinox Hotel
Resort & Spa
Stowe: Golden Eagle Resort; Stowflake Inn & Resort;
Topnotch at Stowe Resort & Spa
Stratton Mountain: New Life Spa

371 VIRGINIA
Hot Springs: The Homestead
Williamsburg: Spa at Kingsmill Resort

375 WASHINGTON
Bellevue: The Spa at Bellevue Club Hotel
Orcas Island: Rosatio Resort & Spa
Snoqualmie: The Alish Lodge & Spa

376 WEST VIRGINIA
Berkeley Springs: Coolfront Resort
White Sulphur Springs: The Greenbrier

378 WISCONSIN
Lake Geneva / Fontana: Fontana Spa at
The Abbey Resort; Interlaken Resort & Country Spa
Osceola: Aveda Spa Retreat

375 WYOMING
Jackson: The Spa at Grand Targhee Ski & Summer Resort
Thermopolis: Holiday Inn of the Waters

376 VENEZUELA
Cumanagoto: Sofite Cumanagoto
Margarita Island: Ista Bonita Golf & Beach
Hotel; La Samanna Hotel & Thalassotherapy Center
Puerto La Cruz: Golden Rainbow Maremares

380 VIRGIN ISLANDS (U.S.A.)
St. Croix: The Bucaneer
St. Thomas: Bolongo Bay Beach Club Villas;
Marriott Frenchman's Reef & Morningstar Resort

381 SPAS AT SEA (CRUISE SHIPS)

386 INTERNATIONAL DAY SPAS

387 U.S.A. DAY SPAS

396 MAKETPLACE

400 SPA GLOSSARY

A DISCLAIMER

Although every effort was made to ensure the accuracy of the information in this guide, B.D.I.T., Inc. and its editors are not responsible for any errors or inaccurate information for the spa programs, treatments, services offered, prices or advertising statements of the individual spas, or hotels. Programs, treatments, services and prices are the responsibility of each establishment and may change due to management changes. Prices depend on various factors that affect the international travel industry including inflation, exchange rate fluctuations, and price increases. When selecting a spa that offers dietary programs, strenuous exercise, or medical treatments, it is strongly recommended to seek the advise of a physician to determine the appropriate programs as they relate to your individual state of health.

The fifth edition of the International Spa Guide has been thoroughly revised and updated to include new information, and keep up with global changes that occurred since the printing of the fourth edition. This edition includes 76 countries worldwide and new Spas from Andorra to the Virgin Islands. No other Spa guide has so much information to offer with equal abundance of high quality Spas and unlimited wellness holidays choices. This guide truly address itself to need of the modern Spa aficionados who demand reliable information. We hope that **Spas - The International Spa guide**© (5th edition) will help you make positive changes in your life, achieve your health and fitness goals and reward your body and soul with the exotic treatments that you deserve.

SHORT HISTORICAL BACKGROUND: Ancient civilizations such as the Greeks, Romans, Chinese and Japanese had a special place in their culture for the unique therapeutic benefits provided by bathing in mineral waters and hot springs. It is not known when the tradition first started as a way to promote or restore good health, but it is certain that during Greek and Roman times it became a part of their medical routine and hydrotherapy was an integral part of their lifestyle. Heracles, in ancient Greece contributed to the dissemination of the knowledge attributed to the therapeutic power of mineral waters. Greeks and Romans pumped pure mountain waters into their towns' water supply for drinking or bathing purposes. Thermal baths were essential to the Roman's daily life and local spring waters were developed for their health-giving properties.

SPAS: After the fall of the Roman Empire, popular towns with hot springs continued to invest in their natural resources. The town of Spa in Belgium, for example, became known for its "miraculous" springs and was fashionable with kings, statesmen, writers, poets, doctors and physicians from the 15th century on. Peter the Great of Russia went to Spa for a cure and a plaque, commemorating this event testifies that he felt much better for it. Spas remained popular in Europe until the outbreak of the First World War. After the war, and with the institutionalization of health care programs they lost their appeal. Most doctors were inclined to tell their patient that anything that waters can do, pills can do better. But, since the early 1970's there has been a notable change of attitude towards the benefits of Spas. More and more doctors and individuals rediscover the advantage and benefits of the natural heal-

ing properties of hot springs, mineral and sea water spas. The town of Spa donated her name as a generic term to a new breed of health resorts world wide ever since.

MODERN SPAS: Unlike the traditional European spas which originally evolved around thermal mineral waters and hot springs, the U.S.A., and other countries with no similar tradition have expanded the definition of spa to include health resorts, centers and institutes that promote and educate how to achieve healthier lifestyles based on exercise, fitness , balanced nutrition, and a variety of pampering and beauty treatments. The modern spas major philosophy is that a spa should teach healthy lifestyle and not just focus on the cure. Most modern spas respond to a contemporary need of individuals who wish to loose weight, get in shape, or just luxuriate in exotic body pampering treatments to regenerate, re-energize and revitalize their body and soul.

New discoveries by prominent researchers in West Germany, Switzerland and Romania helped develop new drugs and techniques to fight the aging process and restore good health. These new techniques known as the Aslan therapy, or fresh cell therapy add new dimension to the term spa in the respect that they too hold the promise of the legendary "Fountain of Youth". Modern Spas cover a wide range of retreats, resorts, and specialized centers. The common denominator for all the spas is that they are live-in places where guests usually stay for at least a few days or for the duration of the spa program. Some offer serious health programs with professional and medical supervision, others will do the most to pamper you and relieve you from stress, or unwanted weight. Some are classic spas in the sense that they provide thermal and/or mineral water therapy.

HOW TO CHOOSE A SPA: This guide contains information on more than 900 Spas in 75 countries around the world including the USA. The Spas are classified according to seven categories: 1. **Hot Springs/Mineral Water Spas**, 2. **Diet and Fitness Spas**, 3. **Beauty Spas**, 4. **Medical Spas**, 5. **Revitalization Clinics**, 6. **New Age Spas** and 7. **Holistic Spas**. A spa may offer one or more of thesecategories. You can choose your spa by geographical location: continent, region or country, or by the benefits you are looking for: medical treatments, health and diet programs, or beauty treatments. When selecting a spa that offers medical benefits it is recommended to check with your physician.

This guide provides information about each spa's facilities, programs and treatments. You will also find rates for spa packages when available. The rates are only indicative and represent the price range that you can expect. Rates do change due to inflation, foreign exchange fluctuations, and season. Therefore, you should confirm rates with the spas, their representatives, or the travel agents that offer specialized spa packages. We hope that this guide will assist you in selecting the Spa which is best for you, and help you discover a new world of an exciting healthful vacation.

HOTEL / SPA CATEGORIES: The guide contains star symbols to describe the standard category of each spa or spa hotel. The stars reflect an overall standard that includes the hotel's category, amenities, Spa facilities and services as follows which may vary among countries:

❤❤❤❤❤ Deluxe
❤❤❤❤+ Superior First Class
❤❤❤❤ First Class
❤❤❤ Tourist Class
❤❤ Budget Class

SPA PROGRAMS & TREATMENTS:
The spas are classified according to the programs and treatments that they offer. Each symbol stands for one category as follows:

 Medical programs or treatments with medical supervision

 Thermal, mineral, hot springs and Thalassotherapy programs

 Fitness, exercise and diet programs

 Beauty, cosmetic, aesthetic & pampering programs

 Revitalization program and rejuvenation treatments

 New Age program

Holistic Program

Holistic Health Spas
The Body, Mind & Spirit Work Out

A holistic spa is a place where you can exercise not only your body, but also your mind and spirit. In Webster's Dictionary, the word holistic is defined as relating to the whole or complete system rather than the analysis or treatment of the parts. And at a holistic spa, the emphasis is not limited to one part, but extends to the whole being: the body, mind and spirit. A visit to a holistic spa can leave you feeling relaxed, rejuvenated, and a bit more confident about handling life.

Spas can generally be divided into two main categories; the resort spa and the all-in-one spa. The resort spa is often located inside a hotel, with a spa program in addition to its other tourist activities. This can be a good idea if your traveling companion prefers golfing instead of rolfing. One drawback to the resort spa is that at dinner time the person next to you maybe eating a high fat, steak and potato dinner while you are dining on brown rice, lean fish, vegetables and mineral water.

At an all-in-one spa you will find that the people you meet are not tourists but health conscious spa guests with similar food and exercise tastes. The facilities and accommodations for the all-in-one spa maybe anything from a tent to an estate.

The holistic spa comes under the all-in-one heading and can be healthy, fun alternative to the traditional spa. Outdoor activities, such as cross country skiing, horseback riding and hiking are often part of the curriculum. The philosophy behind the holistic spa is one of teaching self-love, which stems from harmony between the body, mind and spirit. This is believed to be the secret to radiant good health.

Eastern world techniques such as meditation, yoga and T'ai Chi are used to teach centering of one's body, thoughts and actions. Body work sessions such as Swedish massage, aromatherapy (massage with essential oils) and accupressure are also used to help heal the body, eliminate toxins and achieve peace of mind. Educational lectures are often given on topics such as self-esteem, nutrition and stress management. Meals are usually vegetarian and often quite tasty with items ranging from stir-fry vegetables to veggie burgers. This type of diet helps the body eliminate toxins that can accumulate in the body from elements ranging from an improper diet to stress to environmental pollution. The holistic spa approach is based on the theory that proper eating, relaxation techniques and exercises not only cleanse the body, but also the mind and spirit.

European Health Spas
balneotherapy for revitalization
or preventive medicine

European health spas offer rejuvenating and medicinal treatments based on the world's most ancient natural resource - water. A spa in the classic European sense is a place where a mineral spring (hot or cold) has an unusually high mineral content, and where spa establishments and therapy centers were built to make the benefits of the curative water accessible to the public.

The spa water is what makes it so unique. The water composition varies from one spa location to the other. The particular water composition at the spa is what makes its reputation. Typically, the major mineral components in the spa water are: sodium, calcium, magnesium, bicarbonate and sulfate. Many springs are actually radioactive, although not to the point that they can be dangerous. The mild degree of the radioactivity combined with the mineral content is part of the therapeutic effect of the spa treatment.

The medicinal treatments at the spas are always conducted under medical supervision by health professionals and have no side effects. They can be considered in some cases as an alternative to surgery or powerful drugs.

Hydrotherapy is the main theory behind all the different forms of therapies at the spa. The theory is that during bathing in thermal water, small amounts of minerals or radioactivity will enter your system through the skin or mucous membranes. The absorption of the minerals and low dose of radioactivity by the body will help your system to reenergize and reach a healthier state.

Balneotherapy plays an important role in the cure of various illnesses; in general chronic types of illnesses draw a great benefit from this treatment. The waters are effective in the treatment or cure of hypertension, tumors, hepatic cirrhosis and all disorders in the acute phase.

The therapeutic value of balneotherapy varies in accordance to the water temperature, the length of the immersion, and the mineral content of the thermal water.

Drinking cure is one of the oldest spa treatments and it is most effective in the treatment of the digestive tract, the kidneys and urinary, tract-kidney stones, the metabolism - gout, some forms of diabetes and obesity.

Mud therapy is popular in many European spas. Mud treatment consists of covering the patient with mud compresses while he is lying down. The mud compress is left for about 20 minutes and than it is removed. After the mud application there is a hot mineral bath that causes the skin to sweat and eliminate toxins. Mud is beneficent in many forms of rheumatism, consequences of fractures and neuritis. However, it is also useful in gynecology, chronic-inflammatory forms, and is widely used today in beauty and cosmetic treatments.

Inhalation is a modern treatment based on mineral water. It allows to treat almost any form of inflammatory forms of the respiratory tract (except tuberculosis). Typical indications for inhalation are: asthma, bronchitis, and many respiratory problems in children.

In Europe the spas are considered an important component of the health system. In most of the European countries like Germany, Italy and France spa treatments are covered by the government health insurance. However, the emphasis is now shifting from the short term cure at the spa to a long term change in the individuals lifestyle. This new approach introduces the American concept that more than the need for a cure, the individuals can profit from lectures, and advise from experts on how to be more relaxed, intimate with one's own body and soul, for a healthier and more enjoyable life.

European Spas are not for medicinal purposes only. Many European spas have modern beauty departments which offer world famous cosmetic products, and health and fitness centers with state-of-the-art fitness equipment and techniques. The combination of thermal springs, hydromassage, beauty products based on mineral water and mud reinvigorate the skin, detoxicate the body and adds to a sense of revitalization and well being.

European Spas may not be the legendary 'Fountain of Youth', but they sure can get you a little closer to it.

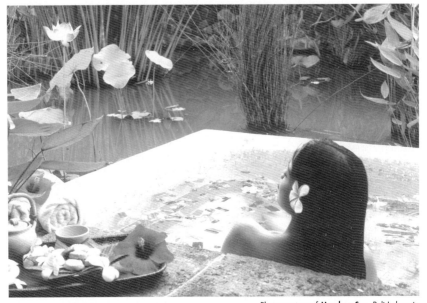

Photo courtesy of **Mandara Spa**, Bali Indonesia

HOW TO REACH US

Should you wish to contact our office to include your spa or spa related service in the 6th edition of **Spas - The International Spa Guide**™ write to:

BDIT Inc., International Spas Department, PO Box 1405, Port Washington NY 11050 (USA).

Tel: (516) 944-5508.
Toll Free (800) 257-5344.
Fax: (516) 944-7540.
Email: bditusa@aol.com
Web: http://www.bdit.com

We would like to hear from the readers of this guide about their personal experiences at the spas that were included in this edition. If you know of any spa that should be included in our next edition, please let us know about it. We need the name of the spa, mailing address, phone, fax and email address. We welcome any material such as brochures, press releases, photographs and news articles relating to the international spa industry and individual spas. However, any material sent to **BDIT Inc.** becomes the property of **BDIT Inc.** and will not be returned to its sender. If we find the information you sent us to be useful in the production of the 6th edition of **Spas - The International Spa Guide**™ we will send you a complimentary copy of the 6th edition.

Spa Reservations: If you need assistance with reservations of spas outside of the USA and Canada, you can call our travel department:

International Spa Guide Travel
Toll Free (800) 257-5344 • Fax: (516) 944-7540
email: bditusa@aol.com

We will be happy to assist you with your reservations and travel arrangements. We pay 10% commission to travel agents.

ANDORRA

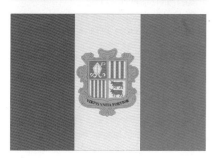

Andorra is a small principality in the Pyrénées mountains nestled between France and Spain. The capital Andorra la Vella, the highest capital in Europe, offers clean air, scenic landscapes, fine hotels and great restaurants.

Andorra attracts international tourists with its favorable climate, world class skiing, sports, fairs and the famous duty-free-shops for luxury goods at bargain prices. Andorra is accessible by car from France or Spain. From France take route N 20 from Toulouse south and cross the border at Pas de la Casa, from Spain take route 145 from Lérida and cross at the Spanish border town of Farga de Moles.

AREA: 188 sq. mi. (487 sq. km.)
POPULATION: 65,000
CAPITAL: Andorra La Vella
OFFICIAL LANGUAGE: Catalan
CURRENCY: Spanish Peseta (Pts)
EXCHANGE RATE: 1 US$ = Pts 138
COUNTRY CODE: 376

Andorra Bureau for Tourism
c/o Gilberto Garcia Sr., 6800 N. Knox Ave.
Lincolnwood, IL 60646
Tel: (847) 674-3091/ Fax: (847) 329-9470

ESCALDES

(no area code)

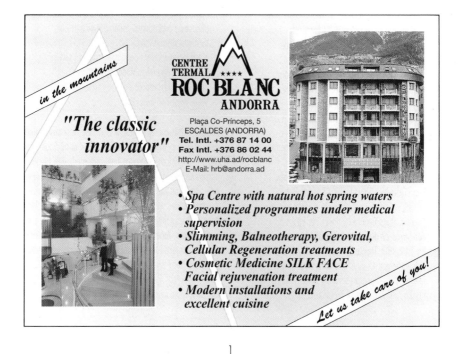

✈ Blagnac Airport (TLS) France
Barcelona Airport (BCN) Spain

A charming resort village in the mountains just outside of the Capital city Andorra La Vella with natural hot springs and wonderful ski slopes. The temperature of the hot springs is 55.3°c / 131°F and the water are rich in minerals: sulfates, fluorides, calcium, magnesium, sodium, potassium, strontium, lithium, and are used for curative treatments at the Centre Thermal Andorra in Roc Blanc.

Centre Thermal Andorra
♥♥♥♥

c/o Hotel Roc Blanc, Plaça Co-Princeps 5, Escaldes. Tel: 00-376-871400. Fax: 00-376-860244. TYPE: Deluxe Hotel & Thermal Center. LOCATION: Alpine setting in the center of Andorra near thermal springs, and duty free shopping centers. SPA CLIENTELE: Men, Women.

* Rooms: 180 w/private bath. Suites: 4 w/jacuzzi
* Telephone, CTV, minibar, hairdryer
* Restaurant: 2 restaurants; "**El Pi**" delicious dishes from the region and abroad; "**L'Entrecote**" beautifully prepared dishes and more functional service
* Airport: Barcelona 190 km. / 118 mi. or Toulouse Airport (France) closer to Andorra
* Train Station: l'Hospitalet 45 km. / 28 mi.
* Airport/Train Transportation: taxi
* Reservations: required
* Credit Cards: VISA/AMEX/MC/DIS/EC
* TAC: 10% (travel agents) (to 20% tour operators)
* Open: Year round
* SPA on premises: **Centre Thermal Roc Blanc**
* Spa Packages: Short Break (2 days) Pts 35,900; Beauty & Relaxation Pts 84,200; Facial & Body Beauty (5 days) Pts 182,100; Anti-Stress (7 days) Pts 168,900; Slimming (7 days) Pts 212,400; Thymus Therapy (7 days) Pts 237,900; Balneotherapy (7 days) Pts 169,900; Thermal Water Treatment for Upper Respiratory Tract (7 days) Pts 161,700; Executive Program (2 days)

Pts 120,500; Gerovital (7 days) Pts 169,900; Basic Cellular Regeneration (7 days) Pts 367,700; Duo Form (2 days) Pts 42,000; Silk Face (facial Rejuvenation - 11 days) Pts 772,000. Prices are per person per day, single supplements and high season supplements apply
* **Spa Facilities**: Thermal pool, Sauna, Turkish bath, Scottish shower, hydrotherapy baths, massage therapy & relaxation rooms, beauty salon
* **Spa Programs**: Revitalization, Anti Stress, Anti Rheumatism, Weight Loss & Beauty, Gerovital, Cellular Regeneration, Cosmetic Medicine
* **Spa Treatments**: Aquagym, aerobic, stretching, sauna & Turkish bath, Scottish shower, hydromassage, hydrotherapy with carbon dioxide, algae & mud packs, foot & hand shower, massages, manual lymphatic drainage, shiatsu, foot reflexology, antalgic ultra sounds, anti-cellulitis ultrasound, pressure therapy, electrolifting, thermoslim, body toner, basic cell regeneration (Dr. P. Niehans method); Asthmology, Thymus therapy, Gerovital H3
* **Indications**: loss of vitality, fatigue, premature aging, depression, arterial hypertension, impotence, liver diseases, skin and intestinal diseases, rheumatic diseases, Parkinsonism, chronic bronchitis and pulmonary emphysema
* **Medical Supervision**: permanent medical service
* **Treatments Approval**: Medical Center
* **Email**: hrb@andorra.ad
* **Web**: www.rocblanc.com

DESCRIPTION: Roc Blanc Hotel is a first class resort and thermal Spa in the heart of Andorra. The hotel is elegant with a magnificent entrance hall decorated with luscious plants and waterfall. Accommodations are in comfortable in well appointed rooms and palatial suites. The world class Thermal Center with its own natural thermal source, features European revitalizing and preventive therapies for premature aging. An expert team of professionals offers up-to-date personalized health programs. A spa vacation at the Roc Blanc Hotel is recommended for relaxation, beauty and stress reduction. Recreation: duty free shopping, golf, skiing, swimming and tourism.

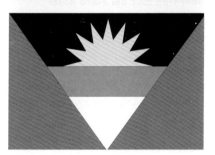

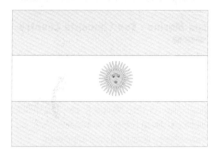

AREA: 108 sq. mi. (280 sq. km.)	**AREA**: 1,072,070 sq. mi. (2,776,661 sq. km.)
POPULATION: 66,000	**POPULATION**: 29,000,000
CAPITAL: Saint John's	**CAPITAL**: Buenos Aires
OFFICIAL LANGUAGE: English	**OFFICIAL LANGUAGE**: Spanish
CURRENCY: Eastern Caribbean Dollar (EC$)	**CURRENCY**: Argentina pesol (ARS)
EXCHANGE RATE: 1 US$ = EC$2.70	**EXCHANGE RATE**: 1 US$ = ARS 1.00
TELEPHONE COUNTRY CODE: 268	**TELEPHONE COUNTRY CODE**: 54

Antigua is a tiny Eastern Caribbean island with beautiful beaches and warm weather year round. For shoppers there are bustling markets to explore in the colonial capital Saint John's. Flying time from New York is approximately 4 hrs. 45 min., and from Miami 3 hrs. 15 min.

 Antigua & Barbuda Dept. of Tourism
610 5th Avenue, Ste 311, New York NY 10020
Tel: (212) 541-4117. Fax: (212)757-1607

SAINT JOHN'S

⅂ (no area code)

✈ V.C. Bird Int'l Airport (ANU)

Sandals Antigua Resort & Spa
♥♥♥♥

🏊 🏃

Dickenson Bay, St. John's. Tel: 462-0267, Fax: 462-4135. TYPE: Resort & Spa. LOCATION: On the beach in tropical setting. DESCRIPTION: All inclusive resort complex with full-service European spa and fitness center. 191 rooms.

❗ Argentina Govt. Tourist information
12 West 56th St.
New York NY 10019
Tel: (212) 603-0443. Fax: (212) 315-5545

BUENOS AIRES

⅂ 1

✈ Ezeize/Ministro Pistarini Int'l AP (EZE)
Jorge Newbery Int'l Airport (AEP)

Tamara di Tella
♥♥♥

🏊 🏃

Lapride 1120, Ciudada de Buenos Aires (Cap Federal), Tel: (1) 961-6727 or 5324. DESCRIPTION: Anti-cellulitis treatments.

Club Olympus
♥♥♥

🏊 🏃

c/o Park Hyatt, Posadas 1086/88. Ciudada de Buenos

Aires (Cap Federal). Tel: (1) 326-1234. Fax: (01) 326-3736. TYPE: Fitness Center & Spa. LOCATION: Heart of Buenos Aires at de Deluxe Park Hyatt Hotel. 165 rooms.

Spa Marino - San Clemente Country
❤❤❤

Ruta de Acceso y Av, XVII, San Clemente de Tuyu (Buenos Aires). Tel: (1) 774-6107, Fax: (1) 252-21679. TYPE: Health Spa. CLIENTELE: Women & men. DESCRIPTION: Health spa offering programs for Anti-stress, weight loss, thalassotherapy, aromatherapy and fangotherapy.

MAR DEL PLATA
) 23

✈ Camet Airport

Club de Mar
❤❤❤

c/o Hotel Torres de Manantiales - Alberti 453, Mar del Plata 7600, Tel: (23) 861388, 861999. Fax: (23) 862-877. TYPE: Hotel & Health Spa. DESCRIPTION: Health Spa offering programs of Thalassotherapy, Weight Loss, Anti-Stress. 224 rooms.

Sheraton Mar del Plata Hotel
❤❤❤❤

Av Alem 4221, Mar del Plata 7600.Tel: (23) 999000. Fax: (23) 999009. TYPE: Hotel & Spa. LOCATION: Near port, shops and beaches. DESCRIPTION: Elegant hotel with Health Club and spa offering massages, aerobics, saunas and gym. 195 rooms.

COLON (Entre Rios)
) 447

✈ Buenos Aires 310 km. / 194 mi.
Jorge Newbery Int'l Airport (AEP)

Quirinale Spa
❤❤❤

c/o Hotel Quirinale, Av. Quiros 185, Colon (Entre Rios). Tel: (447) 21133, 21247. Fax: (447) 21532. TYPE: Revitalization Center. LOCATION: Picturesque river setting 350 km. / 218 mi. from Buenos Aires. DESCRIPTION: 5 star hotel with health spa and casino.

ARUBA

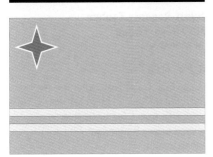

AREA: 70 sq. mi. (180 sq. km.)
POPULATION: 85,000
CAPITAL: Oranjestad
OFFICIAL LANGUAGE: Dutch, Papiamento
CURRENCY: Aruban Guilder (Afl)
EXCHANGE RATE: 1 US$ = Afl 1.80
TELEPHONE COUNTRY CODE: 297

Aruba is the smallest and westernmost of the Dutch "ABC" islands (Aruba, Bonaire, Curaçao) that lie just off the coast of Venezuela. Aruba is one of the fastest-growing destinations in the Caribbean with beautiful hotels, casinos and a new Health & Fitness spa at the elegant Radisson Grand on the beautiful Palm Beach, a five-mile stretch of pure white sand beach. Recreation: duty free shopping, casinos, water sports, scuba, tennis, golf and fishing.

Aruba Tourism Authority

One Financial Plaza, Ste 136, Ft. Lauderdale FL 33394
Tel: (954) 767-6477. Fax: (954) 767-0432

PALM BEACH

(no area code)

Queen Beatrix Int'l Airport (AUA)

Radisson Grand
♥♥♥♥♥

J.E. Irausquin Blvd. #81. Palm Beach. Tel: (297) 866555. Toll Free (800) 333-3333. Fax: (297) 863260. TYPE: Deluxe Hotel, Spa & Casino . LOCATION: Beachfront location on Palm Beach Aruba's best beach. SPA CLIENTELE: Men, Women.

* Rooms: 326 w/priv. bath. Suites: 32
* Telephone, CTV, A/C, C/H
* In room iron, ironing board, refrigerator, safe
* Restaurants, bars & casino
* Reservations: required
* Credit Cards: VISA/AMEX/MC/DIN/DIS
* Open: Year round
* SPA on premises
* Year Established: 1999
* SPA Programs: Beauty, Fitness, Stress Reduction
* SPA Treatments: massages, facials, wraps
* SPA Packages: on request
* Email: arubasales@radisson.com
* Web: www.radisson.com/palmbeachaw

DESCRIPTION: The spectacular Radisson Grand resort provides the upscale traveler with a truly memorable experience in Aruban charm in a luxurious yet relaxed setting. Elegant guest rooms and suites with spacious balconies feature clean architectural lines with accents on colonial West Indian design. An 8,500 sq. ft. / 772 sq. m. spa and fitness facility provides an expansive array of personal services to reduce stress and pamper the most deserving traveler. A comprehensive fitness facility feature the newest cardiovascular and weight training equipment. Beauty treatments include massages and facials.

Wyndham Aruba Beach Resort & Casino - La Spa
♥♥♥♥

J.E. Irausquin Blvd. 77, Palm Beach. Tel: 8-64466, Fax: 8-63403. TYPE: Resort Hotel & Casino. LOCATION: Palm Beach. DESCRIPTION: Large resort hotel with 3500 sq. ft. (318 sq. m.) Health Club offering massages and beauty services.

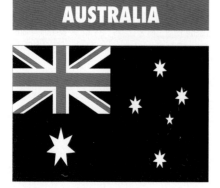

AREA: 2,966,136 sq. mi. (7,682,300 sq. km.)
POPULATION: 14,600,000
CAPITAL: Canberra
OFFICIAL LANGUAGE: English
CURRENCY: Australian Dollar (A$)
EXCHANGE RATE: 1 US$ = A$1.60
TELEPHONE COUNTRY CODE: 61

Australia is a large and diverse country/continent about the size of the continental USA. Americans travelling to Australia will find many things in common: English is spoken, though the accent is definitely Australian, and many values are shared. Located less than a day away from North America, the Land Down Under offers cosmopolitan cities, and magnificent South Pacific and Indian Ocean beaches, just perfect for soaking up the Southern sun. Australia is the home of dramatic sights and the oddest animals on earth.

ⓘ Australian Tourist Commission
2049 Century Park East, Ste 1920,
Los Angeles CA 90067
Tel: (310) 229-4870. Fax: (310) 552-1215

COOLUM (QLD)
ㄣ **7**
✈ Maroochy Airport, 7 km. / 4 mi.

Coolum is located on the Sunshine Coast, 20 km. (13 mi.) south of Noosa. The climate is subtropical, and the weather is sunny and warm year round. Coolum can be reached by car in 10 minutes from the Maroochy airport, or in 1 hr.

20 minutes from Brisbane. By air - flight time from Sydney is 1 hr. 20 minutes, and 2 hrs. from Melbourne.

Hyatt-Regency Coolum
Int'l Resort & Spa
❤❤❤❤❤

Warran Road, Coolum Beach, G.P.O. Box 78, Coolum Beach, QLD 4573. Tel: (7) 5446-1234. Fax: (7) 5446-2957. TYPE: Resort & Spa. LOCATION: On the rolling hills of the picturesque Sunshine Coast. SPA CLIENTELE: Men, women, family.

* Rooms: 330 w/priv. bath; Villas: 150
* Restaurants, wine bar, cafe, deli
* Airport: Moroochy Airport 7 km. / 4 mi.
* Train Station: Nambour (45 minutes)
* Airport/train St'n Transportation: free pick up
* Reservations: credit card guarantee
* Credit Cards: VISA/AMEX/EC/JCB/BC
* Open: Year round
* Rates: on request; TAC: 10%
* SPA on premises
* **Spa Facilities**: Spa and Medical Center, gym, aerobic room, whirlpool baths & sauna rooms, massage and sun court center, large lap pool, squash, beauty salon for men and women
* **Spa Programs**: Lifestyle improvement Health Management, Beauty and Fitness, Executive Health Programs, Revitalization
* **Spa Treatments**: aerobics, herbal wrap, bubbling mineral baths, massages, rejuvenation, body composition analysis, facials, body peeling, cellulite treatment, complete range of tests to evaluate risk of cardiovascular heart disease at the Health Management Center, physical fitness assessment
* **Indications**: revitalization, relaxation, stress reduction, executive health management
* Medical supervision: 3 MD, 3 RN
* Treatments Approved: Australian Medical Association (AMA)

DESCRIPTION: Lifestyle Resort & Spa on the beautiful

Sunshine Coast. The resort spreads over 151 hectares along 1 km. (600 yards) of Pacific Ocean Beach. The emphasis is on healthy and balanced attitude to life, combined with pampering, relaxation and personalized exercise program. The Health Management Center offers professional assessment of your current fitness and health levels and recommendations for health and lifestyle improvement. Recreation: 18 hole golf course, Beach Club, Tennis Club, and Creative Arts Center.

BRISBANE (QLD)
🤙 **07**
✈ Brisbane Int'l Airport (BNE)

Clear Mountain Health Spa
💙💙💙

Clear Mountain Rd, Clear Mountain, QLD 4500. Tel: (0)7-3298-5100, Fax: (0)7-3298-5435. TYPE: Health Retreat. SPA CLIENTELE: Women & men. LOCATION: Mountaintop resort near Brisbane. DESCRIPTION: Peaceful health resort offering fitness activities and spa treatments. Rates from A$125 (room only).

DAYLESFORD (VIC)
🤙 **03**
✈ Essendon Airport (MEB)
   Melbourne Int'l Airport (MEL) 60 mi. / 96 km.

Daylesford is in Victoria's Spa country, 80 min. north of Melbourne. With 75 mineral springs the region known as the Spa Capital of Australia, boasts the largest concentration of naturally occurring springs on the continent. The mineral springs are cool, effervescent with healthful properties.

Lake House
💙💙💙💙

King Street, Daylesford, VIC 3460. Tel: (3) 5348-3329. Fax: (3) 5348-3885. TYPE: Spa Hotel. LOCATION: On several hectares of gardens on the shores of Lake Daylesford. DESCRIPTION: Elegant retreat with an award winning

gourmet country restaurant offering relaxing massages and some soaking in their spa/sauna room.

KINGSTON (TAS)
🤙 **03**

Anubha Mountain Retreat
💙💙

710 Summerleas Rd., Kingston, TAS 7050, Tel/Fax: (0)3-6239-1573. TYPE: Health Retreat. LOCATION: Tasmania with views of Mt. Wellington. SPA CLIENTELE: Women & Men. DESCRIPTION: Intimate retreat offering meditation, hypnotherapy, massages and facials.

KATOOMBA (NSW)
🤙 **02**
✈ Kingsford-Smith Int'l AP (SYD) 69 mi. / 110 km.

Lilianfels Blue Mountains
💙💙💙

Lilianfels Avenue, Echo Point, Katoomba, NSW 2780. Tel: (0)2-4780-1200, Fax: (0)2-4780-1300. TYPE: Resort with Health Spa. CLIENTELE: Women & men. LOCATION: Overlooking National Park. DESCRIPTION: Elegant European style Country House with Health & Beauty Spa.

KURRAJONG (NSW)
🤙 **02**
✈ Kingsford-Smith Int'l AP (SYD) 60 mi. / 96 km.

Kurrajong Heights Health Farm
💙💙💙

1537 Bells Line Rd., Kurrajong Heights, NSW 2758. Tel: (0)2-4567-7100, Fax: (0)2-4567-7575. TYPE: Health Spa. SPA CLIENTELE: Women & men. LOCATION: One hour drive from Sydney. DESCRIPTION: Health Farm to loose weight with delicious low cal cuisine and exercise. Indoor pool for hydrotherapy. Rates from A$85/day (room only).

SURFERS PARADISE (QLD)
) 07
✈ Coolangata Airport (OOL)

Radisson Watermark
♥♥♥

♨ 𝒽 🕴

3032 Highway, Surfer's Paradise 4217 QLD. Tel: (0)7-5588-8333, Fax: (0)7-5588-8300. TYPE: Resort Hotel. LOCATION: Heart of Surfer's Paradise, near beach, nightlife & Shopping. DESCRIPTION: Beach resort hotel with Japanese style Health & Beauty Spa. 411 rooms.

SYDNEY (NSW)
) 02
✈ Kingsford-Smith Int'l AP (SYD) 6 mi. / 10 km.
Palm Beach Seaplane Base (LBH) 20 mi. / 32 km.

Sydney, population 3,600,000, is a great cosmopolitan city made up of many exciting areas, each with its own unique flavor and personality. The Sydney Opera House is the most widely recognized landmark of urban Australia. Sydney is known for its vibrant nightlife, great shopping and festivals. Sydney will host the Olympic Games in the year 2000.

The Observatory Hotel
Day Spa, Health & Leisure Club
♥♥♥♥

♨ 𝒽 🕴 ❀ ☆ ◉

89-113 Kent St., The Rocks, Sydney NSW 2000. Tel: (61-2) 9256-2229. Fax: (61-2) 9256-2235. TYPE: First Class Hotel & Spa. MANAGING DIRECTOR: Mr. Patrick Griffin. SPA DIRECTOR: Deborah Mangum. LOCATION: Historic Rocks district of Sydney. SPA CLIENTELE: Men, women, teenagers and children accepted.

* Rooms: 100 w/priv. bath. Suites: 21
* Phone, CTV, A/C, minibar, hairdryer, CD/Video player

* 24 hrs room service, laundry service
* Restaurant (modern Australian/Italian), bar lounge
* Airport: 12 km. / 8 mi. taxi, bus
* Train Station: 10 minutes walk
* Reservations: required
* Credit Cards: VISA/AMEX/MC/DIN
* TAX: 10%
* Open: Year round
* SPA on premises: The Observatory Hotel Day Spa
* Year established: 1993
* **Spa Packages**: from US$210
  Accommodation packages available on request
* **Spa Facilities**: Total Body Wellness day spa, 7 treatment rooms including wet rooms for hydrotherapy & thalassotherapy, 20 m. heated swimming pool w/jacuzzi, sauna, steam room, fully equipped gym
* **Spa Programs**: one hour or more, full day and up to 7 day programs
* **Spa Treatments**: massages, aromatherapy, body wraps, masks, nutritional consultation, personal training, European & eclectic beauty treatments
* **Indications**: beauty, stress reduction, well being
* **Contraindication**: recent surgery
* Medical Supervision: 1 MD
* Maximum Number of Guests: 220
* Documentation required from doctor: for fitness assessment and fitness program design
* Email: observatory@mail.com
* Web: www.observatoryhotel.com.au

DESCRIPTION: The Observatory Hotel, reminiscent of a 19th century Australian home, has built it's outstanding reputation on a combination of personalized service, exceptional facilities and faultless professionalism. The luxurious rooms and suites are beautifully furnished with antiques, original paintings and tapestries. The Observatory Hotel offers a total body wellness day spa with personalized programs of health, beauty and fitness. *Member: Small Luxury Hotels, Orient- Express Hotels, Leading Hotels of the World, Amex Platinum cardmember.*

AUSTRIA

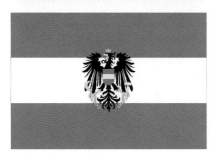

AREA: 32,375 sq. mi. (83,851 sq. km.)
POPULATION: 7,507,000
CAPITAL: Vienna
OFFICIAL LANGUAGE: German
CURRENCY: Schilling (AS)
EXCHANGE RATE: AS 11.40 = US$1
TELEPHONE COUNTRY CODE: 43

Austria is a classic Spa destination with more than a hundred Spas and Health resorts to choose from. The health resorts provide a variety of medical and health care programs according to each Spa's particular curative agents and thermal springs. Most of the Austrian Spas and Health Resorts are medically supervised with state-of-the-art clinics and equipment. Treatments can be considered as a complement to western medical care. Located in the countryside amidst natural beauty, high mountains and lakes, they offer opportunities for relaxation, recreation and tourism. In addition to traditional thermal treatments, Spa enthusiasts can take advantage of the "Kneipp Cures" a natural medicine that is widely administered in Austria as a curative technique.

ℹ Austrian Tourist Information Center
500 5th Avenue
New York, NY 10110
Tel: (212) 944-6880, Fax: (212) 730-4568

ACHENKIRCH (Tyrol)
☏ 5246
✈ Kranebitten Airport (INN) Innsbruck

Posthotel Achenkirch
♥♥♥♥

A-6215 Achenkirch. Tel: (5246) 6522, 6271. Fax: (5246) 6205468. TYPE: Health Spa. LOCATION: Scenic Alpine setting. SPA CLIENTELE: Women and men. DESCRIPTION: Health spa, the largest aquatic and hotel complex in the Tyrol, specializing in the use of Tyrolean stone oil to treat circulatory and metabolic disorders. Programs: weight loss; beauty and pampering using Gertaud Gruber's holistic methods. Recreation: tennis, squash.

BAD AUSSEE (Styria)
☏ 3622
✈ Salzburg Airport (SZG) 80 km. / 50 mi.

Bad Aussee, population 5,000, is an old health spa resort in one of Austria's most beautiful regions. The spa is located between 650 and 850 m. (2,000 - 2,500 ft.) above sea level; it offers outstanding natural health resources, combined with mild healthy climate. The town boasts 800-year-old history. Brine baths were first mentioned in the 16th century and local physicians administered spa cures for sufferers from liver, stomach and gallbladder ailments. Balneology was introduced in 1868, when the town was officially recognized as a Kurort (spa), and since 1911 it became a full-service Bad or spa town for wealthy patrons.

The Kurzentrum (Spa Center) is in the heart of the town. Mineral baths are effective in the cure of: circulatory and regulatory disturbances, pediatric disorders, rheumatism, female disorders, and hyperthyroidism. The Glaubert Salt Spring is effective in the treatment of digestive disorders and may be effective in weight loss regime. Inhalation treatments are recommended for: catarrh, asthma, and emphysema. Brine fango mud is applied for injury of the joints, and the spinal column. Also available at the Health Center: underwater therapy, electrotherapy and Kneipp in the Brine mineral indoor pool with water temperature maintained at 30°c (86°F).

Bad Aussee is an excellent summer resort with good hiking and climbing trails, and fine tennis courts. In the winter the spa offers several ski lifts nearby for ski enthusiasts. If you are interested in fine arts, crafts, porcelain and antiques visit the Galerie Schlob Weyer in Gmunden am Traunsee (near Bad Aussee). Situated in the heart of Austria, Bad Ausee can be easily reached by train, car, or plane (from Salzburg).

Hotel Erzherzog Johann
♥♥♥♥

Kurhauspolatz 62, Bad Aussee (Styria), A-8990. Tel: (3622) 52507. Fax: (3622) 52507-680. TYPE: Hotel & Spa. SPA CLIENTELE: Women & men. LOCATION: Town center near train station. DESCRIPTION: First class Hotel. Covered walk to spa with swimming pool, sauna and mineral baths. Recreation: tennis, skiing & water sports.

Villa Kristina
♥♥♥♥

Prawnfalk 54, A-8990 Bad Aussee. Tel: (3622) 2017. Fax: (3622) 52017-1. TYPE: Spa Hotel. MANAGER: Friedl Raudschl. LOCATION: City garden side. SPA CLIENTELE: Family Oriented.

* Rooms: 15 w/priv. bath; Suites: 3
* Phone, CTV, hairdryer, central heating
* 24 hrs room service
* Wheelchair Accessible
* Restaurant: low fat diet menu available
* TV Lounge & Bar
* SPA off premises: 300 m. / yards away
* Airport: Salzburg, 80 km. / 50 mi.
* Train Station: Bad Ausse, 2 km. / 1 mi.
* Airport/Train Transportation: taxi, bus
* Reservations: required
* Credit Cards: MC/VISA/AMEX/DC/CB
* Open: Year round
* Rates: AS 900 - AS 1,350/day (room only); TAC: 15% Spa treatments available at the Kurzentrum
* **Spa Facilities:** thermal facilities at the Kurzentrum
* **Spa Programs:** Health, diet, fitness
* **Spa Treatments:** See Kurzentrum
* Medical Supervision: 8 MD, 6 RN
* Treatments Approved: Austrian Government

DESCRIPTION: A family run traditional hotel and pension in the center of Bad Aussee. Guest rooms are comfortable and furnished with antiques. A pleasant hotel with Austrian hunting lodge atmosphere. Spa treatments are available at the nearby Spa Center (Kurzentrum).

BAD HALL (Upper Austria)
🌙 **7258**
✈ Horsching Airport (LNZ) Linz

Herzog Tassilo Kurhotel
♥♥♥♥

Park Str. 4, Bad Hall (upper Austria), A-4540, Tel: (7258) 26110, Fax: (7258) 26115.TYPE: Resort Hotel & Spa. LOCATION: In Spa gardens. DESCRIPTION: Hotel with spa facilities, indoor thermal pool using potent iodine springs, low cal diet menu.

BAD HOFGASTEIN (Salzburg)
🌙 **6432**
✈ Salzburg Airport (SZG) 55 mi. / 88 km. North

Bad Hofgastein, population 5,500, is Badgastein's sister spa resort 5 miles (8 km.) to the north. Bad Hofgastein is smaller and somehow less expensive than Badgastein, but share the same thermal source and offer the Gastein radon thermal cures and treatments. In the heart of Bad Hofgastein near the Alpine Kurpark is the spa's own Institute for Rheumatology, Rehabilitation and Sports Medicine. The institute is under the direction of a specialist for internal medicine. A Separate Holiday Unit with thermal pools, solarium, saunas, massages, gym, extensive lawn for relaxation, café and restaurant is available for recreation and holidays.

ℹ For information on the thermal water properties and curative powers see Badgastein.

Grand Park Hotel
♥♥♥♥

Kurgartenstraße 26a, 5630 Bad Hofgastein. Tel: (6432) 63560. Fax: (6432) 8454. TYPE: Deluxe Resort Hotel & Spa. LOCATION: Centrally located in a private park near ski facilities. SPA CLIENTELE: Women and men, Mixed.

* Rooms: 92, 73 w/private bath, 12 shower
* Phone, radio and private balcony
* Restaurant & Cocktail Lounge
* Airport: Salzburg 90 km. / 56 mi.
* Train Station: Badgastein 4 km. (2.5 mi.)
* Train Station Transportation: taxi, bus
* Reservations: suggested
* Credit Cards: AMEX/DC/EC/VISA
* Open: Year round
* Rates: AS 1,300 - AS 4,800/day; TAC: 10%
* Spa on premises
* **Spa Facilities**: Largest indoor thermal swimming
  pool in Austria with water temperature of 32°c
  (90°F), fitness center, sauna, solarium, thermal baths
* **Spa Treatments**: Gastein radon thermal treatments,
  all massages, inhalations, exercises,
  kinebalneotherapy, low calorie meals
* **Indications**: same as Badgastein
* Medical Supervision: 1 MD
* Treatments Approved: Austrian Ministry of Health

DESCRIPTION: Elegant chalet style hotel offering comfort
and service according to high international standards. The
emphasis here is on radon thermal water cure. Some thermal cures can be taken at the hotel. The food is excellent;
biofare food or diabetic food is available. Recreation: skiing,
skating and tennis courts are all available nearby.

Kur & Sporthotel Moser
❤❤

Kaisier-Franz-Platz 2, Bad Hofgastein (Salzburg), A-5630,
Tel: (6432) 6209, Fax: (6432) 620988. TYPE: Spa
Hotel. CLIENTELE: Women & men. LOCATION: Central loca-
tion. DESCRIPTION: Tourist class hotel with Thermal baths,
cure facilities, indoor pool, sauna, gym and sun terrace.
Rates: AS 830 - AS 2,000 (room only).

Kurhotel Germania
❤❤❤

Kurpromenade 14, Bad Hofgastein (Salzburg), A-5630,

Tel: (6432) 6232-0, Fax: (6432) 6232-65. TYPE: Spa
Hotel. LOCATION: On the Kurpromenade. SPA CLIENTELE:
Women & Men. DESCRIPTION: Chalet style hotel with
rooms and suites and Spa facilities. Amenities: Restaurant
(diet menu), indoor pool, solarium and sauna.

Norica Kur & Sporthotel
❤❤❤❤

Bachbauergaße, Bad Hofgastein, Salzburg A-5630. Tel:
(6432) 8391. Fax: (6432) 7187. TYPE: First Class Hotel
& Spa. MANAGER: Hans J. Pernitsch. LOCATION: Heart of
the Gastein Valley surrounded by mountains. SPA CLIEN-
TELE: Men, Women.

* Rooms: 80 w/private bath
* Central heating, phone, color TV
* Train Station: Bad Gastein 5 km. (3 mi.)
* Reservations: suggested
* Credit Cards: MC/VISA/AMEX/DC/EC
* Open: Year round
* Rates: AS 990 - AS 1,290/day (room only); TAC: 10%
* Spa on premises
* **Spa Facilities**: Private hospital in the form of
  independent ambulatory clinic, indoor swimming
  pool, Spa facilities, fitness room, solarium,
  massage rooms
* **Spa Treatments**: A variety of thermal curative
  water baths treatments, body massages,
  underwater therapy, exercises, Gerovital H3,
  Aslan Therapy, diet menu
* **Spa Packages**: 2 weeks inclusive Spa package ;
  Gerovital H3 Aslan therapy
* **Indications**: all rheumatic and degenerative
  illnesses of the joints, peripheral circulatory
  disturbances, fertility and potency disorders,
  geriatric complaints
* Medical Supervision: 1 MD
* Treatments Approved: Austrian Health Ministry

DESCRIPTION: A modern first class hotel with spacious and
comfortable accommodations offering medically oriented spa
treatments based on Radon which is contained in the hot
water of Gastein and is applied in the thermal treatments.

Other treatments include Gerovital H3, Aslan and weight loss programs. Recreation: golf, tennis, skiing and hiking nearby.

Hotel Palace Gastein
❤❤❤❤

Alexander Moser Allee 13, Bad Hofgastein, Salzburg 5630. Tel: (6432) 67150. Fax: (6432) 6715-402. TYPE: Resort Spa Hotel. MANAGER: Mr. Friedrich Dold. LOCATION: Heart of Bad Hofgastein. SPA CLIENTELE: Mixed, Family oriented.

* Rooms: 200 w/priv. bath
* Phone, CTV, balcony, radio
* Bar: "Viennese Coffee Shop"
* Restaurants: 4 & Night Club
* Train Station: Bad Hofgastein 4 km. / 3mi.
* Airport: Salzburg 88 km. / 55 mi.
* Train Station Transportation: Hotel Bus
* Reservations: required
* Credit Cards: MC/VISA/AMEX/MC/DC
* Open: December 20 - October 30
* Rates: AS 690 - AS 1,460 (room only); TAC: 10%
* Spa on Premises: Gastein-Radon-Cure
* Spa Facilities: In house Cure Center, Indoor thermal pool, hot whirlpool, massage room, saunas. Guerlain Paris Beauty Farm
* Spa Treatments: Radon thermal cure, physiotherapy, psychotherapy, fango cures, phytomer applications, medicinal baths, massages, gymnastics, medical examinations, full range of beauty treatments at the Beauty Farm
* Spa Packages: Gastein-Radon Thermal Cure (3 Week), Natural Fango Cure (2 weeks), Schnupper Cure (1 week), Guarlain Beauty Week (6 days), Guerlain Beauty-Vital week (6 days), Ladies and Gentlemen Beauty Day
* Spa Packages: 3 week Gastein-Radon Thermal Cure; 2 week Natural Fango Cure; 1 week Schnupper Cure
* Indications: see Badgastein, beauty and pampering at the hotel's Beauty Farm
* Contraindications: none
* Medical Supervision: house Doctor on call
* Treatments Approved: State-approved therapists

DESCRIPTION: A sports and spa hotel of the first category with its own in house Cure Center. Weight watchers can enjoy specially prepared low cal gourmet diet food. The Guerlain Beauty Farm features 1-6 day beauty and pampering packages. Recreation: golf, tennis, fishing, hunting, skiing and mountain trails. Fashion shows and folklore evenings provide cultural entertainment.

BAD ISCHL (Upper Austria)
6132
✈ Salzburg Airport (SZG) 60 mi. / 96 km.

Kurhotel Bad Ischl
❤❤❤❤

Voglhuberstr 10, Bad Ischl (Upper Austria), A-4820, Tel: (6132) 204, Fax: (6132) 27682. TYPE: Spa Hotel. LOCATION: Mountain spa region. SPA CLIENTELE: Women and men. DESCRIPTION: Resort hotel with cure facilities, outdoor pool. gym, sauna, jacuzzi. Recreation: tennis, golf, skiing, water sports.

BAD KLEINKIRCHEIM (Crinthia)
4240
✈ Klagenfurt Airport (KLU) 35 mi. / 55 km.

Hotel Romerbad
❤❤❤

Bad Kleinkirchheim (Carinithia), A-9546, Tel: (4240) 82340, Fax: (4240) 823457. TYPE: Spa Hotel. LOCATION: Central location. SPA CLIENTELE: Women and men. DESCRIPTION: Small spa hotel with cure facilities, outdoor pool, gym, sauna, jacuzzi.

Themenhotel Das Ronacher
❤❤❤

Bach 18, Bad Kleinkirchheim (Carinthia) A-9546, Tel: (4240) 282, Fax: (4240) 282-606. TYPE: Spa Resort Hotel. LOCATION: Quiet location above cure center. SPA CLIENTELE: Women and men. DESCRIPTION: First class spa hotel with cure facilities and Beauty Farm, outdoor/indoor pools, gym, sauna, jacuzzi.

BADEN BEI WIEN (Lower Austria)

) 2252

✈ Schwechat Airport (VIE) 15 mi. / 24 km.

Baden bei Wien is a lovely spa town in the Vienna Woods with a beautiful Spa Park and Roman Springs. The famous Beethoven came to Baden to find inspiration for some of his best known compositions. The resort has 15 sulfur thermal springs known for their curative powers since Roman times over 2,000 years ago.

Indications: The thermal waters are used in the treatment of: rheumatic and non-rheumatic affections of the locomotor system, sequels of injuries, forms of neuroglia, paralytic conditions, certain skin diseases, severe metal poisoning, gynecological diseases, diseases of the mouth and gums, constipation and allergic diseases of the intestines, and diseases of the respiratory system.

Contraindications: inflammation of the joints and nerves, rheumatic fever, decompensated cardiac complaints, decompensated high blood pressure, all kind of infectious diseases. A team of 20 doctors at the Baden spa provide medical care and supervision.

Baden has 2 theatres, 3 museums, and occasionally spa concerts. For sports enthusiasts there is tennis, squash, horseback riding and bowling. For shopping, there is a pedestrian zone with several shops, boutiques, and coffee houses. Baden bei Wien is located 25 km. (16 mi.) from Vienna, and can be reached from Vienna by car or taxi.

Parkhotel Baden
♥♥♥♥

Kaiser-Franz-Ring 5, Baden bei Wien (Lower Austria), A-2500, Tel: (2252) 443860, Fax: (2252) 80578. TYPE: Spa Hotel. LOCATION: Centrally located in a park. SPA CLIENTELE: Women & men. DESCRIPTION: First class hotel with Spa facilities and gym, indoor pool and diet menu.

Sauerhof Grand Hotel
♥♥♥♥♥

Weilburgstraße 11-13, Baden bei Wien 2500. Tel: (2252) 412510. Fax: (2252) 48047. TYPE: Deluxe Hotel & Spa. LOCATION: In former 19th century Biedermeier Palace, 5 minutes from downtown. SPA CLIENTELE: Women and men.

* Rooms: 88 w/private bath, Suites: 4
* Wheelchair Accessible
* Phone, color TV, radio, minibar
* Dining Room & Viennese Coffee Shop
* Airport: Vienna Airport, 30 km. (19 mi.)
* Airport Transportation: taxi, limo, bus
* Reservations: one night deposit
* Credit Cards: MC/AMEX/DC
* Open: Year round
* Hotel Rates: AS 1,450 - AS 3,000/day (room only)
* TAC: 10%
* **Spa Facilities**: private sulfur spring at 36°c (97°F), indoor pool, sauna, solarium, gym
* **Spa Programs**: Fitness & Anti Stress, Convalescence & Relaxation
* **Spa Treatments**: sulfur baths, mud packs, massages, sauna, Kneipp Cure, cell therapy
* **Contraindications**: Acute inflammation of the joints and nerves, rheumatic fever, decompensated cardiac complaints
* **Medical Supervision**: yes

DESCRIPTION: A baroque style hotel & Spa located in a romantic 19 century palace. Experience the Austrian tradition of a bygone era where imperial luxury and traditions were the rule. Accommodations offered are spacious, tastefully furnished in classic design with contemporary amenities and comfort. The SPA features a private hot sulfur spring and emphasizes an anti stress and relaxation program. Recreation: gourmet dining, golf and tennis. Opera, Theatre and Casino nearby. *Member: SRS Hotels*

Hotel Schloss Weikersdorf
♥♥♥♥

Schlossgaße 9-11, Baden 2500. Tel: (2252) 48301.

TYPE: Deluxe Hotel & Spa. MANAGER: Rudolf F. Graf. LOCA-TION: Centrally located. SPA CLIENTELE: Family oriented.

* Rooms: 108 w/private bath. Suites: 9
* Phone, CTV, hair dryer, minibar, central heating
* Restaurant & Bar
* Nearest Airport: Vienna 27 km. (16 mi.)
* Airport Transportation: train, bus, taxi
* Reservations: suggested
* Credit Cards: MC/VISA/AMEX/EC
* Open: Year round
* Hotel Rates: AS 785 - AS1,140/day (room only)
* TAC: 8%
* Spa on premises
* **Spa Facilities**: Indoor heated swimming pool, sauna, whirlpool, massage & cure facilities,
* **Spa Treatments**: sulfur baths, massages, inhalations, Kneipp cure, beauty treatments, Gerovital H3, Aslan therapy, weight loss
* **Spa Packages**: 2 weeks all inclusive; Gerovital H3, Aslan therapy
* **Indications**: same as Baden bei Wien plus beauty treatments

DESCRIPTION: An old 13 century castle turned into a Health Resort Hotel with top quality amenities and service. Various cures are offered at the hotel including beauty treatments and weight loss programs based on low calorie gourmet menus. Recreation: tennis courts.

BAD MITTERNDORF (Styria)
🕯 **3623**
✈ Salzburg Airport (SZG) 62 mi. / 100 km.

Bad Mitterndorf is a famous health spa located in one of the most beautiful regions of Austria known as the Styrian Salzkammergut southeast of Salzburg. Austrian call the region the "Green Heart of Austria" because of the vast area covered by evergreen forests. Bad Mitterndorf spa offers Acratic thermal springs, curative mud, and pure Alpine climate. The natural setting near high mountains, valleys, rivers and lakes makes it an ideal destination for those who wish to combine spa vacation with activities such as walking, riding, fishing, swimming, wind-surfing, and mountaineering. The Tauplitz Alm (1,965 m. / 5,800 ft.) guarantees good skiing conditions from late November to early April.

Indications: the curative agents are effective in the cure or treatment of the following ailments: chronic rheumatic conditions, convalescence, gynecological disorders, post-operative and post-traumatic treatment, certain skin diseases, and certain cases of essential hypertension.

Bad Mitterndorf is within easy reach from Salzburg which is 85 km. (53 mi.) northwest by train, car or small planes.

Vital Hotel Heilbrunn
❤❤❤❤

Bad Mitterndorf 8983. Tel: (3623) 2486. Fax: (3623) 248633 TYPE: Spa Hotel. LOCATION: Near Bad Mitterndorf close to a natural lake. SPA CLIENTELE: Family oriented.

* Rooms: 107 w/private bath. Suites: 7
* Phone, minibar, CTV, most with balcony
* Restaurant, Bar & Wine Cellar
* Airport: Salzburg 100 km. (62 mi.)
* Airport Transportation: taxi, train
* Reservations: deposit required
* Credit Cards: MC/VISA/AMEX/DC
* Open: December - October
* Hotel Rates: AS 765 - AS 2,610/day (room only)
* Spa on premises
* **Spa Facilities**: Direct access to thermal facilities, indoor and outdoor thermal pools, mud baths, massage room, beauty parlor, sauna, gymnasium, inhalation rooms
* **Spa Programs**: Single Weeks, Ozon-Aslan Regeneration Program, Slim & Beauty Program, Fitness Program
* **Spa Treatments**: thermal baths, mud cures and mud packs, inhalation, massages, underwater massages, ozon treatments, Aslan injections, Wiedermann Cure, physical training and exercises, sun tanning, beauty and regeneration, weight loss treatments, low cal biological food
* **Spa Packages**: Single Week; Regeneration Cure (21 nights); Slim & Beauty Program (14 nights) Fitness Program (14 nights)

* **Indications**: same as Bad Mitterndorf plus beauty, regeneration, weight loss and fitness
* Medical Supervision: 1 MD
* Treatments Approved: Ministry of Health and

DESCRIPTION: Health Resort amidst forests and mountains with modern comfort and elaborate spa facilities. Everything at the hotel revolves around health. The extensive cure programs are designed to enhance the individual's well being including regeneration cures and fitness programs. All programs are medically supervised. A nourishing and well balanced biological gourmet food is offered. Recreation: horseback riding, tennis, hiking, mountain climbing, golf, swimming, surfing, downhill and cross-country skiing.

BAD TATZMANNSDORF (Burgenald)
) 3353

✈ Schwechat Airport (VIE) 63 mi. / 100 km.

Bad Tatzmannsdorf, population 1,900, is a well-known spa resort town in the easternmost Austrian province of Burgenland near the Hungarian border. This small town takes pride in its old spa tradition. The modern "Kurhaus", in the heart of a charming floral park, offers live entertainment in the summer for the enjoyment of the public.

The spa's four thermal springs are classified under three categories: springs containing calcium-carbonate of hydrogen, springs containing sodium-calcium-carbonate of hydrogen, and springs containing calcium-carbonate of hydrogen with iron. In addition to the thermal springs, curative peat bog is also used in therapy.

Indications: mud-packs and baths have curative effect on rheumatism, arthritis, abrasions of the spine, and inflammations of the nerves. Mud baths are used in the treatment of diseases of the female abdominal organs and have a certain success in treating female sterility.

The following illnesses can be treated in Bad Tatzmannsdorf: cardiac and circulatory diseases, symptoms of exhaustion, need for recuperation, convalescence, diseases of the digestive system, diseases of the respiratory system (chronic bronchitis, asthma), arthritis, healing disorders, burns, forms of dermatitis and eczema, disorders of

sexual functions, gout, uric acid stones, anemia from iron deficiency, diseases of the kidneys and urinal conducts, gynecological diseases, rheumatic diseases, sequels of injuries, exhaustion and depression.

Bad Tatzmannsdorf is 75 miles (120 km.) south of Vienna and is accessible from Vienna or Graz (90 km. / 56 mi.) south of Bad Tatzmannsdorf) by car or rail.

Steigenberger Bad Tazmannsdorf
♥♥♥♥

Am Golfplatz 1, Bad Tazmannsdorf (Burgenland), A-7431, Tel: (3353) 88410. Fax: (3533) 884155. TYPE: Spa Hotel. LOCATION: Between two golf courses among rolling hills. SPA CLIENTELE: Women and men. DESCRIPTION: Elegant resort hotel with Beauty Centre, weight loss and cure treatments. Recreation: golf, horseback riding.

BAD WALTERSDORF (Styria)
) 3333

✈ Thalerhof Airport (GRZ) Graz 65 km. / 40 mi.
Schwechat Airport (VIE) Vienna 150 km. / 94 mi.

Der Steirerhof
♥♥♥♥♥

Wagerberg 125, A-8271 Bad Waltersdorf. Tel: (3333) 32110. Fax: (3333) 3211444. TYPE: Spa Hotel. LOCATION: Thermal region of eastern Styria. SPA CLIENTELE: Women and men. DESCRIPTION: Elegant spa hotel with 1000 sq.m. (11,000 sq.ft.) thermal waterpark. Programs: beauty, weight loss, thalassotherapy.

Steigenberger
Bad Waltersdorf Hotel
♥♥♥♥

Am Wagerberg 125, Bad Waltersdorf (Styria) A-8271, Tel: (3333) 32110, Fax: (3333) 3211-444. TYPE: Spa Hotel. LOCATION: Quiet Park-like setting. SPA CLIENTELE: Women and men. DESCRIPTION: Elegant hotel with Health Club and extensive Spa facilities offering cure treatments.

BADGASTEIN
⟩ 6434
✈ Salzburg Airport (SZG) 60 mi. / 96 km.

Badgastein, population 6,200, is the premier spa of Austria and one of the best in Europe. The healing properties of the thermal water were discovered in the 15th century by the Duke of Styria whose gangrenous wound was cured by the water. Ever since, Badgastein has maintained its position as a healing spa resort. The water, hot radon springs at 45°c (110°F), originate in the foothills of the Graukogel Mountains, and are cooled to 20°c (68°F) for medical treatments.

Indications: therapies are recommended in the treatment of the following diseases or conditions: rheumatic and non-rheumatic affections of the locomotor system, sequels of injuries, circulatory disorders, certain metabolic diseases, mouth cavity, geriatric complaints, fertility and potency disorders, neuroglia and neuritis.

The beautiful location of the town on the slope of the Tauren massif combined with pure air, skiing stations and excellent spa facilities make this spa town one of the most popular spa resorts in Europe. Badgastein can be reached from Salzburg by car or rail. The distance is about 50 miles (80 km.) south.

Best Western Hotel Weismayr
♥♥♥♥

Kaiser Franz Josef Str 6, Badgastein (Salzburg), A-5640, Tel: (6434) 2594, Fax: (6434) 2594-14. TYPE: Spa Hotel. LOCATION: Adjacent to the Casino in town center. SPA CLIENTELE: Women and men. DESCRIPTION: Historic hotel with Thermal baths, sauna, solarium and indoor pool. 70 rooms, 8 suites.

Elisabethpark Hotel
♥♥♥♥♥

Kaiser Franz Josef Str 5, Badgastein (Salsburg), A-5640, Tel: (6434) 25510, Fax: (6434) 255110. TYPE: Spa

Hotel. LOCATION: Center of spa resort area, opposite Casino. SPA CLIENTELE: Women and men. DESCRIPTION: Elegant hotel with thermal pool and health spa facilities. Diet menu available. Recreation: golf, tennis and water sports. 110 rooms, 5 suites.

Europäischer Hof
♥♥♥♥

Miesbichlstraße 20, 5640 Badgastein. Tel: (6434) 25260. Fax: (6434) 2526-262. TYPE: Hotel & Spa. MANAGER: Josef Kronbichler. LOCATION: Bad Bruck at the southeastern outskirts of Bad Gastein. SPA CLIENTELE: Women and men, Mixed.

* Rooms: 129 w/priv. bath. Suites: 14
* Phone, CTV, minibar, private balcony
* Restaurant & Terrace Café
* Airport: Salzburg 95 km. / 60 mi.
* Train Station: Badgastein 3.5 km. / 2mi.
* Airport/Train Transportation: free pick up from train station, taxi or train from airport
* Reservations: suggested
* Credit Cards: MC/VISA/AMEX/DC/EC
* Open: Year round
* Hotel Rates: AS 1,150 - AS 2,910/day (room only)
* TAC: 10%
* Spa on premises
* **Spa Facilities**: swimming pool, therapeutic facilities, thermal pool, fitness room, sauna and solarium, Beauty Center
* **Spa Programs**: Medical, Fitness, Beauty (1- 21 day Spa programs)
* **Spa Treatments**: radon thermal baths, underwater massages, mud packs, thermal inhalations, mouth baths, complimentary daily gymnastics at the thermal water pool or at the fitness center, beauty treatments at the Beauty Center (peeling, facials, herbal baths)
* **Spa Packages**: Gastein Cure (21 days) Beauty Program (1 day or 1 week)
* **Indications**: see above
* Medical Supervision: 3 MD
* Treatments Approved: Salzburg Government

DESCRIPTION: A contemporary resort complex with extensive therapeutic spa facilities. Recreation: golf, tennis, horseback riding, swimming, fishing and skiing (winter).

Hoteldorf Grüner Baum
♥♥♥♥

Koetschachtal 25, Badgastein (Salzburg), A-5640, Tel: (6434) 25160, Fax: (6434) 251625. USA/Canada reservations: (800) 257-5344. TYPE: Spa Hotel. LOCATION: Mountainside location amid beautiful landscapes, 3 km. / 2 mi. from town. SPA CLIENTELE: Women and men.

* Rooms: 80 w/priv. bath
* Phone, CTV, minibar, hairdryer
* Restaurants (3) diet menus, bars (2)
* Airport: Salzburg 100 km. / 63 mi.
* Train Station: 5 km. / 3 mi.
* Airport/Train Transportation: taxi
* Reservations: required
* Credit Cards: VISA/AMEX/MC/DIS/EC
* Open: Year round
* TAC: 10%
* Spa on premises
* **Spa Facilities**: in-house thermal springs, thermal pool, Shiseido Beauty Spa
* **Spa Programs**: Beauty, Anti-Stress, Detoxification, classic Gastein therapy
* **Spa Treatments**: facials, masks, slimming treatments, body wraps, thalassotherapy, exfoliating, Japanese sparkling bath, seaweed bath with essential, relaxing bath, thermal baths, massages, motion therapy, Kneipp founding, lymphatic drainage, Shiatsu, Tuina, mud packs, cold packs
* **Spa Packages**: Beauty Day (5 hrs); Shiseido Beauty Day for him (5 hrs.); Beauty Program (3 days); Cellulite Intensive Program (3 days); Vitality Week; Anti-Stress Week; Shiseido Beauty Week (5 days)
* **Indications**: beauty, pampering, revitalization, anti-stress. Gastein Cure indications: rheumatism, arthritis, arthrosis, polyarthritis, vertebral and intervertebral injuries, chronic circulatory disturbances
* Medical Supervision: medical staff
* Treatments Approval: Austrian Health Ministry

DESCRIPTION: Health Spa in historic hotel, a former royal hunting lodge. Accommodations are in Alpine-style rooms and suites. The Health Spa features health, beauty and vitality treatments based on Shiseido products and classic Gastein healing thermal water with radon.

Kur & Sporthotel Miramonte
♥♥♥

Reitlpromenade 3, Badgastein (Salsburg), A-5640, Tel: (6434) 2577, Fax: (6434) 257791. TYPE: Spa Hotel. LOCATION: Hillside location. SPA CLIENTELE: Women and men. DESCRIPTION: Small spa hotel with sauna, solarium, gym offering low cal diet menu. 36 rooms.

Mozart Hotel
♥♥♥

Kaiser Franz Josef Str 25, Badgastein (Salsburg), A-5640, Tel: (6434) 26860, Fax: (6434) 2686-62. TYPE: Spa Hotel. LOCATION: Central location near ski lifts. SPA CLIENTELE: Women and men. DESCRIPTION: Moderate spa hotel from 1900 with traditionally furnished rooms. Recreation: golf, skiing and skating. 70 rooms.

Slazburgerhof Hotel
♥♥♥♥

Grillparzerstr 1, Badgastein (Salsburg), A-5640, Tel: (6434) 2037, Fax: (6434) 3867. TYPE: Spa Hotel. LOCATION: Panoramic location near thermal springs. SPA CLIENTELE: Women and men. DESCRIPTION: Traditional spa hotel with thermal baths near skiing lift. 108 rooms.

Wildbad Hotel
♥♥♥

Waggerlstraße 20, 5640 Badgastein. Tel: (6434) 37610. Fax: (6434) 376170. TYPE: Spa Hotel. LOCATION: Pleasant location with mountain view. SPA CLIENTELE: Women and men.

* Rooms: 40 w/priv. bath. Suites: 4
* Phone, CTV, C/H
* Train Station: Badgastein: 300 m. / 300 yards
* Train Station Transportation: taxi
* Reservations: required
* Credit Cards: AMEX
* Open: December - October
* Hotel Rates: AS 690 - 1,780/day (room only)
* TAC: 10%
* Spa on premises
* **Spa Facilities**: indoor radon thermal pools and baths, Health Center with solarium, massage-inhalation rooms, sauna
* **Spa Packages**: 1,2, or 3 weeks Gastein Cure
* **Spa Treatments**: radon thermal baths, massages, fango mud packs, thermal swimming, inhalations,underwater therapy massage, low calorie healthy food
* **Indications**: same as Badgastein
* Medical Supervision: 1 MD
* Treatments Approved: Austrian Health Ministry

DESCRIPTION: An attractive hotel providing good standard accommodations, great mountain views and a cozy international bar. The house specializes in medical hot springs cures with extensive facilities under medical supervision. Cosmetic treatments, and well being enhancing cures are available. Weight watchers can enjoy a nutritious well balanced low calorie spa diet menu. Recreation: Skiing nearby.

BLUMAU (Styria)
) **3383**

✈ Thalerhof Airport (GRZ) Graz 60 km. / 38 mi.
Schwechat Airport (VIE) Vienna 150 km. / 94 mi.

Rogner-Bad Blumau
A Rogner Dorint Hotel
♥♥♥♥

♨ 🐎 🚶 ◉

Blumau 100, A-8283. Tel: (3383) 5100-0. Fax: (3383) 5100-808. TYPE: First Class Spa Hotel. MANAGING DIRECTOR: Alfred Hackl. LOCATION: Quiet countryside setting near the village of Blumau. SPA CLIENTELE: Men, women, children and teenagers accepted.

* Rooms: 243 w/priv. bath; Suites 4
  Phone, CTV, minibar, safe deposit
* Apartments: 24 w/bedroom, living area, 2 bathrooms, kitchenette
* Restaurants, bar
* Reservations: required
* Credit Cards: MC/VISA/AMEX/DIN
* Open: Year round
* Hotel Rates: AS 1,250 - 1,600 (sgl)
  AS 1,700 - 2,400 (dbl)
  Apartment: AS 2,500 - 3,300
* TAC: 10%
* Spa on premises: Beauty Farm & Wellness Center
* Year Established: 1997
* **Spa Facilities**: indoor & outdoor swimming pools, saunas, therapy center with massages, meditation island, hot springs, gym
* **Spa Programs**: Beauty, Anti-Stress, Fitness, Relaxation
* **Spa Treatments**: drinking cures, inhalation, sound therapy, sodium hydrogen carbonate spring
* **Spa Packages**: available from AS 4,350 per person (3 nights including treatments)
* Length of stay: 3 nights minimum
* Medical Supervision: 2 MD
* Treatments Approved: Austrian Government
* Email: spa.blumau@rogner.com
* Web: www.rogner.com

DESCRIPTION: Unique art hotel, spa, sports and adventure Center near Graz in Styria's thermal region. The resort was designed by the Austrian artist Friedensreich Hundertwasser and it is billed as "the world's largest work of art". The Spa or wellness center, offers an array of treatments for the mind and spirit. The staff is friendly and always very helpful. The ancient thermal baths are Bad Blumau's major attraction. The Spa's main philosophy is to facilitate harmony with nature and soul. Nowhere else do nature, environment and man's creativity harmonize so perfectly as in Rogner-Bad-Blumau. Amenities: 4 outdoor tennis courts and sports facilities. *A Rogner Dorint Hotel.*

ELBIGENALP (Tyrol)
) **5634**

Vital & Erlebnishotel Alpenrose
❤❤❤❤

Untergiblen 21, A-6652 Elbigenalp / Lechtal. Tel: (5634) 6652. Fax: (5634) 665287. TYPE: Spa Hotel. LOCATION: Alpine setting on 6000 sq.m. (66,000 sq.ft.) of parkland with a natural pool and sunbathing lawn. SPA CLIENTELE: Women and men. DESCRIPTION: Tyrolean style health spa with weight loss, anti-stress and beauty programs. Weekly entertainment and cross-country trails nearby.

ELLMAU (Tyrol)
⟩ 5358

Der Baer Hotel
❤❤❤❤

Kirchbichi 9, Ellmau (Tyrol) A-6352, Tel: (5358) 2395, Fax: (5358) 239556. TYPE: Spa Hotel. LOCATION: High Mountain setting. SPA CLIENTELE: Women and men. DESCRIPTION: Tyrolean mountain style health resort with spa facilities and beauty treatments. 31 rooms, 13 suites some with fireplace.

GASCHURN (Vorarlberg)
⟩ 5558
✈ Zurich Int'l Airport (ZRH) Switzerland
Kranebitten Airport (INN) Innsbruck

Dr. Felbermayer
❤❤❤❤

A-6793, Gaschurn/Montafon. Tel: (5558) 86170. Fax: (5558) 861741. TYPE: Spa Hotel. LOCATION: In the heart of Montafon alpine park, in the Silvretta region of Austria near the Swiss border. SPA CLIENTELE: Women and men. DESCRIPTION: Health spa with 30 years experience in regeneration and fitness plans under medical supervision. Weight loss and Beauty programs.

DORNBIRN (Vorarlberg)
⟩ 5572

✈ Zurich Int'l Airport (ZRH) Switzerland

Rickatsschwende
❤❤❤❤

A-6850 Dornbirn. Tel: (5572) 25350. Fax: (5572) 2535070. TYPE: Health Spa. SPA DIRECTOR: Hans Peter Schroff. LOCATION: Lake Constance, the Rhine Valley and the Swiss Apls. SPA CLIENTELE: Women & men. DESCRIPTION: Wellness center specializing in the original Mayr dietary plan. Programs offered are weight loss and beauty programs based on Ahava Dead Sea products.

HALDENSEE (Tyrol)
⟩ 5675
✈ Kranebitten Airport (INN) Innsbruck

Hotel Liebes Rot-Flüh
❤❤❤❤❤

Seestraße no. 5, A-6673 Haldensee. Tel: (5675) 6431. Fax: (5675) 643646 / 643641. TYPE: Spa Hotel. LOCATION: Mountain setting. SPA CLIENTELE: Women and men. DESCRIPTION: Deluxe spa specializing in body management combining the latest findings from medicine and sport. Enjoy Slim and Beautiful week and indulge in an exotic Cleopatra oil-and-milk bath.

HIRSCHEGG (Vorarlberg)
⟩ 8329
✈ Zurich Int'l Airport (ZRH) Switzerland
Kranebitten Airport (INN) Innsbruck

Ifen Hotel
❤❤❤❤

Kleinwalsertal, Hirschegg (Vorarlberg), A-6992. Tel: (8329) 5071, Fax: (8329) 3475. TYPE: Spa Hotel. LOCATION: Ski area of Kleinwalsertal / Allgau Alps. SPA CLIENTELE: Women and men. DESCRIPTION: Mountain spa hotel with Old World atmosphere. Accommodation in 65 spacious rooms, mostly with separate living area. The Wellness center has its own spring water, Beauty Farm and cure facilities.

IGLS (Tyrol)
☽ 512

✈ Kranbitten Airport (INN) Innsbruck 8 km. / 5 mi.

Kurzentrum Parkhotel
♥♥♥♥

Igler Straße 51, Igls (Tyrol) A-6080, Tel: (512) 377305, Fax: (512) 379225. TYPE: Spa Hotel. LOCATION: In a private park near ski lifts. SPA CLIENTELE: Women and men. DESCRIPTION: Elegant health center with village-like character and magnificent Tyrolean scenery. Programs include: weight loss, beauty and anti-aging. Recreation: golf, ski

Schlosshotel
♥♥♥♥♥

Villersteig 2, Igls (Tyrol) A-6080, Tel: (512) 377217, Fax: (512) 378679. TYPE: Resort Hotel & Spa. LOCATION: In a private park near ski lifts. SPA CLIENTELE: Women and men. DESCRIPTION: Historic castle hotel with cure facilities, gym, sauna, diet menu.

Sporthotel
♥♥♥♥

Hilberstr 17, Igls (Tyrol) A-6080, Tel: (512) 377241, Fax: (512) 378679. TYPE: Resort Hotel & Spa. LOCATION: Center of village near ski lifts. SPA CLIENTELE: Women and men. DESCRIPTION: Attractive resort hotel with health spa, cure facilities, solarium and gym. 80 rooms, 14 suites.

ISCHGL (Tyrol)
☽ 5444

✈ Kranbitten Airport (INN) Innsbruck 8 km. / 5 mi.

Trofana Royal
♥♥♥♥♥

A-6561 Ischgl. Tel: (5444) 600. Fax: (5444) 60090. TYPE: Health Spa. LOCATION: Alpine setting. SPA CLIENTELE: Women and men. DESCRIPTION: The largest wellness, sport and beauty complex in the Alps. Programs include: weight loss, beauty, pampering, anti-stress and fitness. Amenities: Adonis waterpark, fitness centre, and indoor golf.

KITZBÜHEL (Tyrol)
☽ 5356

✈ Munich Airport (MUC) Germany,
81 mi. (130 km.) northwest.
Salzburg Airport (SZG) 57 mi. / 90 km.
Kranbitten Airport (INN) Innsbruck 60 mi. / 95 km.

Kitzbühel, population 11,000, is a fashionable ski resort in Tyrol popular with the international jet-set for skiing or summer holiday. The town started to attract the European "upper crust" after Edward, Prince of Wales, chose Kitzbühel for vacation and recreation in the late 1920's. Skiing is the major attraction here. The famous Kitzbühel Ski Circus allows downhill skiing for more than 50 miles (80 km.). In the evening enjoy gaming and entertainment at the Kitzbühel Spiel Casino in the Hotel Goldener Greif (tel: 2300). Casino games include: roulette, blackjack, and baccarat.

Polly's Vital-Center
♥♥♥♥

c/o Hotel Schloss Lebenberg, A-6370 Kitzbühel. Tel: (5356) 4301. Fax: (5356) 4405. TYPE: Health & Beauty Spa. MANAGER: L. Polly Hillbrunner. LOCATION: At the fashionable Hotel Schloss Lebenberg. SPA CLIENTELE: Women , men, family oriented. (Mostly Women).

* Rooms: 96 w/priv. bath. Suites: 58
* Restaurants (3) & Bar
* Wheelchair Accessibility
* Airport: Salzburg or Innsbruck 90 km. (57 mi.)
* Airport Transportation: train, taxi
* Train Station: Kitzbühel, 1 km. / 1/2 mi.
* Reservations: requested
* Credit Cards: MC/VISA/AMEX/DC/EC/JCB
* Open: December - October
* Hotel Rates: AS 980 - AS 3,000 (room only)

* Spa on premises
* **Spa Facilities**: Modern cure department, indoor swimming pool, sauna, solarium, beauty salon
* **Spa Programs**: Beauty & Health, Weight Loss
* **Spa Treatments**: sauna-wrap cure with herb extracts, vibration-massage, underwater massage, interference-massage, Moor bath, sulfur bath, oxygen bath, stanger bath, peeling, body wraps, breast treatments, skin care 'ampule-cure', natural cosmetics
* **Indications**: slimming, beauty, illness of the joints, lumbago, rheum, common feminine illnesses, blood circulation problems, neuralgia
* Medical Supervision: 1 MD
* Treatments Approved: Austrian Health Ministry

DESCRIPTION: Polly-Vital specializes in beauty and slimming based on products made of natural plants, herbs extracts and oils. After complete medical examination a specially chosen herb extracts are applied to problem areas and massaged in. Medicinal baths are prescribed for medical conditions under a strict medical supervision. Guests can enjoy the attractive accommodations at the Hotel Schloss Lebenberg which is a renovated medieval castle. Recreation: skiing and cross-country skiing, casino, hiking, water sports, bridge club.

LEUTASCH (Tyrol)
ↄ **5214**
✈ Kranebitten Airport (INN) Innsbruck

Hotel Quellenhof
♥♥♥♥

A-6105 Leutasch/Tirol. Tel: (5214) 6782. Fax: (5214) 6369. TYPE: Spa Hotel. LOCATION: In the Tyrolean mountains. SPA CLIENTELE: Women and men. DESCRIPTION: Tyrolean chalet style health resort with weight loss, beauty, pampering and fitness programs. Specialties: Kneipp therapy, outdoor saline whirlpools, thalassotherapy.

MAURACH (Tyrol)
ↄ **5243**
✈ Kranebitten Airport (INN) Innsbruck

Sporthotel Alpenrose
♥♥♥♥

A-6212 Maurach 68. Tel: (5243) 52930. Fax: (5243) 5466. TYPE: Spa Hotel. LOCATION: Lake Achensee in Tyrol. SPA CLIENTELE: Women and men. DESCRIPTION: Home to the Wellness Residence the Spa offers beauty, weight loss and fitness programs. Skiing and cross-country trail nearby.

MIEMING (Tyrol)
ↄ **5264**
✈ Kranebitten Airport (INN) Innsbruck

Wellnes Resort Schwartz
♥♥♥♥

A-6414 Mieming 141. Tel: (5264) 52120. Fax: (5264) 52127. TYPE: Wellness Resort. LOCATION: Alpine setting on Mieming's sunny plateau. SPA CLIENTELE: Women and men, family oriented. DESCRIPTION: Award winning wellness center with weight loss, beauty, fitness and holistic programs.

OBERTAUREN (Salzburg)
ↄ **6456**
✈ Salzburg Airport (SZG)

Kohlmayr Hotel
♥♥♥

Dr. F. Kressse Str 102, Obertauern (Salsburg) A-5562, Tel: (6456) 272, Fax: (6456) 406. TYPE: Spa Hotel. LOCATION: In fine ski area. SPA CLIENTELE: Women and men. DESCRIPTION: Traditional spa hotel with cure facilities, gym, solarium, indoor pool. Ski school nearby. 60 rooms.

PERTISAU (Tyrol)
ↄ **5243**
✈ Kranebitten Airport (INN) Innsbruck

Hotel Fürstenhaus
❤❤❤❤

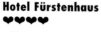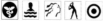

A-6213 Pertisau. Tel: (5243) 5442. Fax: (5243) 6168. TYPE: Spa Hotel. LOCATION: On the shores of Achensee, the largest lake in Tyrol. SPA CLIENTELE: Women and men. DESCRIPTION: First class health resort with 60 rooms, open fireplace and winter garden. Programs: weight loss (1000 calorie diet); Beauty Farm with Gertraud Gruber's holistic beauty care; thalassotherapy, Kneipp facilities.

REUTHE (Vorarlberg)
❩ 5514
✈ Zurich Int'l Airport (ZRH) Switzerland
Kranebitten Airport (INN) Innsbruck

Kurhotel Bad Reuthe
❤❤❤❤

A-6870 Reuthe / Bergenzerwald. Tel: (5514) 22650. Fax: (5514) 2265100. TYPE: Spa Hotel. LOCATION: Bergenz forest area. SPA CLIENTELE: Women and men. DESCRIPTION: Health center offering weight loss and beauty treatments based on natural peat, spring rich in iron, low calorie meals and motion therapy.

SAALFEDEN (Salzburg)
❩ 6582
✈ Salzburg Airport (SZG) 60 km. / 38 mi.

Sporthotel Gut Brandlhof

Hohlwegen 4, Saalfelden (Salsburg) A-5760. Tel: (6582) 7800-0, Fax: (6582) 7800-598. TYPE: Spa Hotel. LOCATION: Scenic location surrounded by mountains. SPA CLIENTELE: Woman and men. DESCRIPTION: Chalet style resort with health spa, Greek sauna village and golf course. Programs: beauty, fitness and weight loss.

SALZBURG (Salzburg)
❩ 662
✈ Salzburg Airport (SZG) 3 mi. / 5 km.

Hotel Kobenzl
❤❤❤❤

Gaisberg 11, Salzburg (Salzburg) A-5020. Tel: (662) 641510, Fax: (662) 642238. TYPE: Deluxe Hotel & Spa. LOCATION: High on Mt. Gaisberg overlooking the city. SPA CLIENTELE: Women and men. DESCRIPTION: Deluxe hotel with spa facilities, indoor pool, sauna, solarium, gym, massage, fitness and beauty treatments. 40 rooms.

Hotel Schloss Fuschl
❤❤❤❤❤

Hof-bei-Salzburg,(Salzburg) A-5322, Tel: (6229) 22530, Fax: (6229) 2253-521.TYPE: Spa Hotel. LOCATION: Near Salzburg on Lake Fuschl. SPA CLIENTELE: Women and men. DESCRIPTION: Deluxe 15th century castle with elegant rooms and suites, private beach, golf course and Shiseido Beauty Farm.

SCHRÖCKEN (Vorarlberg)
❩ 5519
✈ Zurich Int'l Airport (ZRH) Switzerland
Kranebitten Airport (INN) Innsbruck

Hotel Widderstein
❤❤❤❤

A-6888 Schröken 38. Tel: (5519) 4000. Fax: (5519) 4008. TYPE: Health Resort. LOCATION: Alpine setting in the Bergenz Forest. SPA CLIENTELE: Women and men, family oriented. DESCRIPTION: State of the art sports and health centre specializing in weight loss and beauty treatments.

SCHWAZ (Tyrol)
❩ 5242
✈ Kranebitten Airport (INN) Innsbruck

Natur Hotel Grafenast
❤❤❤

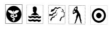

A-6130 Schwaz. Tel: (5242) 63209. Fax: (5242) 6320999. TYPE: Health Resort. LOCATION: On Hochpillberg at 1,330 m. / 4,389 ft. SPA CLIENTELE: Women and men. DESCRIPTION: Mountain health spa with beauty and weight loss programs based on natural products. The spa uses natural mountain spring water, and medicinal herbs from their own garden.

SEEFELD (Tyrol)
⟩ 5519
✈ Kranebitten Airport (INN) Innsbruck

Vital Hotel Royal
♥♥♥♥♥

🐵 ≋ 🏃 🏃 ⊙

A-6100 Seefeld / Reith b. Seefeld. Tel: (5212) 44310. Fax: (5212) 4431450. TYPE: Spa Hotel. LOCATION: Pristine Alpine setting. SPA CLIENTELE: Women and men. DESCRIPTION: Life management resort with Holistic Medical Centre. Programs include: weight loss, beauty and health. Special beauty program for HIM. Combination of Chinese therapies and western medicine.

ST. LEONHARD (Tyrol)
⟩ 5413
✈ Kranebitten Airport (INN) Innsbruck

Sport & Vitalhotel Seppl
♥♥♥♥

🐵 ≋ 🏃 🏃 ⊙

Weißwald 41, A-6481 St. Leonhard, Pitztal. Tel: (5413) 86220 / 86205. Fax: (5413) 86352. TYPE: Spa Hotel. LOCATION: Colorful mountain world of the Pitztal valley. SPA CLIENTELE: Women and men, family oriented. DESCRIPTION: The Spa offers Gertraud Gruber's holistic methods, natural care products and the latest in beauty and slimming treatments. Cross-country trail on the doorstep.

TELFS-BUCHEN (Tyrol)
⟩ 5262
✈ Kranebitten Airport (INN) Innsbruck

Telfs-Buchen are fashionable winter resorts in the heart of the magnificent Tyrolean Alps, near Seefeld and Innsbruck. Recreation: (Winter) Nordic skiing and cross-country ski trails, ice skating, sleigh rides and indoor tennis. (Summer) lake water sports, fishing, tennis and golf.

Interalpen-Hotel Tyrol
♥♥♥♥♥

🐵 🏃 🏃

A-6410 Telfs-Buchen. Tel: (5262) 606194. Fax: (5262) 606190. TYPE: Deluxe Resort & Spa. LOCATION: In a secluded area near Seefeld in the Tyrolean Alps. SPA CLIENTELE: Women and men.

* Rooms: 286 w/priv. bath, Suites: 30
* Restaurants, bars & Cafes
* Wheelchair Accessibility
* Conference Rooms: 10 - 400
* Airport: Innsbruck
* Airport Transportation: taxi
* Open: Dec. 18 - April 1 / May 7 - Oct. 31
* Credit Cards: MC/VISA/AMEX/EC/DC/ACC
* Hotel Rates: AS 1,500 - AS 4,600/day (room only)
* TAC: 8%
* **Spa Facilities**: gym, therapeutic baths, Beauty Farm, indoor swimming pool,whirlpool, solarium
* **Spa Programs**: Beauty, anti-stress, weight loss
* **Spa Packages**: Anti-Stress, Aesthetic, Slimming
* **Spa Treatments**: massages, biosaunas, reflexology, parafango, lymphatic drainage, fitness sessions, hydrotherapy, facials, phytomer
* **Indications**: stress, obesity, pampering
* Medical Supervision: in house MD

DESCRIPTION: Pyramid shaped luxury hotel in a scenic Alpine setting. All public places are tastefully furnished with elegant furnishings, paintings and antiques. The spa offers anti-stress, slimming and revitalizing treatments. Recreation: tennis, golf, hiking, jogging, mountaineering, cross-country skiing, downhill skiing, sleigh rides. Variety of entertainment is provided during the day and in the evenings.

WARMBAD-VILLACH (Carinthia)
⟩ 4242

✈ Klagenfurt Airport (KLU) 38 km. (24 mi.)

Warmbad-Villach, population 64,000, is located on the Drau River in the southern Austrian Alps. It is ideally situated for exploring the magnificent Carinthia's Lake District near the Yugoslav/Italian border. The Acratic thermal hot springs have healing powers that were appreciated centuries ago by the Celts and the Romans. Traditionally a meeting place and playground of the Austro-Hungarian Aristocracy, it is today a modern Spa town where people come to 'take the Waters'; experience modern balneotherapy, revitalization programs, and the pleasant sub-alpine climate.

Indications: rheumatic and non-rheumatic affections of the locomotor system, sequels of injuries and paralysis, symptoms of over-fatigue and exhaustion, functional circulatory disorders, gynecological diseases, neuro-vegetative dystonia.

Warmbad-Villach can be reached from the Klagenfurt Airport via Route 100 going west, or From Salzburg via Hwy A10 going south.

Josefinhof Hotel Im Park
❤❤❤❤

Warmbad-Villach, A-9504. Tel: (4242) 30030. Fax: (4242) 300389. TYPE: First Class Spa Resort Hotel. LOCATION: In a beautifully landscaped private park. SPA CLIENTELE: Men, Women.

* Rooms: 110 w/private bath
* Phone, color TV, radio, balcony
* Restaurants, Lounges, Bar
* Airport: Klagenfurt Airport 38 km. (24 mi.)
* Airport Transportation: taxi, bus
* Reservations: deposit required
* Credit Cards: VISA/MC/AMEX
* Open: Year round
* Rates: AS 890 - AS 1,650/day (full board); TAC: 10%
* Spa on premises
* Spa Facilities: Thermal-Spa Center with private hot spring, 'Long-Evity' Medical Center, Fitness studio, saunas, massage and treatment rooms, medical facilities, whirlpools, jacuzzis

* Spa Programs: Thermal Program, 'Long-Evity' Program with individual emphasis on Fitness, Weight Loss, Diabetes self control
* Spa Treatments: bathing in thermal water, massages, hydrotherapy, wraps, gymnastics, thermal cure, aerobics, stretching, swim-gym, cardio-vascular training, special 500 cal. diet for rapid weight-loss, body composition test
* Spa Packages: Long-Evity Program; Thermal Cure Non-Smoker Training.
* Indications: same as Warmbad-Villach
* Contraindications: cancer
* Medical Supervision: 1 MD
* Treatments Approved: Austrian Health Ministry

DESCRIPTION: Josefinehof Spa Resort Hotel is a modern complex with tastefully appointed rooms, fine service, excellent food, and first class sports and recreational facilities. The Long-Evity SPA emphasizes traditional thermal cures which stimulate all biochemical processes of the human organism, the metabolism of the cell and the nervous system. It also offers a modern medical center featuring various 'Long-Evity' programs under medical supervision of medical professionals from the Vienna University Clinic with particular reputation for its high medical standards. Treatments are available for rejuvenation, revitalization, stress reduction, weight loss etc. The staff speaks English and is used to serve international clientele. Recreation: skiing, tennis, biking and jogging.

WARTH a. ARLBERG (Vorarlberg)
↘ 5583
✈ Zurich Int'l Airport (ZRH) Switzerland
Kranebitten Airport (INN) Innsbruck

Wellnesshotel Warther Hof
❤❤❤❤

Bregenzerwaldstraße 53, A-6767 Warth a. Arlberg. Tel: (5583) 3504. Fax: (5583) 4200. TYPE: Spa Hotel. LOCATION: Alpine setting. SPA CLIENTELE: Women and men, children welcome. DESCRIPTION: Family oriented wellness resort specializing in weight loss, beauty and holistic and Kneipp applications. Ski lifts and ski school nearby.

BAHAMAS

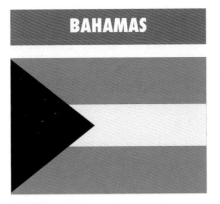

AREA: 5,382 sq. mi. (13,940 sq. km.)
POPULATION: 240,000
CAPITAL: Nassau
OFFICIAL LANGUAGE: English
CURRENCY: Bahamian $ (B$)
EXCHANGE RATE: 1 US$ = 1B$
TELEPHONE COUNTRY CODE: 242

The Bahamas consist of over 700 islands and cays, all blessed with beautiful beaches, and warm sunshine year round. The combination of fine climate, and great beaches makes the Bahamas a perfect destination for outdoor sports and recreation both on water and on the land.

ℹ️ The Bahamas Ministry of Tourism

P.O. Box N3701
Nassau, Bahamas
Tel: (242) 322-7500
Fax: (242) 328-0945

NASSAU

➤ No area code
✈ Nassau Int'l Airport (NAS)

Nassau, the island's capital and main port of entry, is located on the small island of New Providence. Nassau combines Old World charm with a New World glamour. In town you'll find stately colonial buildings, interesting monu-

ments, delightful shops along Bay Street and the side lanes of downtown, and gourmet international restaurants. Nearby Cable Beach and Paradise Island offer world-class resorts and casinos for gambling, entertainment, and fine dining.

The climate in the Bahamas is warm and pleasant year round. The winter's average daily temperature is in the 70°'sF (24°c), and summer's average daily temperature is in the 80°'sF (28°c).

Nassau is the crossroads of the island's air and sea connections. Airlines with direct flights from North American cities to Nassau include: Delta, TWA, Air Canada to mention just a few. Many cruise lines make Nassau their port of call, especially to allow their passengers to spend a night of fun and games at the island's popular casinos.

Sandals Royal Bahamian Resort & Spa
❤️❤️❤️❤️

P.O. B CB-13005, Cable Beach, Nassau. Tel: (242) 327-6400. Fax: (242) 327-6961. TYPE: Deluxe Resort & Spa. LOCATION: Western edge of Cable Beach. SPA CLIENTELE: Women and men.

* Rooms: 196 and 21 villa suites
* Airport: Nassau Int'l 5 mi. (8 km.)
* Season: Year round
* Credit Cards: MC/VISA/AMEX/DC
* Hotel Rates: on request
* SPA on premises
* **SPA Facilities**: Health & Fitness Center
* **SPA Treatments**: Austrian Moor-peat baths, facials, Swedish massages

DESCRIPTION: A gracious Manor House overlooking the ocean with its own private beach and fully staffed health and fitness center. Diet and fitness counselling available. Recreation: golf, tennis, racquetball, squash. Casino, cabaret and nightly entertainment nearby.

BELGIUM

AREA: 11,781 sq. mi. (30,513 sq. km.)
POPULATION: 9,850,000
CAPITAL: Brussels
OFFICIAL LANGUAGES: French, Flemish
CURRENCY: Belgian Franc (BF)
EXCHANGE RATE: 1 US$ = BF 34.06
TELEPHONE COUNTRY CODE: 32

Belgium is famous for the legendary town of Spa, whose name became a world wide accepted generic name for hot springs, health and fitness resorts. Spa is a thermal resort and an important health center.

In addition to Spa, there are three other health resorts in Belgium: Chaudfauntaine - the only natural hot spring resort in Belgium, and two thalassotherapy centers in Oostende and in Knokke.

ℹ Belgian National Tourist Office
Office de Promotion du Tourisme
Rue de Marché Aux Herbes 61, Brussels B-1000 Belgium

BRUSSELS
⟩ 2
✈ Brussels International Airport (BRU) 8 mi. / 13 km.

Metropole Hotel
❤❤❤❤

Place de Brouckere 31, 1000 Brussels. Tel: (2) 217-2300. Fax: (2) 218-0220. TYPE: Hotel with Health Club. LOCATION: City center near train station. DESCRIPTION: Old World style hotel with fitness room. 224 rooms, 12 suites.

Radisson SAS Hotel
❤❤❤❤❤

Rue du Fosse-aux-loups, 1000 Brussels. Tel: (2) 219-2828. Fax: (2) 219-6262. TYPE: Hotel with small Health Club. LOCATION: Downtown near the Grand Place. DESCRIPTION: Deluxe hotel with fitness center, sauna, solarium. 281 rooms, 18 suites, 3 restaurants, 2 bars. Hotel Rate: from BFR 5,500.

CHAUDFONTAINE
⟩ 4
✈ Liege / Bierst Airport (LGG)

Chaudfontaine is a spa town on the edge of the Ardenne Liegeoise about 6 mi. / 10 km. from Liege. This pretty town has its own natural mineral waters, the only natural hot springs in Belgium gushing out from volcanic depths. The thermal waters bubble up from the depths at a temperature of 98°F (26°c). It is pure, chemically neutral and slightly mineralized. As a drinking water "Chaudfontaine-Thermale" and Chaudfontaine-Cristal" help the elimination of excess water, waste and fights constipation. The fluorine content prevents dental decay. Its internal actions complement the external effects of thermal bathing in running water with under water jet showers, which is known to relieve rheumatic pains. A special re-education swimming pool offers great relief for sufferers from rheumatism and injuries.

Palace Hotel
❤❤

Esplanade 2, Chaudfontaine 4050. Tel: (4) 3657508. Fax: (4) 367-4153. TYPE: Hotel. LOCATION: In the center of town. DESCRIPTION: A small well run 2 star hotel convenient to the Thermal Institute and swimming pool.

KNOKKE
✈ 4

✈ Liege / Bierst Airport (LGG)

Knokke is one of three resort towns that make up the Knokke-Het Zoute beach resort area. Knokke offers casino, great beaches, fine shops, restaurants and night spots. The spa facilities are the only ones in Belgium integrated within a luxury hotel. Knokke can be reached by car or train in about one and a half hours from Brussels, twenty minutes from Brugges.

La Reserve Hotel & Thalassa Center
❤❤❤❤

Elisabenthlaan 160, Knokke-Heist, Belgium 8300. Tel: (50) 610606. Fax: (50) 603706. TYPE: Spa Hotel. LOCATION: One block from the beach across from the Casino. SPA CLIENTELE: Men, Women.

* Rooms: 112 w/priv. bath. Suites: 2
* Hotel Facilities: several restaurants, lounge, bar swimming pool, 4 tennis courts
* Train Station: Knokke 1 km. (0.6 mi.)
* Transportation: taxi
* Reservations: required
* Credit Cards: AMEX/DC/EC/VISA
* Open: Year round
* Hotel Rates: from BF 7,500/day
* TAC: 8%
* **Spa on premises**: Thalassotherapy Institute directly linked to hotel
* **Spa Facilities**: swimming pool, baths, showers, balneotherapeutic equipment, gym, consulting rooms
* **Spa Programs**: Rejuvenation, relaxation, general fitness, beauty, medical
* **Spa Treatments**: sea water baths, jet showers, mud packs, massages, electrotherapy, physiotherapy
* Treatment duration: 5 days
* **Indications**: rheumatic diseases, after-effects of bone injuries, orthopedic operations, respiratory illnesses, non-contagious skin diseases, circulatory problems, fatigue

* Medical Supervision: Examinations and tests
* Treatment Approval: Medical Centre

DESCRIPTION: A modern deluxe resort hotel on landscaped grounds, original built in 1949, added onto in 1975, and renovated in 1976, on the shore of the little private Lake Victoria, 200 yards from the beach and casino. One of Belgium's finest hotels with wonderful food, and an extensive art collection adorning the rooms.

LIMELETTE
✈ 10

✈ Brussels Int'l Airport (BRU) 25 km. / 16 mi.

Chateau de Limelette & Centre Thalgo
❤❤❤❤

Rue Charles Dubois 87, Limelette B-1342. Tel: (10) 421999. Fax: (10) 415759. TYPE: Hotel & Spa. LOCATION: Secluded hotel in historic building on 5 landscaped acres. SPA CLIENTELE: Women and men. DESCRIPTION: Elegant hotel with gym, sauna, jacuzzi, indoor pool, tennis, squash, physical therapy and spa treatments. 78 rooms. Hotel rates: from BFR 3,600.

OSTEND
✈ 59

✈ Ostend Airport (OST) 5 km. / 3 mi.

Ostend, population 80,000, is the most important and one of the oldest cities of the Belgian North Sea. It is a year round fishing center, and an important cross channel port of embarkation for steamer's heading to Dover, England. From May to October, it becomes Belgium's most sought after seaside resort with the attractions of a five kilometer beach, the Kursaal-Casino, Whellington Horse Racetrack, Folklore Museum, Marine Museum, golf course, and sports activities.

The "Queen" of the Belgian beach resorts is also a major Spa treatment center with its own Thermal Institute that features state-of-the-art scientific and medical equipment. It is, therefore, the ideal place for those who wish to combine the pleasures of a beach resort with spa treatments.

Iridia Thalassa
♥♥♥

37 Warschuststraat, 8400 Ostend. Tel: (59) 806644. Fax: (59) 805274. TYPE: Spa only. SPA CLIENTELE: Women and men.

Thermae Palace
♥♥♥

Koningin Astridlaan 7, 8400 Ostend, Tel: (59) 806644. Fax: (59) 805274. TYPE: Hotel with Spa. LOCATION: Seafront location within walking distance of downtown and the casino. SPA CLIENTELE: Women and men. DESCRIPTION: Historic Belle-Epoque style Hotel with health spa. 141 rooms, 5 suites, restaurant, bar, nightclub. Tennis and swimming pool nearby.

SPA
↘ **87**

✈ Brussels Int'l Airport (BRU) 120 km. / 75 mi.

Spa, population 12,000, is situated 24 miles (38 km.) southeast of Liege in the Ardenne region. In the 18th and 19th century it became popular when Europe's high society and royalty who flocked to its magical waters for a cure. It was the favored European health resort for many Kings and Queens as well as the highest officials in Europe known as the "Cafe de l'Europe" in the early 18th century. Ever since It has given its name to many health resorts throughout the world.

Hotel Alfa Balmoral
♥♥♥♥

Rte de Balmoral 33, Spa, Belgium 4880. Tel: (87) 772581. Fax: (87) 774174.. TYPE: Hotel with Health Club. LOCATION: Beautiful woodland setting, 2 km. / 1.5 mi. from town. SPA CLIENTELE: Women and men, teenagers and children accepted. DESCRIPTION: First class contemporary style hotel with health club facilities. 98 rooms, 9 con-

dos, restaurant, bar, cafe, heated pool, sauna, solarium.

Domaines des Hautes Fagnes
♥♥♥

Rue des Charmilles 67, Ovifat-Waimes, B-4950. Tel: (80) 446988. Fax: (80) 496919. TYPE: Spa Hotel. CLIENTELE: Women, men. LOCATION: 6 mi. / 10 km. from Spa. 71 rooms, Espace Beauty Thalgo, Thalgo Club (swimming pool, sauna, Turkish Bath, fitness room).

The Thermes de Spa
♥♥♥

2 Place Royale, 4880 SPA. Tel: (87) 772560. Fax: (87) 771363. TYPE: Spa only. LOCATION: Town center. SPA CLIENTELE: Women and men, teenagers accepted.

* Year Established: 1868
* **SPA Facilities**: SPA thermal institute, baths, gym, solarium, sauna, beauty center
* **SPA Treatments**: mineral water baths, massages, showers, peat baths, anti-cellulite, rheumatism, cardial-vascular, nervous tensions natural Carbogazeous baths, peat bath, hydrotherapy, inhalations of carbon-gaseous sulfur water.
* **Indications**: Rheumatic disorders, cardio-vascular disorders, after effects of traumatism - rehabilitation, and infections of the upper respiratory track.
* Medical Supervision: yes

DESCRIPTION: The Thermes de Spa dominates the main square of the town. Treatments at the Spa are administered under medical supervision and prescriptions are written by medical doctors. Thermal cures are effective against stress and various diseases. Those who are interested in a spa cure at the Thermes de Spa can either stay at the "Hotel Cardinal" tourist class hotel opposite the Baths at Place Royale 21-27. Tel: (87) 771064, at the elegant Hotel Alfa Balmoral Tel (87) 772581. Fax: (87) 774174, or at any nearby hotel. July and August are the busiest months at the SPA and early booking is advisable.

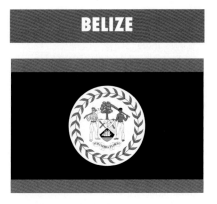

BELIZE

AREA: 8,867 sq. mi. (22,966 sq. km.)
POPULATION: 150,000
CAPITAL: Belmopan
OFFICIAL LANGUAGE: English, Spanish
CURRENCY: Belize Dollar (B$)
EXCHANGE RATE: 1 US$= B$2
TELEPHONE COUNTRY CODE: 501

Belize is a tropical showcase. The northern part is mostly flat, but the Maya Mountains in the western part of the country rise to the height of 1,000 m. / 3,300 ft.

Northern Belize is the famous Mayan country where the ancient Maya prospered and created their legendary civilization. Here you can explore the impressive Mayan ruins and temples at Altun Ha, 55 km. / 34 mi. north of Belize City near the location of the Maruba Resort & Jungle Spa. The Northern region is noted for the jungles and abundance of wildlife, especially many rare species of exotic birds.

The climate is hot and humid day and night during most of the year. In the rainforests of southern Belize the humidity and rainfall is quite substantial. Hurricane season is from July to November with most of the activity from mid-August to mid-September.

ⓘ Belize Tourist Board
421 Seventh Ave., Ste 1110,
New York, NY 10001 U.S.A., Tel: (212) 563-601

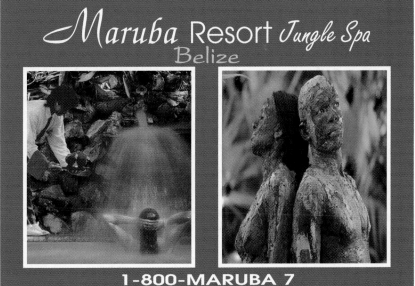

MASKALL VILLAGE

✈ Belize International AP (BZE) 30 mi. / 48 km.

Maruba Resort Jungle Spa
❤❤❤❤

🕴 ❀ ◉

40-1/2 Mile Old Northern Highway, Maskall Village, Belize. Tel: (501) 3-22199. Fax: (501) 2-12049. USA office Tel: (713) 799-2031 Fax: (713) 795-8573, Toll Free 1-800-MARUBA-7. EXECUTIVE DIRECTOR: Veronika Nicholson. MANAGING DIRECTOR: Franziska Nicholson. PROGRAM DIRECTOR: Merickston Nicholson. TYPE: Hotel & Spa. LOCATION: Mayan Jungles of Belize, 40 mi. / 64 km. north of Belize City. SPA CLIENTELE: Mixed, all ages. Teenagers and children accepted. MEDICAL RESTRICTIONS: Must have medical release from physician for exercise and diet program.

* Rooms: 6, suites 10
* Phone, A/C, minibar (in some rooms), priv. bath
* Restaurant, bar
* Reservations: $100 deposit required
* Credit Cards: MC, VISA, AMEX
* Open: Year round
* Rates: (accommodations only) from: $130 - $345
* TAC: 10 - 20%
* Spa on premises
* Year Established: 15 years
* **Spa facilities**: Treatment rooms, swimming pool, Japanese mineral bath, jungle path, weight room
* **Spa Programs**: Health, rejuvenation & relaxation
* **Spa Packages**: 1 day adventure escape

$145 - $155, 1 night $320 - $355, 2 night rejuvenation $470- $540, 5 nights $1,325 - $1,495, 26 day-weight control and rejuvenation $4,145 Adventure and Dive packages available
* **Spa Treatments**: Full-body massage, aromatherapy massage, tropical herbal wrap, seaweed body wrap, sea sulfur and Mood Mud body packs, cellulite treatments, facial, manicure, pedicure, African honey bee scrub, body scrubs, Jungle safari hike, one on one exercise, mineral bath
* Maximum number of guests: 32
* **Email: maruba@flash.net**
* **Web: http://www.maruba-spa.com**

DESCRIPTION: Maruba Resort Jungle Spa ia a unique, private resort nestled in the Mayan Jungles of Belize. Not your traditional spa, Maruba offers an alternative to the regimen and routine. The resort blends various Mayan, Creole, and African designs side by side with a jungle setting. This creates a relaxing and artistically natural environment. The natural products created specifically for the spa treatments are made from ingredients found in the jungle. Our restaurant offers some of the finest menus featured in "Gourmet Magazine". Unique materials from the jungle have been used to make the accommodations comfortable and creative. Each room is decorated differently from the jungle suite set high above the jungle canopy to the rooms and cabanas set amidst pineapple fields, coconut palms, and bird watching areas. Maruba Resort & Jungle Spa believes in blending fitness, beauty, and nutrition with relaxation, informality, and nature. Recreation: horseback riding, canoeing.

BERMUDA

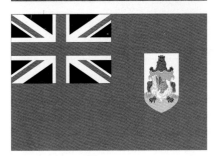

AREA: 21 sq. mi. (54 sq. km.)
POPULATION: 58,460
CAPITAL: Hamilton
OFFICIAL LANGUAGE: English
CURRENCY: Bermuda Dollar (BER$)
EXCHANGE RATE: 1 US$ = BER$1
TELEPHONE COUNTRY CODE: 441

The oldest colony of Great Britain, Bermuda is located about 600 mi. / 960 km. east of the Savannah (GA). This picturesque island, once dubbed by Mark Twain 'the biggest small place in the world' combines a colorful island vacation with a touch of British tradition. Bermuda offers lovely beaches, sports and recreational activities. Due to the island's northern location compared with the Caribbean islands the temperatures are somewhat cooler here and the summer is the best season to take advantage of the marvelous beaches.

ⓘ Bermuda Dept. of Tourism
"Global House", 43 Church St.
Hamilton HM BX Bermuda
Tel: (441) 292-0023

SOUTHAMPTON
⌐ (no area code)
✈ Kindley Field (BER), 16 mi. / 26 km.

Southampton is a popular beach resort on the south shore of Bermuda about 20 minutes by bus or taxi ride from the capital city of Hamilton.

Cambridge Beaches
❤❤❤❤

30 King's Point Rd., Somerset, Sandy's Parish MA 02, Tel: (441) 234-0331, Fax: (441) 234-3352. TYPE: Resort and Spa. LOCATION: On 25 acre peninsula at western tip of the island. SPA CLIENTELE: Women and men. DESCRIPTION: Deluxe resort complex with informal European club atmosphere. The resort offers European style health & beauty spa, outdoor pool, 5 beaches, full service marina. Hotel rates: from US$245.

Sonesta Beach Resort
❤❤❤❤

Southampton Parish, Bermuda. Tel: (441) 238-8463. Fax: (441) 238-8463. TYPE: Resort & Spa. LOCATION: Beach location in Southampton on a private 25 acre landscaped peninsula. SPA CLIENTELE: Men, Women.

* Rooms: 400 w/priv. bath. Suites: 26 beachfront
* CTV, radio, A/C
* Restaurants, bars, nightclub
* Airport: Kindley Airfield, 16 mi. (26 km.)
* Airport Transportation: taxi
* Reservations: 2 night deposit req'd
* Credit Cards: MC/VISA/AMEX/DC
* Open: year round
* Hotel Rates: from US$110 - $280.
* TAC: 10%
* Spa on premises: The SPA at Sonesta Beach
* Year Established: 1984
* **Spa Facilities**: Separate Men's and Women's facilities, 2 whirlpools, 2 saunas, 2 steam rooms, 1 exercise room, universal equipment room, 7 massage rooms, 2 facial rooms, Beauty Salon, indoor and outdoor swimming pool, Spa beach, jogging trail, salt glo room
* **Spa Programs**:The Concentrated Spa Package (min. 4 nights), Spa Refresher Break (3 nights), Mini SPA Vacation Plan (min. 4 nights),

31

Executive Renewal Plan, Sports & Spa Package, Modified Spa Programs, Full & Half Day at the Spa - Day of Beauty, Men's Spa Day, Health & Fitness, Beauty & Relaxation, Weight Loss, Exercise, Diet & Beauty

* **Spa Treatments**: exercise, gym workout, aquatics, whirlpool, Finnish sauna, Turkish steam baths, Rene Guinot facials, Men's facials, cathiodermie, bio-peeling, acne treatments, aromatherapy, salt glo loofa body scrub, body toning, nutrition consultation, 800-1000 calorie per day nutritionally balanced meals
* Documentation required from physician: no
* Medical Supervision: 1 MD

DESCRIPTION: Deluxe resort on a private beach. All the luxurious guest rooms and suites are elegantly appointed, most with water views. The Spa is a European style health & beauty spa featuring a variety of individualized programs in the areas of exercise, fitness, diet and beauty. Weight watchers can select a low calorie meal plan based on 800 - 1000 calories per day. Recreation: beaches, night life, shopping, and island excursions, golf, tennis, fishing, scuba, dinghy races, cricket and horseback riding.

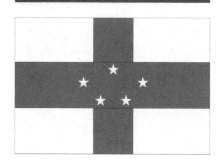

BONAIRE

AREA: 112 sq. mi. (288 sq. km.)
POPULATION: 13,000
CAPITAL: Kralendjik
OFFICIAL LANGUAGE: Dutch, Papiamento
CURRENCY: Bonaire Guilder (BWG)
EXCHANGE RATE: 1 US$ = 1.86 BWG
TELEPHONE COUNTRY CODE: 599

ⓘ Bonaire Gvmt Tourist Bureau
Kaya Simon Bolivar #12, Kralendijk, Bonaire (NA)

Bonaire is a "desert" island with beautiful beaches and Dutch style capital city just 50 mi. / 80 km off the northern shore of Venezuela. The climate is dry and sunny with average high temperatures in the 90's°F (32°c).

KRALENDIJK
☞ **7**

✈ Flamingo Int'l Airport (BON), 4 mi. / 6 km.

Harbour Village Beach Resort
♥♥♥♥♥

Kaya Gobernader North Debrot #72, PO Box 143, Kralendijk, Tel: 7-7500. Fax: 7-507. TYPE: Resort Hotel & Spa. MANAGING DIRECTOR: Jessica Gonzalez. LOCATION: Beachfront within a 100 acre enclave complete with 60 slip marina. SPA CLIENTELE: Women and men. SPECIAL RESTRICTIONS: Must be 16 years or older.

* Rooms: 132 w/ priv. bath; Suites: 26
* Apartments: available
* Phone, CTV, hair dryer, room service
* Spa Cafe, restaurants, bars, retail shops
* Meetings to 150, business services
* 2 outdoor pools, beach, water sports, scuba diving
* Airport: 3 mi. / 2 km., free transfers
* Reservations: 25 % deposit
* Credit Cards: MC/VISA/AMEX/DIS/EC
* Hotel Rates: from $305 (rooms)-$980 (suites)
* TAC: 10%
* Spa on premises: **The Spa at Harbour Village**
* Year Established: 1995
* **Spa Facilities**: 17,500 sq. ft. / 1,590 sq.m spa fitness center, 9 treatment rooms, steam and sauna rooms, outdoor solarium, co-ed whirlpool, separate locker rooms, Roman-style pool and cascade, water aerobics pool, large pool for laps, fitness center, spa shop, spa cafe, beauty salon
* **Spa Programs**: Health, beauty, fitness, wellness
* **Spa Treatments**: Massage, reflrxology, shiatsu, aromatherapy, reflexology, lymph drainage, facials, salt-glow loofahs, bonairian salt exfoliate, body polish, seaweed masks, cellulite relief mask, botanical bath, salt water soak, facials, aloe wraps, depilatory waxing, nail care, hair care, low cal balanced spa cuisine, exercise and fitness classes
* **Spa Packages**: from $1,387-$1,598 per person dbl occupancy including 10 treatments per week Day Spa packages from $95
* Length of Stay Required: 7 nights
* Maximum number of guests: 22

DESCRIPTION: Harbour Village is the one of the best aquatic retreats in the world and a true luxury resort. The resort features full service on-site dive center, water sports and a world class spa and tennis center. The Spa at Harbour Village is a large two-story facility at the entrance to the resort. It is the perfect place to relax and indulge your mind and body. Bask yourself in a spa vacation combining tropical fitness and personalized beauty and pampering services in a natural and relaxing Caribbean setting. Enjoy the perfect spa experience Bonaire style.

BRAZIL

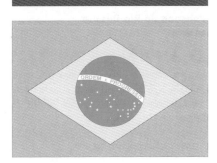

AREA: 3,284,426 sq. mi. (8,506,663 sq. km.)
POPULATION: 157,000,000
CAPITAL: Brasilia
OFFICIAL LANGUAGE: Portuguese
CURRENCY: Real (R$)
EXCHANGE RATE: 1 US$ = R$1.19
TELEPHONE COUNTRY CODE: 55

ⓘ Embratur-Brazilian Tourist Board

Head Office: SCN Quadra 2, bloco G, Brazilia - DF - Brazil
Tel: (55-61) 224-9100, Fax: (55-61) 223-9889
Web: www.embratur.gov.br

CALDAS NOVAS (Goias)

☎ **062**

✈ Brazilia Int'l Airport (BSB)

Caldas Novas, population 26,000, is Goias most famous hot springs region 180 mi. / 290 km. south of the capital Brasilia. Caldas Novas is known for the hot, sulfurous water which is the state's number one tourist attraction. The thermal water flows from the mountains at average temperature between 96°F-104°F (35°c-40°c). The natural springs form thermal pools and offer therapeutic benefits.

Indications: lower blood pressure, eliminate tension and fatigue, increase sexual vigor, disintoxicate and cleanse the system and stimulate the endocrine glands.

To reach Caldas Novas you may either drive from Morrinhos

taking the BR-153 Goiânia-São Paulo highway, or take the bus from Morrinhos.

Pousada do Rio Quente
❤❤❤

Estrada para Morrinhos. USA/Canada reservations: (800) 257-5344. TYPE: Spa Hotel. LOCATION: At the foot of the Caldas Mountains near thermal pools. SPA CLIENTELE: All Welcome.

* Chalets & Suites: 300 w/priv. bath
* Phone, CTV, A/C, minibar, safe deposit box
* Restaurants, Pizza House, bars, live shows, nightclub
* Airport: Brazilia Airport
* Reservations: required
* Credit Cards: MC/VISA/AMEX
* Open: year round
* Hotel Rates: from US$620 (3 nts min.)
* TAC: 10%
* Spa on premises
* **Spa Facilities**: Physiotherapy center, Medical Station, Thermal water pool, Aquatic park
* **Spa Treatments**: bathing in mineral water, physiotherapy
* **Medical Supervision**: yes

DESCRIPTION: Village style thermal water resort complex with modern amenities and recreational facilities. Special events are held throughout the year, in the Nations Festival celebrating countries and cultures from around the world. Recreation: soccer, tennis, electronic games, movie theatre.

FLORIANOPOLIS (Santa Catarina)
ㄱ **051**

✈ Hercillio Luz Airport (FLN)

The Brain Spa
❤❤❤❤

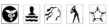

c/o Plaza Itapema Hotel, BR 101 km 145, Santa Catarina 88220. USA/Canada reservations: (800) 257-5344. Tel: (516) 944-5508. Fax: (516) 944-7540. TYPE: Health

Spa. LOCATION: On the Atlantic Ocean near Florianopolis, on 800 m / yards of private beach on the coast of the state of Santa Catarina. SPA CLIENTELE: Family oriented.

* Rooms: 112 w/priv. bath. Suites: 44
* Telephone, CTV, A/C, minibar
* Restaurants, snack bar, games room
* Reservations: required
* Credit Cards: VISA/AMEX/MC/DIS/EC
* Open: Year round
* TAC: 10%
* Spa on premises
* **Spa Facilities**: Health Spa, thermal pools, flotation tank, sauna, Modern equipment for stress control and brain stimulation.
* **Spa Programs**: Anti-stress, relaxation, health recovery
* **Spa Treatments**: Flogiston chair - produces deep steady relaxation; Neurostimulation - audio visual meditation; Oasis Flotation Tank; Alphastim 100 - generates liberation of endorphin, which releases pain and causes feeling of euphoria; Infratonic QGM - Chinese device that recreates the vibrations used by the masters of ching chong; Cooper Biocircuit - for inner peace filling; Hypnagogic Cassette Tapes & CD - sound effects on the brain functioning, massages, thalassotherapy, low calorie food, beauty treatments, exercise, meditation
* **Indications**: Stress-release, relaxation, meditation. inner peace, stress control and brain stimulation

DESCRIPTION: Located in one of the most beautiful sites in the State of Santa Catarina, the Plaza Itapema Resort offer the Brain Spa, a new concept in beauty associated with health, food reeducation, physical conditioning and thalassotherapy. The spa also uses modern equipment, unique in South America, for stress control and brain simulation. Recreation: golf field (9 holes), soccer field, marina for watersports, games room, tennis.

SÃO PAULO
ㄱ **011**

✈ Congonhas Airport (CGH) 8 mi. / 13 km.
   Guarulhos Int'l AP (GRU) 16 mi. / 26 km.
   Viracopos Int'l AP (VCP) 60 mi. / 96 km.

São Paulo, population 16,000,000, is the largest and most cosmopolitan city in Brazil. It is Brazil's leading industry and commercial center. Sitting on a high plateau it gets cold during the winter, and hot in the summer. Avenida Paulista is a landmark avenue with high rise buildings, shops and theatres.

The Maskoud Plaza
❤❤❤❤❤

Alameda Campinas 150, São Paulo 01404-900. Tel: (11) 253-4411. Fax: (11) 253-4544. TYPE: Hotel with Spa. LOCATION: Heart of São Paulo, 1 block from Paulista Ave. SPA CLIENTELE: Mostly women. DESCRIPTION: Deluxe atrium-style hotel with elegant rooms and suites. The hotel features a complete physiotherapy and fitness center and La Prarie Spa with beauty treatments, sauna, massages and a pool. Hotel amenities: gourmet restaurants, bars (5), bingo club. 416 rooms, 45 suites. Hotel rates: from US$345.

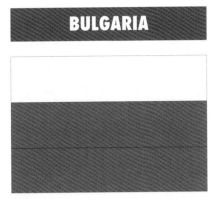

BULGARIA

AREA: 47,000 sq. mi. (110,000 sq. km.)
POPULATION: 8,472,000
CAPITAL: Sofia
OFFICIAL LANGUAGE: Bulgarian
CURRENCY: Lev (BGL)
EXCHANGE RATE: 1US$ = BGL
COUNTRY TELEPHONE CODE: 359

Bulgaria has an age old Spa tradition of water cure and climatic treatments that can be traced back to Tharacians and Roman times. But the recent rebirth of the Bulgarian health resorts and spas began only at the turn of the last century, with major development occurring during the past three or four decades. The major Spas are: Kyustendil and Sandansky in the southwest, famous for their mineral waters, and healthy climate; the Black Sea resorts - Albena, Golden Sands and St. Constantine with beautiful beaches, pleasant sea climate, thermal Spa facilities and luxury hotels; and Sandansky in the south with its rich mineral springs and fine climate.

🛈 Balkan Tourist USA
20 E. 46th St., Ste. 1003, New York, NY 10017, USA
Tel: 800-822-106 or 212-338-6838

🛈 Balkan Tourist
1 Vitosha Blvd., Sofia 1000, Bulgaria
Tel: (359) 43331

ALBENA
🛉 57

✈ Varna Int'l Airport (VAR) 19 mi. / 32 km.

Albena, the most picturesque of the Bulgarian Black Sea resorts is 5 miles (8 km) south of Balchik, 9 miles (14 km.) north of the Golden Sands, and 19 miles (32 km.) north of Varna. Its greatest asset is the 4 miles (7 km.) long very fine sand beach, and clean and shallow sea. The climate is typically coastal. The average annual temperature is 55°F (13°c). The winter is comparatively mild. The temperature in July averages 72°F (22°c) rarely reaching 86°F (30°c). Gentle sea breezes keep the air fresh and the nights cool. Characteristic to Albena is the intensive solar radiation with numerous days of clear skies.

The mineral water is slightly mineralized, hypothermal, hydrocarbonic, chloride, sulfuratic, sodium, with a slightly alkaline reaction. The mineral water is widely used in the open-air pool with a temperature of 76°F (24°c) by thousands of vacationers.

Dobroudja Hotel & Spa
❤❤❤❤

Varna BG-9620. Tel: (57) 2220200. Fax: (57) 222216. TYPE: First Class Hotel & Spa. LOCATION: At the foot of a hill overlooking the black Sea. SPA CLIENTELE: Men, Women.

* Rooms: 227 w/private bath
* Restaurant, night club, folk tavern
* Tennis, golf, horseback riding
* Airport: Varna, 19 miles / 32 km.
* Airport Transportation: taxi, bus
* Open: Year round
* Rates: from $455/week (land only)
* Spa on premises
* **Spa Facilities**: hypothermal pool, balneotherapeutic equipment, gym, consulting rooms, polyclinic
* Treatment duration: 2 or 3 weeks
* **Spa Programs**: Rejuvenation, relaxation, general fitness, diet, beauty and neuropsychic relaxation
* **Spa Treatments**: Sea water baths, massages including underwater massage, electrotherapy, kinetic therapy, physical therapy
* **Indications**: Locomotor disturbances, peripheral nervous system diseases, cardiovascular and chronic non-specific respiratory ailments
* Medical Supervision: Examinations and laboratory tests
* Treatments Approved: Polyclinic and National Institute for Resort Study, Physiotherapy and Rehabilitation

DESCRIPTION: The Dobroudja Hotel and Health Spa at the Albena International Resort is one of the largest resorts complexes in the Balkan peninsula.

Hotel Imperial
❤❤❤❤❤

Ferienklub Riviera, Varna BG-9006. Tel: (52) 855215. Fax: (52) 855101. TYPE: Deluxe Hotel & Spa. LOCATION: Directly on the beach in park like grounds. SPA CLIENTELE: Men, Women.

* Rooms: 56 w/private bath; Presidential Suite
* Phone, CTV, minibar & terrace
* Restaurant, cafe, 3 bars
* Tennis, golf, horseback riding
* Airport: Varna, 19 miles / 32 km.
* Airport Transportation: taxi, bus
* Open: Year round
* Rates: from $765/week (land only)
* Spa on premises
* **Spa Facilities**: Maritime Club, Fitness Center, Balneological Center, swimming pool, latest balneotherapeutic equipment, gym, consulting rooms, polyclinic
* Treatment duration: 2 or 3 weeks
* **Spa Programs**: Rejuvenation, relaxation, general fitness, diet, beauty and neuropsychic relaxation
* **Spa Treatments**: Sea water baths, massages including underwater massage, electrotherapy, kinetic therapy, physical therapy, phythotherapy, phytobalneology, Gerovita treatments
* **Indications**: Locomotor disturbances, peripheral nervous system diseases, cardiovascular and chronic non-specific respiratory ailments
* Medical Supervision: Examinations and laboratory tests

* Treatments Approved: Polyclinic and National Institute for Resort Study, Physiotherapy and Rehabilitation

DESCRIPTION: The Imperial hotel is a five-story resort hotel, part of the Holiday Club Riviera. Located on a private beach it features Health Club and extensive Health & Spa programs.

GOLDEN SANDS (ZLATNI PYASSUTSI)
➲ 52

✈ Varna Int'l Airport (VAR) 20 mi. / 16 km.

Golden Sands, one of the biggest resort complexes on the Black Sea, is situated 10 miles (17 km.) north of Varna. The resort takes its name from the beach, almost 2.5 miles (4 km.) of golden sand 330 feet (100 meters) wide. It lies on the same latitude as the Mediterranean French and Italian resorts. The climate is warm and mild. The average July temperature is 73°F (22°c). The water temperature from June to September never falls below 68°F (20°c) and can reach 81°F (27°c).

The mineral springs of Golden Sands are hypothermal, temperatures of 75°F - 79°F (24°c - 26°c), slightly mineralized, bicarbonic sodium, calcium and magnesium chloride and slightly sulfitic with an alkaline reaction. These active mineral waters and the local sea climate create unique conditions for prophylaxis treatment, rehabilitation and rest to hundreds of citizens from Bulgaria and abroad.

Hotel International
❤❤❤❤

Zlatni Pyassatsi, Bulgaria 9006. TYPE: First Class Hotel & Spa. LOCATION: Overlooking the golden beach and Black Sea. SPA CLIENTELE: Women and men.

* Rooms: 370 w/private bath. Suites: 37
* Radio, TV and balcony in each room
* Restaurant: 2, coffee shop, Night club, bars
* Tennis, squash, bowling, casino, pools
* Airport: Varna, 10 mi. / 17 km. taxi, bus
* Open: Year round
* Hotel Rates: from $100 day
* Spa on premises

* Spa Facilities: indoor thermal swimming pool, balneotherapeutic equipment, sauna, gymnasium, consulting rooms, varied sports facilities
* Treatment duration: 2 or 3 weeks
* Spa Programs: Rejuvenation, vitalcure, relaxation, fitness, anti-stress, diet, beauty, medical
* Spa Treatments: Sea water baths, inhalation, paraffin baths, massages including underwater massage, electrotherapy, kinetic therapy, physical therapy; classical, laser and electric acupuncture; phytotherapy and phytobalneology, sonotherapy, magnetotherapy
* Indications: Chronic or subchronic arthroskeletal inflammation, peripheral nervous system diseases, central nervous system functional disturbances, cardiovascular ailments, chronic non-specific respiratory ailments, over-weight conditions, male sexual disfunction
* Medical Supervision: Examinations and laboratory tests
* Treatments Approved: National Institute for Resort Study, Physiotherapy and Rehabilitation

DESCRIPTION: The Hotel International is a treatment and recreation Spa. It is a lively international resort popular with younger clientele.

KYUSTENDIL
➲ 78

✈ Sofia Int'l Airport (SOF) 50 mi. / 85 km.

Kyustendil, is situated 51 miles (85 km.) southwest of Sofia and has almost the same altitude 1740 feet (530 meters). The town lies in the fertile Kyustendil valley at the foot of Ossogovo Mountain, and is a point of departure for trips to the Zemen Gorge and Osogovo, Konyavska and Lissets mountains. Kyustendil is Bulgaria's "orchard" offering tasty fruits: cherries, apples pears, plums, etc. The climate is continental with a Mediterranean influence. Low mountain ranges shield Kyustendil from the north, west and east. The average annual temperature is 50°F (10°c) with 2,200 hours of sunshine annually and an average precipitation of 14 inches (608 mm).

The curative factors of Kyustendil are in its mineral waters which gush forth from many mineral springs. The chemical composition is almost uniform with equal temperature and sulfide composition. The waters are clear, colorless, with a slight smell of hydrogen sulfide. They contain sulfide, silicium, fluorine, sodium sulfates and are hyperthermal, slightly mineralized, with an alkaline reaction.

Velbazd Hotel & Spa
❤❤❤

🗣 ⚕ 🐎 🏃

4 Boul G. Dimitrov Blvd., Kyustendil. Tel: (78) 20246 or (78) 20248. TYPE: First Class Hotel & Spa. LOCATION: In the immediate vicinity of the Spa Polyclinic. SPA CLIENTELE: Men, Women.

* Rooms: 146 w/private bath. Suites: 10
* Restaurant, Coffee Shop, Bar, Night club
* Sports Hall, Meeting rooms, parking
* Airport: Sofia 51 mi. / 85 km. taxi, bus
* Open: Year round
* Hotel Rates: from $80/day
* Spa off premises; Polyclinic nearby
* **Spa Facilities**: Thermal swimming pool, balneotherapeutic equipment, tubs sauna, gym, consulting rooms, sports facilities
* Treatment duration: 2 or 3 weeks
* **Spa Programs**: Rejuvenation, relaxation, general fitness, diet, beauty and medical
* **Spa Treatments**: Peat mud baths, inhalation, mineral baths, massage, electrotherapy, kinetic therapy, physical therapy
* **Indications**: Degenerative and inflammatory rheumatoidal and infectional arthritis, muscle and tendon diseases, post injury conditions, nervous system disorders, gynecological diseases, skin diseases, occupational poisoning
* Medical Supervision: Examinations and laboratory tests
* Treatments Approved: National Institute for Resort Study, Physiotherapy and Rehabilitation

DESCRIPTION: Opened in 1983, the Velbazd Hotel is a 13 story hotel near the central Polyclinic.

SANDANSKI
🔤 74

✈ Sofia Int'l Airport (SOF) 100 mi. / 160 km.

Sandanski, population 22,500, is situated 103 miles (172 km.) south of Sofia, near the border with Greece at an altitude 735 feet (224 meters). The resort lies in the valley on the Sandansk Bistritsa River in the southeastern foothills of the Pirin Mountains. It is linked with Sofia via Blagoevgrad by the international motorway E-79.

The winter is mild with an average January temperature of 39°F (4°c). The average July temperature is 77°F (25°c). Spring comes early and the autumn is warm and long last. The relative humidity is low. There are no more than 5 to 6 foggy days during the year. The sunshine is intensive and prolonged with 2436 hours of sunshine annually.

The air quality at the resort is good and well protected from northerly winds. Thus the resort has won a reputation as a treatment center for non-specific chronic ailments of the lungs, especially bronchial asthma. In addition to the favorable microclimate the local mineral springs have therapeutic value. The mineral springs are slightly mineralized, hydrocarbonic sulfuratic sodium calcium, fluorine and silicic, hyperthermal, with a weak alkaline reaction.

Worth visiting are the remains of a temple dedicated to water curing baths which have been carefully preserved over the centuries.

Sandanski Hotel
❤❤❤

🗣 ⚕ 🐎 🏌

Sandanski BG-2800. Tel: (74) 65000. Fax: (74) 65271. TYPE: First Class Hotel & Spa. LOCATION: Convenient to all the activities of the spa. SPA CLIENTELE: Family oriented.

* Rooms: 299 w/private bath. Suites: 5
* Restaurant, Coffee Shop
* Bar, Night club, meeting rooms, parking
* Airport: Sofia 103 mi. / 172 km. limo, bus
* Reservations: required
* Open: Year round
* Hotel Rates: from $75 /day
* Spa on premises

* **Spa Facilities**: balneotherapeutic equipment, sauna, tub baths, swimming pools, gym, sports facilities, consulting and diagnostic rooms
* Treatment duration: 2 or 3 weeks
* **Spa Programs**: Rejuvenation, relaxation, general fitness, diet, beauty and medical
* **Spa Treatments**: Aerotherapy, heliotherapy, inhalation, mineral baths, paraffin baths, massage, electrotherapy, kinetic therapy, physical therapy, acupuncture
* **Indications**: Chronic rheumatic and arthritic conditions, muscle and tendon diseases, post injury conditions, peripheral nervous system disorders, gynecological diseases, non-phythisic conditions of the upper respiratory tract & lungs
* Medical Supervision: Examinations and laboratory tests
* Treatments Approved: National Institute for Resort Study, Physiotherapy and Rehabilitation

DESCRIPTION: Opened in 1984, the Sandanski Hotel is a luxury four star balneic treatment center. It is recommended for people suffering from allergies or lung conditions.

ST. CONSTANTINE
〕 **52**
✈ Varna Int'l Airport (VAR) 6 mi. / 9 km.

St. Constantine, is a small Black Sea resort with beautiful sandy beaches and hidden rocky coves.

Grand Hotel Varna
♥♥♥♥♥

St. Constantine, BG-9006. Tel: (52) 861491. Fax: (52) 861929. TYPE: Deluxe Hotel & Spa. LOCATION: In a large park near the Black Sea. SPA CLIENTELE: Men, Women.

* Rooms: 304 w/priv. bath. Suites: 37
* Radio, TV and balcony in each room
* Restaurant, taverna - "Melnik", cake shop
* Night club, 4 bars, conference rooms
* Tennis, squash, bowling, casino
* Airport: Varna 6 miles (10 km.), taxi, bus
* Reservations: required
* Credit Cards: ACC, BC, CB, DC, EC, JCB, MC, VISA
* Open: Year round
* Hotel Rates: from $460 pp/week (land only)
* Spa on premises
* **Spa Facilities**: Indoor and outdoor pools, latest balneotherapeutic equipment, sauna, gymnasium, consulting rooms, sports facilities
* Treatment duration: 2 or 3 weeks
* **Spa Programs**: Rejuvenation, longevity, relaxation, general fitness, anti-stress, body building, diet, beauty and medical
* **Spa Treatments**: Sea water baths, massages including underwater massage, electrotherapy, kinetic therapy, physical therapy, algae therapy, magnetic therapy, acupuncture, phytotherapy and phytobalneology, aerobics
* **Indications**: Chronic or subchronic arthroskeletal inflammation, peripheral nervous system diseases, central nervous system functional disturbances, cardiovascular ailments, chronic non-specific respiratory ailments, over weight conditions, physical & psychic asthenia of the elderly
* Medical Supervision: Examinations and laboratory tests
* Treatments Approved: National Institute for Resort Study, Physiotherapy and Rehabilitation

DESCRIPTION: This Swedish built resort hotel is the best on the Black Sea coast. The Spa has an impressive range of facilities including a complete balneological center with a wide range of curative treatments. A quiet place favored by writers, professionals and older people.

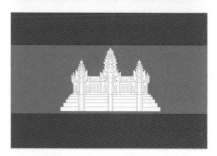

CAMBODIA

AREA: 69,898 sq. mi. (181,036 sq. km.)
POPULATION: 5,200,000
CAPITAL: Phenom Penh
OFFICIAL LANGUAGE: Khmer (Cambodian)
CURRENCY: Riel
EXCHANGE RATE: 1 US$ =
TELEPHONE COUNTRY CODE:855

ⓘ Cambodia Ministry of Tourism
447 Monivong Blvd., Phenom Penn
Tel: (23) 2107.

PHENOM PENN
〕 23
✈ Phenom Penn Airport

Hotel Le Royal
♥♥♥♥

92 Rukhak Vithei Daun Sangkat, Wat Phnom, Phnom Penh.
Tel: (23) 981-888, Fax: (23) 981-168. TYPE: Hotel with
Spa. LOCATION: In the heart of the city. DESCRIPTION:
Landmark French Colonial-style hotel, reopened in 1997,
210 rooms & suites, 3 restaurants 2 bars, meeting facilities,
business center, pool. Fully equipped spa with sauna,
jacuzzi, steam room, gym, beauty salon.

SIEM REAP
〕 63
✈ Siem Reap Airport

Grand Hotel D'Angkor
♥♥♥♥

1 Vithei Charles de Gaulle, Khum Svay, Dang Kum. Tel:
(63) 963-888, Fax: (63) 963-168. TYPE: Hotel with
Spa. LOCATION: On the edge of Siem Reap, 2 km. to the
airport, 8 km. to the Angkor Temple Complex. DESCRIP-
TION: Historic 1929 Hotel reopened in 1997. 131 rooms,
suites, and villas, 3 restaurants, 5 bars, business center,
library/map room, 2 tennis courts, pool. Full health club
with spa treatments.

CANADA

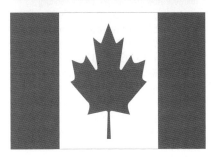

AREA: 3,851,787 sq. mi. (9,976,139 sq. km.)
POPULATION: 25,309,000
CAPITAL: Ottawa
OFFICIAL LANGUAGES: English, French
CURRENCY: Canadian Dollar (CAN $)
EXCHANGE RATE: 1 US$ = 1.54 CAN$

Spa vacation in Canada makes a lot of good sense. The country offers a variety of scenic locations, temperate climate, pure air, high quality of service and facilities, and above all the cost of a Spa vacation in Canada is at a discount to US travelers.

🛈 Canadian Tourist Information
British Columbia: 800-663-6000
Ontario: 800-ONTARIO; **Quebec:** 800-363-7777

ALBERTA

BANFF
ꓕ **403**
✈ Calgary Int'l Airport (YYC) 75 mi. / 120 km.

The Banff and Jasper National parks are fascinating alpine style nature reserves in the Canadian Rockies with green forests, blue lakes, and world class skiing.

Banff Springs Hotel
❤❤❤❤

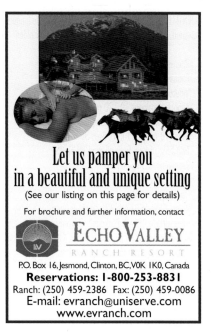
405 Spray Ave., Banff T0L 0C0. Tel: (403) 762-2211. Fax: (403) 762-5755. TYPE: Resort Hotel & Spa. LOCATION: Heart of the Canadian Rockies. DESCRIPTION: European style chateau resort hotel, 770 rooms, 17 restaurants.

BRITISH COLUMBIA

CLINTON
ꓕ **250**
✈ Kamloops Airport 120 mi. / 192 km.

Echo Valley Ranch Resort
❤❤❤❤

P.O. Box 16, Clinton, BC V0K 1K0. Tel: (250) 459-2386. Fax: (250) 459-0086. Reservations Toll Free 1-800-253-8831 (Canada and USA). TYPE: Guest Ranch Resort. LOCATION: BC's Cariboo region, 130 mi. / 208 km. north of Vancouver B.C. MANAGING DIRECTOR: Norm Dove. SPA

CLIENTELE: Women and men, adult oriented. Teenagers accepted. AGE RESTRICTION: Must be 13 years or older.

* Rooms: 15 deluxe w/priv. bath. Cabins: 3
* Phone, CTV, C/H, minibar, jacuzzi
* Video/Satellite TV, outdoor games
* Airport: Kamloops AP 120 mi. / 192 km.
  private airstrip at ranch (summer only)
* Train: 18 mi. / 29 km., Bus: 30 mi. / 48 km.
* Transfers: pick-up from all drop off points
* Reservations: required
* Credit Cards: VISA
* Open: Year round
* Rates: CAN$150-CAN$325/night/person
  rates include "Ranch Package" - accommodations,
  all meals, use of ranch/spa facilities. CAN$220 and up
  include many "soft adventure" activities. À la carte
  services and treatments available
* TAC: 10%
* Spa on premises
* Year Established: 1995
* **Spa Facilities**: treatment rooms (4), beauty salon,
  steam rooms (3), hydrotherapy tub, hot tubs, sauna,
  very well equipped exercise room, indoor heated
  swimming pool, massage services also available in
  guest rooms.
* **Spa Programs**: "Pamper Time" - during the winter
  months the focus is to "Pamper" guests in a beautiful
  and unique environment. Guests are pampered every
  day with spa and beauty treatments and may create
  their own "Pamper Package" from an array of services
  or choose from pre-packaged suggestions. The six night
  package includes 250 points that can be applied to over
  twenty hours of treatments. US$1,950 (6 nts).
* **Spa Treatments**: beauty, pampering, wellness,
  revitalization and fitness
* **Spa Packages: Total body wellness Package -**
  The deluxe treatment for skin and body! Relax and
  begin with Hydro-Active mineral salt scrub for the body.
  Then enjoy our aromatherapy facial boosted by a body
  massage with aromatic oils. Finish with complete
  reflexology foot massage with herbal soak and paraffin
  wax bath treatment. CAN$199.- (3 hrs).
  Day Spa Package - Experience the wonderful feeling
  of freshness as we brush away the dry cells from the

surface of your body. Feel the warmth of the essential oils as they calm your nerves. Quietly relax while the massage eases your muscles. Enjoy a cleansing gommage over your feet with a pedicure. We will continue with a manicure and file and finish your fingertips. We will finish this session with hydrating facial treatment. CAN$210.- (4 hrs.)

E.V. Ranch Retreat Package - biological facial with revitalizing and relaxing massage of the scalp, Relaxing body massage. We will massage away all the stress, using our own special blend of essential oils. Foot reflexology with rehydrating paraffin wax bath treatments. CAN$185 (3 hrs. 30 min.)

* **Indications**: anti-stress, pampering, well-being
* Length of Stay Required: 3 nights minimum
* Maximum number of guests: 20
* Email: evranch@uniserve.com
* Web: www.evranch.com

DESCRIPTION: Echo Valley Ranch is a year-round luxury wilderness resort located amidst four distinct Biomes on a working ranch in the Canadian wilderness. The first-class resort-style ranch features five star accommodations, gourmet food, complete spa facilities, and a diversity of outdoor experiences second to none. The environment is free of water, air, sound and light pollution. To ensure personalized service the number of guests at the ranch are limited to twenty and the staff guest ratio is 1 to 1. Recreation: outdoor games, unguided walk/hikes, bird watching, falcon training, plus we are a working ranch - you can be a cowboy for a day.

FAIRMONT HOT SPRINGS
⟩ 250
✈ Calgary Int'l Airport (YYC)

Fairmont Hot Springs is a family oriented ski resort in British Columbia's Rocky Mountains 305 km. (190 mi.) west of Calgary and 416 km. (260 mi.) north of Spokane (WA).

Fairmont Hot Springs Resort
♥♥♥♥

Box 10, Fairmont Hot Springs, BC V0B 1L0. Tel: (250)

345-6311, Fax: (250) 345-6616. TYPE: Resort Complex. LOCATION: British Columbia's Rocky Mountains ski resort area. SPA CLIENTELE: Family oriented.

* Rooms: 139 w/priv. bath
* Suites: 18, Cottages: 5
* Nearest Airport: 6,200 ft. paved runway
* Airport: 2 km. (1.5 mi.), free pick up
* Reservations: CAN$50 deposit req'd
* Credit Cards: MC/VISA/AMEX
* Open: Year round
* Hotel Rates: from CAN$69 - CAN$144/day
  Rates include use of hot pools; TAC: 10%
* Spa on premises
* **Spa Facilities**: Clear odor less mineral hot-pools at temperature ranging from 35°c - 45°c (95°F - 113°F), Sports Center, Exercise Room, saunas, hydra fitness equipment, indoor and outdoor jacuzzis
* **Spa Programs**: Ski & Swim Packages, Fitness - aerobics and aquacise classes
* **Spa Treatments**: bathing in hot mineral water, massage, exercise

DESCRIPTION: A family oriented vacation complex featuring the largest natural hot mineral pools in Canada. The 10,000 sq. ft. of steaming hot mineral pools draw people to the resort from all over the world for their therapeutic value. The deluxe sports Center has two international racquetball courts, one international squash court, and golf course. Located in a popular ski area guests can enjoy Alpine and Cross country skiing (day and night). The vicinity of lakes and rivers make all water sports accessible. A new complex includes 75 five stars luxury villas near the golf course.

HARRISON HOT SPRINGS
﹚ 604
✈ Vancouver Int'l Airport (YVR)

Harrison Hot Springs is located at the southern point of Harrison Lake about 80 mi. (120 km.) east of Vancouver. To get there by car take the Trans-canada Highway (Hwy 1), or the scenic Hwy 7 from Vancouver. Canadian Pacific Railway stops at Agassiz Train Station. A seaplane landing runaway exists near the hotel.

Harrison Hot Springs Hotel
♥♥♥♥

100 Esplanade, Harrison Hot Springs, BC V0M 1K0. Tel: (604) 796-2244, Fax: (604) 796-9374. TYPE: Resort Hotel & Spa. LOCATION: On Harrison lake. CLIENTELE: Family oriented.

* Rooms: 280 w/priv. bath. Suites & Bungalows
* Restaurants, Lounge & Pub with entertainment
* Train Station: Agassiz, 5 mi. (8 km.), taxi
* Reservations: suggested
* Credit Cards: MC/VISA/AMEX/DC/CB
* Open: Year round
* Hotel Rates: CAN$110 - CAN$250/day; TAC: 10%
* Spa on premises
* **Spa Facilities**: Indoor/outdoor hot sulfur pools, gym, health pavilion, Roman baths, whirlpools, massage rooms, jacuzzis, sauna, beauty salon
* **Spa Programs**: fitness, beauty
* **Spa Treatments**: bathing in mineral water, massages, beauty treatments, exercises

DESCRIPTION: A family oriented Hot Springs resort. The emphasis is on relaxation, exercise and general well being. No special diet program is available. Recreation: golf at the nearby 9-hole Golf Course, and water sports.

ONE HUNDRED MILE HOUSE
﹚ 250
✈ Williams Lake Airport 50 mi. / 80 km.
Vancouver Int'l Airport 250 mi. / 400 km.

One Hundred Mile House, population 2,500, is a popular summer and winter cross-country ski and health resort 290 miles (465 km) northeast of Vancouver B.C., and 1 hour from Williams Lake Airport (4 flights daily by Air Canada). This unspoiled cowboy land is known as the "Cariboo Region" with lovely lakes, small mountains and green valleys. The peaceful Canadian West location is inductive for a stress free and a healthy vacation.

The Hills Health & Guest Ranch can be reached by rail,

road, or air via the nearby Williams Lake Airport. For those who are not in a hurry, a train trip from Vancouver offers a scenic ride through a spectacular terrain.

The Hills Health Ranch
❤❤❤❤❤

🦌 🏃 ✿ ✪

Box 26, 108 Mile Ranch, 100 Mile House, B.C. VOK 2Z0. Tel: (250) 791-5225. Fax: (250) 791-6384. TYPE: Health Resort Complex. MANAGING DIR: Juanita Corbett. PROGRAM DIRECTOR: Monique Cornu. LOCATION: Hwy 97, 108 Mile Ranch, northeast of Vancouver B.C. in a true Canadian West wilderness setting. YEAR ESTABLISHED: 1983. SPA CLIENTELE: Men & women, children and teenagers accepted.

* Rooms: 26 w/private bath, Suites: 2, Cottages: 20
* C/H, phone, CTV, cooking facilities, Restaurant, Bar
* Spa on premises: **The Canadian Wellness Center**
* Train Station: 100 Mile House 8 mi. /13 km.
* Transportation: free pick up from train station
* Reservations: deposit required
* Credit Cards: MC/VISA/AMEX
* Rates: from CAN$1,000/dbl (per person per week)
* TAC: 10%
* **Spa Facilities**: 12 treatment rooms, seminar room, fitness and exercise studio, 200 km hiking trails, therapy pools.
* **Spa Programs**: Weight Loss, Stress Reduction, Inches-Off, Wellness, Education Workshops,Lifestyle Analysis, Fitness Testing and Assessments, Walking holidays
* **Spa Packages**: Weight Loss (10 nts/30 nts); Executive Renewal (6 nts); Inches-Off (6 nts); Smoking Cessation; Successful Aging; Athletic Recovery, Spa Spoiler
* **Spa Treatments**: massage, facials, herbal wraps, reflexology, manicure & pedicure, waxing, mud packs, aromatherapy, paraffin
* **Indications**: lifestyle adjustments, obesity, hypertension, diabetes, osteoarthritis, elevated cholesterol, fubromyalgia, chronic fatigue syndrome,clinical disorders, skin disease, menopause, asthma/lung, low back pain, blood pressure, nutrition

* **Medical Supervision**: 1 MD / 2 RN Kinesiologist certified fitness instructors
* **Maximum Number of Guests**: 80
* Documentation from Physician: not required
* **Email**: thehills@bcinternet.net
* **Web**: http://www.grt-net.com/thehills/

DESCRIPTION: The Hills is Canada's leading renewal and rejuvenation center. The Canadian Wellness Center at the ranch is a complete lifestyle adjustment center. During winter months the resort operates as cross-country ski and health resort (Dec/Jan/Feb/Mar). In the summer the resort operates as a true Canadian west Guest Ranch. Accommodations are in deluxe country style chalets with bedroom, living room, kitchen and a balcony. Nutritious Spa meals are prepared by a Swiss chef. The food is 60% complex carbohydrates, 25% protein, low in fat, and free of salt, sugar, alcohol and caffeine. The gourmet meals consist of fresh fruits, fine cheeses, and organically grown vegetables and grains. Non reduced calorie meals are available. The Spa offers extensive fitness, wellness, beauty, weight loss, and pampering packages that last from 2 to 10 nights. Classes and workshops are conducted on topics of nutrition and lifestyle. Recreation: cross country and downhill skiing (from December 1 - March 31), horseback riding (April to October), nature trails, golf, hay ride and sing-a-long parties, and folklore evenings. The Spa was awarded the title "Specialty Spa of the Year" in 1993, 1995, 1996, & 1997 by Spa & Fitness peers internationally.

ONTARIO

CAMBRIDGE
🕽 **519**
✈ Lester B. Pearson Int'l AP (YYZ) 45 mi. / 70 km.

Langdon Hall Country House Hotel & Spa
❤❤❤❤

🏃 🦌

RR 33, Cambridge ON N3H 4R8. Tel: (519) 740-2100. Toll Free (800) 268-1898. Fax: (519) 740-8161. TYPE: Country Inn with Health Spa. LOCATION: Cambridge (ON),

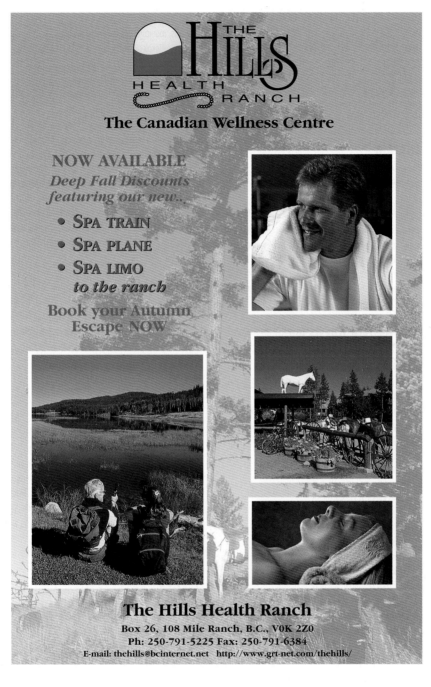

THE HILLS HEALTH RANCH

The Canadian Wellness Centre

NOW AVAILABLE
Deep Fall Discounts featuring our new...

- SPA TRAIN
- SPA PLANE
- SPA LIMO
  to the ranch

Book your Autumn Escape NOW

The Hills Health Ranch

Box 26, 108 Mile Ranch, B.C., V0K 2Z0
Ph: 250-791-5225 Fax: 250-791-6384
E-mail: thehills@bcinternet.net   http://www.grt-net.com/thehills/

45 min. from Toronto. SPA CLIENTELE: Women and men. DESCRIPTION: Country house with heated outdoor pool, tennis, croquet, card room and health spa. Spa treatments: hydrotherapy, massotherapy, esthetic care, algotherapy, fangotherapy, balneotherapy, body exfoliation, herbal wraps. Recreation: golf, ballooning, antiquing, horseback riding. Spa package: from CAN$219.

CHATAM
⟩ 519
✕ Windsor Airport (YQG)

Chatam (ONT), population 41,000, is a commercial center and the seat of the Kent County in southwestern Ontario. It is graciously situated along the banks of the Thames River, which flows into Lake St. Clair, half way between London and Windsor. Chatam is located 65 miles (104 km.) southwest of London (ONT) and 1 hour by car from Detroit/Windsor via Hwy 401 (exit 81).

Best Western Wheels Inn
♥♥♥♥

615 Richmond St., Chatam (ONT) N7M 5K8. Tel: (519) 351-1100. Fax: (519) 436-5541. TYPE: Inn & Fitness Club. LOCATION: In the heartland of Southwestern Ontario, corner of Keil Dr. & Richmond in Chatam. SPA CLIENTELE: Mixed, Family Oriented.

* Rooms: 350 w/priv. bath
* Air-conditioning, color TV, telephone
* Dining Room & Coffee shop
* Airport: Windsor/London 1 hour, taxi
* Reservations: deposit required
* Credit Cards: MC/VISA/AMEX
* Open: Year round
* Hotel Rates: CAN$85 - CAN$152/day
* TAC: 10% (on room rate only)
* Spa on premises: Wheels Country Spa
* Spa Facilities: Fitness Club, gym, saunas, whirlpools, indoor/outdoor pools, fitness pool, massage and therapy rooms, Beauty Salon
* Spa Programs: fitness, beauty

* Spa Treatments: therapeutic massages, facials, manicures, herbal wrap, salt-glo loofa, reflexology, therapeutic clay, low calorie meals
* Spa Packages: 1-5 day packages
* Indications: revitalization, pampering
* Contraindications: high blood pressure, heart problems (for heat related services)

DESCRIPTION: A country resort complex offering Best Western standard rooms and amenities. The Country Spa offers European style revitalizing body and skin treatments, and the Fitness & Racquet Club provides opportunities for sports and fitness activities. Recreation: ping-pong, putting greens, tennis. A supervised day care center provides plenty of fun and organized activities for young children while their parents participate in fitness and spa programs.

GRAFTON
⟩ 905
✕ Lester B. Pearson int'l Airport (YYZ) Toronto
Toronto Island Airport (YTZ) Toronto

Ste-Anne's Country Inn & Spa
♥♥♥

RR#1, Grafton ON K0K 2G0. Tel: (905) 349-2493. Toll Free (888) 3-INN-SPA. Fax: (905) 349-3531. TYPE: Inn & Spa. LOCATION: Resort area 1-1/4 hrs. from Toronto. SPA CLIENTELE: Women & men. DESCRIPTION: Luxury Inn with outdoor pool, tennis & spa. Spa treatments: hydrotherapy, massotherapy, body exfoliation, herbal body wraps, Moor mud baths, meditation, fitness, aromatherapy. Recreation: golf, cross-country skiing. Hotel rate: from CAN$195.

McKELLAR
⟩ 705
✕ Lester B. Pearson int'l Airport (YYZ) Toronto
Toronto Island Airport (YTZ) Toronto

McKellar is a lake side summer resort about 150 mi. / 250 km. north of Toronto near Parry Sound.

The Inn at Manitou
❤❤❤❤❤

McKellar, Ontario P0G 1C0. Tel: (705) 389-2171. Fax: (705) 389-3818. Winter address: 77 Ingram Drive, Suite #200, Toronto ON M6M 2L7. Tel: (416) 245-5606. Fax: (416) 245-2460. Reservations: Toll free (800) 571-8818. TYPE: Luxury Retreat & Spa. LOCATION: On the shores of the unspoiled Manitouwabing Lake, 150 mi. / 240 km. north of Toronto. SPA CLIENTELE: Women and men.

* Rooms & suites: 33 w/priv. bath
* Phone,CTV, C/H, priv. bath
* Restaurant: gourmet cuisine and healthful spa menu
* Reservations: deposit required
* Credit Cards: MC, VISA, AMEX, DISC
* Open: May - October
* TAC: 10%
* Spa on premises
* Name of Spa: **The Spa at Manitou**
* Year Established: 1999
* **Spa facilities**: $1 million fully staffed spa, hydrotherapy baths, gym, beauty salon,
* **Spa Programs**: fitness, health and beauty
* **Spa Packages**: 3,4 and 7 day packages; Pamper Day (for non resident guests).
* **Spa Treatments**: hydrotherapy, massages (holistic, swedish, shiatsu), body wraps (algae, moor mud), body loofah polish, salt glow loofah, hydrotherapy plus, facials, aerobics, health walks, reflexology, low cal gourmet spa cuisine, fitness classes
* **Indications**: beauty, anti-stress, weight loss
* **Cost of Treatments**: from CAN$70
* **Web**: www.manitou-online.com

DESCRIPTION: Luxurious 500-acre retreat on the shores of one of Ontario's most beautiful unspoiled lakes. The Spa at Manitou is an oasis of health, beauty, fitness and rejuvenation offering a wide range of American and European body and pampering treatments. The inn's tennis and golf clinics are some of the best in North America. Spa packages combined with golf and tennis are available. Ladies golf is a specialty with special attention given to the needs of female guests. Recreation: golf, tennis, horseback riding, water sports. Cooking classes are offered by guest chefs. Member: *Relais & Chateaux.*

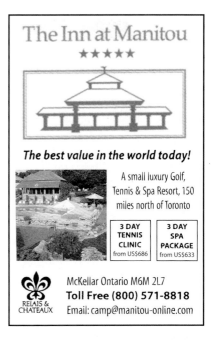

The Inn at Manitou
★★★★★

The best value in the world today!

A small luxury Golf, Tennis & Spa Resort, 150 miles north of Toronto

| 3 DAY TENNIS CLINIC from US$686 | 3 DAY SPA PACKAGE from US$633 |

RELAIS & CHATEAUX

McKellar Ontario M6M 2L7
Toll Free (800) 571-8818
Email: camp@manitou-online.com

ZEPHYR
〕 **905**

✈ Lester B. Pearson int'l Airport (YYZ) Toronto
Toronto Island Airport (YTZ) Toronto

High Fields Country Inn & Spa
❤❤❤

11570 Concession 3, R.R. #1, Zephyr ON L0E 1T0. Tel: (905) 473-6132. Fax: (905) 473-1044. MANAGING DIRECTOR: Norma Daniel. TYPE: Country Inn & Spa. LOCATION:On 175 acres of rolling fields and woodlands just 45 minutes from Metro Toronto. SPA CLIENTELE: Men & Women, adults only.

* Accommodations: 3 rooms, 1 suite, 2 apts.

* Reservations: deposit required
* Credit Cards: MC, VISA, AMEX, DIN
* Open: Year round
* Rates: CAN$130-$250 (rooms)
  Spa Packages: from CAN$250
* Spa on premises
* Year Established: 1989
* **Spa Facilities:** 8 treatment rooms, hot tub, Swedish sauna, state-of-the-art exercise room with certified fitness trainer, swimming pool, nature walks
* **Spa Programs:** Pampering, Revitalization, Rest, Relaxation & Rejuvenation
* **Spa Treatments:** specialized body treatments, Swedish massage, aromatherapy, reflexology, Eastern Western meditation, Barborand Aveda facials, hydrotherapy
* **Indications:** stress
* **Contraindications:** depends on treatments, H.B.P. & heart disease
* **Length of Stay Required:** one day or evening; 2 nights on weekend
* **Medical Supervision:** not available
* **Maximum number of guests:** 14
* **Documentation from Doctor:** only if chronic medical condition exists
* Email:norma@inforamp.net
* Web: www.highfields.com

DESCRIPTION: A secluded and intimate adult, non-smoking, facility, offering day spa services, fitness training, deluxe accommodations, dining, riding, sports facilities.

QUEBEC

CARLETON-SUR-MER
🕭 **418**
✈ Charlo (NB) or Bonaventure (QC) Airport

Acqua-Mer Thalassotherapie
❤❤❤❤

🧖 🧍 🏊 ☆

868 Boul. Perron, Carleton-Sur-Mer, QC G0C 1J0. Tel: (418) 364-7055, Toll Free (800) 463-0867. Fax: (418) 364-7351. MANAGING DIRECTOR: Jules Corriveau. PROGRAMS

DIRECTOR: Yolande Dubois. SPA DIRECTOR: Ginette Cote. TYPE: Thalassoptherapy Center. LOCATION: Nestled amid the sea and the mountains in the heart of the Gaspésie's baie-de-Chaleurs. SPA CLIENTELE: Men & Women.

* Accommodations: 54 rooms, 2 cottages
* Phone,CTV, C/H, priv. bath
* Restaurant, Café Santé, Jacuzzi
* Reservations: deposit required
* Credit Cards: MC, VISA, AMEX, DISC
* Open: Year round
* TAC: 10%
* Spa on premises
* Name of Spa: **Aqua-Mer Thalassothérapie**
* Year Established: 1985
* **Spa Facilities:** Aqua-Gym, warm sea water pool, treatment rooms, Boutique de la Mer, Café Santé - health cuisine
* **Spa Programs:** cellulitis cure, heavy legs cure, anti-backache cure, anti-rheumatic pain cure, nasal hygiene, anti-tobacco cure
* **Spa Packages:** One-week of thalassotherapy, Return to Fitness Marine Cure; Weekend Package; Daily Packages from CAN$215
* **Spa Treatments:** sea water spray, underwater shower, affusion shower, hydrotherapy, underwater jet, rain massage, seawater baths, algotherapy, exothermic mud, thermal ball, marine product treatments, lymphatic drainage, hand massage, pressotherapy, vertebral
* **Indications:**nasal hygiene, addiction to smoking, allergies, bursitis, tendonitis, back & hip pain, stress & circulatory problems, muscular relaxation, relief of rheumatic and back pain
* **Contraindications:** dermatose, recent heart conditions
* **Length of Stay Required:** minimum one week
* **Medical Supervision:** physical therapists, professional aestheticians, registered nurses (3)
* **Maximum number of guests:** 100
* **Cost of Treatments:** from CAN$125-$140
* **Thalasso Package:** 6-7 nights from CAN$1191
* Email: aquamer@globetrotter.qc.ca

DESCRIPTION: Aqua-Mer is a fashionable seaside marine

cure center combining the beneficial treatments of sea water, algae, sea mud and marine climate, with first class resort amenities. The objective of your stay at Aqua Mer is to achieve superior fitness, renewed energy and new habits to improve the quality of your life.

EASTMAN
⟩ 514
✈ Dorval Int'l Airport (YUL)
Mirabel Int'l Airport (YMX)

Centre de Santé d'Estman
❤❤❤❤

895, chemin de Diligences, Eastman QC J0E 1P0. Tel: (514) 297-3009. Toll Free (800) 665-5272. Fax: (514) 297-3370. TYPE: Health Spa. LOCATION: Resort area facing Mt. Orford east of Montréal SPA CLIENTELE: Women and men. DESCRIPTION: Intimate spa with 19 rooms, fine health restaurant, outdoor pool and health spa. Spa treatments: hydrotherapy, massotherapy, esthetic care, algotherapy, body cleansing, weight loss, massages, aquafitness. Recreation: cross-country skiing, golf, horseback riding. Hotel Rates: from CAN$155.

MAGOG-ORFORD
⟩ 819
✈ Dorval Int'l Airport (YUL) (Montréal)
Mirabel Int'l Airport (YMX) (Montréal)

Clinique Algothérapie
❤❤❤❤

c/o Manoir de Sables Resort, 90 ave des Jardins (RR#2), Magog-Orford QC J1X 3W3. Tel: (819) 847-3838. Toll Free (800) 663-9848. Fax: (819) 847-3838. TYPE: Resort with Spa. LOCATION: Resort area on private lake 1 hour east of Montréal. SPA CLIENTELE: Women and men. DESCRIPTION: Resort hotel with 117 rooms, indoor/outdoor pools, golf, private lake, game room, tennis, skating, cross-country skiing, sleigh rides, health spa. Spa treatments: hydrotherapy, massotherapy, reflexology, esthetic care, pressotherapy, holistic face massage. Hotel rates: from CAN$173.

Spa Chéribourg
⚕ 🏇 🚶

2603, chemin de Parc Orford, C.P. 337, Magog-Orford QC J1X 3W9. Tel: (819) 868-0101. Toll Free (800) 567-6132. Fax: (819) 843-2639. TYPE: Resort & Health Center. LOCATION: Between Lake Memphremagog and Mount Orford, 1 hour east of Montréal. SPA CLIENTELE: Women and men. DESCRIPTION: Resort with 97 rooms, restaurant (diet cuisine), indoor/outdoor pools, indoor golf driving, tennis, squash, health spa. Health treatments: hydrotherapy, massotherapy, reflexology, algotherapy, fangotherapy, body exfoliation, kinesitherapy, stretching, muscle stimulation. Hotel rates: from CAN$175.

MONTRÉAL
⟩ 514
✈ Dorval Int'l Airport (YUL) (Montréal)
Mirabel Int'l Airport (YMX) (Montréal)

Relais Santé Effi-Corp
❤❤❤❤

475, Président-Kennedy Street West, Montréal QC H3A 2T4. Tel: (514) 284-4357. Fax: (514) 284-4342. TYPE: Hotel with health Spa. LOCATION: Downtown Montréal between Place des Arts and McGill stations. SPA CLIENTELE: Women and men. DESCRIPTION: 453 room luxury hotel with indoor/outdoor pools. sauna, whirlpool, and health spa. Spa treatments: hydrotherapy, massotherapy, reflexology, algotherapy, body exfoliation, beauty treatments, moor mud, mud packs, mineral packs, aroma-steam, pressotherapy. Spa package (with lodging): from CAN $169.

MONTPELLIER
⟩ 819
✈ Uplands Int'l AP (YOW) Ottawa (ON)

Château Les Beaulne
❤❤❤

218, montée Lafontaine, Montpellier QC J0V 1M0. Tel:

(819) 428-2244. Toll Free (888) 428-2244. Fax: (819) 428-2564. TYPE: Inn with Spa. LOCATION: Lakeside resort area 1 hour from Ottawa in the Outaouais region. DESCRIPTION: 15 room inn with restaurant (vegetarian cuisine) and health spa. Spa treatments: hydrotherapy, massotherapy, algotherapy, fangotherapy, body exfoliation, massages, aromatherapy. Recreation: cross-country skiing, water sports, golf. Spa package: from CAN$ 195.

NOTRE DAME DE LOURDES
☽ 514

✈ Dorval Int'l Airport (YUL) (Montréal)
  Mirabel Int'l Airport (YMX) (Montréal)

Station Santé - Maison d'Orient
♥♥♥♥

5331 rue Principale, Notre-Dame-de-Lourdes QC J0K 1K0. Tel: (514) 759-4264. Toll Free (888) 271-4264. Fax: (514) 759-6925. TYPE: Resort Hotel & Spa. LOCATION: Resort area in the heart of the Lanaudière region 45 min. north of Montréal. SPA CLIENTELE: Women and men. DESCRIPTION: Maison d'Orient offer a variety of spa treatments including: hydrotherapy, massotherapy, esthetic care, algotherapy, fangotherapy, balneotherapy, body exfoliation, pressotherapy. Recreation: golf (9 holes), tennis, cross-country skiing, mountain biking, skating, snowmobiling. Hotel Rates: from CAN$150.

PIEDMONT
☽ 514

✈ Dorval Int'l Airport (YUL)
  Mirabel Int'l Airport (YMX)

Relais des Monts
♥♥♥♥

890 boul des Laurentides, Piedmont QC J0R 1K0. Tel: (514) 227-5181. Toll Free (800) 851-7289. Fax: (514) 227-5181. TYPE: Motel with health Spa. LOCATION: In the Laurentians near Saint-Sauveur, 45 min. from Montréal.

DESCRIPTION: 15 room motel with outdoor pool and health spa. Spa treatments: hydrotherapy, massotherapy, esthetic care, algotherapy, fangotherapy, physiotherapy. Recreation: cross-country and down hill skiing, golf, tennis. Spa package: from CAN$165.

POINTE-AU-PIC
☽ 418

✈ Québec City Airport (YQB) 90 mi. / 140 km.

Manoir Richelieu
♥♥♥♥

181, rue Richelieu, Pointe-au-Pic (QC) G0T 1M0. Tel: (418) 665-2600. Toll Free (800) 699-RELAX. Fax: (418) 665-7299. TYPE: Resort Hotel, Casino & Spa. SPA CLIENTELE: Women and men. LOCATION: On the shores of the St. Lawrence river. DESCRIPTION: Legendary Manor with popular casino. 390 rooms, restaurant (diet cuisine), indoor/outdoor pools, health spa. Spa treatments: massages, algotherapy, aquamassage, flotation tankpressotherapy. Recreation: cross country skiing, gambling, hiking, horseback riding. Hotel rates: from CAN$160.

QUÉBEC CITY
☽ 418

✈ Québec City Airport (YQB) 12 mi. / 19 km.

Château Bonne Entente
♥♥♥♥

3400 chemin Sainte-Foy, Québec City QC G1X 1S6. Tel: (418) 650-4575. Toll Free (800) 463-4390. Fax: (418) 653-3098. TYPE: Hotel with Spa. SPA CLIENTELE: Women and men. LOCATION: In a lovely park 5 min. from downtown Québec City. DESCRIPTION: 170 room Château hotel with restaurant, bar and swimming pool, health spa. Spa treatments: hydrotherapy, massotherapy, reflexology, algotherapy, flotation tank, aquamassage, pressotherapy. Hotel Rates: from CAN$160. Recreation: skiing, downhill skiing, fishing, horseback riding.

SAINT-FAUSTIN
819
✈ Dorval Int'l Airport (YUL)
Mirabel Int'l Airport (YMX)

Centre de Santé - Sonia Blancard
♥♥♥

272, chemin Domaine Lauzon, Saint-Faustin QC J0T 2G0. Tel: (819) 688-6640. Toll Free (800) 347-6011 (Canada); (800) 688-1036 (USA). Fax: (819) 688-6011. TYPE: Health Spa. LOCATION: Rural resort area near Mt. Tremblant, 1-1/4 hrs from Montréal. DESCRIPTION: Small 5 room inn with outdoor pool, restaurant (natural cuisine with white meat), and health spa. Spa treatments: hydrotherapy, massotherapy, esthetic care, algotherapy, fangotherapy, body exfoliation, Japanese hot tub, Oriental Biorythms, aromatherapy. Recreation: tennis, golf, cross-country skiing. Spa package: from CAN$189.

SAINT-GEORGES DE BEAUCE
418
✈ Saint-Georges Airport
Québec City Airport (YQB) 60 mi. / 96 km.

Hôtel le Georgesville
♥♥♥

300, 118th St., Saint-Georges de Beauce QC G5Y 3E3. Tel: (418) 227-7127. Toll Free (800) 463-3003. Fax: (418) 228-4110. TYPE: Resort Hotel & Spa. SPA CLIENTELE: Women and men. LOCATION: Downtown in a semi-urban setting. DESCRIPTION: Elegant hotel, 98 rooms, French restaurant, bar, indoor pool, health spa. Spa treatments: hydrotherapy, massotherapy, algotherapy, aqua-massage. Recreation: tennis, hiking, golf, fishing, cross-country skiing, snowmobiling. Hotel rates: from CAN$145.

SAINT-PAULIN
819
✈ Dorval Int'l Airport (YUL)
Mirabel Int'l Airport (YMX)
Québec City Airport (YQB)

Le Baluchon
♥♥♥♥

3550 chemin de Trembles, Saint-Paulin QC J0K 3G0. Tel: (819) 268-2555. Toll Free (800) 789-5968. Fax: (819) 268-5234. TYPE: Resort hotel with Spa. LOCATION: Nestled in a lovely natural site in the Rivière-du-Loup islands, 1-1/2 hrs from Montréal, 1-3/4 hrs from Québec City. DESCRIPTION: 60 room resort hotel with restaurant (diet cuisine), indoor/outdoor pools, and health spa. Spa treatments: hydrotherapy, massotherapy, esthetic care, aquafitness, massage, body exfoliation, stretching. Recreation: exercise, health workshops, nature watching, cross-country skiing. Hotel rates: from CAN$175.

SHAWINIGAN
819
✈ Québec City Airport (YQB) 60 mi. / 96 km.

L'Escale Santé
♥♥♥

c/o Gouverneur Auberge, 1100, Promenade du Saint-Maurice, Shawinigan QC G9N 1L8. Tel: (819) 537-6000. Toll Free (888) 922-1100. Fax: (819) 537-6365. TYPE: Hotel with Spa. SPA CLIENTELE: mostly women. LOCATION: Heart of the Mauricie Region with panoramic view of the Saint-Maurice River, 35 km. / 22 mi. from Trois Riviéres. DESCRIPTION: 72 room inn, restaurant (healthy cuisine), pool, beauty spa. Spa treatments: paraffin bath, hydrotherapy, massotherapy, esthetic care, algotherapy, aromatherapy, phytotherapy, kinesitherapy, pressotherapy. Recreation: golf, cruises, waterfalls park. Hotel rates: from CAN$115.

CAYMAN ISLANDS

CHILE

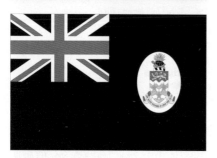

AREA: 96 sq. mi. (249 sq. km.)
POPULATION: 32,000
CAPITAL: George Town
OFFICIAL LANGUAGE: English
CURRENCY: Cayman Dollar (C$)
EXCHANGE RATE: 1 US$ = C$ 0.82
TELEPHONE COUNTRY CODE:345

ℹ Cayman Islands Dept of Tourism
PO Box 67, George Town, Cayman Islands
Tel: (345) 949-0623. Fax: (345) 949-4053

GEORGE TOWN
✆ No area code
✈ Owen Roberts Airport (GCM)

The Beauty Spa
❤❤❤❤
🏃 💆

c/o Hyatt Regency Grand Cayman, Seven Mile Beach, PO Box 2185, Georgetown, Grand Cayman, BWI, Hotel Tel: 949-1234, Fax: 949-8528. Spa Tel: 945-4673, Fax: 949-0520. TYPE: Resort Hotel & Spa. LOCATION: On landscaped grounds across from Seven Mile Beach. DESCRIPTION: Deluxe resort hotel, 236 rooms, restaurants, bars, pools, tennis, health Spa. Spa treatments: Full service spa with body treatments, wraps, hydrotherapy, facial, massage, salon. Hotel Rates: from US$190/day.

AREA: 292,257 sq. mi. (756,946 sq. km.)
POPULATION: 12,961,000
CAPITAL: Santiago
OFFICIAL LANGUAGES: Spanish
CURRENCY: Chilean Peso (Clp)
CURRENCY EXCHANGE: 1 US$ = Clp 464
TELEPHONE COUNTRY CODE: 56

MAITENCILLO
✆ 32
✈ Viña del Mar Airport

Marbella Resort
❤❤❤❤
🏃 💆

klm 35 Con Con, Zapallar Rd. Region V. Tel: (32) 772020. Fax: (32) 772030. TYPE: Resort Complex & Spa. LOCATION: 100 mi / 160 km from Santiago and 40 min. from Viña del Mar. SPA CLIENTELE: Men & Women. DESCRIPTION: Mediterranean-style resort situated beachfront. 78 rooms w/sea view, optional jacuzzi and fireplace, restaurants, bars, 18-hole golf course, polo field, swimming pools, tennis courts. Spa for physical conditioning, and rejuvenation. Hotel rates: from US$195.

PATAGONIA
✆ 2 (Santiago)
✈ Coihaique/Balmaceda Airport

52

Termas de Puyuhuapi Hotel & Spa
❤❤❤

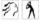

Puerto Puyuhuapi, Tel: (2) 724-1515. Fax: (2) 460267. TYPE: Small resort & Spa. LOCATION: Southern Chilean fjord of Northern Patagonia. SPA CLIENTELE: Men & Women. DESCRIPTION: A remote native wood hotel & spa with thermal hot spring baths, hot sea-water jacuzzi, steam showers, seaweed wraps, massages, facials, weight & cardic equipment. A great base to explore Queulat National park to view the Hanging Glacier, and fish in Dorita Bay.

SANTIAGO
ʔ 2

✈ Arturo Merino Bentez Airport

San Cristobal Tower & Neptuno Spa
❤❤❤❤

Av. Santa Maria 1742, Providencia (Santiago), Tel: (2) 707-1000, Fax: (2) 707-1010. TYPE: Elegant Hotel & Spa. LOCATION: In the residential Providencia area of Santiago, 40 km. to Arturo Merino Benitez Airport. SPA CLIENTELE: Men & Women. DESCRIPTION: 139 rooms & suites, 2 restaurants, lounge, bar, entertainment, meeting facilities, business center, tennis courts & 2 outdoor pools. Neptuno Spa & Fitness center offers massage, aromatherapy, reflexology and shiatsu treatments, heated indoor pool, gym, exercise equipment, sauna & steam room. Hotel rates: from US$390.

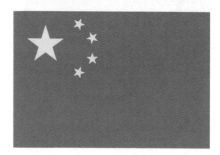

CHINA

AREA: 3,691,000 sq. mi. (9,559,690 sq. km.)
POPULATION: 1,133,682,501
CAPITAL: Beijing
OFFICIAL LANGUAGES: Chinese, Chuang, Uigur, Yi, Tibetan, Miao, Mongol, Kazakh
CURRENCY: yuan (Y)
CURRENCY EXCHANGE: 1 US$ = Y 8.50
TELEPHONE COUNTRY CODE: 86

ℹ China National Tourist Office
No. 9A Jian Guo Men Nei Ave.
Beijing 100740. China

BEIJING
ʔ 10

✈ Capital Int'l Airport (NAY) 14 mi. / 22 km. NE

Beijing, population 5,531,000, is the capital of the People's Republic of China. It is a great dynamic metropolis where the ancient monuments coexist with the contemporary. Beijing consists of 3 quite symmetrical layouts. **The Forbidden City**, the residence of China's Emperors is the innermost rectangle. The 2nd rectangle outlines the former boundaries of the Imperial City. The outermost rectangle in the area between the Inner City and the Outer City Walls is where the government buildings, market districts and old residential area are located. With a history of over 3,000 years, Beijing is famous for its ancient sites and cultural relics.

The Palace Hotel
❤❤❤❤❤

8 Goldfish Lane, Beijing 100006 . Tel: (10) 6512-8899. Fax: (10) 6512-9050. TYPE: Deluxe Hotel & Spa. LOCATION: In Wangfujing shopping district near the Diplomatic Quarter and business district. Walking distance from the Forbidden City. SPA CLIENTELE: Men & Women.

* Rooms: 530 w/priv. marble bath
* Suites: 18 duplex suites w/spectacular view
* Phone, CTV (24 hrs. news channel, movies), radio, minibar, hair dryer
* Rooms for non smokers
* Restaurants: Chinese, Japanese, German
* Karaoke bar, lounges, disco
* Airport: Beijin Int'l 35 km. / 22 mi.
* Train Station: Beijing Central 2 km. / 1 mi.
* Reservations: required
* Credit Cards: MC/VISA/AMEX/DC/CB
* Open: Year round
* Hotel Rates: from $190
* TAC: 10%
* Spa on premises: **The Palace Spa**
* **Spa Facilities**: Full health club, gym, saunas massage rooms, solarium, steam room, jacuzzi, Beauty salon
* **Spa Programs**: Health, diet, fitness
* **Spa Treatments**: therapeutic massages, martial arts and aerobic classes

DESCRIPTION: The elegant Palace Hotel Beijing in the heart of the Chinese Capital near the famous Forbidden City has a striking Atrium-style incorporating ancient Chinese architecture. **The Palace Spa**, located on the third floor of the

hotel offers heated indoor pool, fully equipped gymnasium, whirlpools, saunas and a solarium. Spa treatments: fitness, beauty and pampering therapies based on European and ancient Chinese traditions.

SHANGHAI
🌙 **21**

✈ Hongqiao Airport (SHA) 10 mi. / 16 km.

Hotel Sofitel Hyland
❤❤❤❤

505 Nan Jing Rd. East, Shanghai 200001. Tel: (21) 6351-5888. Fax: (21) 6351-4088. TYPE: Hotel with Spa. LOCATION: Downtown in the city center. DESCRIPTION: Attractive downtown hotel, 321 rooms, 68 suites, nonsmoker rooms, 3 restaurants, 3 bars, lounge, pub with mini-brewery, meeting facilities, business center. Fitness spa with gym, jacuzzi, sauna, beauty salon.

TIANJIN
🌙 **22**

✈ Tianjin Int'l Airport

Hyatt Tianjin
❤❤❤❤❤

219 Jie Fanf N. Rd., Tianjin 300042. Tel: (22) 2330-1234. Fax: (22) 2331-1234. TYPE: Deluxe hotel with Spa. LOCATION: City center on the banks of the Hai River. DESCRIPTION: Neo-classic hotel, 450 rooms, Regency Club floor, nonsmoker rooms, 5 restaurants, bar, lounge, entertainment, meeting facilities, business center. Health spa with gym, sauna, steam room, massage, plunge pools.

CHINA (HONG KONG)

AREA: 403 sq. mi. (1,044 sq. km.)
POPULATION: 5,761,000
CAPITAL: Victoria
OFFICIAL LANGUAGES: Chinese, English
CURRENCY: Hong Kong Dollar (HK$)
CURRENCY EXCHANGE: 1 US$ = HK$ 7.75
TELEPHONE COUNTRY CODE: 852

KOWLOON

✎ No area code

✈ Hong Kong Int'l Airport Kowloon (HKG)

Gold Coast Hotel - Balinese Spa
♥♥♥♥

1 Castle Peak Rd., Castle Peak Bay, Kowloon, Hong Kong. Tel: 2452-8888, Fax: 2440-7368. TYPE: Resort hotel & Spa. LOCATION: On 10 beachfront acres in Kowloon. DESCRIPTION: Superior first class resort with Health & Beauty spa, fitness center, outdoor pools, restaurant, cafe, lounge. 450 rooms, 10 suites. Hotel rates: from HK$ 1,480

The Peninsula Hotel & Spa
♥♥♥♥♥

Salisbury Rd., Tsimahatsui, Kowloon, Hong Kong, Hotel Tel: 2366-6251. Fax: 2722-4170. Spa Tel: 2315-3135. Fax: 2315-3124. TYPE: Hotel & Spa. LOCATION: Facing the harbor in the heart of the shopping area. DESCRIPTION: Superior deluxe hotel with Health Club and Spa. 300 rooms, 54 suites, 7 restaurants, lounge, bar, meeting facilities, business center, indoor pools, shops. Hotel rates: from HK$ 2,700.

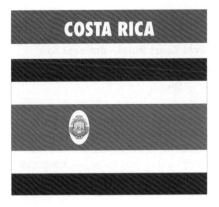

COSTA RICA

AREA: 19, 575 sq. mi. (50,700 sq. km.)
POPULATION: 2,959,000
CAPITAL: San José
OFFICIAL LANGUAGE: Spanish
CURRENCY: Cólon (C)
EXCHANGE RATE: 1US$ = C
TELEPHONE COUNTRY CODE: 506

Costa Rica is a small country in central America with a unique history, colorful villages, sunny beaches, and beautiful resorts. The country has a long tradition of democracy and peacefully coexistence with its central american neighbors.

The climate is temperate tropical year round with temperature averaging 70°F (21°c). All these qualities make Costa Rica an ideal destination for fun and relaxation. There are four spas in metropolitan San José area.

ⓘ Inst. Costarricense de Turismo
Calle 5-7 Avenida 4, San José, Costa Rica
Tel: (506) 223-8423. Fax: (506) 223-5452

SAN JOSE
🕎 No area code
✈ Juan Santamaria Int'l Airport (SJO)
12 mi. / 19 km. northwest of San José

San José, population 215,000, is located in a broad valley at an altitude of 1,150 m. (3,795 ft.). The city is cos-

mopolitan, clean and modern with old public buildings and manicured parks. It is the cultural and the commercial center for the whole country. San José can be reached by many international airlines either direct or via Miami, New Orleans or Los Angeles in the USA.

Melia Comfort Corobici Hotel
❤❤❤❤

Highway General Cañas, Sabana Norte, P.O. Box 2443-1000 San José. Tel: 232-8122. Fax: 231-5834. TYPE: Hotel with Spa. LOCATION: Heart of San José 5 min. to business district. SPA CLIENTELE: Women and men.

* Rooms: 200 w/priv. bath. Suites: 4
* Restaurant, Bar, Coffee Shop
* Airport: 20 min. bus, taxi
* Open: Year round
* Credit Cards: MC/VISA/AMEX
* Hotel Rates: from US$110/day
* TAC: 10%
* Spa on premises
* **Spa Facilities**: gym, swimming pool, sauna
* **Spa Treatments**: weight training, massages, low calorie meals

DESCRIPTION: Multistory business hotel 1 block from La Sabana Park with complete health & fitness spa. Recreation: casino, golf, tennis, nightclub.

El Tucano Hotel
❤❤

P.O. Box 114-1017, San José 2000. Tel: 460-1822. Fax: 460-1692. TYPE: Hotel. LOCATION: 20 mi. / 32 km. from the airport. 90 rooms, sauna, gym, restaurant, thermal hot springs. Hotel Rates: from US$55.

San José Palacio Spa & Casino
❤❤❤❤

El Robledal, P.O. Box 458, La Uruca 1150. Tel: 220-2034. Fax: 231-2325. TYPE: Spa & Casino Hotel. LOCATION: 5

mi. / 8 km. from Juan Santamaria AP in a natural forest. 254 rooms, spa with gym, sauna, massage parlor. Hotel rates: from US$130.

Tara Resort Hotel
❤❤❤❤

Aptdo Postal 1459, 1250 Escazù. Tel: 228-6992. Fax: 228-9651. TYPE: Resort & Spa. LOCATION: In Escazù with a breathtaking view of San José's Central Valley. 14 rooms, suites and bungalows, gourmet restaurant, bar, sauna, massage, rejuvenation treatments. Hotel Rates: from US$125/day.

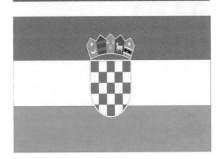

CROATIA

AREA: 22,050 sq. mi. (56,538 sq. km.)
POPULATION: 4,600,000
CAPITAL: Zagreb
OFFICIAL LANGUAGE: Croatian
CURRENCY: Croatian Dinar (CRD)
EXCHANGE RATE: 1 US$= CRD
TELEPHONE COUNTRY CODE: 38

Croatia has mineral, thermal and radio-active springs in various areas. Their spas are traditionally linked to the Romans who were the first to experience the great healing powers of Croatian thermal and mineral waters.

The spas and health resorts are well developed and equipped with teams of qualified experts. They are easily accessible and connected to major towns by a good communication system.

ℹ Croatia Ministry of Tourism
Ulica Girada Vukovar 78, 41000 Zagreb
Tel: (41) 613347 / 612653. Fax: (41) 6113246

DUGA UVALA
☎ **52**
✈ Pula Airport. 9 mi. / 15 km.

Duga Uvala is a resort set at the end of a deep inlet surrounded by lush Mediterranean vegetation. It is 25 km. northeast of Pula, the largest town in Istria Peninsula.

Hotel Croatia Duga Uvala
❤❤❤

52208 Krnica/Pula, Tel: (52) 553-256, Fax: (52) 553-277. TYPE: Hotel Health & Recreation Center. CLIENTELE: Men & women. DESCRIPTION: Spa facilities with cardio-vascular diagnostic equipment, rheumatological diagnostic & treatment equipment, indoor heated sea water pool, fitness studio. Programs: early preventive health care & rehabilitation courses dealing with back & neck pain, osteoporosis, stress management, slimming & stop smoking.

OPATIJA
➲ 51

✈ Rijeka Airport. 15 mi. / 25 km.

Opatija, population 29,000, is situated on the shores of Kvarner Bay of the Adriatic coast. It is one of the leading seaside resorts in Croatia. It has a long tradition of luxury and medical excellence with more than 30 hotels, restaurants, parks, and an attractive promenade along the waterfront. A special role in the development of health tourism can be attributed to the **Thalassotherapia** an institute for the rehabilitation and treatment of heart, lung and rheumatic diseases.

Thalassotherapia
❤❤❤

M. Tita 232, Opatija CR-51410, Tel: (51) 712-322, Fax: (51) 271-424. TYPE: Thalassotherapy Centre. SPA CLIENTELE: Women and men.

* Rooms: 120 with private bath, restaurant
* Airport: Rijeka, taxi
* Open: Year round
* Treatment duration: 2 weeks
* Spa on premises

* Spa Facilities: indoor warm salt water pool, balneotherapeutic equipment, gym, consulting rooms, diagnostic laboratories, x-ray
* Spa Programs: Rejuvenation, relaxation, general fitness, beauty, medical
* Spa Treatments: salt water bathing, mud applications, mineral and bubble baths, massages, electrotherapy, kinesitherapy
* Indications: heart disease - coronary insufficiency, rehabilitation following infarction, angina pectoris, pre-infarct conditions, vegetative disorders of the heart and circulation, conditions following heart surgery, prevention of arteriosclerotic conditions, compensated myocardiopathia, disorders of the peripheral arteries; pulmonary disease - chronic bronchitis, pulmonary emphysema; rheumatism - chronic inflammatory and degenerative
* Medical Supervision: Specialists doctors
* Treatments Approved: Medical Institute

DESCRIPTION: The Thalassotherapia provides extensive care for seriously afflicted patients. A team of over 25 specialists handle diagnosis and therapy.

SIBENIK
➲ 59

✈ Zadar or Split Airports. 31 mi. / 50 km.

Thalassotherapy Institute, Hotel Ivan
❤❤❤

Sibenik CR-59000. Tel: (22) 363-970 or 999. Fax: (22) 361-800 or 801. TYPE: *Beachside Spa Complex*. LOCATION: Solaris Hotel Complex set in Pine Woods with 1,283 rooms. Thalassotherapy & Sports center. Indications: Diseases of the bones, joints, muscles, ligaments. peripheral nervous system & vascular system. Special treatments with curative mud. Rates: on request.

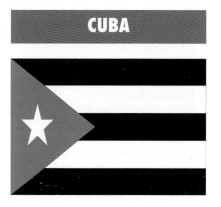

CUBA

AREA: 43,261 sq. mi. (110,922 sq. km.)
POPULATION: 11,000,000
CAPITAL: Havana
OFFICIAL LANGUAGE: Spanish
CURRENCY: Cuban peso (Cp)
EXCHANGE RATE: 1 US$= 21Cp
TELEPHONE COUNTRY CODE: 53

ℹ️ Cuba Tourist Board
55 Queen St. E, Ste 705
Toronto ON M5C 1R5 Canada
Tel: (416) 362-0700. Fax: (416) 362-6799

PIÑAR DEL RIO
🔾 **7**

✈️ Jose Marti Int'l Airport (HAV)

Piñar Del Rio is located in northwestern Cuba. it is the center of the most famous and rich tobacco producing region of Cuba. San Diego Spa uses mud found at the mouth of the river for diverse medical and beauty treatments. The thermal water are low radioactive mineral-medicinal waters containing: calcium, sulfides, sulfates, magnesium, fluorine, at temperatures between 30°c and 40°c (86°F-104°F). The thermal water are effective against dermatological and osteomyoarticulatory conditions.

San Diego de los Baños
❤️❤️❤️

Calle 23 final, San Diego de los Baños, Los Palacios, Piñar del Rio. Reservations: Turismo de Salud. Tel: (7) 225511. Fax: (7) 202350. TYPE: Spa Resort. LOCATION: Mountainous area surrounded by beautiful landscapes, flora and fauna. SPA CLIENTELE: Women and men.

* Rooms: at the Mirador Hotel***
* Open: year round
* Spa on premises
* **Spa Facilities:** thermal spa, treatment rooms, gym, medical centre, laboratory, pharmacy
* **Spa Programs:** physical medicine, medical cosmetology, weight loss, anti-stress, skin condition, beauty and pampering, fitness
* **Spa Treatments:** medicinal baths, mud therapy, hydrotherapy, inhalation, vaginal irrigations, underwater hydromassage, physiotherapy, electro therapy, heat therapy, kinesiotherapy, full body massage, steam baths, acupuncture, health walks,
* **Indications:** osteomyoarticulatory conditions, skin diseases, stress, obesity, beauty
* Medical Supervision: MD and medical staff

DESCRIPTION: Health Spa with 3-star hotel in a mountainous region of western Cuba. The newly refurbished spa offers traditional services and specialized medical consultations. Recreation: party evenings and excursions.

TOPES DE COLLANTES
🔾 **7**

✈️ Jose Marti Int'l Airport (HAV)

Topes de Collantes is 377 km. / 235 mi. southeast of Havana , 900 m. / 2,970 ft. above sea level atop the Sierra del Escambray Mountains. The temperate mountain and seaside climate is healthy.

Topes de Collantes
❤️❤️❤️

Reservations: Turismo de Salud. Tel: (7) 225511. Fax: (7) 202350. TYPE: Health & Rest Resort. LOCATION: Mountainous area. SPA CLIENTELE: Women and men.

* Rooms: hotels, apartments and cabins and kurhotel
* Open: year round
* Spa on premises
* **Spa Facilities**: treatment rooms, open air gym, sauna, medical centre, laboratory, pharmacy
* **Spa Programs**: climotherapy, physical therapy, medical programs, geriatrics
* **Spa Treatments**: aromatherapy, heliotherapy, thalassotherapy, acupuncture, green medicine, beauty treatments, aesthetic surgery, massages
* **Indications**: stress, recovering before and after surgery, general health
* Medical Supervision: MD and medical staff

DESCRIPTION: Health resort covering an area of 34 sq. km. (13 sq. mi.) with a new Kurhotel. The resort specializes in Climatotherapy, physical therapy and Geriatic care. Recreation: marvelous beaches, natural waterfalls, mountain climbing nearby.

VILLA CLARA
⟩ 42
✈ Jose Marti Int'l Airport (HAV)

Thermal springs area of central Cuba. The medicinal waters at the Elguea Baths reaching a temperature of 50°c (122°F) are rich in minerals (more than 40g per liter) such as: chloride, bromide, radon, and sulfur.

Indications: thermal cure relieves circulatory, neurological, digestive, rheumatic and respiratory problems, as well as skin irritations.

Horizontes Elguea Hotel & Spa
♥♥♥

Corralillo, Villa Clara. Tel: (42) 686290. Fax: (42) 686387. TYPE: Spa Resort Hotel. LOCATION: Near thermal pools of Elguea Baths. SPA CLIENTELE: Women and men.

* Rooms: 139 w/priv. bath
* Phone, A/C, CTV, refrigerator, safe deposit
* Restaurant, cafeteria, pool, tennis, volleyball
* Open: year round

* Spa off premises: 600 m. / yards
* **Spa Facilities**: bathhouse, physiotherapy room
* **Spa Programs**: medical, physical fitness, beauty
* **Spa Treatments**: physiotherapy, heliotherapy, kinetic therapy, electrotherapy, massages, hydrotherapy
* **Indications**: stress, general fitness, see also indications for Elguea Baths
* Medical Supervision: MD and medical staff

DESCRIPTION: Health Resort hotel near the medicinal Elguea Baths offering a perfect combination for health, relaxation and recreation. The hotel also offers excursions to Blanquizel Key, whose sulfuric sand is used for natural beauty masks.

VIÑALES
⟩ 8
✈ Jose Marti Int'l Airport (HAV)

The San Vicente Spa in western Pinar del Rio province is known for its natural beauty. It is located just 5 km. / 3 mi. from Viñales Valley. The spa uses medicinal mud extracted from the mouth of the San Diego River and thermal sulfurous water at 31°c (88°F). The medicinal mud contains algae and sea organisms rich in biologically active substances such as steroids, masculine and feminine hormones, antibiotics and vitamins.

Indications: The medicinal springs and mud are used to cure or alleviate skin, nervous, gastrointestinal and respiratory problems.

Horizontes Rancho San Vicente
♥♥♥

Valle San Vicente, Viñales, Pinar del Río. Tel: (8) 93200. TYPE: Spa Resort Hotel. LOCATION: San Vicente Spa. SPA CLIENTELE: Women and men.

* Cabanas: 20 w/priv. bath
* Phone, A/C, CTV, refrigerator, safe deposit
* Restaurant, nightclub
* Open: year round

* Spa on premises
* **Spa Facilities**: 10 individual thermal baths, thermal sulfur pool, treatment rooms, gym, medical office
* **Spa Programs**: medical, physical fitness, beauty
* **Spa Treatments**: hydrotherapy, mud wraps, massages, acupuncture, digitopuncture, exercise, medical checkups, rehabilitation
* **Indications**: stress, general fitness, see also indications for San Vicente Spa
* **Medical Supervision**: MD and medical staff

DESCRIPTION: Small health Resort hotel offering a perfect combination for health, relaxation and recreation combined with thermal and mud cures at the San Vicente Spa. Recreation: horseback riding and trekking along ecological paths.

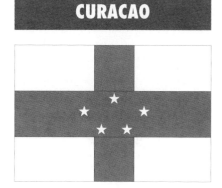

CURACAO

AREA: 183 sq. mi. (474 sq. km.)
POPULATION: 168,000
CAPITAL: Willemstad
OFFICIAL LANGUAGE: Dutch, English
CURRENCY: Antilles Florin (NAf)
EXCHANGE RATE: 1 US$= NAf 1.80
TELEPHONE COUNTRY CODE: 599

🛈 Tourist Information Office
Pietermaii No. 19, Willemstad, Curaçao
Tel: (599) 9-616000, FAX: (599) 9-612305

⟩ 7
✈ Hato Int'l Airport (CUR)

Sonesta Beach Hotel & Casino
♥♥♥♥♥

Piscadera Bay, PO Box 6003, Curaçao. Tel: (7) 368800. TYPE: Resort Hotel. LOCATION: Oceanfront 5 min. from downtown Willemstad. DESCRIPTION: Colonial style beach resort and casino with Health Club and beauty salon. 248 rooms, bar, grill, restaurant, casino, swimming pool with swim up bar. Hotel rates: from US$180.

CYPRUS

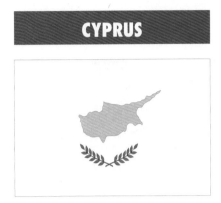

AREA: 3,572 sq. mi. (9,251 sq. km.)
POPULATION: 730,000
CAPITAL: Nicosia
OFFICIAL LANGUAGE: Greek,Turkish
CURRENCY: Cypriot pound (C£)
EXCHANGE RATE: 1US$ = C£ 0.54
TELEPHONE COUNTRY CODE: 357

Cyprus is a beautiful island in the eastern Mediterranean with sandy beaches, cosmopolitan resorts, historic sites, and cool mountains. According to mythology Cyprus was the birth place of the goddess Aphrodite. The climate is balmy Mediterranean. The average winter temperatures in the low 60's°F (17°c); and summer in the high 80's°F (32°c). Cyprus offer 340 days of sunshine a year.

ℹ️ Cyprus Tourism Organization
PO Box 4535, CY 1390, Lefkosia (Nicosia) Cyprus
Tel: (2) 337715. Fax: (2) 331644
Web: www.cyprustourism.org

LARNACA
🕎 04
✈️ Larnaca Int'l Airport (LCA) 5 mi. / 8 km.

Lordos Beach Hotel
♥♥♥♥
🏋️
PO Box 541/542, Larnaca. Tel: (4) 647444. Fax: (4)

645847. TYPE: Resort Hotel with Health Club. LOCATION: On the golden beach of Larnaca Bay close to town and the airport. SPA CLIENTELE: Women and men. DESCRIPTION: Resort hotel with 175 rooms, restaurants, lounge, bars, games room and Leisure Club with sauna, massage room, steam bath, gym, solarium. The Leisure Club offers fitness program and relaxing massages.

LEFKOSIA (Nicosia)
🕎 02
✈️ Larnaca Int'l Airport (LCA) 30 mi. / 48 km.

Lefkosia, population 190,000, is the capital of Cyprus where Government offices and embassies are located. Today it blends a rich historic past, Byzantine churches and monasteries, with the bustle of a modern city. The town is split in two between the Greek and Turkish part of the island.

Cyprus Hilton Hotel
♥♥♥♥♥
🏊 🏋️
Archbishop Makarios III Ave., Lefkosia. Tel: (2) 377777. Fax: (2) 377788. TYPE: Hotel with Spa. LOCATION: Centrally located near business, shopping and entertainment areas. SPA CLIENTELE: Women and men.

* Rooms: 298 w/priv. bath. Suites: 18
* Phone, CTV, A/C, minibar, hairdryer
* Restaurant (2), bar, outdoor pool, tennis & squash
* Airport: Larnaca, taxi
* Reservations: required
* Credit Cards: VISA/AMEX/MC/DIS/EC
* Open: Year round
* Hotel Rates: from C£113
* TAC: 10%
* Spa on premises: **Hiltonia Club**
* **Spa Facilities**: indoor skylit pool, three gym rooms, one with fully equipped body-building equipment, other two for aerobics, two separate Health Clubs for men and women with Spa, sauna, steam bath, beauty salon
* **Spa Programs**: beauty, pampering, general fitness

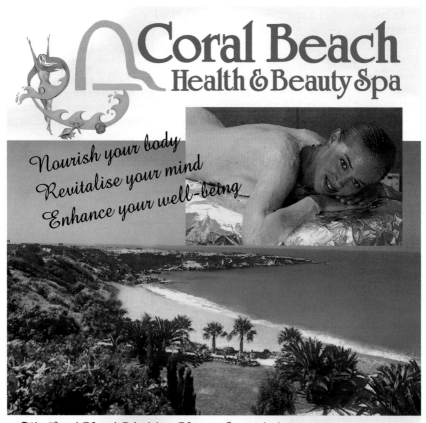

* **Spa Treatments**: aerobics, callanetics, yoga, exercise, beauty treatments, massages

DESCRIPTION: Elegant 5-star business hotel featuring the Hiltonia Club a luxurious haven for relaxation, recreation and exercise. The Hiltonia Club is staffed by qualified instructors, trainers and coaches. A full time receptionist can arrange appointments with on-call doctor and dietician for medical consultation. Qualified beauticians offer aromatherapy, body and facial massage and a series of beauty treatments.

LEMESOS (Limassol)
⟩ 05
✈ Larnaca Int'l Airport (LCA) 38 mi. / 60 km.

Four Seasons Hotel
❤❤❤❤❤

PO Box 7222, Lemessos. Tel: (5) 310222. Fax: (5) 310887. TYPE: Resort Hotel & Spa. LOCATION: On the beachfront with panoramic seaview. SPA CLIENTELE: Women and men.

* Rooms & Suites: 310
* Phone, CTV, A/C, minibar, hairdryer
* Restaurant (3), bars (4), gift shop, shopping Arcade Tennis Courts (2), Squash courts (2)
* Airport: Larnaca, taxi
* Reservations: required
* Credit Cards: VISA/AMEX/MC/DIS/EC
* Open: Year round
* TAC: 10%
* Spa on premises: **Thalassotherapie Spa**
* **Spa Facilities**: Spa, jacuzzi, sauna, gym
* **Spa Programs**: Thalassotherapy, beauty, pampering
* **Spa Treatments**: sea-water, mud wraps and beauty treatments

DESCRIPTION: Luxury beach resort with Thalassotherapy Center. Recreation: water sports, snooker room and games room. For families with children there is a supervised Kindergarten and a Children's pool with water slide.

PAPHOS
⟩ 06
✈ Paphos Airport (PFO) 4.5 mi. / 7 km.

Paphos, population 9,500, is a picturesque beach resort town in western Cyprus. Once the Roman capital of Cyprus, it rich in historical remains. According to Greek Mythology Paphos is where Aphrodite, the Greek goddess of love and beauty, is said to have risen from the waves that crash on its shores.

Coral Beach Hotel & Resort
❤❤❤❤❤

Coral Bay, PO Box 2422, 8099 Paphos. Tel: (6) 621601. Fax: (6) 621742. TYPE: Resort Hotel & Spa. LOCATION: Beachfront in lush gardens and over 300 m. / yards of natural sandy beach. SPA CLIENTELE: Women & men.

* Rooms: 304 w/priv. bath, Suites: 66
* Phone, CTV, A/C, minibar, hairdryer
* Restaurants (5), bars/lounges (4)
* Reservations: required
* Credit Cards: VISA/AMEX/MC/DIS/EC
* Open: Year round
* Hotel Rates: from C£72
* TAC: 10%
* Spa on premises
* **Spa Facilities**: indoor heated pool, whirlpool, state of the art gym, aerobics studios, computerized fitness assessment treatment rooms
* **Spa Programs**: Anti-Stress & Relaxation, Rejuvenating & Re-energizing, Body toning & firming
* **Spa Treatments**: beauty and body treatments, reflexology, aromatherapy, massages
* **Spa Packages**: flexible and designed to fit in with your own vacation plans
* **Indications**: stress, sports injuries, cervical and lumber problems

DESCRIPTION: A Mediterranean Oasis with an idyllic setting on a beautiful beach yet close to the mountains. The Coral Beach Hotel & Resort offers superbly appointed rooms, garden suites and studio suites, all furnished and equipped to the highest standards. The Coral Beach Health & Beauty Spa is the most up to date and extensive resort spa in Cyprus, blending fitness and exercise, indulgent beauty and body treatments, including reflexology and aromatherapy. Recreation: water sports, Art & Crafts Workshop, international theme nights.

Paphos Amathus Beach Hotel
❤❤❤❤❤

Poseidon Ave., PO Box 2381, 8098 Paphos. Tel: (6) 264300. Fax: (6) 264222. TYPE: Resort Hotel. LOCATION: On the seashore just 2 km. / 1 mi. from Paphos' fishing harbor. DESCRIPTION: Elegant resort with 257 rooms, 21suites, restaurants (3), cocktail lounge, bars (3), free-form swimming pool. Health & Leisure Center includes gym, sauna, steam bath, solarium and health bar. Treatments at the Spa include: hydromassage, body massage and pampering. Recreation: tennis, squash, golf.

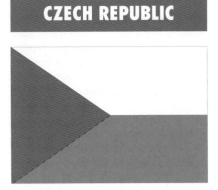

CZECH REPUBLIC

AREA: 30,449 sq. mi. (78,864 sq. km.)
POPULATION: 10,450,000
CAPITAL: Prague
OFFICIAL LANGUAGES: Czech
CURRENCY: Koruna (CSK)
EXCHANGE RATE: 1 US$ = CSK 28
TELEPHONE COUNTRY CODE: 420

The history of Czech Spas dates back to Roman times when they were discovered by Marcus Aurelius and his legions. There are several spas in the Czech Republic with health restoring mineral springs, some with a unique chemical composition that makes them famous and attract thousands of spa goers from all over the world. Most of the Spas are concentrated in the western region of the Czech Republic, in and around **Karlovy Vary**, the largest and the best-known Czech Spa with its unique thermal springs.

FRANTISKOVY LAZNE
166
✈ Karlovy Vary Airport 58 miles / 97 km.

Frantiskovy Lazne (Franzenbad), situated in the westernmost corner of the Czech Republic, is the oldest of the four West Bohemian spas. Its position on a upland plain is ideal; endowing it with a pleasant climate of warm summers, temperate autumns and springs, and mild winters. Its climate and clean air free of dust and smoke is due to its forest setting and long distance from industrial areas. Treatment at Frantiskovy Lazne is based mainly on the rich sources of mineral waters, ferrous sulfide peat, and gas.

Nature has provided Franzenbad with over 24 springs of hydrocaronate-sodium-calcium composition, 12 of which are used for baths, drinking cures and irrigations. Natural carbonic baths are the chief therapeutic procedure. Frantiskovy Lazne has been known for its success in treating gynecological disorders. It also treats cardio-vascular disorders. There is also a unique children's sanatorium.

Today, Frantiskovy Lazne with its classical architecture is a protected cultural reservation. Colonade concerts, plays, operas and operettas with prominent domestic and international artists are held in the town. There are many opportunities for brief excursions or short walks. Either choice will reward you with scenic beauty, historical discovery, or simple harmony with nature. The historic town of Cheb is just 3 miles (5 km.) away and Marianske Lazne is 10 miles (17 km.) away. Tours are available to each town.

Imperial Hotel
❤❤❤

Spa Sanatory Imperial, Sady Bedricha Smetany, 351 01 Rantiskovy Lazne. Tel: (166) 542971-3, fax: (166) 542973. TYPE: Hotel and Spa Sanatorium. LOCATION: Garden of the spa quarter. SPA CLIENTELE: Men, Women.

* Rooms: singles & double w/private bath
* Restaurant, bar
* Airport: Karlovy Vary, taxi, bus
* Open: Year round
* Rates: on request
* Treatment duration: 14 - 21 days
* Spa on premises
* **Spa Facilities**: Indoor swimming pools, latest balneotherapeutic equipment, sauna, gymnasium, consulting rooms, varied sports facilities
* **Spa Programs**: Rejuvenation, relaxation, general fitness, medical
* **Spa Treatments**: Carbon dioxide baths, bubble, mud and spring gas baths, mud packs & vaginal tamponade, inhalation therapy, subcutaneous injection of mineral spring gas, electrotherapy, hydrotherapy, reflex massages, exercises, acupuncture, diet, Gerovital H3
* Indications: Cardio-vascular disorders, heart valve,

defects, ischematic heart disease, post myocardial infarction; hypertension disorders, myocarditis, artherosclerosis, conditions after thrombosis and thrombophlebitis, primary and secondary sterility, infertility, ovarian function and inflammatory ailments, menopausal syndrome
* Medical Supervision: doctors examinations and laboratory tests
* Treatments Approved: Czech Spas and Mineral Springs, Balnea

DESCRIPTION: A modernized, classical hotel and sanatorium.

Reservations for all spa houses through town's spa management: **Lazne Frantiskovy Lazne a.s.**, Jiraskova 17, 35101 Frantiskovy Laazne, Czech Republic. Tel: (166) 542225. Fax: (166) 542970.

JACHYMOV
➐ **164**

✈ Karlovy Vary Airport, 24 miles (40 km.)

Jachymov, situated in the wooded northern area of the Czech Republic near Karlovy Vary, became famous in 1906 for the establishment of the first radioactive spa in the world. Jachymov is a popular winter resort with a 1,630 m. / 5,380 ft. long cable lift running from the town to the peak of the Ore Mountains Klinovec. Excursions can be arranged to Bozi Dar and its peat bogs. Located 1020 meters above sea level, the town has the highest altitude in Central Europe. The spring waters of the Spa are composed of saline-alkaline mineral water with natural radon and such rare elements as molbdenum, titanium and baryllium. The springs have been used for treatment for over 75 years. Their effect is based on the favorable influence of repeated small doses of alpha radiation on the human organism.

Indications: diseases of the motor apparatus and certain nervous disorders are treated. The basic therapeutic agents used are the thermal springs and their natural radioactivity.

Akademik Behounek
❤❤❤

362 51 Jachymov. Tel: (164) 831111, fax: (164) 911444. TYPE: Hotel and Spa Sanatorium. LOCATION: On a slope overlooking the center of town. SPA CLIENTELE: Women and men.

* Rooms: singles & double w/private bath
* Restaurant, bar
* Airport: Karlovy Vary, taxi, bus
* Reservations: required
* Open: Year round
* Rates: on request
* Spa on premises
* **Spa Facilities**: Indoor swimming pools, latest balneotherapeutic equipment, sauna, gymnasium, consulting rooms, sports facilities
* **Spa Programs**: Rejuvenation, relaxation, general fitness, medical
* **Spa Treatments**: Radon and galvanic baths, electrotherapy, hydrotherapy, classical and reflex massages, remedial exercises, acupuncture, diet, x-ray therapy, radium therapy, Gerovital H3
* Treatment duration: 14-21 days
* **Indications**: Rheumatic disease (progressive polyarthritis, Bechterev's diseases), arthrosis, vertebral disc syndrome, diseases of the muscles, tendons and ligaments, conditions following injury to the joints and surgery, neuralgia especially with radicular syndrome and polyneuropathy
* Medical Supervision: doctors examinations and laboratory tests
* Treatments Approved: Czech Spas and Mineral Springs, Balnea

DESCRIPTION: A modern hotel and sanatorium equipped with diagnostic and laboratory facilities to assure integrity of all procedures and the monitoring of the patient's progress.

Spa Sanatory Radium Palace
❤❤❤

T.G. Masaryka 413, 362 51 Jachymov. Tel: (164) 811511. Fax: (164) 831743. TYPE: Hotel & Spa Sanatorium. LOCATION: Overlooking the center of town. SPA CLIENTELE: Women & men. DESCRIPTION: Spa sanatorium.

Reservations for all spa houses through town's spa management: **Lecebne Lazne Jachymov a.s.**, 362 51 Jachymov, Czech Republic. Tel: (164) 911208; Fax: (164) 911730.

KARLOVY VARY
) **17**
✈ Karlovy Vary Airport

Karlovy Vary (Carlsbad), the largest and best known Czech spa, has long been a favorite retreat for kings, writers and musicians. The Spa is situated along the Tepla River in the forested West Bohemian hills. There are 12 major springs at Karlovy Vary with a hydrocarbonate-sulfate-chloride-sodium composition. The oldest and warmest spring is Vridlo with a temperature of 160°F (71°c) and an emission of 2000 liters per minute. Each spring can benefit the particular patient as prescribed by the physician.

Bristol Spa Hotel
❤❤❤

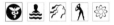

19 Sadova St., Karlovy Vary 36098. Tel: (17) 3113111. Fax: (17) 3226683. TYPE: Superior First Class Spa Hotel. LOCATION: In the Spa Quarter. CLIENTELE: Men & Women.

* Rooms: 127 with full bath
* Phone, CTV, radio, refrigerator
* Restaurant, bar
* Season: Year round
* Rates: from $75 per day based on doubled occupancy and include accommodations, full board, daily treatments except Sundays with complete physical
* Length of Stay Required: 14 - 28 days
* SPA on premises
* **SPA Facilities**: All services under one roof, modern treatment center with constant medical service, beauty and cosmetic salon.
* **SPA Treatments**: Classical, reflex and underwater massage, baths, Scotch showers, electro-procedures, acupuncture, acupressure, exercise therapy, sauna and thermal swimming pool
* **Indications**: Gastric, intestinal and metabolic disorders,

and allergies as the result of digestive diseases

DESCRIPTION: Quality spa hotel in the Spa district area. Walk to thermal springs and casino.

Elwa Sanatorium
❤❤❤❤

🗿 ♨

Zahradní 29, 360 21 Karlovy Vary. Tel: (17) 3228472-5, Fax: (17) 3228473. TYPE: First Class Spa Hotel. LOCATION: In the valley of the river Teplá. SPA CLIENTELE: Women and men, family oriented. MEDICAL RESTRICTIONS: Treatment of disorders of the metabolism and gastric diseases only.

* Rooms: 17 w/priv. bath. Suites 2. Apartments 5
* Phone, CTV, C/H, minibar
* Restaurant, bar
* Airport: Prague 120 km. / 75 mi.
* Train Station: Karlovy Vary
* Reservations: Required
* Credit Cards: MC, VISA, AMEX
* Open: Year round
* Rates: on request; TAC: 10%
* Spa on premises
* **Spa Facilities**: Latest equipment for health procedures and facilities for fitness and relaxation
* **Spa Programs**: Medical, fitness
* **Spa Packages**: on request
* **Spa Treatments**: hydrotherapy, thermal waters, carbonic waters, alkaline waters and saline waters
* **Indications**: Disorders of the digestive system, metabolic disorders, disorders of the the endocrine glands
* Medical Supervision: 2 MD, 11 RN
* Length of Stay Required: 14 - 28 days

DESCRIPTION: Elwa is a traditional spa hotel.

Grandhotel Pupp
❤❤❤

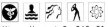

Mirove Namesti 2, 360 91 Karlovy Vary. Tel: (17) 3109111, Fax: (17) 3224032. TYPE: Hotel & Spa. LOCA-

TION: In Spa Quarter. SPA CLIENTELE: Women and men. DESCRIPTION: First class spa hotel, 265 rooms, 15 suites, restaurants, outdoor cafe, bar. Hotel rates: from CZK 4000.

Hotel Dvorak
❤❤❤❤

🗿 ♨ 🎐 🚶 ❀

Nova Louka 11, Karlovy Vary 36021. Tel: (17) 3224145, Fax: (17) 3222814. USA/Canada Reservation: (800) 257-5344. Fax: (516) 944-7540. TYPE: Elegant Spa Hotel. LOCATION: Downtown in the Spa district area. CLIENTELE: Women and men.

* Rooms: 77, Suites: 3 all w/priv. bath
* Phone, CTV, A/C, radio, minibar, hairdryer
* Restaurant, piano bar, Opera Café
* boutique, laundry, parking, tennis
* Free admission to the nearby Casino
* Open: Year round
* Hotel Rates: from $110/day; TAC: 10%
* Spa on premises: Treatment Center
* **Spa Facilities**: Latest equipment for medical procedures, indoor pool, sauna, beauty salon,
* **Spa Treatments**: massages, physiotherapy, Dr, F.X. Mayr regenerative treatments, Karlovy Vary mineral water cure, balneotherapy, bubbling-water and carbon-dioxide baths, Multiplex - Geriatric treatments, Oxygen therapy, movement therapy, electrotherapy, beauty treatments,fitness work-outs, massages: classical, reflex, underwater
* **Spa Packages**: Complex Therapy; F.X. Mayr treatments; Oxygen Therapy; Multiplex Geriatric Treatment; Treatments for the Locomotive System, Beauty Treatments, Relaxation treatments. Packages are from 1-3 weeks and start at about $1,200/week
* **Indications**: Gastric, intestinal and metabolic disorders, allergies as the result of digestive diseases, rejuvenation, well-being
* Medical Supervision: medical specialists

DESCRIPTION: Superior first class Spa hotel within walking distance of Karlsbad Springs. All rooms are air-conditioned with private bath. The hotel is equipped with its own treatment center. Treatments and dietary programs are tailored to the individual needs of the patient. The Treatment Center specializes in regenerative treatment program devised by Dr. F.X. Mayr and complex therapy program in which primarily digestive and metabolic problems are treated with Karlovy Vary mineral water cures.

Spa Hotel Imperial
♥♥♥

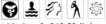

Libuina 18, 361 21 Karlovy Vary. Tel: (17) 3227541. Fax: (17) 3225647. TYPE: Hotel & Spa. LOCATION: In Spa Quarter. SPA CLIENTELE: Women and men. DESCRIPTION: First class spa hotel, restaurant, sauna. Hotel rates: from CZK 4000.

Spa Hotel Central
♥♥♥

Divadelní námìstí 17, 360 68 Karlovy Vary. Tel: (17) 3182111. Fax: (17) 3229086. TYPE: Hotel & Spa. LOCATION: In Spa Quarter. SPA CLIENTELE: Women and men. DESCRIPTION: First class spa hotel, restaurant, sauna. Hotel rates: from CZK 4000.

Spa Hotel Sirius
♥♥♥

Zahradní 3, 360 01 Karlovy Vary. Tel: (17) 3222310, Fax: (17) 3223469. TYPE: Hotel & Spa. LOCATION: In Spa Quarter. SPA CLIENTELE: Women and men. DESCRIPTION: First class spa hotel, restaurant, sauna. Hotel rates: from CZK 4000.

Spa Hotel Kolonáda
♥♥♥

I.P.Pavlova 8, 360 01 Karlovy Vary. Tel: (17) 3131111, Fax: (17) 3222670. TYPE: Hotel & Spa. LOCATION: In Spa Quarter. SPA CLIENTELE: Women and men. DESCRIPTION: First class spa hotel, restaurant, sauna. Hotel rates: from CZK 4000.

At the Karlovy Vary, reservation can be made directly with each hotel, or through your travel agent.

LAZNE BEOHRAD
Ƨ 434

 Ruzyne Airport (PRG) 63 mi. / 100 km.

Lazne Belohrad (White Castle Spa), is a little town set in a picturesque environment at the foot of the Krkonose Mts. The town is surrounded by pine forests, at 300 m. / 1000 ft. above sea level. The climate is mild and the air is pollution free. The Spa was founded in 1885 by the Prussian duchess Anna von Asseburg and was named "Anenske slatinne lazne" (Ann's peat spa). The spa is a sulphide peat spa known for the healing effect of the local peat (mud) and its climate.

Indication: disorders of the motoric system - rheumatism, disorders of the spine, Bechterew's disease, arthrose, states following orthopedic surgery or injury, sciatica, weak forms of peripheral paralysis, disorders of peripheral arteries, painful syndromes of tendons, subskin tissue, fat and skeleton muscles; skin disorders - treatment of injury or burn deforming scars. Also available: beauty and weight loss programs.

Ann's Peat Spa
♥♥♥♥

Annenske Slatinne Lazne, Lazenska 165, 50781 Lazne Belohrad. Tel: (434) 667111. Fax: (434) 667443. TYPE: Health Spa. SPA DIRECTOR: Ing. Radim Kalfus. LOCATION: Central location in the spa area. SPA CLIENTELE: Women and men.

* Rooms: at the three hotels in the Spa Complex Grand Hotel, Hotel Janecek, Hotel Anne-Marie
* Reservations: required
* Open: Year round
* SPA on premises
* **SPA Facilities:**
* **SPA Programs:** Medical, Beauty, Weight Loss
* **Spa Treatments:** thermotherapy, peat pack, peat baths, paraffin packs, hydrotherapy, water massages, Hubbard bath, physiotherapeutic pool, electrotherapy, magnetotherapy, diathermy, laser, infra-red radiations, ultrasound, physiotherapy,

classical and reflex massages, manipulation treatment, gas injection, acupuncture, hippotherapy for children, climatic treatments, health food, natural curative source.

* **Spa Packages**: Medical, Weight Loss, Beauty
* **Indications**: see Lazne Belohrad
* Medical Supervision: medical staff

DESCRIPTION: Health spa with 100 years of spa tradition. Accommodations are offered in a three hotels on the complex. The new spa hotel Anne Marie offer rooms and apartments with shower, toilet, phone and CTV. The hotel has a pleasant bar with terrace. The spa specializes in Peat (mud) treatments for chronic ailments, but also features programs for weight loss and beauty.

LUHACOVICE
˩ 67
✈ Ruzyne Airport (PRG)

Hotel Adamantino
❤❤❤

Pozlovice 337, 763 26 Luhaèovice. Tel: (67) 7131082. TYPE: Spa Hotel. CLIENTELE: Women and men.

Hotel Zalesi
❤❤❤

Zatloukalova alej 858, 763 26 Luhaèovice. Tel: (67) 9319067. Fax: (67) 932935. TYPE: Health Spa. SPA CLIENTELE: Women and men.

Sanatorium Palace
Spa house Morava
Spa house Bedricha Smetany
❤❤❤

Reservation: Lazne Luhacovice, a.s., Lazenske nam. 436, 763 26 Luhacovice. Tel: (67) 9311. Fax: (67) 933214. Reservation: Directly with hotels or your travel agent.

MARIANSKE LAZNE
˩ 165
✈ Marianske Lazne Airport

Marianske Lazne (Marienbad), "Pearl Among the Czech Spas", is the youngest and second largest of the West Bohemia spas. There are about 140 mineral springs in and around the spa, but only 39 are used for healing purposes. The springs are cold and considerably carbonated composed of hydrocarbonate-calcareous-saline-ferrous acidulous and hydrocarbonate-sulfate-saline waters. Spa treatments include: drinking cure, heat and physical therapy, and diet.

Hotel Excelsior
❤❤❤

Hlavní 121, 353 01 Marianske Lazne. Tel: (165) 622705, 622706. Fax: (165) 625346. CLIENTELE: Women and men.

Spa hotel Centralni lazne
❤❤❤

Goethovo nam. 1, 35353 Marianske Lazne. Tel: (165) 635080 (Under management of Lecebne lazne Marianske Lazne Bohemia, Hlavní tøída 100, 353 01 Marianske Lazne. Tel: (165) 623251, 623252, Fax: (165) 622753. TYPE: Spa Hotel. CLIENTELE: Women and men.

Spa Hotel Hvizda
❤❤❤

Goethovo nan. 7, 353 52 Marianske Lazne. Tel: (165) 631114. TYPE: Hotel & Spa Sanatorium. LOCATION: Near town center. SPA CLIENTELE: Women and men.

* Rooms: w/private bath
* Restaurant & bar
* Airport: Karlovy Vary, 48 miles (80 km.) limo, bus
* Reservations: required
* Open: Year round
* Hotel Rates: from CZK 4000
* Spa off premises: nearby

* **Spa Facilities**: indoor pool, latest balneotherapeutic equipment, sauna, solarium, gym, consulting rooms, sports facilities
* **Spa Programs**: Rejuvenation, relaxation, general fitness, diet, medical
* **Spa Treatments**: Carbon dioxide baths & subcutan injections, mineral water baths, hydrotherapy, heat therapy w/ mud packs, compresses, electrotherapy, inhalation, physical therapy,reflex massage, remedial exercise, medication, drinking cures, Gerovital H3
* Treatment Duration: 2 - 3 weeks
* **Indications**: Bronchitis, asthma allergies of respiratory tract; kidney and urinary tract ailments; neurological and metabolic diseases
* Medical Supervision: doctor examinations and laboratory tests
* Treatment Approval: Czech Spas and Mineral Springs, Balnea

DESCRIPTION: A gracious modernized spa.

Spa Hotel Palace
♥♥♥

Hlavní 67, 353 01 Marianske Lazne. Tel: (165) 622222. Fax: (165) 624262. TYPE: Spa Hotel. CLIENTELE: Women and men.

Spa Hotel Royal
♥♥♥

Lesní 345, 353 01 Marianske Lazne. Tel: (165)625446 - 8. Fax: (165) 622346. TYPE: Spa Hotel. LOCATION: 1/2 mi / 800 m north of town center in a natural forest park. CLIENTELE: Women and men. DESCRIPTION: 30 rooms, French restaurant, indoor pool, gym, sauna, complete Spa treatments. (Under management of Lecebne lazne Marianske Lazne).

At the **Marianske Lazne**, reservations can be made directly with the hotels, through your travel agent, or through spa management office: **Lecebne lazne Marianske Lazne**, Masarykova 22, 353 29 Marianske Lazne, Czech Republic. Tel: (165) 655550. Fax: (165) 655500. Spa management office manage 6 spa houses: Hvezda; Labe; Pacifik; Centralni lazne; Svoboda; Vltava.

PODEBRADY
🦢 **324**

✈ Ruzyne Airport (PRG)

Hotel Bellevue Tlapak
♥♥♥

Nam T. G. Masaryka 654/III, 290 01 Podebrady. Tel: (324) 5900. Fax: (324) 4584. TYPE Spa Hotel. CLIENTELE: Women & men. There is a Balneo Centre at the hotel.

Spa Hotel Libensky
♥♥♥

Nam. T.G. Masaryka 637/III, 290 01 Podebrady. Tel: (324) 2664 - 5. Fax: (324) 2664. TYPE: Spa Hotel. CLIENTELE: Women & men. There is a Balneo Centre at the hotel

TREBON
🦢 **333**

✈ Ruzyne Airport (PRG)

Spa Sanatory Aurora
♥♥♥

379 01 Trebon. Tel: (333) 724711. Fax: (333) 724710. Reservation: **Statni lecebne lazne**, s.p. 379 13 Trebon, Czech Republic. Tel: (333) 724711. Fax: (333) 724710.

DOMINICAN REPUBLIC

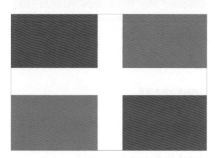

AREA: 19,120 sq. mi. (49,520 sq. km.)
POPULATION: 6,290,000
CAPITAL: Santo Domingo
OFFICIAL LANGUAGE: Spanish
CURRENCY: Dominican peso (DOM$)
EXCHANGE RATE: 1 US$ = DOM$13.30
TELEPHONE COUNTRY CODE: 809

The Dominican Republic is a tropical show case in the Caribbean. This island country is the oldest settlement in the western hemisphere where tourists can find interesting historical buildings, restored quarters, museums and churches. The island offers sunny beaches, natural streams, and lush tropical forests. The island is big enough to offer fine golf courses, tennis courts, scuba and water sports facilities.

LA ROMANA
⟩ No area code
✈ Las Americas Int'l AP (SDQ)

La Romana, is a beach resort near the famous Boca Chica beach, some 25 km. / 16 mi. east of Santo Domingo. An international artist villa in mock-Italian style has been established nearby and is worth a visit. La Romana can be reached by air or bus.

Casa de Campo
♥♥♥♥♥

P.O. Box 140, La Romana. Tel: (809) 523-3333. Fax:

(809) 523-8548. TYPE: Resort Complex & Spa. LOCATION: Along the southeast coast. SPA CLIENTELE: Women and men. DESCRIPTION: A large self-contained 7000-acre resort complex with an ambience created by Oscar de la Renta. Health club with outdoor pool, sauna and gym. Recreation: tennis, golf, water sports, deep-sea fishing.

SAN JOSÉ DE LAS MATAS
⟩ No area code
✈ Las Americas Int'l AP (SDQ)

Hotel Club Spa La Mansion
♥♥♥♥

Parque Turistico Los Pinos, San José de Las Matas 1546. Tel: (809) 581-0393. Fax: (809) 532-4494. TYPE: Mountain Retreat & Spa. LOCATION: Surrounded by hills and pine trees, 30 km. / 19 mi. from Santiago. SPA CLIENTELE: Women and men. DESCRIPTION: First class mountain retreat, 64 rooms, restaurants, bar, outdoor pool, gym, sauna. Hotel Rates: from US$100/day.

SANTO DOMINGO
⟩ No area code
✈ Las Americas Int'l AP (SDQ) 18 mi. / 29 km.

Santo Domingo, with population of over 1,600,000, is a chief seaport and the bustling capital of the Dominican Republic. Santo Domingo was founded in 1496 by Columbus' brother and is the oldest settled city in the western hemisphere which explains the richness of its historic buildings, churches, monuments and traditions.

Renaissance Jaragua Hotel & Casino
♥♥♥♥♥

Avenida George Washington No. 367, Santo Domingo. Tel: (809) 221-2222. Fax: (809) 686-0528. TYPE: Deluxe Hotel, Casino & European Spa. LOCATION: Waterfront location in the heart of the city. SPA CLIENTELE: Women and men.

* Rooms: 310 w/private bath. Suites: 8

* Phone, CTV, A/C, private balcony with sea view
* Restaurants (5), bar, casino, cabana club
* 24 hrs. room service & Valet Service
* Airport: 15 km. / 10 mi., taxi, limo
* Reservations: suggested
* Credit Cards: VISA/AMEX/DC
* Open: Year round
* Hotel Rates: from $150/day
* TAC: 10%
* Spa on premises
* **Spa Facilities**: swimming pools (2), saunas, Turkish Baths, fully equipped gym, Fitness center, whirlpool, Beauty Salon
* **Spa Programs**: fitness, beauty
* **Spa Treatments**: massages, facials, loofa, herbal wraps, sauna, Turkish bath, hot-cold showers, exercise, aerobics, European beauty treatments, salt glo

DESCRIPTION: A World Class Hotel Casino and European Spa in the tropical setting of Santo Domingo. The hotel features deluxe rooms, fine service, choice of gourmet restaurants, nightly entertainment, and a spa for body pampering, exercising or relaxation. Recreation: casino, tennis, golf, sight seeing, and beaches.

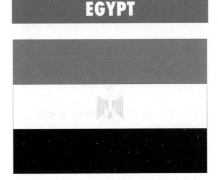

AREA: 386,659 sq. mi. (1,001,447 sq. km.)
POPULATION: 53,080,000
CAPITAL: Cairo
OFFICIAL LANGUAGE: Arabic
CURRENCY: Egyptian Pound (E£)
CURRENCY EXCHANGE: 1US$ = E£ 3.40
TELEPHONE COUNTRY CODE: 20

Egypt attracts millions of visitors to its fascinating historical sites, Pharaonic treasures and monuments. Yet, there are a few sulfur springs in different parts of the country, but they have not been developed as health resorts to provide adequate amenities for Spa cure or recreation.

Helwan, about 15 mi. (24 km.) south of Cairo is the only Spa town that has developed around the town's six hot sulfur springs, but heavy industrialization makes it rather unattractive for international Spa travelers.

The only internationally recommended Spa in Egypt is located at the five star Hotel Aswan Oberoi in Aswan. It is a charming desert winter oasis some 600 mi. (960 km.) south of Cairo. Aswan is a perfect location to combine health vacation and explore the magnificent sites of the Pharaonic era. Other desert Oases famed for their therapeutic tourism include: Fayoum, Kharga, Dakhla, Farafrah, Bahereya and Siwa.

ASWAN
☎ **97**
✈ Daraw Airport (ASW) 25 mi. / 40 km.

Aswan, population 50,000, is one of the most exciting destinations in Egypt. Most tourists stay in Aswan on their way to visit the magnificent ancient monuments of Abu Simbel, but the town is a wonderful winter resort with an excellent climate for those who suffer from asthma or skin diseases. However, summers can be extremely hot with temperatures topping 104°F (40°c).

Hotel Aswan Oberoi Hotel & Spa
❤❤❤❤❤

P.O. Box 62, Aswan, Egypt. Tel: (97) 314666. Fax: (97) 313538. TYPE: Deluxe Resort Complex & Spa. MANAGER: Kripa Shankar, GM. LOCATION: On the Elphantine Island in the middle of the River Nile, 100 yards away from downtown. SPA CLIENTELE: Men, Women.

* Rooms: 180; 96 w/priv. bath. Suites: 54
* Cottages: 10
* Phone, CTV, A/C
* Private balcony with view of the Nile
* Private Gardens, restaurants, Bar, Night Club
* 24 hrs. room service & Valet Service
* Airport: Aswan Airport 17 km. / 10 mi. taxi
* Reservations: 25% deposit required
* Credit Cards: MC/VISA/AMEX/DC
* Season: Year round
* Hotel Rates: $95 - $485/day
* TAC: 10%
* Spa on premises
* **Spa Facilities**: Whirlpools, sauna, steam baths, gym, large swimming pool, solar heated outdoor swimming pool, jogging trails, 'sand pit'
* **Spa Programs**: health & fitness, beauty
* **Spa Treatments**: steam/sand baths, body massage, short wave treatments, special exercises for the lungs, special diets with calculated calories, loofa bath & massage with herbal soap and cream
* Medical Supervision: MD for check ups
* **Indications**: diseases of the bones, joints,

rheumatic diseases, stiff joints, allergic diseases, bronchial asthma, skin diseases, obesity, convalescence, post operative, vascular diseases and varicose veins
* Medical Supervision: 2 MD, 1 RN
* Number of Customers per Dr.: 1-7
* Treatments Approved: Egyptian Medical Assoc.

DESCRIPTION: Hotel Aswan Oberoi, secluded among the gardens of the Elphantine Island, offers a unique spa program based on Aswan's dry air with a high ozone content, and hot sand enriched with iron content. The spa food is completely natural and farmed without the use of fertilizers, or chemical additives. Spa program are offered to hotel guests who wish to relax, shed a few pounds and keep healthy. Some of the spa treatments are medically oriented and bring relief to certain form of ailments. Recreation: tennis and sailing. Member: *The Leading Hotels of The World.*

HURGHADA
〉 65

✈ Hurghada Airport

Hurghada is a resort town on the Red Sea. El Gouna is nestled between the majestic red mountains of the Eastern Desert and the crystal clear waters of the Red Sea, 22 km. / 14 mi. north of Hurghada.

Dawar El Omda
❤❤❤❤

Kafr El Gouna, El Gouna Resort, Red Sea. Tel: (65) 545060. Fax: (65) 545061. TYPE: Resort Hotel & Spa. LOCATION: Red sea Resort area near Hurghada. SPA CLIENTELE: Women and men. DESCRIPTION: Elegant resort hotel, 52 rooms, 6 suites, restaurant, bar, disco, swimming pool, beauty farm, solarium, massages. Amusement park and casino are under construction. Hotel Rates: from US$44.

FINLAND

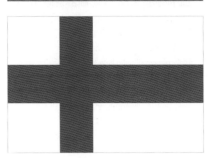

AREA: 130,128 sq. mi. (337,032 sq. km.)
POPULATION: 4,973,000
CAPITAL: Helsinki
OFFICIAL LANGUAGE: Finnish, Swedish
CURRENCY: Marka (FM)
EXCHANGE RATE: 1 US$ = FM 5.19
TELEPHONE COUNTRY CODE: 358

Finland is famous for its arctic health Spas. Many visitors come to Finland each year from to enjoy the full range of health spas and resorts that this country has to offer in a pure environment and spectacular surroundings.

Health spas range from the rustic to the most sophisticated. The Sauna which is universally associated with health spas is the most Finnish of all pleasures. In Finland there is one sauna for every 4.5 Finns.

Most Spas in Finland feature a sauna, steam bath, and relaxing pools. Treatments vary according to the location of the spas. Coastal spas offer maritime salt baths and thaslassotherapy, while others may offer mud therapy. Beauty and cosmetic treatments are available too.

ℹ Scandinavian Tourist Board
655 Third Avenue, New York NY 10017
Tel: (212) 949-2333

IKAALINEN
�’ 3
✈ Tampere-Pirkkala Airport (TMP), 55 km. / 35 mi.

Ikaalinen is a rural community on a lake with a Health Spa, casino and summer theatre and ski slopes (winter). Ikaalinen is easy to reach by car or public transportation. The Spa resort is located near the Tampere-Vaasa main road, 5 km. / 3 mi. north of the intersection to Ikaalinen.

Ikaalinen Spa
❤❤❤

Ikaalinen SF-39510. Tel: (3) 451-2100. Fax: (3) 451-2032. TYPE: Spa Resort Hotel. LOCATION: Lakeside in a rural setting. CLIENTELE: Women and men.

* Rooms: 411 w/priv. bath, 4 suites
* Phone, CTV, some w/balcony
* Restaurant, cafeteria, lounges
* Airport: Tampere 55 km. / 35 mi.
* Hotel Rates: from FM 590/day (room only)
* TAC: 10%
* Spa on premises
* **Spa Facilities**: Water park with swimming pools; Health Spa & gym, saunas
* **Spa Programs**: Fitness, Pampering
* **Spa Treatments**: massages, cosmetics

DESCRIPTION: Ikaalinen Spa is mostly a recreational Spa with a Water Park atmosphere. The air and water temperatures are kept at a constant 30°c (86°F). Ski slopes are located nearby during the winter season.

KUUSAMO
�’ 8
✈ Kuusamo Airport

Kuusamo Tropical Spa
❤❤❤

Kylpylantie SF-93600. Tel: (8) 85960. Fax: (8) 852-1909. Fax: (212) 599-0380. TYPE: Tropical Spa Resort Hotel. LOCATION: On the shore of Lake Petajanlami near the Arctic Circle. SPA CLIENTELE: Women and men.

* Rooms: 120 w/priv. bath, 2 suites

* Rooms for allergy sufferers
* Phone, CTV, hair dryer
* Restaurant, bars, outdoor Summer terrace
* Airport: Kuusamo 5 km. / 3 mi.
* Hotel Rates: from FM 650/day (room only)
* TAC: 10%
* Spa on premises
* **Spa Facilities**: Tropical Pool Area, waterfall, saunas, gym, massage rooms, solar grove
* **Spa Programs**: Beauty & Fitness
* **Spa Treatments**: exercise in the pool, water massage, clay pack, aroma massage, facials, relaxation exercise, herbal bath, nutrition lectures

DESCRIPTION: A tropical spa in the middle of the wilderness of the Arctic Circle on a beautiful lake. Perfect for sporting people and nature lovers who enjoy outdoor activities.

LAPLAND
〉 8

✈ Rovaniemi Airport (RVN)

Lapland covers the northern third of Finland, almost all of it is above the Arctic Circle. This is the most beautiful wilderness, where 200,000 reindeer roam its icy landscape. The Land of the Midnight Sun offers 70 straight days of uninterrupted daylight that begin in mid-May. At the end of November the sky gets dark and the Northern Lights illuminates the Arctic landscape.

Spa Hotel Levitunturi
♥♥♥

FIN-99130 Sirkka, Lapland. Tel: (16) 646-301. Fax: (16) 641-434. TYPE: Arctic Spa Resort. LOCATION: Some 100 km. / 63 mi. north of the Arctic Circle. SPA CLIENTELE: Women and men.

* Rooms: 80 family rooms for 4 w/mini-kitchen 37 dbl rooms, 4 suites
* Phone, CTV, hair dryer
* Restaurant, cafeterias, licensed bars
* Airport: Rovaniemi Airport 170 km. / 106 mi.
* Hotel Rates: from FM 650/day (room only)

* TAC: 10%
* Spa on premises
* **Spa Facilities**: Finnish Sauna, Turkish Bath, Main pool & children pool, gym, Beauty Salon
* **Spa Programs**: Health & Beauty
* **Spa Treatments**: Swedish massage, Thalassotherapy, Turbo bath, Acu bed, reflexology, herbal bath, herbal bubble bath, Clarins baths, fango pack, paraffin, facials, make up and other cosmetic treatments

DESCRIPTION: This unique Arctic Spa is the northernmost spa and recreation center in the world. Located at the Levitunturi Hotel, the complex consists of the main hotel building and seven other annexes including the health spa department, all built with solid round Finnish logs. The spa specializes in soothing massages, thalassotherapy and beauty treatments. Recreation: indoor - tennis, badminton, squash, table tennis, golf-simulator, Europe-bowling. Outdoors - hiking, fishing, canoe and boat trips, downhill skiing (31 slopes), cross-country skiing, snowmobile, reindeer sleigh riding, husky-dog safaris.

NAANTALI
〉 2

✈ Turku Airport (TKU), 14 km. / 9 mi.

Naantali is a traditional Spa town in Southwestern Finland near Turku. It is a charming little town by the sea. The town still conserves a whole quarter from the 17th and 18th century. The curative powers of the Spa waters were discovered in 1723 when people began to take the health-giving waters of the spring at Viluluoto under the instructions of professor Elfving.

In 1863 the first Spa building was opened and the the Spa began to flourish at the turn of the century. The tradition was revived again in 1984 with the opening of the new town spa, designed according to the latest European standards.

Naantali Spa is now the largest spa in the Nordic countries. The new Spa center has been planned to be entirely devoted to relaxation, rehabilitation, and holiday enjoyment. "The Waters" are the essential elements in the cures.

Naantali Spa Hotel
♥♥♥

Matkailijantie 2, Naantali SF-21100. Tel: (21) 857-711. Sales Office: (21) 857-740. Fax: (21) 857-791. TYPE: Spa Hotel. LOCATION: Centrally located. CLIENTELE: Women and Men.

* Rooms: 209 w/priv. bath, 6 suites
* Mini-suites: 110 (32 sq. m. / 352 sq. ft.)
* Phone, CTV, hair dryer, some w/balcony
* Restaurant, cafeteria, bars, summer terrace
* Airport: Turku 15 km. / 10 mi.
* Hotel Rates: from FM 610/day (room only)
* TAC: 10%
* Spa on premises
* **Spa Facilities**: Spa department, Finnish sauna, Turkish bath, hot-water Roman pool with jacuzzi, swimming pool, fitness training hall, solariums, laboratory, The Belleza beauty parlor, hairdressing salon
* **Spa Programs**: Beauty, Fitness & Medical
* **Spa Treatments**: water and brush massage, balneotherapy - remedial, galvanic, exchange baths, underwater massage, water gymnastics; physiotherapy - massage, thermal, galvanic and electric; hot natural clay, aromatherapy, manipulation, rehabilitation
* **Spa Packages**: Weekend (3 days) Diet Week (8 days); Spa Holiday (6 days)
* **Indications**: stress, traumatic injuries, muscular maladies, insomnia, obesity, tiredness
* Medical Supervision: specialized doctors, nurses
* Treatments Approved: Bureau of Medicine

DESCRIPTION: The Naantali Spa is devoted to both holiday makers and intensive rehabilitation. The Spa's baths, with their hot Roman pools and cool swimming pools are a true water paradise. A wide range of healing massages, soothing water treatments, fragrant steam baths, and mud baths using the famous Naantali clay will make your spa experience unforgettable. If you need to loose weight the Spa offers a special Diet Week that includes 1000 calories controlled diet, bodytrim, seaweed wrap, and various massages. Light Spa holiday packages are available from 3 days to 2 weeks. Recreation: children activities, sailing, windsurfing, water skiing, fishing, ice-skating rink, skiing, horseback riding, golf, theme parties, excursion programs.

NOKIA
↰ **3**

✈ Tampere - Pirkkala Airport (TMP) 15 mi. / 24 km.

Nokia is a suburb of Tampere, the second largest city in Finland on the banks of the Tammer River.

Nokia Spa Hotel Eden
♥♥♥

Paratiisikatu 2, FIN-37120 Nokia. Tel: (3) 280-1111. Fax: (3) 342-1800. TYPE: Spa Resort Hotel. LOCATION: On the banks of the river golf surrounded by natural forest. CLIENTELE: Women and men, Family oriented.

* Rooms: 109 rooms, 250 beds
* Restaurants, 3 summer terraces
* Airport: Tampere-Pirkkala 15 min.
* Credit Cards: VISA/AMEX/DC/CB/EC
* Open: Year round
* Hotel Rates: from FM 760
* Spa on premises
* **Spa Facilities**: swimming pool, Finnish, Turkish & Roman Irish saunas, fitness studio, beauty parlor, solarium,
* **Spa Programs**: Health, Beauty, Fitness
* **Spa Treatments**: herb bath, water massage, clay treatment, zonetherapy, polariatherapy, aromatherapy, shiatsu, physiotherapy
* **Spa Packages**: Refreshing Break (3 days) Beauty Holiday (2 days); Relaxing Holiday (5 days) à la carte treatments available
* Medical Supervision: yes

DESCRIPTION: Nokia Spa Hotel Eden is a tropical paradise under a huge glass roof covering an area of 1,500 sq.m. (16,500 sq.ft.) with large swimming pool, saunas and whirlpools. The air temperature is kept at a constant 30°c (86°F). Staying overnight at the hotel is reasonable. The price of the room includes unlimited use of the spa, gym and sauna facilities. This is mostly a recreational spa for relaxation and body pampering, but medical rehabilitation treatments are available. Recreation: squash, gym, bowling golf, children's playroom, golf practice course (summer) and cross-country ski tracks (winter).

PORVOO
⟩ 19
✈ Helsinki-Vantaa Int'l Airport (HEL)

Porvoo is a quaint city with an intact town plan from the 18th century. The town's layout gives it a southern European flavor, but the old pastel wooden houses are distinctly Scandinavian. Porvoo is located 31 mi. / 50 km. east of Helsinki.

Haikko Manor Spa
❤❤❤❤

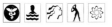

FIN-06400 Porvoo. Tel: (19) 57601. Fax: (19) 576-0399. TYPE: First Class Hotel & Spa. MANAGER: Veikko Vuoristo. SALES MANAGER: Leena Åkerberg. LOCATION: Gulf of Finland, 6 km. / 4 mi. from the town of Porvoo. SPA CLIENTELE: Women and men.

* Rooms: 244 w/priv. bath. Suites: 4
* Phone, CTV, C/H, minibar
* 27 Manor rooms
* Restaurant, bar, nightclub
* Airport: Helsinki-Vantaa 40 km. / 25 mi.
* Train Station: Helsinki 46 km. / 29 mi.
* Airport/Train Station Transfers: limo, taxi
* Credit Cards: VISA/MC/AMEX
* Open: Year round
* Hotel Rates: from FM 750/day (room only)
* TAC: 10%
* Spa on premises
* **Spa Facilities**: Biotherm Studio, indoor and outdoor pools, sauna bath, jogging trails
* **Spa Programs**: Health & Beauty individual and group programs
* **Spa Treatments**: relaxing baths, beauty treatments for men and women, physiotherapy, Heat treatments - clay pack, paraffin pack,

health counselling; Baths - carbonated, galvanic bubble & medical, turbo; Electric; Stretching; Motion - group and individual physiotherapy Facials - Bioenergic, massage, treatments for men; Body Treatments - mechanic lymph, algae, body peeling, anticellulite cure

* **Spa Packages**: several packages are available from one day to one week. Feeling Good (5 days) Stress Releasing (3 days); Beauty Package (2 days) à la carte treatments available
* Medical Supervision: 2 MD, 1 RN
* Maximum number of guests: 400
* Number of clients per doctor: 30
* Documentation required from physician: in case of heart problems specification recommended

DESCRIPTION: Health Spa set on 25 acre estate. Haikko Spa is a Biotherm Spa. The Biotherm cures and products were developed by French physicians to rejuvenate the body and enhances the metabolism of the skin. The resort offers restaurants, nightclub and ski tracks in the winter.

TAMPERE
⟩ 3
✈ Helsinki-Vantaa Int'l Airport (HEL)

Tampere, population 170,000, is the second largest city in Finland on the banks of the Tammer River. There are about 180 lakes within the city limit.

Spa Hotel Tampere
❤❤❤

Lapinniemenranta 12, Tampere SF-33180. Tel: (3) 2597111. Fax: (3) 2597400. TYPE: Spa Hotel. LOCATION: On the shore of lake Nasijärvi, 15 min. walking distance from city center. SPA CLIENTELE: Women and men.

* Rooms: 42 duplex suites w/priv. bath, sauna, microwave, coffee maker, dishwasher
* Phone, CTV, minibar, jacuzzi
* Restaurant, bar
* Airport: Tampere 15 min.
* Season: Year round

* Hotel Rates: from FM 680 (room only);
  Spa package rates on request.
* TAC: 10%
* Spa on premises
* **Spa Facilities**: Fitness room, relaxation room
  with pool, Roman & Finnish saunas,
  Swiss showers
* **Spa Programs**: Health, Fitness, Beauty
* **Spa Treatments**: Hydrotherapy, fango, phyiotherapy,
  Dead Sea & Mineral water baths, ultra sound,
  reflexology, Shiatsu, all massages,
  acupuncture, beauty treatments
* **Indications**: arthritis, rheumatism, gout,
  post-operative recuperation
* Medical Supervision: 1 MD
* Documentation required from physician: no

DESCRIPTION: Spa Hotel housed in an old textile mill on the shore of Lake Näsijärvi near the center of Tampere. This is the only spa in Finland to operate under agreement with the famous "Les Thermes de Spa" from Belgium. Enjoy exercise in the lovely countryside. The Treatment Department offers a wide range of health and beauty treatments. Recreation: ski tracks right at the doorstep.

TURKU

ᔆ 2

✈ Turku Airport (TKU) 4 mi. / 6 km. North

Turku, population 162,000, is an historic seaport and the provincial capital of the province. It is the oldest city of Finland, the home of two universities and a major technology center. The city offers interesting museums, including the famous Turku Art Museum with turn-of-the-century classics and contemporary art; The Botanical Garden at the University of Turku is a showplace of over 5,000 species of aromatic herbs and medicinal plants.

Turku can be reached by flights from Helsinki, Stockholm and Hamburg via SAS, Lufthansa or Finnair flights. There are also good train and bus connections to and from Helsinki.

Health Spa Ruissalo
♥♥♥

Ruissalo Island, Turku SF-20100. Tel: (2) 44540. Fax: (2) 4454590. TYPE: First Class Spa Hotel. LOCATION: In the southwestern part of Ruissalo Island, about 10 km. / 6 mi. from the City of Turku. SPA CLIENTELE: Family oriented.

* Rooms: 132 w/priv. bath
* Phone, CTV, w/sea view
* Restaurant, cafeteria, summer terrace
* Airport: Turku 22 km. / 14 km.
* Credit Cards: VISA/AMEX/DC/CB/EC
* Open: Year round
* Hotel Rates: from FM 610 (room only)
* Spa on premises
* **Spa Facilities**: saunas, pool, solarium, beauty
  parlor, hairdresser salon, laboratory, medical
  rehabilitation & convalescent departments
* **Spa Programs**: medical (at the Sanatorium);
  Fitness, weight loss, beauty, well being at the
  Spa Hotel
* **Spa Packages**: Spa Holiday (7 days)
* **Spa Treatments**: physiotherapy, balneotherapy,
  exercise therapy, treatments for insomnia
* **Indications**: injuries and illnesses of the
  musculo-skeletal system, rheumatic ailments,
  chronic aches and pains, stress, sports
  injuries, weight problems, rehabilitation
* Medical Supervision: yes

DESCRIPTION: Ruissalo Spa is a modern and completely renovated health resort. It offers a variety of rehabilitation, recreational and health holidays. The Sanatorium functions as a medical department for the treatment of injuries and serious medical problems. The Spa Hotel offers fitness, beauty and weight loss programs. Spa treatments and services are available to all without a doctor prescription. Ruissalo Island is a peaceful and scenic island with Old-World charm and atmosphere. The serene surrounding and the beautiful sea views make this place an ideal location for recovery after illness or relaxation.

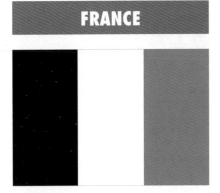

FRANCE

AREA: 210,038 sq. mi. (543,998 sq. km.)
POPULATION: 56,160,000
CAPITAL: Paris
OFFICIAL LANGUAGE: French
CURRENCY: Franc (FF)
EXCHANGE RATE: 1 US$ = FF 5.70
TELEPHONE COUNTRY CODE: 33

France is a favorite destination for Spa enthusiasts thanks to the variety of Spas one can find, the quality of the thermal waters, and the facilities offered. Today, about 40 Spas and health resorts operate in different parts of the country.

The most acclaimed Spas Are: Evian in the French Alps, Deauville in the Normandie coast, Quiberon in Bretagne, and La Baule - a Thalassotherapy Center in southern Brittany (near Nantes).

Traditional spa towns are: Vichy with its famous "Institute de Vichy", and Contrexville in the Vosges which is known for its climactic and thermal spa. For additional information about Spas and spa vacations in France contact:

ℹ️ French Government Tourist Office
444 Madison Ave, New York NY 10022
Tel: (212) 838-7800. Fax: (212) 838-7855

AJJACIO (Corsica Island)
✈ 4
✈ Campo Dell Oro AP (AJA) 5 mi. / 8 km. SE

Best Western Eden Roc
❤❤❤

Rte des Sanguinaires, Ajaccio, Corsica Island F-20000, Tel: (4) 9551-5600, Fax: (4) 9552-0503. TYPE: Hotel & Spa. LOCATION: On spacious landscaped grounds near the sea. DESCRIPTION: Resorts hotel with fitness center, sauna, hammam, jacuzzi, thalassotherapy and gym. 40 rooms, 5 suites, restaurant, bar. Hotel rates: from FF 410.

Sofitel Thalassa Porticcio
❤❤❤❤

Domaine de la Pointe Golfe d'Ajaccio, Porticcio, Corsica Island F-20166. Tel: (4) 9525-0555, Fax: (4) 9525-1170. TYPE: Spa Hotel. LOCATION: In the bay of Ajjacio. SPA CLIENTELE: women and men. DESCRIPTION: Superior first class spa hotel with direct access to Thalassotherapy Center, indoor and outdoor pools, gym, solarium, private beach. 98 rooms, restaurant, bar, lounges, Hotel rates: from FF 630.

ARZON
✈ 2
✈ St. Nazaire Airport
Chateau-Bougon AP (NTE) Nante

Hotel Miramar Port Crouesty
❤❤❤

Port Crouesty, Arzon F-56640, Tel: (2) 9767-6800. Fax: (2) 9767-6899. TYPE: Hotel & Spa. LOCATION: On the lake between the marina and the beach. DESCRIPTION: Modern hotel built like an ocean liner linked to Louison Bobet Seawater Therapy Institute. Hotel rates: from FF 850.

LA BAULE
✈ 2
✈ St. Nazaire Airport
Chateau-Bougon AP (NTE) Nante

La Baule, population 14,000, is a resort town in southern Brittany near Nantes. The resort's major attraction is a long stretch of sandy beach which is 3 miles (5 km.) long. In the resort you will find elegant hotels, fashionable boutiques, gourmet restaurants, tennis courts, and a superb golf course. For entertainment there is an elegant European style casino Beach Casino (Tel: 4060-2023) which operates from May to September and offers various casino table games, nightclub, brasserie, and a shopping center.

La Baule has a unique Thalassotherapy Center - **Thalgo - La Baule**. The center is directly linked to the charming Hôtel Royal and offers a variety of therapeutical and preventive treatments or programs for relaxation, beauty/pampering, and medical purposes.

La Baule can be accessed by air to its Saint-Nazaire airport (15 km./ 10 mi.), or to the Nantes Airport (75 km. / 47 mi.). By train to the La Baule-Escoublac Railway Station, and By car via the Paris-Nantes-La Baule route.

Hotel Royal Thalasso
♥♥♥♥

6 Ave. Pierre Loti, B.P. 17H, F-44504 La Baule. Hotel - Tel: (2) 4011-4848. Fax: (2) 4011-4845. SPA - Tel: (2) 4011-9999. Fax: (2) 4060-5517. MANAGING DIRECTOR: Roland Muntzer. TYPE: Hotel & Thalassotherapy Center. LOCATION: In a private park overlooking the Atlantic. SPA CLIENTELE: Women and men. SPECIAL RESTRICTIONS: Children under 16 not admitted to the Spa.

* Rooms: 100 w/priv. bath; Suites: 6; Apartments: 5
* Phone, CTV, A/C, mini-bar
* Restaurant, bar, nightclub
* Airport: Saint-Nazaire, 15 km. (10 mi.)
* Airport Transportation: taxi
* Credit Cards: AMEX/DC/EC/CB
* Open: Year round
* Hotel Rates: from FF 890 (room only); TAC: 10%
* Spa on premises: **Centre Thalgo La Baule**
* Year established: 1988
* **Spa Facilities**: Seawater Treatment Center, swimming pools for remedial physiotherapy and underwater massage-jets, gym, sauna, hammam, jacuzzi, beauty salon, solarium
* **Spa Programs**: 'Thalgo Beauty', Physicals and Myocardial fitness programs, weight loss, antismoking
* **Spa Treatments**: Thalassotherapy, algotherapy, electrotherapy, reflexology, pressure jet pool/showers, balneotherapy, massages, anti-cellulitis massages, aquagym, seaweed wraps, essential oil baths
* **Spa Packages**: Diamond back to health cure, Thalgo Back, Special Man, Anti Stress, Stop Smoking, Poor Blood & Lymphatic Circulation, Menopause Problems, Cellulite Treatments, Slimming, Thalassotherapy, Dietetics, New Mothers, Back to Heart, Sleep Program. All programs are for 6 days.
* **Indications**: cardio-vascular problems, tobacco addiction, rheumatological disorders, sports related disorders, blood circulation problems, stress, nervous tension, excess body weight, neurovegetative problems, venous problems, sore joints, skin problems, genito-urinary problems, osteoporosis,
* Maximum number of guests: 200
* Number of clients per doctor: 30/35

DESCRIPTION: A Thalassotherapy Center in the impressive sea-front surroundings of the Royal-Thalasso Hotel with a full range of Spa facilities and treatments. The spa specializes in treatments based on sea water and sea products. It also offers a specially developed AQUAMEDIC formula based on the principles of preventive treatments with a special emphasis on cardio-vascular illnesses. Also available a wide range of beauty and pampering treatments for relaxation. Recreation: heated salt water pool, sailing, windsurfing, golf, tennis, riding, 2 yacht harbors, casino.

BIARRITZ
🌙 **5**
✈ Biarritz-Bayonne Anglet AP (BIQ)
2 mi. / 3 km. northwest of Biarritz

Biarritz, population 27,000, is a fashionable year round beach resort full of local colors and authentic Basque folklore. It is located on the Atlantic Ocean in the south west of France near the Spanish border. Besides the fine beaches, the town has a casino, recreational and sports facilities, gourmet restaurants, and a romantic tiny fishing port. Nearby St-Jean-de-Luz is a delightful harbor and a summer resort. Biarritz can be reached by car from Bordeaux via highway A63 south.

Miramar Hotel
❤❤❤❤

13, Rue Louison Bobet, 64200 Biarritz. Tel: (5) 5941-3000. Fax: (5) 5924-7720. TYPE: Deluxe Hotel & Spa. LOCATION: On the beach. SPA CLIENTELE: Women and men.

* Rooms: 126 w/priv. bath. Suites: 17
* Phone, CTV, A/C, wet bars, private balcony
* Restaurants: 2, gourmet and dietetic
* Airport: Biarritz (Parme) 3 km. / 2 mi.
* Train St'n: La Negresse 3 km. / 2 mi.
* Reservations: 2 night deposit
* Credit Cards: MC/VISA/AMEX/DC/CB/DIS/EC
* Season: Year round
* Hotel Rates: from FF 725; TAC: 8%
* Spa on premises
* **Spa Facilities**: Institute of Thalassotherapy "Louison Bobet" (SPA & Fitness Center), seawater heated swimming pool, gym room, sauna, Hammam, solarium, Spa restaurant
* **Spa Programs**: Special Health Package (min. 6 nights), Fitness & Weight Loss
* **Spa Treatments**: hydrotherapy, algotherapy, thalassotherapy, jet showers, under water showers, massages, kinesitherapy, ionisation
* **Indications**: stiffness, impotence due to rheumatic diseases or following injury, fatigue, convalescence, reactional depression
* Medical Supervision: 3 MD, 27 physiotherapists (medical institution)
* Treatments Approved: French Health Ministry

DESCRIPTION: An elegant L-shaped hotel with balcony set back facade on a prime beach location near the famous "Louison Bobet" Institute of Thalasso-therapy. Accommodations consists of spacious and contemporary designed rooms. Two fine restaurants for excellent dining, one specializing in gourmet/ dietetic menus. The Spa specializes in sea water and sea based product treatments and medical cures. Diet and beauty programs are offered at the hotel. Recreation: golf, tennis, water sports and tourism.

CAPVERN-LES-BAINS
〕 5

✈ Lourdes Int'l AP (LDE)

Capvern-les-Bains is a small spa town in the southwest of France near the town of Lourdes which is a pilgrimage destination for many Catholics. Nestled between high mountains, lakes and waterfalls, the spa has a specialized medical center which uses the mineral water to cure kidney, liver, and gallbladder disorders and after effects of tropical illnesses, nutrition troubles, gout, rheumatism, arthosis and associated diseases. Visitors can explore nearby medieval abbeys and absorb the local tradition. Capvern-les-Bains is located 35 km. (22 mi.) from Lourdes and has a local train station.

Hotel Le Laca
❤❤❤

Capvern-les-Bains 65130. Tel: (5) 6239-0206. TYPE: Spa Hotel. LOCATION: Near thermal station. CLIENTELE: Family oriented.

* Rooms: 60 w/priv. bath
* Restaurant & Bar
* Airport: Tarbes-Lourdes, 35 mi. (22 km.)
* Airport Transportation: Hotel shuttle
* Reservations: suggested
* Credit Cards: VISA/AMEX/DC
* Open: May - October
* Hotel Rates: FF 595 day
* Spa on premises
* **Spa Facilities**: Heated indoor swimming pool, solarium, near thermal center
* **Spa Treatments**: At the Thermal Center: medicinal plants, diet, acupuncture, mesotherapy, hydrotherapy, gymnastics, baths, pressotherapy, ionisation, saunas
* **Spa Programs**: Visa Biophytoforme, Visa Minceur (slimming Visa), Visa Bioenergetique (Bioenergetic Visa),

Visa Detente (Relaxing Visa);
all programs are for 3 or 7 days.
* Medical Supervision: 4 paramedics, 11 MD at
  the center

DESCRIPTION: Chalet style hotel near the Thermal Center offering medical cures at the center and diet and beauty programs at the hotel.

CONTREXVILLE
ﬧ 3
✈ Mirecourt-Juvaincourt AP 30 km. (19 mi.) NE

Contrexville, is a small Alsatien village near Vittel in the northeast of France. This is the heart of the verdant Vosge Mountains between Nancy and Basel (Switzerland), a rolling countryside with quaint villages, famous white wine, and distinguished cuisine. Contrexville is a climactic and thermal Spa. The mineral springs gush out naturally and contain: sulphur, calcium and magnesium.

The thermal Establishment in Contrexville specializes in Weight Loss and promises to help individuals to loose weight safely under medical supervision in 10 days and teaches how to keep in shape without weight gain. There are two Thermal Establishments in Contrexeville, one of which The Aquarius operates at the Hotel Cosmos (see description below).

Indications: urinary infections, high cholesterol, high blood pressure, obesity, relaxation, and stress reduction.

Contrexeville can be reached by domestic flights to the Mirecourt-Juvaincourt airport some 30 km. (19 mi.) north-east, or via SNCF trains to the Gare de Contrexville. By car take the A31, Dijon-Metz highway, exit Bulgneville. Contrexeville is located about 320 km. (200 mi.) from Paris.

Hotel Cosmos
♥♥♥

Rue Metz, 88140 Contrexéville (Vosges). Tel: (3) 2908-

1590, 2908-1991. TYPE: Spa Hotel. LOCATION: Near the Casino and Thermal Baths. SPA CLIENTELE: Women and men. SPECIAL RE-STRICTIONS: No Pets.

* Rooms: 70
* Restaurant: low calorie menus
* Airport: Mirecourt-Juvaincourt, 30 km. (16 mi.)
* Airport Transportation: taxi, bus
* Reservations: required
* Credit Cards: VISA/AMEX/DC
* Open: April - September
* Spa on premises
* **Spa Facilities**: Aquarius Thermal Establishment, massage rooms, thermal bath, shower rooms, exercise and aerobic rooms, gymnasium, jogging trails
* **Spa Programs**: Medical, Weight Loss, Fitness
* **Spa Treatments**: massages, underwater massage, thermal showers, jet stream baths, fango mud applications, mineral water drinking cure, low cal diets, exercises, yoga, aerobics
* **Spa Packages**: 10 days SPA Package, rates include: accommodations, 3 meals, 27 treatments, drinking cure, exercise & yoga, dietetic cooking classes, entertainment
* **Indications**: obesity, metabolic problems, high cholesterol, gout, urinary and renal problems, post-operational rehabilitation
* Medical Supervision: Doctors, nurses
* Treatments Approval: Medical Institute

DESCRIPTION: First Class hotel decorated in Classic Old World motives. Excellent elegant restaurant serves gourmet Alsatian cuisine or low calorie menus. There is a thermal establishment in the hotel - The Aquarius offering a variety of medical programs and treatments. A special weight reduction program is available. Recreation: jogging, archery, tennis, biking, afro-jazz dance classes, nature or archeological walks. There is a gambling casino nearby, and some interesting international tourist destinations are within easy reach (Switzerland, and West Germany).

DEAUVILLE
ﬧ 2
✈ Saint Gatien AP (DOL), 4 mi. / 6.5 km. east

Deauville, population 5,700, is a fashionable beach resort on the Côte Fleurie in northwestern France. During the summer it is bustling with many Parisians who come to the beach to escape the heat and crowds of the capital. Deauville is famous for its Grand Prix horse race, and the famous wooden promenade that runs along the beach. There is plenty going on in Deauville during the high season, including exciting night life, world class casino gambling at the newly refurbished Casino de Deauville, fine restaurants, and a Festival of American Films.

Deauville has an excellent Spa and Thalassotherapy Center - **Biotherm Deauville** specializing in health, fitness, weight loss and anti-aging beauty treatments under medical supervision. The Biotherm Center is located on Boulevard de la Mer and occupies 2,000 sq. m. of luxurious Spa facilities facing the sea. Treatments at the center include: jet showers, hot whirlpools, electrotherapy, pressotherapy, dietotherapy, vitaminotherapy. Special beauty and anti-aging treatments include: wrinkle elimination, and Bio-lift. There is a special anti-aging program for men - "Special Hommes" to improve aesthetic appearance and conditions of the skin.

Although the Biotherm Center does not have accommodations, participants in the programs can use the luxurious **Hotel Normandy** Tel: (2) 3198-6622 and **Hotel Royal** Tel: (2) 3198-6633. Deauville is only 90 minutes from Paris via Highway A13, or 20 minutes by air flight.

EUGENIE-LES-BAINS
5

✈ Biarritz-Bayonne Anglet AP (BIQ)

Eugenie-les-Bains is a small spa town in the Southwest of France, just north of the Pyrenees, virtually equal distance from Biarritz, Toulouse and Bordeaux. It is 33 miles (53 km.) from Pau and 43 miles (69 km.) from Dax. It has been a health center since the days of Henri IV. However it has come to prominence through the effects of what one eats rather than drinks or bathes in. This is the home of Les Pres d'Eugenie created by Michel and Christine Guerard. It is the mecca for all gastronomy lovers. Michel is the creator of nouvelle cuisine and cuisine minceur, which he developed specifically to complement the water cures.

Les Pres d'Eugenie
♥♥♥♥

Eugenie-les-Bains 40320. Tel: (5) 5805-0607. Fax: (5) 5851-1359. TYPE: Hotel & Spa. LOCATION: In a garden setting. SPA CLIENTELE: Women and men.

* Rooms: 12 w/priv. bath. Suites: 7
* Phone, CTV, radio, refrigerator
* Restaurant: Gourmet Nouvelle Cuisine and cuisine minceur. Bar
* Airport: Pau Uzein 30 mi. / 50 km.
* Airport Transportation: limo, taxi
* Credit Cards: AMEX/DC
* Open: March - November
* Hotel Rates: rooms from FF 990; TAC: 8%
* Spa on premises
* **Spa Facilities**: Thermal baths, sauna, swimming pool, gym tennis courts
* **Spa Treatments**: baths, diet, hydrotherapy, physical exercise, saunas
* **Spa Programs**: Visa Biophytoforme, Visa Minceur (slimming Visa), Visa Bioenergetique (Bioenergetic Visa), Visa Detente (Relaxing Visa); all programs are for 3 or 7 days.
* Medically Supervised Health Program

DESCRIPTION: Intimate country mansion and spa with some areas dating from 1820. Michel Guerard and his wife Christine have developed the spa and its cuisine minceur - gastronomically delicious and low in calories (1,300 calorie). Member: *Relais et Chateaux and Traditions et Qualite Hotels.*

EVIAN LES BAINS
4

✈ Geneva Int'l Airport (GVA)

Evian-les-Bains is a lakeside spa resort in the scenic French Alps near the border with Switzerland. The cosmopolitan city of Geneva is only 40 km. (25 miles) away. Evian became an international spa resort after the discovery of the curative effects of its mineral waters. Evian mineral waters are the leading bottled water in France and are considered to have a beneficial effect in the diet of babies, salt free diets, and in cases of gout and arthritis.

Indications: diseases of the urinary system and metabolism problem, diseases of the digestive system, rheumatology and after effects of bone-joint damage.

Evian can be reached by high speed trains (TGV) from Paris or from Geneva by car, bus, taxi or helicopter.

Royal Club Evian
❤❤❤❤

South Shore Lake of Geneva, 74500 Evian. Tel: (4) 5026-8500. Fax: 5075-6100. TYPE: Resort & Spa. LOCATION: South bank of Lake Geneva on a 27-acre landscaped park. SPA CLIENTELE: Women and men, Family oriented. SPECIAL RESTRICTION: No dogs in restaurant, Spa Institute and Swimming Pools.

* Rooms: 156 w/priv. bath, Suites: 29
* 5 Restaurants, Bar & Lounges
* Phone, CTV, C/H, minbar, jacuzzi
* Restaurant, bar, casino, cabaret-disco
* Airport: Geneva International, 45 km. (28 mi.)
* Airport Transportation: Free pick up, taxi, limo, bus, helicopter
* Train Station: Evian 1 mi. / 2 km. free shuttle
* Reservations: 25% deposit required
* Credit Cards: MC/VISA/AMEX/DC/EC/JCB
* Open: Feb. 15 - Nov. 30
* Hotel Rates: from FF 990; TAC: 8%
* Name of Spa: **The Better Living Institute**
* Year Established: 1985
* SPA Facilities: The Better Living Institute; Hydrotherapy Center, pool, sauna, muscular exercise room, music gym, jogging trails, Beauty Salon for women and men.
* **Spa Programs**: Dietetic , Better Living, Super Better Living for Ladies and Men, Biological Cure, Cellular Treatment, Face Care for Women & Men, Fitness & Health, Golf Program, Tennis & Relaxation
* **Spa Packages**: Dietetic; Body Remodeling (6 days);

Super Better living for Ladies or Men (6 days), Slimming (6 days), Back Fitness (6 Days), Harmony (6 days), Sleep (5 days), Cellular Regeneration (6 days) à la carte programs available.
* **Spa Treatments**: hydrotherapy, ozone and oxygen baths, ionization, laser sessions, multi-jet shower, algae bath, sea mud wrap, lymphatic, draining, hydromassage, bubbling baths, underwater showers, massages, balanced dietetic meals of 1,500 calories per day, algae sheathing, Evian water mist treatment, facial care, beauty masks, biological cure, esthetic treatments; phytotherapy, neuraltherapy, homeotherapy, aromatherapy, sophrology
* **Medical Supervision**: guidance by top level professionals, doctors, dietician, physical therapists, beauticians

DESCRIPTION: Palatial Hotel with views of Lake Geneva and the Swiss Alps. All rooms and suites are spacious and individually decorated. The famous "Institut Mieux Vivre" (Better Living Institute) with its ultra modern spa facilities offers a wide array of treatments. Their specialty is the Biological Cure Program based on synergy to regain physical fitness by combining the physical with the psychic. The Biological Cure treats both general conditions and "fields of disturbance" such as stress, suppressed psychic problems, chronic infections, falls and operations. Cellular Treatment or application of fresh cells by cryotherapy is available, rates on request. Member: *The Leading Hotels of the World*.

PARIS
つ 1

✈ Orly Airport (ORY) 9 mi. / 14 km. South
Charles de Gaulle (CDG) 14 mi. / 22 km. NE

Paris, population 10,073,000 metro area, is the Capital of France and a major industrial, cultural and financial center. Known as the 'City of Light' or 'Paname' by the Parisians, Paris epitomizes the chic of international fashion, perfumes, gourmet cuisine and 'Joie de Vivre'. Whether you come to Paris for business or pleasure you can always be sure of a great time. Paris is easily accessible via International flights to 'Orly' or 'Charles de Gaulle' Airports.

Royal Monceau Hotel
❤❤❤❤

37 Avenue Hoche, 75008 Paris. Tel: (1) 4299-8800. Fax: (1) 4299-8990. TYPE: Deluxe Hotel & Spa. LOCATION: Avenue Hoche, 5 minutes from Champs Elysées and the Arc de Triumph. SPA CLIENTELE: Women and men.

* Rooms: 219 w/private bath, Suites: 39
* Phone, CTV, A/C, video films, radio & minibar
* Wheelchair Accessibility
* 3 Restaurants & Bars
* Airport: Orly, Charles de Gaule, 30 km. (19 mi.)
* Airport Transportation: bus, taxi
* Reservations: 1 night prepaid
* Credit Cards: MC/VISA/AMEX/DC/DIS/EC
* Open: Year round
* Hotel Rates: from FF 2,200
* Spa on premises: **'Les Thermes'**
* **Spa Facilities**: gym, exercise room, pool with an inverted current heated to 28°c (82°F), sauna, Turkish baths, Roman Baths, Jacuzzi, Beauty Salon, Hair and Skin Care Salon
* **Spa Treatments**: balneotherapy, exercise, gymnastics with music, stretching, jazz exercises, body and face care using 'la Prairie' products, lymph drainage, cellulotherapy, high pressure tan, pure U.V.A., bathing therapy, steam bath, massages, underwater jet massage, dietetic low, calorie gastronomic meals
* **Spa Programs**: Exercise, weight loss, Beauty programs for men and women
* Medical Supervision: available

DESCRIPTION: Deluxe hotel in a fashionable area of Paris. The hotel offers deluxe rooms, suites and apartments. The Spa - 'Les Thermes du Royal Monceau' is an elegant fitness and beauty center with scheduled fitness classes, and a Beauty Salon offering treatments based on the 'La Prairie' products. Medical and balneotherapy treatments are available. Special low calorie meals are offered.

QUIBERON
🌙 2

✈ L'Orient Airport

Quiberon, is a summer resort on the tiny Presqu'île de Quiberon in the northwestern Province of Morbihan. The Institut de Thalassoterapie de Quiberon is a medical Clinic that specializes in cures and treatments based on the basic elements of thalassotherapy: sea water, algaes, and the marine climate. Both deluxe hotels - **Sofitel Diététique** and the **Sofitel Thalassa** are directly connected to the Medical Institute and share the facilities and know how with the center. Sofitel Diététique specializes in nutrition and weight loss programs.

Sofitel Diététique
❤❤❤❤

Pointe de Goulvars, P.O. Box 170, Quiberon 56170. Tel: (2) 9750-2000. Fax: (2) 9730-4763. TYPE: Health Spa. LOCATION: At the southern tip of the Quiberon peninsula overlooking the ocean. SPA CLIENTELE: Women and men.

* Rooms: 78 w/priv. bath, Suites: 2
* Phone, CTV, balcony, radio
* Wheelchair Accessibility
* Restaurant & Bars
* Airport: Orient, 45 km. (28 mi.)
* Airport Transportation: taxi, bus
* Reservations: deposit req'd
* Credit Cards: AMEX/CBL/DC/EC
* Open: Year round (closed January)
* Hotel Rates: from FF 1,900/day; TAC: 8%
* Spa on premises: directly connected with the Institute of Thalassotherapy
* **Spa Facilities**: Linked to the Thalassotherapy Institute, Medical Center with radiology and laboratories, baths, gymnasium, indoor swimming pool with heated sea water, solarium,
* **Spa Treatments**: thalassotherapy, health diets prepared by nutritional experts, boiling baths, jet showers, underwater massages, inhalations and exercises
* **Spa Programs**: Nutritional and diet programs
* **Indications**: stress management, cardiovascular problems, arthritis, sinuses
* **Contraindications**: bad blood circulation
* Treatments Approved: Institute of Thalassotherapy of Quiberon

* Medical Supervision: 6 MD, 1 R
* No. of Customers per Doctor: 40
* Treatments Approved: Medical Institute

DESCRIPTION: The elegant Hotel Sofitel Diététique is linked directly to the Institute of Thalassotherapy of Quiberon; it offers specialized treatments in weight loss and nutrition under strictly supervised medical supervision. Seafood lovers can enjoy the gourmet 900 calories per day diet featuring fresh oysters from the Bay of Biscay, fresh lobsters, clams, mussels and crabs. All the leisure facilities are shared with the nearby Hotel Sofitel Thalassa.

Sofitel Thalassa Hotel
♥♥♥♥

Pointe de Goulvars, P.O. Box 170, Quiberon 56170. Tel: (2) 9750-2000. Fax: (2) 9730-4763. TYPE: Beachfront Resort Hotel & Spa. LOCATION: At the southern tip of the Quiberon peninsula overlooking the ocean. SPA CLIENTELE: Men and Women.

* Rooms: 133 w/priv. bath, Suites: 17
* CTV, radio, balcony
* Wheelchair Accessibility
* Restaurant & Bars
* Airport: Lorient Airport, 60 km. (38 mi.)
* Airport Transportation: taxi, bus
* Train Station: Auray, 2 km. (1 mi.)
* Train Station Transportation: taxi, bus
* Credit Cards: MC/VISA/AMEX/DC/EC/CB
* Open: Year round
* Hotel Rates: from FF 1,100/day
* TAC: 8%
* Spa on premises
* **Spa Facilities**: Linked to the Thalassotherapy Institute, Medical Center with radiology and laboratories, baths, gymnasium, indoor swimming pool with heated sea water, solarium,
* **Spa Treatments**: thalassotherapy, hydrotherapy, algotherapy, physiotherapy, electrotherapy, baths, showers, underwater massages, inhalations, exercises
* **Spa Programs**: Marine hydrotherapy
* Indications: stress management, cardiovascular problems, arthritis, sinuses, back aches, rheumatism

* Treatments Approved: Institute of Thalassotherapy of Quiberon
* Medical Supervision: Medical Institute

DESCRIPTION: The Sofitel Thalassa is connected by an indoor passage to the Institute of Thalassotherapy . The Spa emphasizes treatments and cures based on sea water and sea products. The minerals, and algaes in sea water provide excellent therapy for rheumatism and post operation recuperation. All the treatments are medically supervised. Recreation: golf, tennis, water sports, sight seeing excursions.

TOULOUSE
⌐ 5

✈ Blgnac Airport (TLS) 4.8 mi. / 8 km.

Grand Hotel de L'Opera
♥♥♥♥

1 Place du Capitole, Toulouse F-31000. Tel: (5) 6121-8266. Fax: (5) 6123-4104. USA/Canada reservations: (800) 257-5344. TYPE: Deluxe Hotel & Spa. LOCATION: In Ville Rose the historic center of Toulouse facing the Opera. SPA CLIENTELE: Women and men.

* Rooms: 49 w/priv. bath, Suites: 9
* Phone, CTV, A/C, C/H, minibar, balcony
* Wheelchair Access
* Restaurant & Bar in Greenhouse
* Airport: Balgnac Airport, taxi, bus
* Credit Cards: MC/VISA/AMEX/DC/EC/CB
* Open: Year round
* Hotel Rates: from FF 650/day; TAC: 8%
* Spa on premises: L'Opera Club
* **Spa Facilities**: health club center, jet-wave pool, sauna, hammam, body building gym, indoor pool
* **Spa Treatments**: massages, watergym, beauty care with "Les Complexes Biotechniques" products
* **Spa Programs**: fitness, beauty care

DESCRIPTION: Elegant hotel in a former 17th century Abbey with opulent and fanciful public areas. The L'Opera Club is a health center with Turkish bath, sauna and fully equipped gym.

VICHY
⟩ 4
✈ Charmeil Airport

Vichy, population 36,000 is a spa resort with a tradition dating back to Roman times. Located between the mountains and the plains of the Massif Central, it offers foreign travelers an insight into one of the most authentic regions of France. Vichy, is known for its bottled mineral waters from twelve springs. The cure at the Vichy Spa is based on the drinking of the appropriate thermal water based on a medical prescription. The thermal water belong to a group of sodic bicarbonate waters, containing 4.50 to 5.60 g mineral salts: sodium bicarbonate, ion sodium, potassium, calcium, magnesium, iron as well as lithium, fluorine, silica, iodine, and carbon dioxide and radon gases.

There are two Public Spa establishments in Vichy: **Grand Etablissement Thermal**, located at 1, Avenue Thermale, and includes the famous "Institute De Vichy", and the recently renovated **Bains Caillou**, on Square F. Glénard. Both establishments offer complete range of thermal baths, mud treatments, Vichy showers, sulfurous baths, massages, physiotherapy etc. under complete medical supervision.

Indications: migraines, after-effect of toxic or medicinal viral hepatitis, painful functional disorders, non infectious of the gallbladder and biliary tract, gastritis and hiatus hernias, allergic disorders, nutritional complaints; excess of cholesterol and blood lipides, diabetics, obesity, gout, and rheumatism.

The Novotel Thermalia Hotel (see below) is the only hotel directly linked to the "Vichy Institute". The elegant Pullman Palace Hotel is scheduled to reopen in June 1991.

Vichy offers beautiful parks, and many recreational activities. It can be accessed by domestic flights or SNCF trains from Paris or Lyon.

Hotel Les Celestins
❤❤❤

111 Ave. des États-Unis, Vichy F-03201. Tel: (4) 7030-8200. Fax: (4) 7030-8201. TYPE: Hotel & Cure Center.

LOCATION: In Park near 18-hole golf course. SPA CLIENTELE: Women and men. DESCRIPTION: Deluxe hotel with Cure Center, massages and beauty treatments. 131 rooms, 11 suites, restaurants, bar, indoor & outdoor pools. Hotel rates: from FF 730.

Novotel Thermalia
❤❤❤

1, Avenue Thermale, Vichy 03200. Tel: (4) 7031-0439. Fax: (4) 7031-0867. TYPE: Spa Hotel connected with the "Institut De Vichy". LOCATION: Central location near the Grand Etablissement Thermal and Bains Caillou. SPA CLIENTELE: Women and men, Family Oriented.

* Rooms: 128 w/priv. bath. Suites: 3
* Phone, CTV, A/C
* Wheelchair Accessible
* Restaurant, Grill Room & Bar
* Airport: Vichy, 20 minutes
* Credit Cards: AMEX/DC/CB/EC
* Open: Year round
* Hotel Rates: from FF 500/day (room only); TAC: 8%, Special Spa packages and rates on request
* **Spa Facilities**: directly linked to the famous "Institute De Vichy" and the Grand etablissement Thermal with their International Migraine Center, Thermal Hospital, & surgical private clinics; at the hotel - reeducation thermal pool, meconotherapy room, gym, hydrotherapy care rooms
* **Spa Programs**: individualized thermal based medical programs
* **Spa Treatments**: drinking cure, thermal baths, mud, massages, hydrotherapy, physiotherapy, aerosols, inhalations, pulverizations
* Treatments Approved: Institut De Vichy
* Medical Supervision: Medical Institute

DESCRIPTION: The only hotel directly linked to the famous Thermal Establishments of Vichy allowing guests to have direct access to medical or recreational Spa treatments. Accommodations are comfortable with good service. Nearby recreational activities include: casino gambling, tennis, water skiing, yacht club, golf, and horse racing.

GERMANY

AREA: 137,753 sq. mi. (356,780 sq. km.)
POPULATION: 79,000,000
CAPITAL: Berlin
OFFICIAL LANGUAGE: German
CURRENCY: Deutch Mark (DM) also Euro
EXCHANGE RATE: 1 US$ = DM 1.70
TELEPHONE COUNTRY CODE: 49

Germany has over 90 health Resorts. Many of them were already known for their healing powers centuries ago when they were discovered by the Romans. There are four types of spas - mineral and moorland spas, climatic health resorts, seaside spas and Kneipp Spas. The spas offer traditional spa cures; some include sophisticated applications of the Kneipp method and regenerative cell therapy in their programs. Most of the spa towns are attractive with casinos, restaurants, and lovely scenery.

ℹ️ DZT- German National Tourist Office
Beethovenstraße 69, D-60325, Frankfurt am Main
Tel: (069) 75720. Fax: (069) 751903

BAD ALEXANDERSBAD
✈ 9232
✈ Nueuremberg Airport 50 km. / 31 mi.

Hotel Alexandersbad
❤❤❤❤

Markgrafenstraße 24, Bad Alexandersbad D-95680. Tel:

(9232)8890. Fax: (9232) 889461. TYPE: Spa Hotel. CLIENTELE: Women and men. DESCRIPTION: Spa hotel with fitness room, solarium and restaurant. 110 rooms. Hotel rates: from DM 160.

BAD BEVENSEN
✈ 5821
✈ Fuhlsbuttel Airport (HAM) 100 km. / 62 mi.

Grünings Landhaus Hotel
❤❤❤

Haberkamp 2, Bad Bevensen D-29549. Tel: (5821) 98400. Fax: (5821) 984041. TYPE: Spa Hotel. DESCRIPTION: Spa hotel with Beauty Farm, swimming pool, and solarium in a quiet forest location. 20 rooms. Hotel rates: from DM 140.

BAD BRUCKENAU
✈ 9741
✈ Frankfurt Int'l Airport (FRA) 150 km. / 92 mi.

Dorint Hotel
❤❤❤

Heinrich-Von-Bibra Str. 13, Bad Brueckenau D-97769. Tel: (9741) 850. Fax: (9741) 854-25. TYPE: Resort Hotel & Spa. LOCATION: Center of town near the Kurpark with direct access to the Spa House. 146 rooms, garden cafe, pub, bar, dancing, pool, sauna, solarium, tennis. Rates: from DM 210/day (room only).

BAD DUERKHEIM
✈ 6322
✈ Frankfurt Int'l Airport (FRA) 30 km. / 19 mi.

Kurparkhotel
❤❤❤

Schlossplatz 1-4, Bad Duerkheim D-67098. Tel: (6322) 7970. Fax: (6322) 797-158. TYPE: First Class Spa Hotel.

LOCATION: 1 km from city center, 300 m. from train station. 112 rooms, restaurant, bar, indoor pool, sauna, fitness room, roof terrace. Rates: from DM 180/day (room only).

BAD EMS
⟩ 2603
✈ Frankfurt Int'l Airport (FRA) 100 km. / 62 mi.

Bad Ems, population 10,500, is located east of Koblenz on both banks of the river Lahn. The region is a famous wine country with beautiful vine-covered hills, colorful small villages, century old castles and fortresses. Within a radius of about 80 miles (128 km) are the major cities of Heidelberg, Frankfurt, Wiesbaden, Mainz, Cologne and Bonn. Bad Ems is easily accessible from Bonn, or Frankfurt. Bad Ems offers 18 hot springs with health giving properties. The mineral water combined with modern medical science provide cures and reliefs for various ailments.

Indications: catarrh, asthma, cardiac and circulatory disorders, rheumatism, arthritis, allergies, and ailments of the joints and vertebrae.

Atlantis Kurhotel
❤❤❤❤

Romerstrasse 1-3, Bad Ems 5427. Tel: (2603) 7990. Fax: (2603) 799252. TYPE: First Class Hotel & Spa. LOCATION: A lovely riverside location. SPA CLIENTELE: Women and men.

* Rooms: 113 w/priv. bath, Suites: 4
* Radio, phone, color TV, hair dryer, trouser press
* Restaurant, bar
* Train Station: Koblenz 10 km. / 6 mi. taxi
* Credit Cards: MC/VISA/AMEX/DC/EC
* Open: Year round
* Hotel Rates: from DM 170/day; TAC: 8%
* Spa on premises
* **Spa Facilities**: Thermal pool fed by mineral springs (88°F - 31°c); Spa and health center - Kurmittelhaus directly opposite
* **Spa Treatments**: medical treatments at the nearby Kurmittelhaus; mineral baths, massages at the hotel

* **Spa Programs**: health, fitness, beauty
* Medical Supervision: Spa physicians
* Treatments Approved

DESCRIPTION: The spa's leading hotel with a refined palatial resort style. The rooms are elegantly appointed with breathtaking views of the Lahn River. The Hotel amenities include in house spa and a nearby complete medical Kurmittelhaus for specialized treatments under medical supervision.

BAD FÜSSING
⟩ 8531
✈ Munich Airport (MUC) 140 km. / 88 mi.

Hotel Garni Villa Fortuna
❤❤❤

Thermalbadstraße 19, Bad Füssing D-08531. Tel: (8531) 9546. Fax: (8531) 954700. TYPE: Kurhotel. LOCATION: Near thermal baths. DESCRIPTION: Small spa hotel with thermal cure facilities, solarium, beauty treatments, 30 rooms, restaurant. Hotel rates: from DM 85.

BAD GRIESBACH
⟩ 8532
✈ Munich Airport (MUC) 160 km. / 100 mi.

Bad Griesbach, located in the Lower Bavarian Forest near Passau is the youngest thermal spa in Germany. The Spa has three bubbling thermal springs at water temperature of 68°c, 38°c and 30°c (154°F, 100°F and 86°F). All are rich in fluoride, sodium, and hydrogen-carbon-chloride.

Indications: for a cure at the Bad Griesbach thermal Spa include: Rheumatism, sciatic nerve complaints, lumbago, joint diseases, and rehabilitation after sickness.

Gulfhotel Maximilian
❤❤❤

Kuralle 1, Bad Griesbach D-94086. Tel: (8532) 7950. Fax: (8532) 795151. TYPE: Spa Hotel. LOCATION: Edge of the town. SPA CLIENTELE: Family Oriented. 232 rooms, sauna, Spa facilities including a Beauty Farm. Rates: from DM 210/day.

Parkhotel
❤❤❤❤

🐵 ⚓ 🐎 🏃

Am Kurwald 10, Bad Griesbach D-94086. Tel: (8532) 280. Fax: (8532) 28204. TYPE: Spa Hotel. LOCATION: In the Spa area, 5 km. / 3 mi. from train station. 162 rooms, therapy center for baneology, indoor thermal pools, physical and sports medicine, thermal spring grotto. Rates: from DM 260/day.

Hotel Fürstenhof
❤❤❤❤

🐵 ⚓ 🐎 🏃

Thermalbadstraße, Bad Griesbach D-94086. Tel: (8532) 9810. Fax: (8532) 981135. TYPE: Spa Hotel. LOCATION: In the Spa area, 5 km. / 3 mi. from train station. 240 rooms, therapy center for baneology, indoor thermal pools, physical and sports medicine, thermal spring grotto. Rates: from DM 260/day.

BAD HARZBURG
🌙 5322

Seela Hotel
❤❤❤

🐵 ⚓ 🐎 🏃

Nordhaeuserstr. 5, Bad Harzburg D-38667. Tel: (5322) 7960. Fax: (5322) 796199. TYPE: Spa Hotel. LOCATION: Centrally located in the Spa area., 120 rooms, gym, sauna, health & beauty treatments. Rates: from DM 230/day.

BAD-KISSINGEN
🌙 971

✈ Frankfurt Int'l Airport (FRA)

Bad-Kissingen, population 22,000, is an attractive health resort in the Franconian Basin of northern Bavaria. The town is also known for its medieval romantic Baroque architecture and features Bavaria's only historical casino, many parks and gardens. Bad Kissingen can be reached via Frankfurt and Würzburg. From Würzburg take the motorway via the Hammelburg exit.

Indications: The municipal Kurhaus baths offer treatments for the following ailments - stomach, intestine, liver, gallbladder, heart and circulatory system, metabolic disorders (supportive treatment of obesity and diabetes), disorders of the nervous system, rheumatic illnesses and gynecological ailments. Mineral water cures are Rakoczy, Pandur, Maxbrunnen and Luitpoldsprudel. The bathing cures include naturally carbonated brine and mineral baths, mud baths and packs with natural High-Rhön mud from the area of the 'Red Moor'.

Additional treatments include Roman-Irish steam baths, dry carbon-dioxide baths, underwater massages, body-training, natural brine bubble baths (at local clinics and sanatoriums) physical exercises, inhaling exercises, tension releasing exercises, brush baths and massages. Spa facilities include whirlpool with natural spa water at 32°c (90°F), recreation rooms, drinking and promenade halls, inhaling rooms, open-air brine inhalations, outdoor exercise complex, clinic for internal complaints and gastric disorders.

Bristol Hotel
❤❤❤

⚓ 🐎 🏃

Bismarckstr. 8-10, Bad-Kissingen D-97688. Tel: (971) 8240. Fax: (971) 8245824. TYPE: Spa Hotel. LOCATION: Directly on Rosegarten at the entrance to Luitpoldpark. 82 rooms, sauna, solarium, gym, Beauty Farm. Hotel Rates: from DM 180.

Steigenberger Kurhaushotel
❤❤❤❤❤

⚓ 🐎 🏃

Kurgarten 3, Bad-Kissingen D-97688. Tel: (971) 80410. Fax: (971) 80410. Fax: (971) 8041597. TYPE: Deluxe Hotel & Spa. DIRECTOR: Mr. Michael Kain. LOCATION: Quietly situated in the pedestrian and spa garden area. SPA CLIENTELE: Women and men.

* Rooms: 141 w/private bath
* Municipal Kurhaus 50 m. / 150 ft. away

* Train Station: Bad-Kissingen 800 m. / 1/2 mi.
* Train Station Transportation: taxi
* Credit Cards: MC/VISA/AMEX/DC/EC
* Open: Year round
* Hotel Rates: from DM 240/day; TAC: 8%
* Spa on premises
* **Spa Facilities**: Indoor swimming pool, fitness room, sauna, solarium, massage rooms, sun terrace; direct access to the municipal Kurhaus with its extensive spa cure facilities, Beauty Farm
* **Spa Treatments**: Kurhaus spa treatments; in house diet, low calorie meals, solarium, full massage, massage of the connective tissue
* **Spa Packages**: Discover Bad Kissingen (2 nts); The Kissingen Diet (7 nts); Winter in 7th Heaven (30 nts)

DESCRIPTION: A distinguished Spa hotel, built in the mid 19th century where European dignitaries and celebrities used to socialize and 'take the water'. Accommodations are spacious and comfortably furnished; public meeting rooms are elegant, serene, and well decorated. The emphasis at the hotel is on the cures available at the Kurhaus, but the hotel offers wonderful French Haute Cuisine with dietary modifications, if requested, and a special Kissingen Diet program.

BAD KREUZNACH
⟩ 671

✈ Frankfurt Int'l Airport (FRA) 80 km. / 50 mi.

Hotel Der Quellenhof
♥♥♥

Nachtigallenweg 2, Bad Kreuznach D-55543. Tel: (671) 838330. Fax: (671) 35218. TYPE: Spa Hotel. LOCATION: In Kurpark area. SPA CLIENTELE: Women and men. DESCRIPTION: Spa hotel with thermal & cure facilities, Finnish sauna, Hammam, massages. 30 rooms. Hotel rates: from DM 130.

Park Hotel Kurhaus
♥♥♥

Kurhausstraße 28, Bad Kreuznach D-55504. Tel: (671) 8020. Fax: (671) 35477. TYPE: Spa Hotel. LOCATION: In

Kurpark area on an island in the Nahe River. SPA CLIENTELE: Women and men. DESCRIPTION: Grand Spa hotel with thermal indoor/outdoor pools, sauna, massage, cosmetic studio, homeopathic therapy. 108 rooms, 4 suites, international restaurant. Hotel rates: from DM 145.

BAD LAUTERBERG
⟩ 5524

✈ Hannover Int'l Airport (HAJ) 100 km. / 63 mi.

Bad Lauterberg, population 15,000, is a spa town in Lower Saxony, a few miles southeast of Goslar and about 45 km .(28 mi.) northeast of Göttingen, at the foot of the Hartz Mountains. This area has interesting villages; many still conserve their old medieval style. Nearby Göttingen is the hometown of the oldest and most revered University in Germany. Bad-Lauterberg is accessible by car or train via Göttingen.

Indications: the Bad-Lauterberg spa offers cure programs for the following disorders - Illnesses of the stomach, intestinal, liver and biliary ducts, illnesses of the metabolism, women diseases, Cardiovascular disease, rheumatic diseases, illnesses of the locomotion and post-injury recuperation.

Kneipp Kurhotel Heikenberg
♥♥♥

Heikenbergstraße 19-21, Bad Lauterberg D-37431. Tel: (5524) 8570. Fax: (5524) 6741. TYPE: Hotel & Spa. LOCATION: In a pleasant residential area. SPA CLIENTELE: Women and men.

* Rooms: 60 w/priv. bath
* Airport: Hannover, 100 km. (62 mi.)
* Airport Transportation: train than taxi
* Reservations: suggested
* Credit Cards: MC/VISA/AMEX
* Open: Year round
* Hotel Rates: from DM 130/day
* TAC: 8%
* Spa on premises
* **Spa Facilities**: mineral bath, sauna, solarium, fitness center, cosmetic center, exercise room, Sanatorium, Diet Spa Restaurant

* **Spa Treatments**: cosmetic and skin care based on pure natural biologic ingredients - aromatherapy, massages, peeling, lymph drainage, cellulite reduction, low calorie nutritional meals; medical treatments at the Sanatorium
* **Spa Programs**: Standard, Regeneration, Diet
* **Medical Supervision**: Dr. Moser MD
* **Treatments Approved**: by Sanatorium

DESCRIPTION: Moderate spa hotel with well appointed rooms. There is plenty of activities to keep you busy and entertained. The hotel offers an intensive cosmetic and skin care program and access to the Sanatorium for serious medical cures. Recreation: bowling, tennis, & cross-country skiing in the winter.

BAD MERGENTHEIM
⟩ 7931
✈ Frankfurt Int'l Airport (FRA) 120 km. / 75 mi.

Maritim Parkhotel
❤❤❤❤

Lothar-Daiker Str. 6, Bad Mergentheim D-97980. Tel: (7931) 5390. Fax: (7931) 539100. TYPE: Spa Hotel. LOCATION: Center of Kurpark, 600 m. / yards from train station. 116 rooms, bar, diet menu, pool, sauna, medical and therapy treatments. Hotel Rates: from DM 190/day.

BAD NEUENAHR-AHRWEILER
⟩ 2641
✈ Cologne-Bonn Int'l AP (CGN) 53 km. / 33 mi.

Giffels Goldener Anker
❤❤❤❤

Mittelstraße 14, Bad Neuenahr D-53474. Tel: (2641) 8040. Fax: (2641) 804400. TYPE: Spa Hotel. LOCATION: Center of town near casino. SPA CLIENTELE: Women and men. DESCRIPTION: Elegant Spa hotel with fitness room, indoor thermal pool, special diets, massage and mud baths, international restaurant, 82 rooms, 4 suites. Hotel rates: from DM 160.

Steigenberger Hotel
❤❤❤❤

Kurgartenstraße 1, Bad Neuenahr D-53474. Tel: (2641) 9410. Fax: (2641) 7001. TYPE: Spa Hotel. MANAGER: Dr. Michael Hattenhauer. LOCATION: Center of town near the resort park. SPA CLIENTELE: Women and men. DESCRIPTION: International resort spa hotel with indoor thermal pool, cure facilities and special diets. 224 rooms, 13 suites, restaurant, bar, cafe. Hotel rates: from DM 230.

BAD ORB
⟩ 6052
✈ Frankfurt Int'l Airport (FRA) 60 km. / 38 mi.

Steigenberger Bad Orb
❤❤❤❤

Horststraße 11, Postfach 1420, Bad Orb D-63619. Tel: (6052) 880. Fax: (6052) 881-35 TYPE: Spa Hotel. LOCATION: In the Kurpark. SPA CLIENTELE: Women and men.

* Rooms: 104 w/private bath
* Public Spa facilities: 200 m. (600 ft.)
* Airport: Frankfurt, 60 km. (38 mi.) taxi, bus
* Credit Cards: MC/VISA/AMEX/DC/CB
* Open: Year round
* Hotel Rates: from DM 290/day
* TAC: 8%
* Spa on premises
* **Spa Facilities**: indoor/outdoor thermal pools, gym, sauna, spa baths available; other spa facilities are located at the public Leopold-Koch-Bads nearby
* **Spa Treatments**: in hotel - sauna, solarium, fitness massages; other more intensive treatments are available at the public Leopold-Koch-Bads
* **Spa Programs**: Stress Management (7 nts) Winter in 7th Heaven (30 nts)
* Medical Supervision: 1 MD

DESCRIPTION: Spa hotel with an elegant public lobby, comfortable rooms, in a charming garden setting. The focus is on spa cures at the nearby Leopold-Koch-Bads (a sophisticated spa complex). Some fitness treatments and massages are available at the hotel.

BAD REICHENHALL
) 8651

✈ Munich Airport (MUC) 15 km. / 10 mi.
Salzburg Airport (SZG) Austria

Bad Reichenhall, population 16,000, is one of the few German spas that are called Staatsbaad for their excellence. Nestled in the foothills of the Bavarian Alps, the Spa is known for its salt-laden springs containing as much as 24% salt. The most saline concentrated springs in Europe. Bad Reichenhall's air and water quality is protected by Federal law that prohibits industrial pollution in the region. In addition to its famous water, visitors can enjoy excellent skiing within easy reach; ice skating facilities are available in town. Salzburg with its old churches, castles and world famous music festival is only 15 km. (10 mi.) northeast. Bad Reichenhall can be reached by train from Munich. The train trip takes about 2 hours. If driving by car, take the Alpine Road. From Salzburg take the E14 to E11.

Indications: the following ailments can be treated at Bad Reichnhall - asthma and illnesses of the respiratory system, women's diseases, cardiovascular diseases, rheumatic diseases, children's ailments.

Parkhotel Luisenbad
♥♥♥♥

Ludwigstraße 33, Bad Reichenhall D-83435. Tel: (8651) 6040. Fax: (8651) 62928. TYPE: Spa Hotel. LOCATION: Cental location in landscaped gardens. SPA CLIENTELE: Women and men. DESCRIPTION: Traditional hotel with cure house, beauty farm, fitness center and sauna. 83 rooms, 8 suites, indoor pool, parking. Hotel rates: from DM 190.

Steigenberger Axelmannstein
♥♥♥♥♥

Salzburger Straße 2-6, 8230 Bad Reichenhall D-83435.

Tel: (8651) 7770. Fax: (8651) 5932. TYPE: Deluxe Spa Hotel. MANAGER: Dr. Klaus Brand. LOCATION: On 8 acres of private park in Bad Reichenhall. SPA CLIENTELE: Women and men.

* Rooms: 151 w/private bath
* Suites: 9; Apartments: 5
* Park Restaurant: International cuisine; Axel-Stübel: Bavarian cuisine
* Airport: Salzburg (Austria), 12 km. (8 mi.)
* Airport Transportation: taxi, bus
* Credit Cards: MC/VISA/AMEX/DC
* Open: Year round
* Hotel Rates: from DM 179/day; TAC: 8%
* Spa on premises
* **Spa Facilities**: Balneotherapy department, Hairdressing & Beauty Salon, Fitness Center, sauna, solarium, indoor swimming pool, direct access to mineral bathing facilities
* **Spa Treatments**: therapeutic bathing, showers, inhalations, affusions, packs, physiotherapy, respiratory exercises, compresses, rubdowns, therapeutic massages; beauty treatments at the beauty salon operated by Charles of the Ritz; Fitness - exercise,
* **Spa Programs**: Fitness Program, Beauty Program, Weight Loss Program
* **Spa Packages**: Slim Program (12 night); Cure & Vacation (7 nights); Winter in 7th Heaven (30 nights)

DESCRIPTION: The hotel, known as "Axel" for short, offers luxurious accommodations, breathtaking views of the Bavarian Alps and a Spa center known as one of the best in Europe. The Spa stresses the importance of health, beauty and fitness. Many guests prefer to use the hotel facilities as they combine advanced curative treatments with the atmosphere, and service of a first class hotel.

BAD SAAROW
) 33631

✈ Tegel Airport (TXL); Tempolhof Airport (THF)
Schoenfeld Airport (THF) Berlin

Kempinsky Hotel
Sporting Club Berlin
❤❤❤❤

Parkallee 1, Bad Saarow D-15526. Tel: (33631) 60, Fax: (33631) 62000. TYPE: Spa & leisure hotel. LOCATION: On the banks of Lake Scharmutzel. DESCRIPTION: Health center, spa/beauty treatments, massage, solarium, whirlpool, Finish sauna, steam bath, indoor & outdoor pools. Hotel rates: from DM 290.

BAD SALZUFLEN
Ↄ 5222

✈ Hannover Airport (HAJ) 90 km. / 57 mi.

Maritim Staatsbadhotel
❤❤❤❤

Parkstr. 53, Bad Salzuflen D-32105. Tel: (5222) 181-0, Fax: (5222) 18-600. TYPE: Spa hotel. LOCATION: Adjacent to Kurpark. DESCRIPTION: Attractive Spa hotel. Therapeutic department with beauty regimen, fitness programs, physical therapy, sauna, solarium. Hotel rates: from DM 280.

BAD URACH
Ↄ 7125

✈ Stuttgart Airport (STR) 35 km. / 22 mi.

Hotel Graf Eberhard
❤❤❤❤

Bei den Thermen 2, Bad Urach D-72574. Tel: (7125) 1480. Fax: (7125) 8214. TYPE: Spa Hotel. LOCATION: Central near Thermal Baths. SPA CLIENTELE: Women and men. DESCRIPTION: Elegant Spa hotel offering thermal cure and diet cuisine. 70 rooms. Hotel rates: from DM 180.

BAD WIESSE
Ↄ 8022

✈ Munich Airport (MUC) 94 km. / 60 mi.

Hotel Graf Eberhard
❤❤❤❤

Im Sapplfeld 8, Bad Wiesse D-83707. Tel: (8022) 98470. Fax: (8022) 83560. TYPE: Spa Hotel. LOCATION: Central location, 2 km. / 1 mi. from train station. SPA CLIENTELE: Women and men. DESCRIPTION: Elegant 4-star Spa hotel with pool, sauna, solarium and cure facilities. 15 rooms. Hotel rates: from DM 162.

BAD WILDBAD
Ↄ 7081

✈ Stuttgart Airport (STR) 50 km. / 31 mi.

Badhotel Wildbad
❤❤❤

Kurplatz 5, Bad Wildbad D-75323. Tel: (7081) 1760. Fax: (7081) 176170. TYPE: Spa Hotel. LOCATION: Mountain resort area. SPA CLIENTELE: Women and men. DESCRIPTION: Health resort with fitness room, Palais Thermal, cure facilities and diet cuisine. 60 rooms, pool, bar, sauna. Hotel Rates: from DM 145.

Sommerberg Hotel
❤❤❤❤

Heermannsweg 5, Bad Wildbad D-75313. Tel: (7081) 1740. Fax: (7081) 174612. TYPE: Spa Hotel. LOCATION: Mountain resort. 90 rooms, restaurant, bar, pool, gym, sauna, physio-therapeutic treatments, cosmetic studio, winter sports nearby. Rates: from DM 160/day.

BAD WILDUNGEN
Ↄ 5621

✈ Frankfurt Int'l Airport (FRA) 100 km. / 63 mi.

Maritim Badehotel
❤❤❤

Dr. Marc Str. 4, Bad Wildungen D-34537. Tel: (5621)

7999. Fax: (5621) 799-699. TYPE: First Class Traditional Spa Hotel. LOCATION: Spa garden setting. 250 rooms, bar, lounge, therapeutic baths, solarium, jogging track, tennis, minigolf, horseback riding. Rates: from DM 270/day.

BAD WÖRISHOFEN
⟍ 8247

✈ Munich Int'l Airport (MUC) 85 km. / 53 mi.

Kneipp-Kurhotel Kreuzer
❤❤❤

Kneippstr. 4, Bad Woerishofen D-86817. Tel: (8247) 3530. Fax: (8247) 353138. TYPE: Inclusive Spa Resort. LOCATION: Central location, 500 m. / yards from train station. 100 rooms, restaurant, wine cellar, special diets, fitness room, massage, golf course and tennis nearby. Rates: from DM 180/day.

Kurhotel Eichwald
❤❤❤❤

Eichwaldstraße 20, Bad Wörishopen D-86825. Tel: (8247) 6094. Fax: (8247) 6679. TYPE: Spa Hotel. LOCATION: Central location. SPA CLIENTELE: Women and men. DESCRIPTION: Elegant spa hotel with fitness room, diet program and cure facilities. Hotel rates: from DM 110.

BADEN-BADEN
⟍ 7221

✈ Stuttgart Airport (STR) 120 km. / 75 mi.

Baden-Baden, population 50,000, is a health spa, vacation and convention resort on the edge of the Black Forest. The town lies 800ft. (270m) above sea level amidst woodland, valleys and mountains. Thanks to its location, Baden-Baden is considered one of the most beautiful towns on the upper Rhine. It ranks at the top of all German spas in popularity with international tourists.

One of the oldest thermal establishments is **Friedrichsbad** with its famous Roman Irish Baths. The atmosphere is elegant and reminiscent of the "belle époque". The bathing experience starts with a luxurious shower followed by hot-air bath and then a soap-and-brush massage for a unique healthful and relaxing experience. Treatments include co-ed thermal bath, thermal spray bath, exercise pools and cool and warm pools. A complete spa experience at Friedrichsbad detoxicates the body, assists the metabolism, stimulates blood circulation and gives an unsurpassed sensation of well being. Certain ailments such as rheumatism, sinus, and glandular disorders can benefit from a spa experience at the Roman Irish Baths. **The Augustabad** includes outdoor pools, hot and cold water cave, whirlpool, sauna, solarium and massage department. **The Caracalla** Therme, a large thermal bath was recently added to the Augustabad. Treatments at the Caracalla include: thermal exercising baths, therapeutic baths, Fango-mud bath, aerosol inhalations. The Trinkhalle / Pump room was built in the early 19th century and contains 14 romantic frescoes that depict the legends of Baden-Baden. Visitors often drink the radioactive chloride water from local springs and learn about mineral water and juice treatments. Baden-Baden can be reached from Stuttgart, Pforzheim or Strasbourg (France).

Badhotel Zum Hirsch
❤❤❤

Hirschstraße 1, Baden-Baden D-76530. Tel: (7221) 9390. Fax: (7221) 38148. TYPE: Spa Hotel. LOCATION: City Center, pedestrian area, 5 minutes to Casino, Kurhaus and Kurpark. SPA CLIENTELE: Women and men.

* Rooms: 58 w/priv. bath
* Airport: Stuttgart 120 km. / 75 mi.
* Train Station: Baden-Oos 5 km. / 3 mi.
* Airport/Train Transportation: taxi, bus
* Reservations: required
* Credit Cards: MC/VISA/DC/AMEX/DC/EC
* Open: Year round
* Hotel Rates: from DM 200 (room only); TAC: 8%. A la carte treatments at the Medical Bath Ward.
* Spa on premises
* **Spa Facilities**: thermal baths, hydroelectric full baths, thermal pools, massage rooms
* **Spa Programs**: intensive thermal cure
* **Spa Treatments**: thermal water baths, mud

baths, hydroelectric complete bath, ultrasonic bath, massages, underwater pressure-jet massage, physiotherapy, fango-compress
* Treatments Approved: German medical insurance authorities

DESCRIPTION: 300 year old hotel with spa facilities. Each room equipped with period style furniture. All bathrooms have thermal water. The hotel features its own thermal bathing department, and is recommended for guests who want to take an intensive cure. Member: *SRS Hotels*

Brenner's Park Hotel & Spa
❤❤❤❤❤

An der Lichtentaler Allee, 76530 Baden-Baden. Tel: (7221) 9000. Fax: (7221) 38772. TYPE: Deluxe Hotel & Spa. LOCATION: A private park location in the center of the spa area. SPA CLIENTELE: Women and men.

* Rooms: 100 w/private bath
* Junior Suites and Suites: 20
* Phone, CTV, A/C, C/H, minibar
* Restaurants, bars, entertainment
* Airports: Strasbourg (75 km. / 47 mi.), Stuttgart (110 km. / 68 mi.), Frankfurt (180 km. / 112 mi.)
* Train Station: Baden-Baden (10 min.)
* Airport Transportation: taxi, limo, train.
* Reservations: required
* Credit Cards: AMEX/VISA/MC/JBC
* Open: Year round
* Hotel Rates: from DM 360
* TAC: 8% (on room only)
* Spa on premises (also off premises)
* Distance to Public Spa: 500 m/yards
* **Spa Facilities**: Lancaster Beauty Spa, indoor pool, saunas, work-out room, solarium; Black Forest Clinic in Villa Stephanie, private clinic for internal medicine with physiotherapy. Public spas and clinics nearby
* **Spa Programs**: Beauty, Sports & Fitness programs. Preventive medicine, rehabilitation, check-up; institute for two-day-check-up program; natural medicine
* **Spa Packages**: Beauty week á la carte services available

* **Spa Treatments**: At the Lancaster Beauty Spa: beauty treatments, aroma-therapy, cellulite cure, depilation, color and style counseling, color therapy, massages (full, partial, reflexology), iontophorese, body pack with brush massage, body peeling, lymph drainage, sea algae body treatment, modeling, thermo dyn treatment shiatsu. Relaxation training, water gymnastics, pool cycling, exercises, yoga, jogging, mountain-biking.
At the Villa Stephanie: Orthodox medicine and natural, biological healing treatments, balneo therapy, physical therapy, therapeutic treatments, nutrition physiology (diet kitchen), medical baths, packs and compresses, electrotherapy
* Medical Supervision: 3 MD, 3 RN
* No. of Customers per Doctor: 12 - 37
* Treatments Approved: licensed Clinic

DESCRIPTION: A distinguished landmark Hotel & Spa and the favorite of many spa connoisseurs. Guest rooms are large and decorated in classic style. The elegant public rooms are lavishly decorated with fine objets d'arts and antiques. The **Lancaster Beauty-Farm** offers beauty, pampering and cosmetic treatments. The **Ausava Club** is an exclusive bath club; it is the Roman word for the river Oos, which can be seen from the pool. The **Villa Stephanie** specializes in internal medicine. Recreation nearby: Tennis, golf, horseback riding, hiking, fishing, hunting. Member: *The Leading Hotels of the World, Preferred Hotels & Resorts Worldwide, Relaix and Chateaux.*

Quisisana Privathotel
❤❤❤❤

Bismarkstrasse 21, 7570 Baden-Baden. Tel: (7221) 3690. Fax: (7221) 369269. TYPE: Spa Hotel. LOCATION: Central near the Spa. SPA CLIENTELE: Women and men.

* Rooms: 60 with private bath, Suites: 9
* Phone, CTV, C/H, minibar, private safe
* Restaurant, bar, winter garden
* Airports: Frankfurt (170 km. / 106 mi.), Stuttgart (120 km. / 75 mi.); Straßourg (60 km. / 38 mi.)

* Train Station: Baden-Baden
* Reservation: Required
* Credit Cards: MC, VISA, AMEX, DC
* Open: Year round
* Hotel Rates: from DM 360 (room only)
* TAC: 10%
* Spa on premises
* **Spa Facilities**: Pool, sauna, steam bath, fitness area, whirlpool, solarium, beauty salon
* **Spa Programs**: Medical & Beauty
* **Spa Treatments**: massage, Kneipp, showers

DESCRIPTION: Small Spa hotel in ornamental old villa with modern extensions. Winter garden & enclosed pool & spa facilities.

Schlosshotel Bühlerhöhe
Beauty Farm - Health Spa
❤❤❤❤❤

Schwarzwaldhochstrasse 1, 77815 Baden-Baden / Bühl. Tel: (7226) 550, Fax: (7226) 55674. TYPE: Deluxe Resort Spa. LOCATION: On a hilltop surrounded by parks and forests, In the Northern Black Forest, 15 km. / 10 mi. from Baden-Baden. SPA CLIENTELE: Men & Women.

* Rooms: 90 with private bath, Suites: 21
* Phone, CTV, C/H, minibar, private safe
* Restaurant, bar
* Airports: Frankfurt (170 km. / 106 mi.), Stuttgart (120 km. / 75 mi.); Strassbourg (60 km. / 38 mi.)
* Train Station: Baden-Baden
* Reservation: Required
* Credit Cards: MC, VISA, AMEX, DC
* Open: Year round
* Hotel Rates: Rooms only from DM 490, one-bedroom from DM 1,300; TAC: 10%
* **Spa Facilities**: Pool, sauna, steam bath, fitness area, whirlpool, solarium, beauty salon
* **Spa Programs**: Relaxation, Beauty Care, Recovery
* **Spa Packages**: beauty stay de luxe (3 day) , Intensive treatment de luxe (7 day), Thalgo-sea algae therapy (7 day),

Aromatherapy vitalization treatment (7 day)
* **Spa Treatments**: Thalassotherapy, Kneipp showers, aromatherapy, herbal wraps, lymph drainage, loofah scrub, anti-cellulite, anti-age, Chinese energetical lifting, shiatsu, pointmassage, body peeling, sea-wave bath, body massage, facials; algae pack, Gelatine Verveine, ampoule and make-up, deep cleansing, collagen-fleece, massage, masks on face, eyes, neck and cleavage. manicure, pedicure, body brushing massage, whey bath, creamy body pack, sea salt bath, lymph drainage, reflexology, Tai-Chi-Chuan

DESCRIPTION: The Schlosshotel Bühleröhe is a baronial style palace hotel with a luxurious and cosy atmosphere. The beauty farm offers service for vitality, health and beauty. Recreation: downhill and cross-country skiing, tennis, horseback riding and golf.

Steigenberger Avance
Badischer Hof
❤❤❤❤❤

Lange Straße 7, 7570 Baden-Baden. Tel: (7221) 9340. Fax: (7221) 934470. TYPE: Deluxe Hotel & Spa. LOCATION: City center, at the beginning of the pedestrian area, near the Kurpark Casino. SPA CLIENTELE: Women and men.

* Rooms: 134 w/priv. bath. Suites: 5
* Phone, CTV, C/H, A/C, minibar
* Restaurant, bar, atrium lobby
* Credit Cards: MC/VISA/AMEX/ACC
* Open: Year round
* Hotel Rates: from DM 190; TAC: 8%
* Spa on premises
* Name of Spa: **Institut Mireille**
* **Spa Facilities**: Thermal bath, Swimming pool with diluted thermal water, sauna, solarium, massage dept, relaxing rooms, medical bathing dept. Institut Mireille (Beauty Farm & Health Center)
* **Spa Programs**: Fitness, Anti-Stress, Slimming, Beauty, Balneotherapy
* Spa Packages: 1-3 week packages available Fitness, Anti-Stress, Slimming, Health Course Vacation for Beauty

* **Spa Treatments**: biodynamic treatments, stretching and aquatic gymnastics, reflex-zonal treatments with seawater algae, massage and water massage, foot reflex-zonal treatments, reduced-calorie health menu (1,000 - 1,200 calories), aromatherapy
* **Medical Supervision**: 1 MD

DESCRIPTION: A recuperative Oasis in the midst of a magnificent park-like grounds. This classic spa hotel is located in a renovated 19th century Capuchin Monastery, with modern wing and luxuriously furnished rooms and suites. Hot thermal water is supplied to hotel bathrooms which can be transformed into private spas. Medically supervised programs are available for sufferers from rheumatic and circulatory ailments. The Institute Mireille offers a wide range of beauty and cosmetic treatments. Member: *SRS Hotels*

BADENWEILER
⟩ 7221
✈ Stuttgart Airport (STR) 120 km. / 75 mi.

Hotel Römebad
♥♥♥
🐵 ⚕ 🏇 🚶 ⚛

Schlossplatz 1, Badenweiler D-79410. Tel: (7632) 700. Fax: (7632) 70200. TYPE: Spa Hotel. LOCATION: In beautiful landscaped grounds near Baden-Baden. SPA CLIENTELE: Women and men. DESCRIPTION: Distinguished spa hotel with health club and Estee Lauder Beauty Salon. 84 rooms, 11 suites, indoor and outdoor thermal pools, sauna, gym, solarium, tennis. Hotel rates: from DM 240.

BERGISCH GLADBACH (Cologne)
⟩ 2202
✈ Cologne-Bonn Int'l AP (CGN)

Lancaster Beauty Farm
♥♥♥♥♥

c/o Schlosshotel Lerbach, Lerbacher Weg, 51465 Bergisch Gladbach. Hotel - Tel: (2202) 2040. Fax: (2202) 32702. Spa Tel: (2202) 204604. TYPE: Beauty Spa. MANAGING DIRECTORS: Mrs. Althof & Mrs. Schneider. LOCATION: In an old Castle style hotel on 70 acres private park, 20 km / 13 mi from Cologne. SPA CLIENTELE: Women and men.

* Rooms: 54 w/priv. bath
* Phone, CTV, safe, minibar, hair dryer
* Restaurants (2), bar
* Train Station: Cologne / Bergisch Gladbach
* Reservations: required
* Credit Cards: MC/VISA/AMEX
* Open: Year round
* Rates: from DM 195
* TAC: 8%
* Spa on premises
* Year established: 1993
* Spa Facilities: beauty center, treatment rooms, indoor pool, sauna, solarium, jogging track
* **Spa Treatments**: sea-wave bath, lifting, collagen fleece, masks, bust treatments, relaxation training (Jacobsen, Bublitz), water gymnastics, treatments after aesthetic surgery, beauty injections, La Prairie treatments
* **Spa Programs**: Beauty, thalassotherapy, aromatherapy, relaxation
* **Spa Packages**: from DM 195-285 (day program) to DM 2,650 (5 day program); weekend program from DM 990; body special program from DM 1,990; Thalassoprogram from DM 350
* **Medical Supervision**: part-time on request

DESCRIPTION: Famous Beauty Farm just outside of Cologne offering a variety of beauty, cosmetic and anti-aging treatments in the deluxe Schlosshotel Lerbach. The 5-day Beauty Spa programs are on half-board basis. Day programs and Thalassaprogram do not include accommodations.

BERLIN
⟩ 30
✈ Tegel Airport (TXL); Tempolhof Airport (THF) Schoenenfeld Airport (SXF)

Hotel Berlin
♥♥♥♥
🐵 ⚕ 🏇 🚶

Luetzowplatz 17, Berlin D-10785. Tel: (30) 26050. Fax: (30) 26052716. TYPE: Hotel & Spa. LOCATION: Quiet location 1 km / 1/2 mi. from Zoo Station. SPA CLIENTELE: Women and men. DESCRIPTION: Large distinguished hotel, 701 rooms, 21 suites with Health Club & Beauty Spa. Hotel Rates: from DM 350.

FREUDENSTADT
➲ 7441
✈ Stuttgart Airport (STR) 100 km. / 62 mi.

Freudenstadt, population 21,000, is a sunny resort in the Black Forest region of Germany. The town has an old character, with many buildings from the 16th and 17th century. The town's main attraction is its favorite location amidst the best hiking, camping and skiing areas of the Black Forest. Freudenstadt can be reached by car from Stuttgart, or Strasbourg (France). The town is linked to German and European railroad system. It is easily accessible by trains from Stuttgart, Frankfurt, Strasbourg and Basel.

Schwartzwaldhof Hotel
♥♥♥

Hohenriedersraße 74 , Freudenstadt D-72250. Tel: (7441) 86030. Fax: (7441) 860330. TYPE: Spa Hotel. LOCATION: In a secluded park in Freudenstadt in the Black Forest. SPA CLIENTELE: Women and men.

* Rooms: 42 w/priv. bath. Suites: 3
* Phone, C/H, balcony
* Restaurants: 2, Bar & TV Lounge
* Airport: Stuttgart Airport, 85 km. / 53 mi.
* Airport Transportation: taxi, train
* Train Station: Freudensdtadt 300 m. / yards
* Reservations: deposit required
* Credit Cards: MC/VISA/AMEX/DC
* Open: Year round
* Rates: from DM 120/day; TAC: 10%
* **Spa on premises**: also 300 m. away
* **Spa Facilities**: indoor pool, medicinal baths, sauna, solarium, gym
* **Spa Treatments**: natural treatments,massages, diet, thermal baths, fango mud, medical
* **Spa Program**: Diet & Fitness

* Medical Supervision: 2 MD, 2 RN
* No. of customers per doctor: 18

DESCRIPTION: Small spa hotel with cure and sports facilities. The spa offers a special 7 nights Diet Program based on natural treatments.

HINDELANG
➲ 8324
✈ Munich Airport (MUC) 160 km. / 100 mi.
Zürich Int'l Airport (ZRH) Switzerland

Hindelang or Prinz-Luitpold-Bad is a small Bavarian spa on a mountain slope overlooking Bad Oberdorf. Situated at an altitude of 2,943 ft. (892 m) above sea-level, it is the highest Sulfur-Mud-Bath in Germany. The spa's reputation as a cure center goes back to the 17th century. The Spa features a modern medical section for the diagnosis of heart ailments, and circulation of the blood, and lung diseases. Hindelang is located 70 km. / 44 mi. from Lake Constance, and 160 km. (100 mi.) south of the Munich Airport, it can be reached by car via the Immenstadt-Sonthofen-Hindelang highway, or by train to Sonthofen Train Station.

Indications: The water's healing power is recommended in the treatment of: diseases of the bile system, arthritis, rheumatism, and various disturbances of the digestive system. The highly active mud is used in combination with the spa water as a cure in the treatment of rheumatism, chronic infections, female abdominal complaints, convalescence following operations, accidents, and sport injuries. In addition to its thermal water, and mineral rich mud, the spa uses extracts of the mountain fir tree as special baths for strengthening the nervous system, as well as nervous disturbances. A combination of sulfuric baths with natural carbonic acid is used in the treatment of heart diseases.

Hotel Prinz-Luitpold-Bad
♥♥♥♥

Orsteil Bad Oberdorf, D-87541. Hindelang, Bavarian Alps. Tel: (8324) 8900. Fax: (8324) 890379. TYPE: Mountain Hotel & Spa. MANAGER: A. Gross family. LOCATION: In the Bavarian Alps overlooking Bad Oberdorf. SPA CLIENTELE:

Women and men. Teenagers and children accepted.

* Rooms: 110 w/priv. bath
* Phone, CTV, C/H, radio
* Restaurant, bar, terrace café, jacuzzi
* Airport: Munich Airport, 160 km. (100 mi.)
* Airport Transportation: car, bus, train
* Train Station: Sonthofen, 9 km. (6 mi.)
* Credit Cards: Visa
* Open: Year round
* Hotel Rates: from DM 160; TAC: 8%
* Spa on premises
* Year Established: 1864
* Spa Facilities: indoor and outdoor thermal pools (at 86°F / 30°c), mud baths, sauna, mud grotto, whirlpool, solarium, gym, medical center, aerosol-station; Beauty Salon
* Spa Treatments: therapeutic mineral, mud and aerotherm baths, underwater massage, under-water intestine bath, inhalations, Kneipp therapy
* Spa Program: Medical programs for heart, lung and blood circulation; Diet/Fitness, Beauty
* Medical Supervision: 1 MD, 1 RN
* Number of customers per Doctor: about 30
* Treatments Approved: by all German health insurance plans, and by the government

DESCRIPTION: Prinz-Luitpold-Bad is a family run health resort in the Bavarian Alps amidst magnificent mountains. The Spa hotel (built in 1864) has a typical rustic Bavarian style, and it caters mainly to a mature clientele. The spa offers a private sulfur spring and curative mud bath. Those who are in a perfect good health can enjoy the revitalizing effects of mineral rich mud baths and thermal spa water. Kneipp treatments, as well as beauty treatments and mas-sages are available for relaxation and revitalization.

Romantik Hotel Bad-Hotel Sonne
❤❤❤❤

Markstraße 15, Hindelang D-87541. Tel: (8324) 8970. Fax: (8324) 899143. TYPE: Spa Hotel. LOCATION: In the Bavarian Alps. SPA CLIENTELE: Women and men. DESCRIP-TION: Elegant Spa hotel with cure facilities and diet cui-

sine.60 rooms, bar, restaurant. Hotel rates: from DM 122.

JUIST
⤷ **4935**
✈ Bremen Airport (BRE) 7 km. / 4 mi.

Nordsee-Hotel Freese
❤❤❤❤

Wilhelmstraße 60/61. Juist D-26571. Tel: (4935) 8010. Fax: (4935) 1803. TYPE: Spa Hotel. LOCATION: Quiet location in private park. SPA CLIENTELE: Women and men. DESCRIPTION: Elegant spa hotel with solarium, massages, and beauty treatments. Diet cuisine available. 80 rooms, indoor pool. Hotel rates: from DM 165.

KASSEL
⤷ **561**
✈ Kassel Calden Airport 35 km. / 22 mi.

Parkhotel Emstaler Höhe
❤❤❤❤

Kissinger Straße, Bad Emstal-Sand D-34308. Tel: (5624) 5090. Fax: (5624) 509200. TYPE: Spa Hotel. LOCATION: Bad Emstal-Sand. SPA CLIENTELE: Women and men. DESCRIPTION: Elegant spa hotel with thermal springs, cure facilities, fitness room, solarium. Hotel rates: from DM 180.

RODACH bei Coburg
⤷ **9564**
✈ Nürnberg Airport (NUE) 95 km. / 60 mi.

Kurhotel am Thermalbad
❤❤❤❤

Kurring 2, Rodach bei Coburg D-96476. Tel: (9564) 207/208. Fax: (9564) 206. TYPE: Spa Hotel. LOCATION: Quiet scenic location. SPA CLIENTELE: Women and men. DESCRIPTION: Elegant spa hotel with cure facilities and beauty treatments. 50 rooms. Hotel rates: from DM 120.

SCHLANGEBAD
⏳ 6129

✈ Frankfurt Airport (FRA) 20 mi. / 32 km. NE

Parkhotel Schlangebad
♥♥♥♥

Rhingauer Str. 47, Schlangebad D-65388. Tel: (6129) 420. Fax: (6129) 41420. TYPE: Spa Hotel. LOCATION: On private park. SPA CLIENTELE: Women and men. DESCRIPTION: Traditional spa hotel with health club, solarium and beauty farm. 84 rooms, 4 suites, restaurant, weinstube, indoor and outdoor pool. Hotel rates: from DM 190.

SCHLIERSEE
⏳ 8026

✈ Munich Airport (MUC) 50 km. / 31 mi.

Annabella Alpenhotel
♥♥♥♥

Spitzingstraße 5, Schliersee D-83727. Tel: (8026) 7980. Fax: (8026) 798879. TYPE: Resort & Spa. LOCATION: Bavarian Alps. SPA CLIENTELE: Women and men. DESCRIPTION: Popular Bavarian Chalet resort with Beauty Farm, Fitness Center and glass enclosed brine thermal pool. 122 rooms, restaurant, bar. Hotel rates: from DM 245.

SEESEN
⏳ 5381

✈ Hannover Airport (HAJ) 50 km. / 31 mi.

Hotel Seesen mit Beautyfarm
♥♥♥

Lauthenthaler Str. 70, Seesen D-38723. Tel: (5381) 5381. Fax: (5381) 2090. TYPE: Spa Hotel. LOCATION: Hartz mountains. SPA CLIENTELE: Mostly women. DESCRIPTION: Intimate Spa hotel with a Beauty farm. Hotel rates: from DM 120.

SPEYER
⏳ 6232

✈ Frankfurt Airport (FRA) 44 mi. / 70 km.

RR Binshof Resort
♥♥♥♥♥

Binshop 1, Speyer D-67346. Tel: (6232) 6470. Fax: (6232) 647199. TYPE: Resort Hotel & Spa. SPA CLIENTELE: Women and men. LOCATION: Frankfurt area off A61by the Rhein river.

* Rooms: 80 w/priv. bath
* Phone, CTV, minibar, hairdryer
* Restaurant: fitness & health bistro
* Reservations: required
* Credit Cards: VISA/AMEX/MC/DIS/EC
* SPA on premises
* **SPA Facilities**: thermal baths, sauna, beauty farm, gym, medical and treatment facilities
* **SPA Programs**: Thalassotherapy, beauty & pampering fitness, medical, anti stress
* **Spa Treatments**: aromatherapy, full body massage, foot massage, manual lymphdrainage, natural mudpacks from the Dead Sea, moor mud packs, algae packs, cleopatra bath, creme bath, movement therapy, electrotherapy, ice therapy, acupuncture, pain reduction therapy, beauty treatments of Borghese.
* Medical Supervision: medical clinic

DESCRIPTION: Elegant resort with first class atmosphere offering thermal cures with medical service and beauty and pampering treatments at the Beauty Farm.

TIMMENDORFER STRAND
⏳ 4503

✈ Fuhlsbuttel Airport (HAM) 53 mi. / 85 km.

Maritim Seehotel
♥♥♥♥

An der Waldkapelle 26, Timmendorfer Strand D-23669.

Tel: (4503) 6050. Fax: (4503) 2932. TYPE: Resort Hotel & Spa. LOCATION: Forest area near the Baltic Sea. SPA CLIENTELE: Women and men. DESCRIPTION: Elegant resort hotel with fitness room, solarium, massages, therapeutic baths, natural health center, and beauty farm. 194 rooms, restaurant, pub, coffee shop, 36 holes of golf, 5 tennis courts. Hotel rates: from DM 370.

WIESBADEN
⅃ 611

✈ Frankfurt Airport (FRA) 20 mi. / 32 km. NE

Wiesbaden, population 250,000, is a world famous spa town occupying a sheltered position between the Rhine and the Taunus Mountains. Wiesbaden is only 20 min. by car from Frankfurt, and can be reached by regular train service.

The history of the spa is traced back to Roman times when the healing powers were first discovered. Today there are 26 mineral springs with temperature of 67°c (150°F). Public spa facilities include: **Opelbad**, one of Germany's finest open-air thermal pools situated in the fresh mountain air and the Aukamm Thermal Baths that include indoor and outdoor open-air pools, massage rooms, solariums, sauna and gymnasium. During the winter you may take a dip in the warm pools (34°c/85°F) while the snow is falling.

Indications: the following illnesses can be treated at Wiesbaden Spa - illnesses of the respiratory organs, rheumatic diseases, illnesses of the locomotorium, and after treatment of accident injuries.

Aukamm Hotel
♥♥♥♥

Aukamm Allee 31, 6200 Wiesbaden. Tel: (611) 5760. Fax: (611) 576264. TYPE: Spa Hotel. LOCATION: In a fashionable residential area, across from the Spa Gardens, next to the Clinic for Diagnostic, 5 min. from downtown Wiesbaden. SPA CLIENTELE: Women and men.

* Rooms: 158 w/priv. bath & balcony. Suites: 12
* Restaurants, Beer Pub, nightclub

* Airport: Frankfurt International, 25 km. (16 mi.)
* Airport Transportation: taxi, limo, train
* Credit Cards: MC/VISA/AMEX/DC/CB
* Open: Year round
* Hotel Rates: from DM 290
* Spa off premises
* Distance to the Spa: 100 m. (100 yards)
* Spa Facilities: 5 saunas, Roman-Irish baths, Extensive spa gardens with hiking and jogging trails, cosmetic studio
* Spa Treatments: massages, beauty treatments (at the hotel); thermal pools, sauna, solarium, gym at the nearby spa
* Spa Program: fitness program

DESCRIPTION: Modern deluxe hotel with comfortable rooms, balconies, in house video (English available), meeting rooms, and spectacular views over Wiesbaden. Conveniently located to all the spa activities.

Hotel Baeren
♥♥

Baerenstrasse 3, 6200 Wiesbaden. Tel: (611) 301021. Fax: (611) 301024. TYPE: Spa Hotel. LOCATION: Centrally located near the Kurhaus and the theatre. SPA CLIENTELE: Women and men, family oriented.

* Rooms: 60 w/private bath
* Airport: Frankfurt Airport, 30 km. / 19 mi.
* Airport Transportation: train
* Reservations: not required
* Credit Cards: MC/VISA/AMEX/DC
* Rates: DM 90 - DM 220/day; TAC: 8%
* Spa on premises
* **Spa Facilities**: Own thermal baths, Massage rooms; other spa facilities are available at the public Wiesbaden spas
* **Spa Treatments**: balneotherapy, massages
* Medical Supervision: yes

DESCRIPTION: An old historic hotel built in the early 17th century with its own thermal hot springs featuring mainly in house medical spa treatments.

Schwarzer Bock Hotel
❤❤❤❤

12 Kranzplatz, 6200 Wiesbaden. Tel: (611) 1550. Fax: (611) 155111. TYPE: Spa Hotel. LOCATION: Downtown near spa facilities. SPA CLIENTELE: Women and men.

* Rooms: 150 w/priv. bath, Suites: 20
* Phone, CTV, mini-bar, radio
* Roof Garden Restaurant
* Airport: Frankfurt 30 km. / 19 mi.
* Train Station: Wiesbaden 2 km. / 1 mi.
* Train/Airport Transport: pick up on request
* Credit Cards: AMEX/VISA/MC/DC/EC
* Season: Year round
* Rates: from DM 375/day
* TAC: 10%

* Spa on premises
* **Spa Facilities**: Wiesbaden spa, in hotel spa facilities - indoor thermal pool, exercise room, massage parlor, thermal tub baths, sauna, solarium, health spa, Japanese therapy bath
* **Spa Treatments**: balneotherapy , carbonic-acid/oxygen bath, mud packs, underwater massage, connective tissue massage, exercise
* **Indications**: rheumatism, arthrose, gout, sciatica, discopathy, neuralgias, accidental injuries, muscular pains, after-treatments, postural disturbances, nervous strain, sleeplessness

DESCRIPTION: The most distinguished hotel in Wiesbaden. The 500 years old hotel is decorated in Teutonic architecture, antiques and valuable objets d'art from different periods. The Schwarzer Bock offers thermal pool, sauna, solarium for physical fitness and spa therapy.

Photo courtesy of the **Lancaster Beauty Spa**

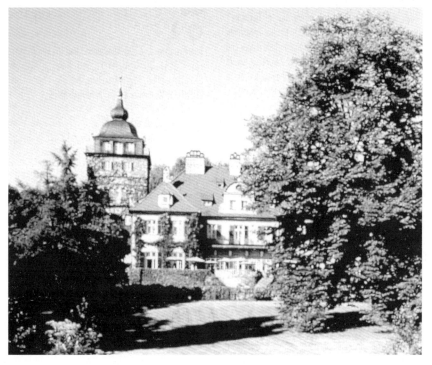

GREAT BRITAIN

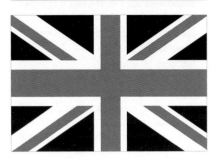

AREA: 94,399 sq. mi. (244,493 sq. km.)
POPULATION: 55,700,000
CAPITAL: London
OFFICIAL LANGUAGE: English
CURRENCY: Pound Sterling (UK£)
EXCHANGE RATE: 1US$ = £0.60
TELEPHONE COUNTRY CODE: 44

ⓘ British Travel Centre
12 Regent's Street, London SW1 England

ⓘ British Tourist Authority
551 Fifth Ave, Ste 701, New York NY 10176-0799
Tel: (212) 986-2200. Fax: (212) 986-1188
Toll Free: (800) 462-2748

BATH
⌁ 1225

 Bristol Airport Lulsgate (BRS)

Bath, population 85,000, is an historic spa town. According to tradition the city was built by the father of Shakespeare's King Lear who found cure for a dreadful disease while bathing in the hot and healing springs of Bath. However, the true history of Bath's spa began much earlier in Roman times like many other great European Spas.

Bath Spa Hotel
♥♥♥♥♥

🝆 🐎 🏃

Sydney Rd., Bath BA2 6JF. Tel: (1225) 444424. Fax: (1225) 444006. TYPE: Spa Hotel. LOCATION: On landscaped grounds 10 min. from the centre of town. SPA CLIENTELE: Women and men.

* Rooms: 98 w/private bath. Suites: 6
* Train Station: Bath, 15 minutes
* Credit Cards: VISA/AMEX/DC
* Open: Year round
* Rates: from £120/day
* Spa on premises
* **Spa Facilities**: sauna, solarium, gym, indoor pool, beauty salon, whirlpool
* **Spa Treatments**: body massage, G5 massage, body wraps, dietary advice, aromatherapy, electrolysis, slendertone, physiotherapy, special diets
* **Indications**: beauty, pampering, weight loss

DESCRIPTION: Beautifully restored 1830's Georgian Mansion featuring Leisure Club with health, beauty and fitness treatments.

Combe Grove Manor Hotel & Country Club
♥♥♥♥

🝆 🐎 🏃

Brassknocker Hill., Monkton Combe, Bath BA2 7HS. Tel: (1225) 834644. Fax: (1225) 834961. TYPE: Spa Hotel. LOCATION: On landscaped grounds 10 min. from the centre of town. SPA CLIENTELE: Women and men.

* Rooms: 40 w/private bath. Suites: 3
* Train Station: Bath, 15 minutes
* Credit Cards: VISA/AMEX/DC
* Open: Year round
* Rates: from £110/day
* Spa on premises
* **Spa Facilities**: Beauty Clinic & Spa complex, hydrospa, steam room, sauna, solarium
* **Spa Treatments**: aromatherapy massage, traditional massage, fitness classes, aerobics
* **Indications**: anti-stress, rejuvenation

DESCRIPTION: Elegant Georgian Manor hotel in building

dated from 1694 situated in a scenic valley. Individually decorated rooms and suites with marble bath, furnished with antiques and period furniture. The Spa specializes in beauty, pampering and relaxation services. Recreation: tennis, golf, jogging.

DROITWICH SPA
〉 1905

✈ Birmingham Int'l Airport (BHX)

Droitwich Spa's unique brine baths are Britain's biggest Spa development in this century. The brine is pumped from an underground lake containing 30% natural salt in a concentration that is similar to that of the Dead Sea in Israel.

In 1985 a Brine Bath was opened in the middle of Droitwich with its pool under the same roof as the Worchestershire Clinic. The Brine Bath is open to the public 7 days a week for recreation and relaxation. Special Spa treatments available at the Brine Bath include: Hydrotherapy under medical supervision of specialized physiotherapists.

Indications: treatments at the spa are beneficial to patients who have difficulty moving their limbs or suffering pains from arthritis, neurological conditions, post-orthopedic operations, or after sport injury. The particular buoyancy of the water allows for easier therapy and rehabilitation. The Spa is also recommended for the general purpose of relaxation and well-being.

Chateau Impney Hotel
♥♥♥♥

Droitwich Spa, Worchestershire LR9 OBN. Tel: (1905) 774-411. Fax: (1905) 772371. TYPE: Luxury Hotel. LOCATION: 1 mi. from Exit 5 M5 Motorway, 1/2 hour from Stratford Upon Avon. CLIENTELE: Family oriented.

* Rooms: 65 w/private bath. Suites: 9
* Train Station: Droitwich, 5 minutes
* Train Station Transportation: pick up
* Credit Cards: VISA/AMEX/DC
* Season: Year round (closed Xmas)

* Rates: from £100/day
* Spa off premises
* Distance to the Spa: 1 mi. (1.6 km.)
* **Spa Facilities**: Brine Pool at the Droitwich Spa
* **Spa Treatments**: Hydrotherapy, bathing in warm mineral water
* **Indications**: see above

DESCRIPTION: Elegant French style Chateau accommodations on 65 acres of parkland and landscaped gardens. The hotel is conveniently located for those who wish to experience the spa facilities at the Droitwich Spa Brine Baths. Other activities include: horseback riding, tennis and fine Continental dining. Member: Impney Hotels.

GRAYSHOTT
〉 1905

✈ Heathrow Airport (LHR) / Gatwick Airport (LGW)

Grayshott, population 2,000, is located in southeast England in the county of Surrey, one of the smallest yet one of the loveliest counties in the country. Surrey, is an ideal place for a peaceful, get-away-from-it-all holidays in an authentic English countryside. Grayshott Hall can be reached by car from London via the A3 to Hindhead. Trains from Waterloo to Halsemere run twice an hour and take 55 minutes.

Grayshott Hall
♥♥♥♥

Grayshott near Hindhead, Surrey. Tel: (142873) 4331. TYPE: Deluxe Health Spa. LOCATION: In the beautiful countryside. SPA CLIENTELE: Women and men.

* Rooms: 8 luxury double/twin rooms w/private bath in the Main house. 72 bedrooms are available at the Main Wing and the Century Wing (single rooms w/showers & private patio)
* Light Diet Room
* Airport: London, 55 minutes, train, taxi
* Reservations: deposit required
* Credit Cards: AMEX/DC/ACC
* Open: Year round

* Rates: About $1,200/week (8 days/7 nights), rates include - accommodations, beauty and selected Spa treatments
* Spa on premises
* **Spa Facilities**: treatment rooms, fully equipped gym, heated indoor pool, jacuzzi, sauna, steam cabinets, variety of beauty and therapy salons
* **Spa Programs**: Fitness, weight loss or weight gain, relaxation, pampering, beauty care
* **Spa Treatments**: exercise, body workout, aerobics, callistenics, yoga, relaxation, weight training, impulse showers, friction rubs, blanket wrap, panthermal, Swedish massage, G5 deep toning massage, slendertone, aromatherapy, reflexology, hair & skin treatments, wholesome and fresh low cal gourmet meals
* **Indications**: see above

DESCRIPTION: Grayshott Hall is one of the oldest health Spas in England. Located on 47 acres of landscaped grounds, the Victorian mansion offers elegant accommodations decorated in Old English Country style. The European hydrotherapy spa features a complete health and beauty programs with emphasis on fitness, weight loss and pampering. Recreation: golf, croquet, tennis and badminton.

HENLOW
☎ 1462
✈ Heathrow Airport (LHR) / Gatwick Airport (LGW)

Henlow is a small village in Mid Bedfordshire north of London. Henlow Grange is accessible by car from London via M1 north to Luton, than A505 east to Hitchin, then A600 to A6001 leading to Henlow.

Henlow Grange Health Farm
💗💗💗💗

Henlow Grange, Henlow, Bedfordshire. Tel: (1462) 811111. Fax: (1462) 815310. TYPE: Health Farm. LOCATION: In a private park overlooking the River Hiz. SPA CLIENTELE: Women and men.

* Rooms: 80 w/priv. bath, Suites: 8
* Phone, CTV, C/H, cooking facilities, jacuzzi.
* Restaurant, bar
* Airport: London Heathrow, 45 minutes
* Reservations: deposit required
* Credit Cards: VISA/DC/MC
* Open: Year round.
* Rates: from £125; TAC: 10%.
* Spa on premises
* **Spa Facilities**: 25m. indoor pool (ozone treated), whirlpool, sauna, steam and plunge pools, Life Fitness gymnasium.
* **Spa Programs**: Exercise, Beauty Care.
* **Spa Packages**: on request
* **Spa Treatments**: Body massage, G5 massages, hydrotherapy, diets, aromatherapy, physiotherapy, reflexology, wax bath, volcanic mud, seaweed baths, electrolysis, facials, bust treatments, body wraps

DESCRIPTION: A Georgian style mansion amidst a huge park along a peaceful river with plenty of fresh air and nature trails. Accommodations are pleasantly decorated with a mixture of classic and contemporary English style. The Health farm features a large gym and a full service beauty salon, and separate male and female spa area. The programs emphasize fitness, general health, as well as beauty and pampering for pleasure and relaxation. Recreation: horseback riding, tennis, canoeing, fishing, and sight-seeing.

HOAR CROSS
☎ 1283
✈ Birmingham Int'l Airport (BHX) 40 mi. / 65 km.

Hoar Cross Hall
Health & Spa Resort
💗💗💗💗

Hoar Cross nr. Voxall, Staffordshire DE13 8QS. Tel: (1283) 575671. Fax: (1283) 575652. TYPE: Health Spa. LOCATION: In the countryside near historic Lichfield. SPA CLIENTELE: Women and men.

* Rooms: 80 w/priv. bath

* Phone, CTV, C/H, whirlpool bath (some)
* Restaurant, Champagne bar
* Airport: Birmingham, 30 min.
* Reservations: deposit required
* Credit Cards: VISA/DC/MC
* Open: Year round.
* Rates: from £125; TAC: 10%.
* Spa on premises
* **Spa Facilities**: hydrotherapy baths, swimming pool, fitness room, sauna, steam room
* **Spa Programs**: Exercise, beauty care, relaxation
* **Spa Packages**: on request
* **Spa Treatments**: flotation therapy, baths, massages, gym pool exercise, jet stream massage
* **Indications**: premature aging, arthritis, depression, loss of vitality

DESCRIPTION: Health spa in historic building with Palatial interiors and elegant period decor. The Spa features a wide range of programs and treatments for health, beauty, fitness and relaxation.

IPSWICH
⟩ 1442
✈ Ipswich Airport, 7 mi. / 11 km.

Ipswich, population 121,500, is an important port and industrial town in the eastern Suffolk county. Suffolk is known for its fishing villages, historic homes, and national monuments. Ipswich is located about 78 mi. (125 km.) northeast of London and can be reached from London by car via the A12, coach or train.

Shrubland Hall Health Clinic
♥♥♥

Coddenham, Ipswich, Suffolk IP6 9QH. Tel: (1473) 830404. TYPE: Health Clinic. LOCATION: 6 miles (10 km.) north of Ipswich and within easy reach of the sea. SPA CLIENTELE: Women and men.

* Rooms: 40; 21 w/private bath, Cottages: 1
* Phone, CTV, C/H
* English Garden, boutique

* Airport: Heathrow/Gatwick, 78 mi. (125 km.), taxi
* Reservations: deposit required
* No Credit Cards
* Rates: on request
* Arrival Days: Sundays & Wednesdays
* Health Clinic on premises
* Clinic Facilities: 2 heated pools, outdoor solarium for Ladies, indoor solarium for sunbathing, fully equipped gym, Physiotherapy Department, Beauty salon, sauna, steam cabinets, Turkish baths
* **Spa Programs**: Medical, Diet/Fitness & Beauty
* **Spa Treatments**: massage, under-water massage, Kneipp water therapy, herbal baths, peat baths, aromatherapy, seaweed baths, colonic irrigation, specialized physiotherapy, manipulative therapies, postural re-education, private instruction in relaxation, exercise classes, spot reducing, diet based on raw food, salads, health food, dairy products
* Medical Supervision: 2 MD, 4 RN
* Treatments Approved: not officially

DESCRIPTION: Shrubland Hall is an historic 18th century chateau style mansion with a spectacular English garden in the style of the Villa d'Este near Rome. Guests accommodations vary in style but all are furnished in Old English Country style with antiques and objets d'arts. The aim of Shrubland Hall Health clinic is to assist in restoring the fullest health potential of each individual. Upon arrival each guest receives a thorough medical examination by staff doctor, which determine the nature of one's program or treatments. The supportive atmosphere and the tranquil English Country elegance help reduce stress, and facilitate the diet and health treatments. Recreation: billiard games, library and music room, tennis, fishing club, horseback riding, and visits to nearby places of interest.

KINTBURY
⟩ 1488
✈ Heathrow Airport (LHR) / Gatwick Airport (LGW)

Inglewood Health Hydro
♥♥♥

Templeton Rd., Kintbury, Berkshire. Tel: (1488) 682022.

Fax: (1488) 682595. TYPE: Health Spa. LOCATION: On the edge of Berkshire Downs. SPA CLIENTELE: Women and men. DESCRIPTION: Health spa in the countryside one hour from London offering massages, aromatherapy, reflexology, peat bath and hydrotherapy.

LIPHOOK
↘ 1428
✈ Heathrow Airport (LHR) / Gatwick Airport (LGW)

Liphook, is located in Hampshire, some 48 mi. (77 km.) southwest of London in a garden setting overlooking a lovely lake. The area lends itself to outdoor recreation, biking, jogging, lake water sports, and fishing.

Forest Mere
♥♥♥♥

Liphook, Hampshire, GU30 7JQ. Tel: (1428) 722051. Fax: (1428) 723501. TYPE: Health Farm. LOCATION: In Hampshire close to the border of Surrey. SPA CLIENTELE: Women and men.

* Rooms: 65 w/priv. bath
* Restaurants: regular & Light Diet Room
* Airport: Heathrow or Gatwick
* Distance to Airports: 48 - 50 mi. / 77 - 80 km.
* Airport Transportation: taxi
* Season: Year round
* Hotel Rates: from £150
* Spa on Premises
* **Spa Facilities**: large indoor pool, thalassotherapy salt water hydrotherapy pool, treatment rooms (70), computerized gym, air-conditioned exercise studios (2)
* **SPA Programs**: Weight Loss, Stress Reduction, Alternative Therapies, Exercise, Beauty & Pampering
* **SPA Treatments**: acupuncture, allergy testing, aromatherapy, bach flower remedies, chinese herbalism, chiropody, feng shui, meditation, osteopathy, podiatry, reiki healing, self relaxation, shiatsu, stress management, thai massage, zen yoga, sauna, hydrother-aquatic exercises, beauty and skin treatments

DESCRIPTION: Forest Mere has reopened following a spectacular refurbishment (1998). It has transformed into one of the largest and most luxurious health spas in Great Britain. The health farm offers well structured programs emphasizing stress reduction, diet and weight management. Their fully trained and dedicated staff offer a wide range of beauty, relaxation and body treatments based on products from the best European cosmetic houses such as Clarins, Guinot, Decleor, Thalgo and their own La Zouche. For those interested in Alternative Medicine, the internationally renowned Dr. Rajendra Sharma, offers advisory services at Forest Mere in holistic health, homeopathy for healthier lifestyle.

NEW MILTON
↘ 1425
✈ Hurn Airport, 10 mi. / 16 km.

Chewton Glen Hotel
♥♥♥♥♥

Christchurch Rd., New Milton, Hampshire BH25 6QS. Tel: (1425) 275341. Fax: (1425) 272310. TYPE: Hotel & Spa. LOCATION: On Parkland acres between the New Forest and the Sea. SPA CLIENTELE: Women and men.

* Rooms: 52 w/priv. bath. Suites: 14
* Phone, CTV, C/H, mini safe, hairdryer
* Restaurant, bar with terrace, lounges (3)
* Airport: Hurn Airport, taxi
* Reservations: Required
* Credit Cards: MC, VISA, AMEX, DC
* Open: Year round
* Hotel Rates: from £210
* Spa on premises
* **Spa Facilities**: sauna, solarium, steam room, gym, exercise rooms, indoor pool, jogging track
* **Spa Programs**: Relaxation, health & fitness, beauty, firm & tone
* **Spa Treatments**: wide range of beauty, relaxation, and body toning treatments, body massage, G5 massage, physiotherapy, osteopathy, acupuncture, chiropody, dietary advice, aromatherapy, reflexology, bust treatments, Shiatsu, body wraps, alternative

therapies by appointment

* **Spa Packages**: Healthy Break packages

DESCRIPTION: Deluxe country house with health spa offering various health, beauty and pampering treatments in private rooms. Special diets available on request.

PACKINGTON
⌇ 1530
✈ East Midlands Airport

Springs Hydro
❤❤❤❤❤

Packington, Nr Ashby-de-la-Zouch, Leicestershire LE65 1TG. Tel: (1530) 273873. Fax: (1530) 270987. TYPE: Health Spa. LOCATION: In the Leicestershire countryside with excellent road links to the rest of the UK. SPA CLIENTELE: Women a nd men.

* Rooms and studios w/priv. bath
* Phone, CTV, C/H, mini safe, hairdryer
* Restaurant, bar
* Airport: East Midlands, taxi
* Reservations: Required
* Credit Cards: MC, VISA, AMEX, DC
* Open: Year round
* Hotel Rates: from £110
* Spa on premises
* Year Established: 1990
* **Spa Facilities**: Life Fitness Gym, exercise studio, spa bath, pool, treatment rooms (30), sauna, steam, indoor pool, plunge pool, whirlpool, flotation room
* **Spa Programs**: Detoxification, relaxation, health & fitness, beauty, firm & tone
* **Spa Treatments**: wide range of beauty, relaxation, and body toning treatments, physiotherapy,cosmetic products (Clarins, Aveda, Guinot, Thalgo, La Zouche) aromatherapy, flotation, hydrotherapy
* **Spa Packages**: on request

DESCRIPTION: Britain's only purpose built health farm set in the heart of England. Springs Hydro offers extensive ranges of health and beauty treatments by skilled and experienced staff. Springs Hydro specializes in calorie controlled healthy eating. Vegetarians, Kosher and special diets are available on request. Recreation: golf, practice range, croquet, tennis and basketball. Member: *Purdew Health Farm Group*

RAGDALE
⌇ 1664
✈ East Midlands Airport

Ragdale Hall
❤❤❤❤❤

Ragdale Village, Near Melton Mobray, Leicestershire LE14 3PB. Tel: (1664) 434831, Fax: (1664) 434587. TYPE: Deluxe Health Resort. LOCATION: Heart of the Leicestershire countryside. SPA CLIENTELE: Women and men. AGE RESTRICTIONS: Must be 16 years old.

* Rooms: 64 Suites: 4 all with private bath
* Phone, CTV, C/H
* Restaurant, bar
* Airport: East Midlands
* Train Station: Melton Mowbray
* Airport/Train Station Transportation: Taxi
* Reservations: Required
* Credit Cards: MC, VISA, AMEX, DC
* Open: Year round
* Hotel Rates: from £90
* Spa on premises
* Year Established: 1970
* **Spa Facilities**: Gym, exercise studio, pool, spa bath, sauna, steam, plunge pool, tennis, hair salon, suncentre
* **Spa Programs**: Detoxification, relaxation, health & fitness, beauty, firm & tone
* **Spa Treatments**: multi method massages, G5 massage, ionithermie, aromatherapy, seaweed baths, body wraps, Shiatsu, flotation, manicure, pedicure, waxing, floatation, hydrotherapy, cathiodermie, reflexology, oesteopathy, cairopody, stress management, computerized fitness assessment, metabolic rate test, diet advice, cholesterol test, slendertone
* **Spa Packages**: Midweek Special; Healthy Holiday (6 nts); Relaxer Break (24 hrs.), Ragdale Day;

Select Day, Luxury Day. Rates: from £79
* Length Of Stay Required: Minimum 2 nights

DESCRIPTION: Ragdale Hall is a converted country house, built in 1785 and set in a beautiful Leicestershire countryside. The spa offers separate Ladies and Men's spa facilities with a wide variety of beauty and health treatments.

TAPLOW (London)
⟩ 1628
✈ Heathrow Airport (LHR), Gatwick Airport (LGW)

Cliveden
❤❤❤❤❤

Taplow, Buckinghamshire SL6 0JF. Tel: (1628) 668561. Fax: (1628) 661837. TYPE: Hotel & Spa. LOCATION: Set in 376 acres of manicured gardens overlooking the Thames. SPA CLIENTELE: Women and men.

* Rooms: 38 rooms w/priv. bath. Suites: 10
* Phone, CTV, C/H
* Restaurants (3), bars (3), lounges (3)
* Airports: Heathrow or Gatwick
* Airport/Train Station Transportation: limo
* Reservations: Required
* Credit Cards: MC, VISA, AMEX, DC
* Open: Year round
* Hotel Rates: from £190
* Spa on premises
* **Spa Facilities**: sauna, solarium, steam room, gym, indoor/outdoor pools
* **Spa Programs**: Beauty & Pampering, Fitness
* **Spa Treatments**: body massage, G5 massage, wax bath, reflexology, electrolysis, facials, bust treatments, body wraps, thalassotherapy, body exfoliation, percussion massage, cellulite treatment, fitness
* **Spa Packages**: The Cliveden Week End

DESCRIPTION: Superior Deluxe hotel in a Stately Home & Country Estate, former residence of three dukes, a Prince of wales and the Astor Family. The health spa with separate salons for women, offer a full range of health, leisure and

sporting activities. Recreation: tennis, golf, fishing.

TAUNTON
⟩ 1823
✈ Bristol Airport Lulsgate (BRS) 40 mi. / 64 km.

Taunton, population 40,000, is a resort town in the warm region of southwest England. The area is attracting many tourists and holiday makers to the Dartmoor National Park, and the popular beach resorts of Torquay and Newquay.

Cedar Falls Health Farm is conveniently located for access by main line rail and motorway networks. Driving time from London is 2-1/2 hours, or 1 hour from Bristol. If you drive from London and South Wales use the M4/M5, and from Bristol/Midlands and Devon use the M5.

Cedar Falls Health Farm
❤❤❤❤

Bishops Lydeard, Taunton, TA4 3HR. Tel: (1823) 433233. Fax: (1823) 432777. TYPE: Health Resort Complex. LOCATION: In the foothills of the Quantock Hill, near the Exmoor National Park. SPA CLIENTELE: Women and men.

* Rooms: 33 w/priv. bath. Suites: 2
* Dining Rooms
* Airport: Bristol, taxi
* Reservations: deposit required
* Credit Cards: VISA/AMEX/ACC
* Open: Year round
* Hotel Rates: from £120/day;
* Spa on Premises
* **Spa Facilities**: Beauty & Clinic departments, indoor/outdoor pools, sauna, steam rooms, solarium, whirlpool, aerobic rooms, gym, walking/jogging trails
* **Spa Programs**: Diet & Weight Management, Beauty & Pampering, Fitness
* **Spa Treatments**: aqua-aerobics, flotation, G5 massage, relaxation classes, yoga, dance and body shaping, calisthenics, Swedish massage, hydrotherapy, aromatherapy,

acupuncture, ostheopathy, reflexology, iridology, 600-700 calorie diet, beauty treatments (Clarins, Guinot, Thalgo), natural therapies
* Medical Supervision: MD on call

DESCRIPTION: An 18th century English country mansion with a complete Health Farm. The Spa specializes in face and body treatments with special attention given to wholesome, natural, and calorie counted menus. All Spa personnel are qualified in their own fields. Recreation: 9 hole golf course, croquet and putting greens, fly fishing in trout lakes, and tennis, gliding, squash, and dry slope skiing nearby.

TORQUAY
⟩ 1803
✈ Exeter Airport (EXT) 30 mi. / 48 km.

Lorrens Health Hydro
♥♥♥

Cary Park, Babbacombe, Torquay TQ1 3NN. Tel: (1803) 323740 or 329994. TYPE: Health Spa. LOCATION: In the famous English Riviera. SPA CLIENTELE: Women and men. DESCRIPTION: Health spa offering massages, beauty treatments and dietary advice. Rates: from £198.

WIGGINTON
⟩ 1442
✈ Heathrow Airport (LHR) / Gatwick Airport (LGW)

Champneys
♥♥♥♥♥

Wigginton, Tring, Hertfordshire HP23 6HY, England. Tel: (1442) 291111, Fax: (1442) 291001. TYPE: Deluxe Health Resort. LOCATION: In the Chiltern Valleys. SPA CLIENTELE: Women and men. SPECIAL RESTRICTIONS: Must be 16 years of age or older.

* Rooms: 63 w/priv. bath. Suites: 3
* Phone, CTV, C/H, minibar, jacuzzi
* Restaurant, bar, nightclub
* Airport: London Heathrow 25 mi. / 40 km. approx. 40 min.
* Train Station: Berkhamsted, 4 mi. / 6 km.
* Airport/Train Station Transportation: taxi, limo
* Reservations: Required
* Credit Cards: MC, VISA, AMEX, ACCESS
* Open: Year round
* Rates: from £160
* TAC: 10%
* Spa on premises
* **Spa Facilities**: sauna, solarium, steam room, steam cabinets, gym. indoor pool, beauty salon, whirlpool, herbal bath, squash, tennis
* **Spa Programs**: Physical fitness, mental health, beauty & pampering, back-care
* **Spa Treatments**: Aromatherapy, aromazone, acupuncture, aerobics, blood pressure checks, bust, bio-peel, body conditioning circuit, cholesterol testing, cathoidermie, chiropody, depilatory waxing, dry float (hay, mud, Cleopatra), eye treatment course, fitness assessment, faradism, facials, galvanism, hydrotherapy, medical consultations & screening, massage, neck treatment course, osteopathy, physiotherapy, paraffin wax treatments, pedicure, seaweed body wrap, salt glow, slendertone, shiatsu, stress management, tai chi chuan, thai massage, underwater & vibro massages, waxing & bleaching
* Length of Stay: Minimum 2 nights / 3 days
* Medical Supervision: MD 1, RN 6

DESCRIPTION: Champneys at Tring is one of the oldest and most respected health spas in Great Britain. Established over 70 years ago it is housed in an elegant Victorian Rothschild Mansion. It occupies 170 landscaped acres above the Vale of Aylesbury on the edge of the Chilterns. Guest rooms are tastefully decorated with facilities that you would expect from a luxury hotel. The rooms offer peaceful views. During your stay you will learn how to have a healthier and more enjoyable life. All meals are calorie counted. The resort recreates a unique ambiance where you can feel good about yourself both inside and out.

SCOTLAND

ⓘ Scottish Tourist Board
23 Ravelston Terrace, Edinburgh EH4 3EU, Scotland UK
Tel: (+44-131) 343-1608. Fax: (+44-131) 343-1844
Email: conventionbureau@stb.gov.uk
Web: www.convention.scotland.net

AUCHTERARDER
⟩ 1764
✈ Glasgow Int'l Airport (GLA)
Edinburgh Int'l Airport (EDI) 35 mi. / 56 km.

Champneys the Health Spa
♥♥♥♥♥

🖐 ✺ ◉

c/o Gleneagles Hotel, Auchterarder, Pertshire PH3 1NF,
Scotland. Tel: (1764) 662231,Fax: (1764) 662134.
TYPE: Luxury Resort & Spa. LOCATION: Set in its own 830
acre estate near Auchterarder. 50 mi. / 80 km. from
Edinburgh. SPA CLIENTELE: Women and men.

* Rooms: 234 w/priv. bath. Suites: 18
* Phone, CTV, minibar, jacuzzi
* Restaurants: Elegant Strathearn (Scottish),
  'The Conservatory' (international)
* Airports: Edinburgh / Glasgow
* Train Station: Gleneagles
* Airport Transportation: taxi, limo
* Reservations: required
* Credit Cards: MC/VISA/AMEX/DC
* Open: Year round
* Hotel Rates: from £130
* TAC: 8% (room only)
* Spa on premise
* Spa Facilities: 22 m. lagoon shaped pool, jacuzzi &
  Canadian hot-tubs, sauna & Turkish bath, fully equipped
  gym, solarium, massage rooms,Beauty Salon
* Spa Programs: Health & Leisure
* Spa Treatments: beauty treatments based on Clarins,
  Christian Dior and Rene Guinot products,
  cathiodermie, steam cabinet and spa bath, body

massage, back massage, G5 massage, aromatherapy.
* Indications: fitness, diet, beauty

DESCRIPTION: A palatial hotel with excellent service, elegant decor and fine international dining. Health & Beauty
programs are available at the Spa for those who wish to
relax, loose a few pounds and improve their appearance.
Gleneagles has gained an international reputation for its
four golf courses. The Country Club features facilities for
tennis, croquet, bowling and shooting clay pigeons.
Member: *The Leading Hotels of the World.*

EAST KILBRIDE
⟩ 13552
✈ Glasgow Int'l Airport (GLA) 15 mi. / 24 km.

Stakis East Kilbride
♥♥♥♥♥

🖐 ✺ ◉

Steartfield Way, Philipshill, East Kilbride, Strathclyde G74
5LA. Tel: (1355) 236300. Fax: (1355) 233552. TYPE:
Hotel & Spa. LOCATION: In town center close to Glasgow.
SPA CLIENTELE: Women and men. DESCRIPTION: First class
traditional hotel with leisure club and spa. Spa facilities:
sauna, solarium, steam room, gym, indoor pool, whirlpool,
plunge pool, aerobics studio. Spa treatments: body massage, aromatherapy, reflexology, waxing, Clarins beauty
treatments. 99 rooms, restaurants, bars. Hotel rates: from
£91.

EDINBURGH
⟩ 131
✈ Edinburgh Int'l Airport (EDI) 6 mi. / 10 km.

The Balmoral Edinburgh
♥♥♥♥♥

🖐 ✺ ◉

Princes St., Edinburgh EH2 2EQ. Tel: (131) 556-2414.
Fax: (131) 557-3747. TYPE: Hotel & Spa. LOCATION:
Right in the heart of Edinburgh overlooking Edinburgh
Castle & Gardens. SPA CLIENTELE: Women and men.
DESCRIPTION: Traditional Edwardian hotel with full service
health & beauty spa, sauna, solarium, steam room, indoor

pool. Spa treatments: body massage, aromatherapy, reflexology, facials. 189 rooms, 22 suites, restaurant, brasserie, bars, tea room. Hotel rates: from £130.

Dalmahoy Hotel Golf & Country Club
♥♥♥♥♥

Nr. Edinburgh, Midlothian EH27 8EB. Tel: (131) 333-1845. Fax: (131) 333-1433. TYPE: Golf Hotel & Spa. LOCATION: Set in 1,000 acres of beautiful lakes, streams and trees, 7 mi. / 11 km. west of Edinburgh. SPA CLIENTELE: Women and men. DESCRIPTION: Magnificent Georgian mansion with Spa, sauna, jacuzzi, swimming pool, steam room, sunbeds, fitness room, squash, tennis court, golf courses. Spa treatments: body massage, G5 massage and vacuum suction, muscle toning, holistic aromatherapy, facials, electrolysis.

PEEBLES
✈ 1721
✈ Edinburgh Int'l Airport (EDI)

Peebles, population 6,700, ia a small, medieval and aristocratic town south of Edinburgh on the river Tweed. nearby Rttrick Forest was once a favorite hunting place for Scottish Royalty. Nearby Edinburgh, population 420,000, is the administrative and cultural capital of Scotland.

Peebles Hydro Hotel
♥♥♥♥♥

Innerleithen Road, Peebles EH45 8LX. Tel: (1721) 720602. Fax: (1721) 722999. TYPE: Hotel & Spa. LOCATION: Set in 35 acres overlooking the Tweed Valley, 20 mi / 32 km south of Edinburgh. SPA CLIENTELE: Women and men. DESCRIPTION: Elegant hotel and conference center with Health & Fitness Spa. Spa facilities: sauna, solarium, steam room, gym, indoor pool, beauty salon. Spa treatments: body massage, G5 massage, aromatherapy, waxing, electrolysis, facials, slendertone. 137 rooms, 2 suites, dining room, coffee shop, putting green, tennis, croquet, golf. Hotel rates: from £55.

ST. ANDREWS
✈ 1334
✈ Edinburgh Int'l Airport (EDI) 40 mi. / 64 km.

The Old Course Hotel Golf Resort & Spa
♥♥♥♥♥

St. Andrews, Kingdom of Fife KY16 9SP. Tel: (1334) 474371. Fax: (1334) 477668. TYPE: Luxury Resort & Spa. LOCATION: Overlooking golf course. SPA CLIENTELE: Women and men.

* Rooms: 125 w/priv. bath. Suites: 17
* Phone, CTV, C/H, minibar, balcony with view
* Restaurants (2), bar, pub, library
* Airport: Edinburgh, taxi, limo
* Reservations: required
* Credit Cards: MC/VISA/AMEX/DC
* Open: Year round
* Hotel Rates: from £195; TAC: 8% (room only)
* **Spa Facilities**: solarium, steam room, saunas, cardio vascular room, weights room, pool, whirlpool, treatment rooms (5)
* **Spa Programs**: Anti Stress, beauty, pampering
* **Spa Treatments**: Swedish body massage, reflexology, aromatherapy, parafin wax, algae/mud wraps, facials, bust treatments, fitness services, swimming lessons
* **Spa Packages**: Spa Taster, Anti Stress, Detoxifying

DESCRIPTION: Stately Golf hotel with health spa. The full service health spa is open to hotel guests, members of the spa and outsiders when on a treatment package. The Duke's course is located 2 mi. / 3 km. from the hotel.

TROON
✈ 1292
✈ Glasgow Int'l Airport (GLA)

Marine Highland Hotel
♥♥♥♥♥

Troon, Ayrshire KA10 6HE. Tel: (1292) 314444. Fax: (1291) 316922. TYPE: Hotel & Spa. LOCATION: Heart of Burns Country overlooking the 18th fairway of the Royal Troon Golf Course. SPA CLIENTELE: Women and men. DESCRIPTION: Traditional luxury hotel with health & beauty spa. Spa treatments: Declear facials, Ultraderm facials, body massage, aromatherapy, reflexology. Spa facilities: sauna, solarium, steam room, indoor pool, spa bath, fitness room, squash courts.

TURNBERRY
⌐ 1655

✈ Glasgow Int'l Airport (GLA)

Ayrshire, a region of western Scotland, is famous for its world class champion golf courses, golden beaches, and Victorian villages. The climate is mild and pleasantly dry year round. Ayr, the major nearby city, is a pretty harbor town and a popular resort with lovely beaches and famous race course.

Turnberry Hotel, Golf Courses & Spa
♥♥♥♥♥

Turnberry, Ayrshire KA2 69LT, Scotland. Tel: (1655) 331000. Fax: (1655) 331706. TYPE: Golf Hotel & Spa. LOCATION: On the west coast of Scotland, 53 mi. / 85 km. from Glasgow. HEALTH SPA MANAGER: Ms. Trina Peters. SPA CLIENTELE: Women and men, teenagers accepted. SPE-

CIAL RESTRICTIONS: Children under 5 are not permitted to use Spa. Under 16 supervision required.

* Rooms: 132 w/priv. bath. Suites: 10
* Phone, CTV, C/H, jacuzzi
* Restaurants (3) with Spa cuisine, classic and casual menus, bar, lounge
* Airports: Edinburgh / Glasgow, taxi, limo
* Train Station: Ayr Station 15 mi. / 24 km.
* Reservations: required
* Credit Cards: MC/VISA/AMEX
* Open: Year round
* Hotel Rates: from £130
* TAC: 10% (room only)
* Spa on premises: opened 1991
* **Spa Facilities:** Gym, squash & tennis courts, 20 m. pool, saunas, solarium, treatment rooms (6)
* **Spa Programs:** Day & Half Day guest programs
* **Spa Treatments:** aromatherapy, hydrotherapy, holistic, facials, mud packs, full body massage
* **Spa Packages:** Turnberry Lifestyle from £360; 3 Day Revitalizer from £480
* Indications: fitness,beauty, revitalization

DESCRIPTION: Stylish Spa in a deluxe, award winning country house hotel. Visitors to the spa are encouraged to take fitness consultation with one of the fully qualified experts who can monitor and develop the progress of those embarking on exercise program. Two world famous championship golf courses are open all year to hotel guests.

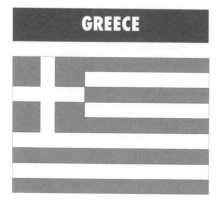

GREECE

AREA: 50,944 sq. mi. (131,945 sq. km.)
POPULATION: 10,000,000
CAPITAL: Athens
OFFICIAL LANGUAGE: Greek
CURRENCY: Greek Drachma (GDR)
EXCHANGE RATE: 1 US$= GDR 285
TELEPHONE COUNTRY CODE: 30

ℹ️ Hellenic Tourism Organisation
2 Amerikis St., PO Box 1017, Athens 10564 Greece
Tel: (1) 322-3111-9. Fax: (1) 322-4148

**ℹ️ Hellenic Association
of Municipalities and communities
of curative springs and spas**
Aristoleous Sqr. 6, 3rd Fl., 546 23 Thessaloniki Greece
Tel: (31) 230-933, 230936. Fax: (31) 285962

KAMENA VOURLA SPA
⟩ 235
✈️ Hellenikon Int'l Airport (ATH)

Astir Hotel Galini
❤️❤️❤️

Galini Beach, Kamena Vourla Spa GR-35008. Tel: (235) 22327. Fax: (235) 22307. TYPE: Hotel & Spa. LOCATION: Beachfront on the Green coast of central Greece. SPA CLIENTELE: Women and men. DESCRIPTION: First class beach hotel with thermal baths, pool, taverna, restaurant, bar, beach disco. 131 rooms, 2 suites w/priv. bath, A/C, phone, CTV. Hotel rates: from GRD 15,000.

LOUTRAKI (Pozar)
⟩ 384
✈️ Thessaloniki Airport (SKG) 120 km. / 75 mi.

The Spa of Loutraki (Pozar) lies on the slopes of Bora mountain, 20 km. / 13 mi. from Aridea and 120 km. / 75 mi. from Thessaloniki in Northwestern Central Macedonia. The Spa water are carbonated hypotonic at 37°c (99°F). Do not confuse this spa with the Loutraki Spa in the Peloponnese.

Loutraki Spa
❤️❤️❤️
😊 ♨️

Municipality of Loutraki GR-57200. Tel: (384) 91300, 91388, 91071. TYPE: Spa & Hotel. LOCATION: near Aridea of Central Macedonia. SPA CLIENTELE: Women and men.

* Rooms: hotel units available
* Reservations: required
* Open: Year round
* Spa on premises
* **SPA Facilities:** thermal springs carbonated mineral hypotonic waters, individual baths, thermal pool, fountains for drinking therapy, swimming pool
* **Spa Treatments:** hydrotherapy, drinking therapy
* **Indications:** diseases of the respiratory and nervous systems, rheumatism, arthritics, gynecological and skin diseases, sciaticas, disturbances of the circulatory system, drinking therapy for infections of the liver, kidney, gall, gastritis, ulcers, chronic colitis, disturbances of digestive, circulatory and urinary systems

DESCRIPTION: Health spa with a full medical centre and hotel facilities specializing in hydrotherapy and drinking cures.

LOUTRAKI SPA
⟩ 744
✈️ Hellenikon Int'l Airport (ATH) 85 km. / 54 mi.

The Spa of Loutraki-Perahore lies in the Peloponnese on the north coast of the Gulf of Corinthos in the foothills of Mt. Gerania. It is famous for drinking therapy. Not far from the spa are the ruins of the temple of Hera Akraia and Limenia.

Hotel Poseidon Club
♥♥♥♥

Loutraki-Perahora GR-20300. Tel: (744) 26411-18. Fax: (744) 26424. TYPE: Resort Hotel & Spa. LOCATION: Beachfront near Loutraki. SPA CLIENTELE: Women and men. DESCRIPTION: Large resort hotel gym, sauna, hydro-massage and massage services. Recreation: tennis, mini-golf, water sports.

Therme Loutraki
♥♥♥

Loutraki-Perahora GR-20300. Tel: (744) 22423. TYPE: Health Spa. LOCATION: Golf of Corinthos. SPA CLIENTELE: Women and men.

* Hotel units available
* Reservations: required
* Open: Year round
* Spa on premises
* **SPA Facilities**: thermal water containing chlorine, sulfur, slightly alkaline and radioactive at 30°c (86°F) three hydropathic units, centres for drinking therapy, sports centre, bottling factory
* **Spa Treatments**: hydrotherapy, drinking cure
* **Indications**: kidney and gall stones, liver insufficiency, hyposthetic dyspasia, psamiasis, chololethiasis, rehumatisms, arthritic, dental and gynecological diseases, drinking therapy for heart ailments, distur-bances of the nervous, circulatory and digest system.

DESCRIPTION: Health spa with sports facilities, congress centre and hotel accommodations.

SIDEROKASTRO
↻ 323

✈ Thessaloniki Airport (SKG)

Siderokastro Spa
♥♥♥

Municipality of Siderokastro GR-62300. Tel: (323) 22422, 22434, 22441. TYPE: Spa Hotel. LOCATION: 26 km. / 16 mi. from Serres. SPA CLIENTELE: Women and men.

* Rooms: 100 w/priv. bath
* Reservations: required
* Open: Year round
* Spa on premises
* **SPA Facilities**: thermal springs containing sulfur, sodium, alkaline at 43°c (110°F), hydropathic units, individual and group baths, medical center
* **Spa Treatments**: hydrotherapy, kinesitherapy
* **Indications**: rehumatism, vertebral diseases, arthritic, gynecological diseases, sciaticas, myalgia, lumbago

DESCRIPTION: Health spa with a full medical centre and modern hotel.

VRAVRONA
↻ 294

✈ Hellenikon Int'l Airport (ATH) 30 km. / 19 mi.

Mare Nostrum Thalasso
♥♥♥♥♥

Thalasso Hotel Club, Vrarvrona, Attica GR-19003. Tel: (294) 48412. Fax: (294) 47790. Head Office: 22 Anagnostopoulou St., Athens GR-10673. Tel: (1) 362-0662. Fax: (1) 364-1391. TYPE: Spa Hotel. LOCATION: Vravrona Bay, 30 km. / 19 mi. southeast of Athens. SPA CLIENTELE: Women and men.

* Rooms: 352 w/priv. bath & Suites
* Phone, CTV, minibar, hairdryer
* Restaurant:
* Reservations: required
* Credit Cards: VISA/AMEX/MC/DIS/EC
* Open: Year round; TAC: 10%
* Spa on premises: **Mare Nostrum Thalasso**
* **SPA Facilities**: Thalassotherapy Centre, large pool,

treatment rooms, aquagym, solarium, fully equipped fitness room, steam room

* **SPA Programs:** Thalassotherapy, medical, beauty & pampering, fitness, rejuvenation
* **Spa Treatments:** thalassotherapy, hydrotherapy, water massage, multi jet massage, aquagym classes, aerosol, Swedish massage, lymphatic drainage, reflexology, Shiatsu, body care, facial care, exfoliation, wax, foot care, manicure, solarium, stretching, aerobics
* **Spa Packages:** on request
* **Indications:** tiredness, depression, cellulite, circulation problems, traumatisms, rheumatism
* **Contraindications:** heart problems, high blood pressure, iodine allergy, cerebral accidents, leg ulcer, evolutive illnesses
* **Medical Supervision:** yes

DESCRIPTION: Elegant Thalassotheapy Center, the first of its kind in Greece, combining the benefits of the seawater with the warm Mediterranean climate of the Athens area.

CRETE ISLAND

LIMIN HERSONISSOS
🕽 **897**

✈ Heraklion Airport (HER) 14 mi. / 22 km.

Royal Mare Thalasso
❤❤❤

Limin Hersonnissos, Crete, GR-70014. Tel: (897) 623-0400, Fax: (897) 808-4392. TYPE: Health Spa. LOCATION: Near Heraklion. SPA CLIENTELE: Women and men. DESCRIPTION: 3,700 sq.m. / 40,700 sq.ft. thalassotherapy center with indoor seawater pools, showers. Algae and mud applications, physiotherapy.

IKARIA ISLAND

AGIOS KIRIKOS
🕽 **275**

✈ Agios Kirikos Airport

The springs of Ikaria are situated at Agios Kirikos, near the beach of Therma and Lefkada on the southeastern coast of Ikaria. The springs are radioactive at 55°c (130°F).

Ikaria Spa
❤❤

Municipality of Agios Kirikos GR-83300. Tel: (275)22202. Fax: (275) 22298. TYPE: Health Spa. LOCATION: Agios Kirikos. SPA CLIENTELE: Women and men.

* Hotel units are available. For accommodations you can also try: **George** (22517); **Anna** (22095).
* Reservations: required
* Open: June 1-October 31
* Spa on premises
* **SPA Facilities:** two hydropathic unit with group and individual baths.
* **Spa Treatments:** hydrotherapy
* **Indications:** rheumatism, arthritis, diabetes, liver and kidney ailments, gynecological diseases, disturbances of the circulatory system, hemopathies, skin diseases

DESCRIPTION: Health spa with hotel units.

LESVOS ISLAND

THERMI
🕽 **251**

✈ Mytilini Airport

The spa of Thermi lies near the beach about 11 km. / 7 mi. from Mitilini the capital of the island. The springs at Thermi are famous since antiquity. Nearby is the famous Monastery of St. Rafael.

Thermi Spa
❤❤❤

Municipality of Thermi, Thermi GR 81100, Lesvos. Tel: (251) 71277. TYPE: Health Spa. LOCATION: Near the beach north of Mitilini. SPA CLIENTELE: Women and men.

* Hotel units are available. For accommodations you can also try: **Blue Beach** (71290); **Vostala** (71231).
* Reservations: required
* Open: June 1-October 31
* Spa on premises
* **SPA Facilities**: hydropathic unit with group and individual baths.
* **Spa Treatments**: hydrotherapy
* **Indications**: rheumatism, arthritis, diabetes, liver and kidney ailments, gynecological diseases, disturbances of the circulatory system, hemopathies, skin diseases

DESCRIPTION: Health spa with hotel units.

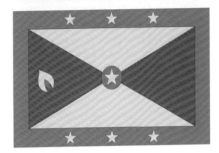

GRENADA

AREA: 133 sq. mi. (344 sq. km.)
POPULATION: 104,000
CAPITAL: St. George's
OFFICIAL LANGUAGE: English, French patois
CURRENCY: East Caribbean Dollar (EC$)
EXCHANGE RATE: 1 US$= EC$ 2.70
TELEPHONE COUNTRY CODE: 473

ℹ Grenada Board of Tourism
PO Box 293, St. George's, Grenada
Tel: (473) 440-2279. FAX: (473) 4406637

☞ No area code
✈ Point Saline Int'l AP (GND)

Allamanda Beach Resort & Spa
❤❤❤❤

PO Box 27, St. George's. Tel: 444-0095, Fax: 4440126.
TYPE: Beach Resort & Spa. LOCATION: On Grand Anse Beach. SPA CLIENTELE: Women and men. DESCRIPTION: Modern resort with health club, gym, sauna, whirlpool, aerobics, massages, beauty salon. 48 rooms, 2 suites, restaurants, pool, poolside lounge, tennis. Hotel rates: from $115.

La Source
❤❤❤❤

PO Box 852, Pink Gin Beach, St. George's. Tel: 4442556. Fax: 4442561. TYPE: Resort Hotel & Spa. LOCATION: On Pink Gin Beach on the southwest of the island. SPA CLIENTELE: Women and men. DESCRIPTION: First class all inclusive beach resort with health spa and beauty salon featuring beauty and relaxation treatments: massages, foot massage, aromatherapy, salt and oil loofah rubs, facials, seaweed wraps, reflexology. 100 rooms, 9 suites, restaurants, terrace bar, swimming pool. Hotel rates: from US$275.

HUNGARY

AREA: 35,920 sq. mi. (93,000 sq. km.)
POPULATION: 10,700,000
CAPITAL: Budapest
OFFICIAL LANGUAGE: Hungarian
CURRENCY: Forint (HF)
EXCHANGE RATE: 1 US$ = HF 220
TELEPHONE COUNTRY CODE: 36

Spas and bathing has a thousand-year-old tradition in Hungary. One can trace back its origins to the Roman who spread the cult of balneology to Pannonia or present day Hungary. In the 12th century, the St. John Knights founded a thermal medical center at the foot of Gellért Hill where the Rudas Baths can be found today. From the 18th century on the development of spas and balneotherapy centers was further accelerated and by the 19th century Hungarian Spas such as Héviz, Balf, Balatonfüred and Harkany became popular among the European nobility.

Budapest became an important center of balneotherapy after the First World War. Today, it is an international research center and the site of many international conferences on the subject of balneology. Hungary offers a convenient geographical location, right in the center of Europe and a mild climate. There is a great variety of thermal and medicinal waters available for therapy according to the individual spa.

Most of the important Hungarian spas have medical facilities and staff at the spa, others are located near hospitals. The ideal period for a spa cure in Hungary is three weeks.

ℹ Hungarian National Tourist Office
Margit krt. 85, H-1024 Budapest, Hungary
Tel: (1) 175-3819. Fax: (1) 375-3819

USA - New York
150 E. 58th St., New York NY 10155-3398
Tel: (212) 355-0240. Fax: (212) 207-4103.

BUDAPEST

↘ 1

✈ Ferihegy Int'l Airport (BUD) 9 mi. / 15 km.

Budapest, population 2,100,000, is the capital of Hungary and one of the most appealing historical cities in Europe. Located in the north central area, the city spreads over the two banks of the Danube River. Buda, on the right - west bank of the river is hilly, while Pest on the left - east bank, is flat with gentle slopes. Budapest is not only the center of government, industry and commerce, it is also one of the largest spa cities in the world.

There are a total of nine spas in Budapest, seven in Buda one in Pest, and one on Margitsziget Island in the middle of the Danube. 123 thermal and mineral springs with proven medical affects are used for Spa cure and recreation.

Danubius Aquincum Hotel
♥♥♥♥

Árpád fejedelem útja 94, Budapest H-1036. Tel: (1) 436-4100. Fax: (1) 436-4156. TYPE: Spa Hotel. LOCATION: On the buda side of Arpad bridge, opposite Margaret Island. SPA CLIENTELE: Women and men.

* Rooms: 312 w/private bath. Suites: 8
* Phone, CTV, A/C, minibar
* Restaurants, cafe, bar, gift shops
* Airport: Budapest 13 mi. / 20 km.
* Train Stn: Budapest West 5 mi. / 8 km.
* Airport.Train Transportation: bus, taxi
* Reservations: full payment
* Credit Cards: MC/AMEX/DC/EC
* Open: Year round
* Hotel Rates: from $140/day

* Spa on premises - water composition: sodium, potassium, calcium, magnesium, iron, manganese, ammonium, hydrocarbonate
* Spa Facilities: medical unit, swimming pool, steam baths, sauna, thermal pools, Scottish shower, beauty salon, fitness center, therapy rooms.
* Spa Treatments: hydrotherapy, massages, physiotherapy, beauty treatments, post-surgery treatments
* Spa Programs: medical, beauty, fitness
* Indications: injuries, post-surgery, dyscopathy, spinal diseases
* Medical Supervision: medical clinic
* Treatments Approved by: Hungarian Health Insurance

DESCRIPTION: Superior first class spa hotel with modern spa therapy facilities in a pleasant environment. A comprehensive locomotor medical unit is available on premises. Member: *Danubius Hotel & Spa Company.*

Danubius Grand Hotel Margitsziget
♥♥♥♥

Margitsziget, Budapest H-1138. Tel: (1) 132-1000. Fax: (1) 153-3029. TYPE: Spa Hotel. LOCATION: In the peaceful northern end of Margitsziget Island, 2 miles (3 km.) from town center. SPA CLIENTELE: Women and men.

* Rooms: 164 w/private bath. Suites: 10
* Restaurants, Cafe & Bar
* Airport: Budapest 13 mi. / 20 km.
* Train Stn: Budapest West 5 mi. / 8 km.
* Airport.Train Transportation: bus, taxi
* Reservations: full payment
* Credit Cards: MC/AMEX/DC/EC
* Open: Year round
* Hotel Rates: from $160/day
* Spa off premises: spa therapy center (direct link) Thermal Package from $590/wk
* SPA Facilities, Treatments & Programs: See Thermal Hotel

DESCRIPTION: Traditional turn of the century hotel opened in 1873, renovated and reopened in the spring of 1987.

Rooms are decorated and furnished in various Baroque and period styles. Hotel guests can use the direct underground link to all the spa facilities of the adjacent Thermal Hotel Margitsziget. Member: *Danubius Hotel & Spa Company.*

Danubius Hotel Gellért
❤❤❤❤

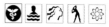

Gellért ter 1, Budapest H-1111. Tel: (1) 185-2200. Fax: (1) 166-6631. Baths: Kelenhegyi ut 4-6, Budapest XI. Tel: (1) 460-760. TYPE: Hotel & Spa. LOCATION: Surrounded by a landscaped park at the foot of Gellért Hill, on the Buda side overlooking the Danube River, 1 mile (2 km.) from town center. SPA CLIENTELE: Women and men.

* Rooms: 239 w/private bath. Suites: 15
* Phone, CTV, A/C, radio, minbar
* Restaurant, Gellért brasserie, bar, night club
* Airport: Budapest 9 mi. / 14 km. taxi
* Train Stn: Budapest East 5 mi. / 8 km. taxi
* Reservations: full payment required
* Credit Cards: VISA/AMEX/DC/CB/EC
* Open: Year round
* Hotel Rates: from $119 (room only)
* Spa on premises: **Gellért Spa**
* **Spa Water Composition**: Ten springs provide radioactive medicinal water containing calcium-magnesium, alkalis, chloride, hydrogen-carbonates, sulfate and fluoride
* **Spa Facilities**: Co-ed Thermal pools; bubble, tub,surf,mud and brine baths, inhalation rooms, massage rooms, gymnasium
* **Spa Programs**: Rejuvenation, relaxation, general fitness, beauty and medical
* **Spa Treatments**: Inhalations and carbon dioxide gas, stimulating baths, massages including underwater jet massage, traction electrotherapy, curative gymnastics
* **Spa Packages**: Pleasure & Beauty (2 wks) from $926, Beauty Week from $528
* **Indications**: Asthmatic and chronic bronchial catarrh; degenerative diseases of the joints and spine, disopathy, chronic and semi-acute arthritic inflammations, gout, conditions after accidents,

neurologia; gynecological disorders, sclerotic and circulatory disorders
* Medical Supervision: yes
* Treatments Approved: Hospital dept.

DESCRIPTION: Neo-classical hotel built in 1918 and restored in 1970. The elegant furnishings, decor and fine service complement its grand style. Most of the rooms and suites have scenic views of the river and the Budapest skyline. It was the premier hotel of the city when inaugurated. However, the mineral springs have been used for medical purposes for nearly 2,000 years. The art deco medical baths - Gellért Spa - adjoins the hotel. Guests can use a special lift to take them to the thermal pools. The thermal pools are open for anyone for an admission fee. Member: *Danubius Hotel & Spa Company*

Danubius Thermal Hotel Margitsziget
❤❤❤❤

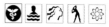

Margitsziget, Budapest H-1138. Tel: (1) 329-2300. Fax: (1) 329-3923. TYPE: Spa Hotel. LOCATION: On the northern part of the island, 2 mi. (3 km.) to town center. SPA CLIENTELE: Women and men.

* Rooms: 206 w/priv. bath. Suites: 8
* Wheelchair Access, Balconies
* Phone, CTV, A/C, minibar, radio
* Restaurant, 2 Bars, Night Club
* Airport: Budapest 13 mi. / 20 km.
* Train Stn: Budapest West 5 mi. / 8 km.
* Airport/Train Transportation: Taxi
* Reservations: Full payment required
* Credit Cards: MC/VISA/AMEX/DC/CB/EC
* Open: Year round
* Rates: $169/day (room only)
* Spa on premises: **Thermal Margitsziget.** Mineral water from 67°c - 70°c, (152°F - 158°F), containing calcium-magnesium-hydrogen-carbonates, chloride and sulfates.
* **Spa Facilities**: Swimming pool (1), thermal medicinal pools (4), sauna, solarium, medical laboratory, sports and exercise facilities

* **Spa Programs**: Rejuvenation, relaxation, general fitness, 1-3-weeks. Full spa therapy or basic balneotherapy
* **Spa Treatments**: Stimulating baths, massages, underwater jet massage, solarium, physiotherapeutic treatments for rheumatic ailments
* **Spa Packages**: 1 Week Thermal; Thermal Special (21 days). A la carte treatments available
* **Indications**: Chronic degenerative locomotor disease, osteoarthritis of the spine, ankylosing spondylitis, chronic and sub-acute arthritis and chronic inflammatory gynecological diseases
* Medical Supervision: Medical Section w/diagnostic center.

DESCRIPTION: A modern 4-star medicinal spa hotel in the middle of the Danube fed by three therapeutic springs. English speaking medical staff. The gastronomic "Platán" restaurant serves excellent diet food. The Havana Night Club recreates the flavors of the Caribbean.

Danubius Thermal Hotel Helia
❤❤❤❤

😀 ⛲ 🐎 🏃 ⚛

Kárpát u. 62-64, H-1133 Budapest, Hungary. Tel: (1) 452-5800. Fax: (1) 452-5801. TYPE: Spa Hotel. MANAGER: Dr. Gábor Galla. LOCATION: On the banks of the river Danube, opposite Margaret Island. SPA CLIENTELE: Women and men, family orientated.

* Rooms: 262; Suites 8; all with private bath
* Phone, CTV, A/C, C/H, minibar, radio
* Restaurants (Hungarian specialties), Hungarian pastries cafe, and Summer Terrace
* Airport: Ferihegy I, 19 km. / 12 mi.
* Train Stn: Nyugati Palyaudvar, 3 km. / 2 mi.
* Airport/Train Station Transportation: Taxi, limo, minibus.
* Credit Cards: MC, VISA, AMEX, DC, JBC, EC
* Open: Year round.
* Hotel Rates: from US$130; TAC: 10%
* Spa on premises - thermal water composition: calcium-magnesium, hydro-carbonic thermal water piped from the Magde spring on Margaret island

* **Spa Facilities**: medical department, fitness facilities, indoor swimming pool, 2 thermal pools, sauna, steam bath, gym, jacuzzi, solarium, beauty salon
* **Spa Programs**: health, fitness, beauty
* **Spa Packages**: Recreation week (7 nights); Duna fortnight (14 nights); Supersaver (21 nights) Helia- D Beauty Package (7 nts); Slimming Special (7 nights); Tennis Package (3 nights) Touch of Budapest (2 nights)
* **Spa Treatments**: Hydrotherapy - carbon dioxide baths, medicinal weight baths, tangentor, steam bath, massages, mud wrap, cream wrap, effervescent bath, jet massage, port, reflex; electrotherapy ultrasound, decimed, iontophoresis, short-wave diathermy, microwave, interference current, vasotrain, vacotron, quarz, sollux, four cells galvanic current; gymnastics, physiotherapy (group or individual), Inhalation - with medicines or medicinal water
* **Indications**: Post operative rehabilitation, locomotor disorders, articular pain, rheumatism, circulatory disorders.
* **Contraindications**: Infectious diseases, acute inflammations, epilepsy, asthmatic attack, pregnancy, tumors, leukemia, thrombosis, cardiac disease, sclerosis multiplex, steady high blood pressure, accumulated angina pectoris, feverish condition, pregnancy
* Length of stay: 2-3 weeks combined therapy.
* Medical supervision: 3 MDs, 3RNs.
* Supervised by: Ministry of Health

DESCRIPTION: Thermal hotel Helia is an elegant 4-star Spa hotel with a refined atmosphere and warm Hungarian hospitality. Most rooms offer a panoramic view of the Danube and the Buda hills. The Spa offers a wide range of diagnostic and therapeutic facilities in the state-of-the-art in house Cure Center under the supervision of qualified, multilingual physicians. Natural healing energy from mineral rich hot springs is used for health improvement, cure or relaxation. A luxurious swimming pool complex with two thermal baths is used for balneotherapy. Each Spa guest receives carefully prepared treatment schedule and exercise program after examination. The hotel features a modern beauty salon and a fashionable Fitness Center to make your stay as enjoyable as possible. Member: *Danubius Hotel & Spa Company.*

BUKFURDO
⟩ 94

✈ Schwechat Airport (VIE) 76 mi. / 122 km.

Bük, one of Hungary's most recently developed spas, is situated in the western part of the country known as Transdanubia on the eastern foot of the Alps, 25 km (16 mi.) from the Austrian border and 122km (76 mi.) from Vienna (Austria). The village is near the Hungarian towns of Köszeg and Szombathely, both have interesting historical sites dating from the Roman period in Szombathely, and the medieval times in Köszeg.

The high pressure thermal water was discovered while doing construction work on the site. The water temperature is 58°c (136°F). The iron rich mineral spring water contains calcium-magnesium and hydrogen-carbonate. Bük can be reached by rail from Vienna or Budapest on the Sopron-Szobathely route.

Danubius Thermal & Sporthotel Bük
❤❤❤❤

Bük H-9740. Tel: (94) 358-500. Fax: (94) 358-620. TYPE: Spa Hotel. LOCATION: Near the Austrian border, 26 km. (16 mi.) from Szombathely and 20 km. (13 mi.) from Köszeg. SPA CLIENTELE: Women and men.

* Rooms: 200 w/private bath, Suites: 15
* Phone, CTV, radio, minibar, balcony
* Airport: Vienna 70 mi. / 112 km.
* Train Stn: Szombathely 20 mi. / 32 km.
* Airport/Train Transportation: bus, taxi
* Reservations: full payment required
* Credit Cards: VISA/AMEX/DC/EC
* Open: Year round
* Hotel Rates: from $90/day
* Spa on premises
* **Spa Facilities:** Therapy Center, Dental Dept., thermal baths, swimming pool, sauna
* **Spa Programs:** Basic one week, Complete two weeks with additional one week extensions
* **Spa Treatments:** balneotherapy, massages, hydrotherapy, mud pack, electrotherapy,

medical gymnastics, underwater jet massage, beauty & cosmetic treatments, drinking cures
* **Spa Packages:** Eve or Adam Beauty Package (7 nts) 1-2 week thermal packages
* **Indications:** Chronic degenerative articular diseases, chronic polyarthritis, osteoarthritis of the spine, rheumatoid arthritis, discopathia, muscular rheumatism, Bechtherew syndrome, chronic gynaecologiocal diseases
* **Medical Supervision:** physical examination and medical care

DESCRIPTION: A modern Spa hotel, built by the Swedish ABV company and opened in 1986. All rooms are comfortable and tastefully furnished. The hotel features medically oriented spa programs based on the thermal water's effectiveness in the treatment of the digestive and respiratory problems. The magnificent countryside location makes it an ideal place for relaxation and tourism. Recreation: 18 hole golf course, tennis, horseback riding, hunting. Member: *Danubius Hotel & Spa Company.*

EGER
⟩ 36

✈ Ferihegy Int'l Airport (BUD) 9 mi. / 15 km.

Eger is located at the southern foot of the Bükk hills. The town is historic with baroque style architecture. The region is famous for its excellent wine production.

Hotel Flóra
❤❤❤

Fürdo út 5, 3300 Eger. Tel: (36) 320211. TYPE: Medicinal Spa. LOCATION: Near the open air thermal springs. SPA CLIENTELE: Women and men.

* Rooms: 60 w/private bath.
* Phone, CTV, minibar, radio
* Wheelchair access
* Airport: Budapest, bus or train
* Open: Year round
* Hotel Rates: from $80/day
* Spa on premises

* **Spa Facilities**: swimming pool, medical center, sauna, solarium, medicinal springs
* **Spa Treatments**: balneotherapy, massage, physiotherapy
* **Spa Programs**: Medicinal Therapy 2-3 wks
* **Indications**: locomotor diseases, rheumatic complaints
* **Medical Supervision**: yes

DESCRIPTION: Medicinal hotel with a covered corridor connecting with the medical unit and the therapy pools. General fitness and conditioning programs are available. Member: *Hungarian National Holiday Foundation*

GYULA
⟩ 66
✈ Ferihegy Int'l Airport (BUD) 220 km. / 138 mi.

Gyula, population 36,000, is a spa town with pleasant climate in southeastern Hungary near Békés on the Romanian border. The **Castle Spa** in town is one of the nicest thermal spas in Hungary. The baths in a castle park are open to visitors who want to receive treatments, ensure relaxation, recreation, regeneration and rehabilitation.

Hotel Erkel
♥♥♥

Vérkert u. 1, 5701 Gyula. Tel: (66) 463555. TYPE: Medicinal Spa. LOCATION: Between the lake and the Mansion. SPA CLIENTELE: Women and men.

* Rooms: 20 w/private bath.
* Phone, CTV, minibar, radio
* Wheelchair access
* Airport: Budapest, bus or train
* Open: Year round
* Hotel Rates: from $80/day
* Spa on premises
* **Spa Facilities**: swimming pool, medical center, sauna, solarium, castle bath medicinal springs
* **Spa Treatments**: balneotherapy, massage, physiotherapy
* **Spa Programs**: Medicinal Therapy 2-3 wks
* **Indications**: locomotor disorders, rheumatic and

articular complaints, gynecological diseases, rehabilitation following heart attack or accidents
* **Medical Supervision**: yes

DESCRIPTION: Spa hotel connected to the castle baths, 20 thermal pools that can be reached via a covered corridor from the hotel. Member: *Hungarian National Holiday Foundation*

HEVIZ
⟩ 83
✈ Héviz charter airport 10 km. / 6 mi.
Ferihegy Int'l Airport (BUD) 9 mi. / 15 km.

Héviz, the jewel of the Hungarian spas, is located among gentle verdant hills only a few miles from the scenic Lake Balaton, a popular resort and recreation area. The 12-acre Thermal Lake at Héviz is known for its therapeutic properties since Roman times, and it is fed by a natural hot spring.

Héviz main attraction is the large, natural, 12 acres thermal lake, which is unique in Europe and the second largest in the world. The lake's water changes completely every two days. The water temperature varies between 32°c - 33°c (89°F - 92°F) and does not drop below 24°c (75°F) during the coldest winter months thus making open-air swimming possible year round. The elliptic shaped medicinal lake is fed by a thermal spring providing about 1 cbm of water per second or 16,000 gallons per minute. The most important curative factors are the lake's thermal water and the radioactive mud covering the bottom. In addition to the lake springs there are also several slightly radioactive thermal wells with water composition similar to that of the thermal lake containing alkali, hydrogen-carbonate and sulfate.

Héviz is located 190 km. / 118 mi. southwest of Budapest, and some 208 km. / 130 mi. southeast of Vienna. Héviz can also be reached by car from Sopron, via route 84, or by rail to Keszthely, and by a regular service bus to Héviz.

Danubius Thermal Hotel Aqua
♥♥♥♥

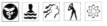

Kossut Lajos u. 13-15, Héviz H-8380. Tel: (83) 341-180.

Fax: (83) 340-666. TYPE: Spa Hotel. LOCATION: In a quite park-like setting on Europe's largest thermal lake. SPA CLIENTELE: Women and men.

* Rooms: 229 w/private bath. Suites: 6
* Phone, CTV, minibar, radio, minibar
* Wheelchair access: 35 rooms
* Restaurant, Brasserie, Bar, Casino nearby
* Airport: Budapest 140 mi. / 88 km.
* Train Station: Kesztely 8 mi. / 13 km.
* Airport/Train Station Transportation: taxi, bus
* Credit Cards: VISA/AMEX/DC/CB/EC
* Open: Year round
* Hotel Rates: from $120/day
* Spa on premises
* **Spa Facilities**: Thermal, Fitness & Therapy Center, indoor thermal pool, swimming pool, gymnasium, sauna, solarium, thermal baths, sun terrace, sauna
* **Spa Treatments**: balneotherapy, massage, physiotherapy, mechanotherapy, electrotherapy
* **Spa Programs**: Spa Therapy 2-3 wks
* **Indications**: locomotor diseases, states of exhaustion, degenerative articular diseases, muscular rheumatism, post-traumatic conditions, disiopathia, gout, osleoarthritis of the spine
* **Medical Supervision**: yes

DESCRIPTION: The Aqua Hotel was built in 1984 to meet the rapidly growing demand for accommodations at this internationally renowned resort. Guests seeking treatment or relaxation can use the curative facilities of either the Thermal Lake of Héviz, or the Aqua's modern equipment.

Danubius Thermal Hotel Héviz
❤❤❤❤

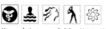

Kossuth Lajos u. 9-11, Héviz H-8380. Tel: (83) 341-180. Fax: (83) 340-666. TYPE: Spa Hotel. LOCATION: On a large thermal lake near Lake Balaton. SPA CLIENTELE: Women and men.

* Rooms: 203 w/private bath. Suites: 7
* CTV, minibar, radio

* Terrace Restaurant, brasserie, bar, game room, casino
* Airport: Budapest 140 mi. / 224 km.
* Train station: Keszthely 8 mi. / 13 km.
* Airport /Train Station Transportation: taxi, bus
* Reservations: full payment required
* Credit Cards: MC/VISA/AMEX/DC/CB/EC
* Open: Year round
* Hotel Rates: from $110/day
* Spa on premises
* **Spa Facilities**: Therapy Center, Indoor and outdoor swimming pools, fitness room, sauna, medical and dental clinic
* **Spa Programs**: Rejuvenation, relaxation, stress reduction, general fitness, recommended programs of 1, 2 and 3 weeks
* **Spa Treatments**: balneotherapy, physiotherapy, hydrotherapy, electrotherapy, medicinal gymnastics, massage, mud packs
* **Indications**: Chronic degenerative articular diseases, muscular rheumatism, polyalgia, post-traumatic conditions, disiopathia, gout, osleoarthrithis of the spine, exhaustion
* **Medical Supervision**: all treatments supervised by physician

DESCRIPTION: The thermal hotel Héviz, constructed in 1976 opened its casino in 1984 to expand its selection of recreational activities. Two restaurants feature gourmet and dietetic meals. Guests seeking treatment can use the extensive facilities of the Thermal Hotel Héviz on the thermal lake. Recreation: 2 tennis courts. Member: *Danubius Hotel & Spa Company*.

Rogner Hotel Lotus Therme
❤❤❤

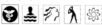

Lotuszvirag Str., Héviz H-8380. Tel: (83) 500-000. Fax: (83) 340-591. TYPE: Spa Hotel. LOCATION: In a peaceful parklike area near thermal lake. SPA CLIENTELE: Women and men. DESCRIPTION: Modern resort hotel with indoor thermal pool, medical treatment center, outdoor swimming pool, sauna, gym, jacuzzi, beauty salon. 235 rooms, 4 suites, restaurants, bar, tennis. Hotel rates: from US$80.

SARVAR

꒛ 95

✈ Schwechat Airport (VIE) 75 mi. / 120 km.

Sárvár, population 15,000, is a small spa town with natural thermal springs, located in the middle of a National Park half way between Lake Balaton and the city of Sopron, population 54,000.

The nearest large city is Szombathely, the oldest town in Hungary with its magnificent Roman and old Medieval sites. Nearby is the Abbey of Ják which is a famous architectural monument, a Hungarian Romanesque masterpiece. Sárvár is located 75 mi. / 120 km. from Vienna, and 130 mi. / 208 km. from Budapest. Sárvár can be reached by rail from Vienna or Budapest, or by car via route 84 from Sopron or Szombathely.

Indications: Sárvár has two different mineral springs - one at 111°F (48°c) is effective in the treatment of rheumatic diseases, and the other at 181°F (83°c) has a high saline concentration which is beneficial for patients suffering from gynecological or respiratory ailments.

Danubius Thermal Hotel Sárvár
❤❤❤

1 Rákóczi ut 1, Sárvár H-9600. Tel: (95) 332-999. Fax: (95) 320-406. TYPE: Spa Hotel. LOCATION: In the middle of a National Park in the historic King's Garden region. SPA CLIENTELE: Women and men.

* Rooms: 136 w/private bath. Suites: 4
* CTV, minibar, radio, balcony
* Wheelchair accessibility
* Terrace Restaurant & Bar
* Airport: Vienna 90 mi. / 144 km.
* Train Station: Sárvár 2 mi. / 3 km.
* Airport /Train Station Transportation: taxi, bus
* Reservations: full payment required
* Open: Year round
* Hotel Rates: from $90/day

* Spa on premises
* **Spa Facilities**: Therapy Center, thermal baths, inhalation rooms, gym, swimming pool, sauna, dental department
* **Spa Treatments**: balneotherapy, underwater jet massage, mud pack, electrotherapy, saline bath, inhalation therapy, hydrotherapy
* **Indications**: Locomotor and gynecological diseases and respiratory disorders
* Medical Supervision: Weekly physical examination and medical care, treatments are specified by physician, medical hostess service

DESCRIPTION: The Spa was completed in 1985 on the site of 2 thermal springs with medically recognized properties. The rural area is ideal for relaxation and sightseeing. Nearby is the historical Nádasdy Castle, the former residence of King Louis III. Member: *Danubius Hotel & Spa Company.*

ZALAKROSI

꒛ 93

✈ Ferihegy Int'l Airport (BUD)

Zalarkarosi, is a small spa town in southern Transdanubia. A tourist region of the Zala province in western Hungary 30 km. / 19 mi. from Lake Balaton. Established in 1965 the village with its special micro-climate lies in the middle of the wine country. The thermal baths are excellent for medicinal purposes or relaxation.

Indications: locomotor disorders, gynecological complaints, post-operative care

Men Dan Thermal Aparthotel
❤❤❤

Gyógyfürdo tér 8, Zalakaros H-8749. Tel: (93) 340-887. Fax: (93) 340-887. TYPE: Spa Aparthotel. LOCATION: In the spa park area. SPA CLIENTELE: Women and men. DESCRIPTION: Nice aparthotel with high standards of service and direct access to the thermal baths.

ICELAND

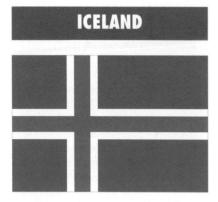

AREA: 39,768 sq. mi. (103,000 sq. km.)
POPULATION: 250,000
CAPITAL: Reykjavík
OFFICIAL LANGUAGE: Icelandic
CURRENCY: Krona (IK)
EXCHANGE RATE: 1 US$ = IK 219
TELEPHONE COUNTRY CODE: 354

Iceland is known for its pure, fresh air and spectacular environment. Swimming in geothermal water is considered a vital activity for the maintenance of good health. The big attraction about swimming in Iceland is the very hot water - maintained at a steady 25°c-30°c (77°F-86°F) all year round. The most famous Health Tourism destination in Iceland is the **Blue Lagoon**, whose near-miracle curative powers for skin disorders were discovered in 1980. Bathing in the Blue Lagoon is beneficial to treat people with psoriasis, eczema, and other skin ailments

ℹ️ Iceland Tourist Board
655 Third Ave., New York NY 10017
Tel: (212) 949-2333. Fax: (212) 983-5260

HVERGERDI

➲ No area code
✈ Reflavik AP (KEF)

Nature Health Association of Iceland
(NLFI) Spa & Clinic, Hveragerdi. Tel: 483-0300, Fax: 483-0320.

RYEKJANES PENINSULA

➲ No area code
✈ Reflavik AP (KEF) 32 mi. / 51 km. from Reykjavik

The Reykjanes Peninsula is the first sight to greet almost every visitor to Iceland. The Peninsula is noted for its diverse lava fields, hikeable mountains, intense geothermal activity and scenic shore. The famous **Bláa Iónió** (The Blue Lagoon) is a lovely geothermal lake with very hot water, 25°c-30°c or 77°F-86°F year round. it is located near Reykjavik with a quick connection to the International airport.

The Blue Lagoon
Hotel & Treatment Center
❤️❤️

🧖

Bláa Iónió. Hotel - Tel: 426-8800. Fax: 426-8888. TYPE: Geothermal Spa, Hotel & Restaurant Complex. LOCATION: Near Reykjavik in southwest Iceland. SPA CLIENTELE: Women and men, family oriented.

* Rooms: with private facilities
* Airport: Reykjavik, 20 min. taxi or bus
* Open: Year round
* Spa on premises: **The Blue Lagoon**
* **Spa Facilities**: Geothermal lake
* **Indications**: skin ailments, psoriasis, eczema

DESCRIPTION: Iceland's best known destination for health tourism. The Blue Lagoon is a deep blue lake with pure mineral rich geothermal brine. The complex caters to local and international visitors for cure or recreation.

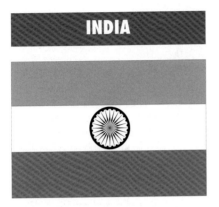

INDIA

AREA: 1,269,339 sq. mi. (3,287,588 sq. km.)
POPULATION: 844,000,000
CAPITAL: New Delhi
OFFICIAL LANGUAGE: Hindi, English + tribal languages
CURRENCY: Indian rupee (IR)
EXCHANGE RATE: 1 US$ = IR 42.50
TELEPHONE COUNTRY CODE: 91

ℹ️ India Dept of Tourism
No. 1 Parliament, New Delhi 110001 India
Fax: (+91-11) 371-0518

GOA
➘ 832
✈️ Dabolim AP (GOI)

Four Seasons Resort Leela Beach
❤️❤️❤️❤️❤️

Mobor, Cavelossim Village, Salcette, Goa 403731. Tel: (834) 746-363. Fax: (834) 746-352. TYPE: Beach Resort Hotel & Spa. LOCATION: Southern tip of Colva Beach, between the Sal River and the Arabian Sea.

* Rooms: 164 with priv. bath. Suites & Villas: 82
* Phone, CTV, minibar, private balcony
* Restaurants, cafe, gaming club, lounges, swimming pool and swim-up bar
* 24 hrs room service

* Open: Year round
* Hotel Rates: from US$175 + Tax: 15%
* TAC: 10%
* Spa on premises
* **Spa Facilities:** fully equipped spa & fitness centre
* **Spa Treatments:** Indian massages

DESCRIPTION: Luxurious beach resort with spa facilities featuring the richness of age-old Indian heritage combined with a unique Portuguese flair. Member: *Four season Resort.*

JAIPUR
➘ 141
✈️ Sanganeer AP (JAI) 8.5 mi. / 14 km.

Rajvilas Jaipur
❤️❤️❤️❤️❤️

Goner Road, Rajasthan, Jaipur. Tel: (141) 364-391. Fax: (141) 364-391. TYPE: Deluxe Hotel & Spa. LOCATION: 12 km. / 8 mi. to the Palace of Jaipur. SPA CLIENTELE: Women and men.

* Rooms: 71 with priv. bath.
* 14 luxury tents, 3 villas
* Phone, CTV, minibar, private balcony
* Restaurants, cafe, private pool & garden
* 24 hrs room service
* Open: Year round
* Hotel Rates: from US$230 + Tax: 10%
* TAC: 10%
* Spa on premises
* **Spa Facilities:** fully equipped spa & fitness centre, whirlpool, steam room, exercise equipment
* **Spa Treatments:** Indian massages, yoga, exercise, aromatherapy, body wraps

DESCRIPTION: Resort hotel designed to look like a traditional royal Rajasthan fort set amidst orchards and gardens. The Health Spa and Beauty Center offer a wide range of relaxing and pampering treatments.

INDONESIA

AREA: 788,430 sq. mi. (2,042,034 sq. km.)
POPULATION: 179,136,000
CAPITAL: Jakarta
OFFICIAL LANGUAGES: Indonesian, Papuan, English
CURRENCY: Rupee (IR)
EXCHANGE RATE: 1 US$ = IR 7,400
TELEPHONE COUNTRY CODE: 62

Indonesia consists of 13,677 islands stretching over a huge territory of 5,120 km / 3,200 mi. from the Pacific to the Indian Ocean. The island of Bali is the country's number one tourist attraction and it is one of the most exotic and fascinating travel destination in the world. Here you can find Indonesia's most developed tourism infrastructure complete with world class resort hotels, beautiful beaches, ancient temples, lovely villages and a friendly population for a peaceful and spiritually fulfilled vacation. The Island of Lombok east of Bali is less developed and not as crowded but it is rapidly becoming popular with international tourism.

ℹ️ Indonesia Tourism Office
13 Sjalan Merdeka Selatan, Jakarta, Indonesia
Fax: (+62-21) 2311801.

BALI ISLAND

JIMBARAN BAY
❯ 361
✈️ Ngurah Rai Airport (DPS) 15 km. / 10 mi.

Four Seasons Bali at Jimbaran Bay
💟💟💟💟💟

Bukit Permai, Jimbaran, Denpasar, Bali 80361. Tel: (361) 701-010. Fax: (361) 701-020. TYPE: Resort & Spa. LOCATION: Beautiful hillside overlooking Jimbaran Bay. SPA CLIENTELE: Women and men. DESCRIPTION: Elegant Balinese-style villas resort complex with an expanded 1,000 sq.m. (10,760 sq. ft.) spa and health club facilities offering traditional Indonesian beauty and massage treatments. Amenities: restaurants, pub, swimming pools, jacuzzi, tennis courts, squash courts, private beach. 147 villas, 2BR Royal villas, villas for non smokers. Hotel rates: from US$475.

LEGIAN/KUTA BEACH
❯ 361
✈️ Ngurah Rai Airport (DPS)

Hotel Imperial Bali
💟💟💟💟

Jalan Abimanyu, Legian Beach, Bali 80361. Tel: (361) 730730. Fax: (361) 730545. TYPE: Resort Hotel & Spa. LOCATION: Next to the exclusive Legian Beach, amidst lush tropical gardens. SPA CLIENTELE: Women and men. DESCRIPTION: Secluded beachfront resort hotel with Spa - **Imperial Spa** - Balinese style spa with sauna, Balinese and international style massages, herbal facials, Indonesian body scrubs created by Mandara spa and beauty treatments. 137 rooms, 11 suites, 16 villas, restaurants, cafe, swimming pools, putting green, private beach. Hotel rates: from US$160.

Hotel & Residence Jaykarta Bali
💟💟💟💟

Jl. Werkudara, Po Box 3244, Denpasar. Tel: (361) 751433. Fax: (361) 752074. TYPE: Beachfront Resort & Spa. LOCATION: Set in landscaped gardens. SPA CLIENTELE: Women and men. DESCRIPTION: Elegant resort with health spa and fitness center, sauna, massages, swimming pools (3), tennis court. 278 rooms, 166 apartments. Hotel rates: from US$120.

The Oberoi Bali
❤❤❤❤❤

PO Box 3351, Legian Beach, Bali 80033. Tel: (361) 730361. Fax: (361) 730791. TYPE: Resort Complex & Spa. LOCATION: Amidst tranquil gardens on Legian. SPA CLIENTELE: Women and men. DESCRIPTION: Intimate Balinese style resort complex featuring Indonesian style health spa with open air massage pavilions, beauty treatments, sauna, gym, beauty salon. 75 rooms, cottages and villas, restaurant, cafe, piano bar, swimming pool, private beach, tennis. Hotel rates: from $255.

The Legian Bali
❤❤❤❤❤

Jalan Kayu Aya, Seminyak, Kuta. Tel: (361) 730-622. Fax: (361) 730-623. TYPE: Resort Hotel & Spa. LOCATION: Beachfront in tropical landscaped gardens. SPA CLIENTELE: Women and men. DESCRIPTION: All-Suite beachfront resort with Health Spa - **The Spa at the Legian** - Balinese style 400 sq.ft. / 36 sq.m. deluxe spa with sauna, variety of massages, herbal facials, reflexology, mineral baths, body scrubs and various Bailese and international beauty treatments. 71 suites, brasserie, restaurant, beach bar, outdoor pool. Hotel rates: from US$180.

White Rose Hotel
❤❤❤❤

Jl. Legian, Kuta, Bali. USA/Canada reservation Tel: (800) 257-5344. Tel: (516) 944-5508. Fax: (516) 944-7540. TYPE: Hotel & Spa. LOCATION: Very heart of Kuta, few minutes walk to the white sands of Kuta Beach. SPA CLIENTELE: Women and men.

* Rooms: 144 w/priv. bath
* Phone, CTV (satellite), in house movies, A/C, coffee/tea maker, hair dryer
* Restaurants, coffee shop, lounges
* Swimming pool, swim up bar
* Airport: Ngurah Rai Int'l AP, 10 min.
* Open: Year round

* Hotel rates: from US90; TAC: 10%
* Spa on premises: **Sehatku Spa**
* **Spa facilities**: sauna, steam, cold dip, hot whirlpool, bar with healthy food, relaxing room, separate facilities for Gents/Ladies, fitness center, poolside massage hut
* **Spa Treatments**: shiatsu massage, aromatherapy, "kawas" sauna/spa massage
* **Spa Programs**: beauty, wellness, anti-stress

DESCRIPTION: Beautiful 4-star hotel , a surprise secret pocket of luxury hidden away behind the hustle and bustle of Kuta's famous main shopping street. Guests can enjoy a special massage followed by a relaxing scented oil massage. Work out exercises are available at the Fitness Center guided by highly professional instructors.

MANGGIS
☎ **363**
✈ Ngurah Rai Airport (DPS) 70 km. / 44 mi.

The Serai Hotel
❤❤❤❤

Buitan, Manggis. Tel: (363) 41011. Fax: (363) 41015. TYPE: Hotel & Spa. LOCATION: Amidst lush coconut grove, private beach, 6 km. / 4 mi. from ancient Tenganan village. SPA CLIENTELE: Women and men. DESCRIPTION: Elegant low-rise traditional Balinese resort with a spa - **Manadara Spa** - open air Balinese spa with sauna, massages and beauty treatments. 66 rooms, 2 spa suites, outdoor pool and poolside massages, cooking school. Hotel rates: from US$150.

NUSA DUA
☎ **361**
✈ Ngurah Rai Airport (DPS) 20 km. / 12 mi.

Aston Bali Resort & Spa
❤❤❤❤

Jalan Pratama 68x, Tanjung Benoa, Nusa Dua, Bali 80363. Tel: (361) 773-577. Fax: (361) 774-954. TYPE: Beach resort & Spa. LOCATION: Amidst lush coconut palms, hibiscus and banana trees 1 mile to Nusa Dua shopping center. DESCRIPTION: Balinese style beach resort with full service spa. gym, sauna, massage and jacuzzi. 187 rooms, 18 1BR ocean front villas, international restaurants, 9000 sq.ft. / 818 sq.m. fresh water pool featuring waterfalls and private caves. Hotel rates: from $110/day.

Club Med Bali
❤❤❤❤

Tuban Bali. Tel: (361) 771521. Fax: (361) 771835. TYPE: Club Med Resort & Spa. LOCATION: on the east coast of the southern tip of Bali. SPA CLIENTELE: Women and men. DESCRIPTION: Self-contained village resort with Health Spa - **Banyan Spa** - includes two deluxe spa villas with private outdoor jacuzzi, a spa with beauty treatments, fitness center, jacuzzi, sauna. 400 rooms and bungalows, restaurants, bar, disco, swimming pools, tennis, squash. Hotel rates: from US$140. Club Med membership required.

Gran Mirage Resort
❤❤❤❤

Jalan Pratama 74, Tanjung Benoa, PO Box 43, Nusa Dua, Bali 80363. Tel: (361) 771888. Fax: (361) 72148. TYPE: Hotel & Spa. LOCATION: Beachfront 12 km. to Ngurah Rai Int'l Airport. SPA CLIENTELE: Women and men. DESCRIPTION: Exotic beachfront resort with thalassotherapy spa and aquamedic pool offering 11 various treatments. 310 rooms & suites, restaurants (3), bars (3), lounge, entertainment, meeting facilities, tennis court, water sports. Hotel rates: from US$180.

Nusa Dua Beach Hotel
❤❤❤❤

PO Box 1028, Denpasar, Nusa Dua, Bali 80001. Tel: (361) 771210. Fax: (361) 772617. TYPE: Resort hotel & Spa. LOCATION: On the southern peninsula 20 minutes to airport. SPA CLIENTELE: Women and men. DESCRIPTION: Traditional Balinese beach resort with Health club & Spa. Spa facilities include: Spa café, gym, aerobics, sauna, massage, plunge pools, steam baths, lap pool. 380 rooms,

swimming pool, pool bar, restaurants. Hotel rates: from US$200.

Nikko Bali Resort & Spa
❤❤❤❤

JL. Raya Nusa Dua Selatan, Nusa Dua, Bali 80363. Tel: (36) 773377. Fax: (361) 773388. TYPE: Hotel & Spa. LOCATION: On a cliff top overlooking the beach. SPA CLIENTELE: Women and men. DESCRIPTION:Balinese & Japanese style resort hotel with health spa. The Spa facilities - **Chavana Spa** - 8000 sq.ft. / 730 sq.m. health spa with six deluxe spa villas for couples, individual beauty treatment rooms, fitness center, jacuzzi, sauna. 395 rooms, 15 suites, restaurants, bars, outdoor pool. Hotel rates: from US$180.

PADMA
➁ 361
✈ Ngurah Rai Airport (DPS) 5 km. / 3 mi.

Bali Padma Hotel
❤❤❤❤

Jl. Padma No. 1, Legian. Tel: (361) 752111. Fax: (361) 752140. TYPE: Hotel & Spa. LOCATION: Seaside village of Padma in Bali. SPA CLIENTELE: Women and men. DESCRIPTION: Beautiful 400 room resort in traditional Balinese style with Health Spa - **Mandara Spa**. The spa offers three ultra deluxe spas with waterfalls, extensive gardens, spa treatment beds, garden showers, private relaxation areas, five single spa treatment rooms on the garden level and full service beauty salon. Also available health club, gym, sauna, steam room, aerobics, swimming pool, tennis and squash. Hotel rates: from US$160.

UBUD
➁ 361
✈ Ngurah Rai Airport (DPS) 55 km. / 35 mi.

Banyan Tree Kamandalu
❤❤❤❤

Jl Tegallalang, Nagi, Ubud 80571. Tel: (361) 975-825.

Fax: (361) 975-851. TYPE: Mountain Retreat & Spa. LOCATION: Peched on Nagi's hill above the Petanu River. SPA CLIENTELE: Women and men. DESCRIPTION: Picturesque village style retreat with spa, herbal massages, and jogging track. 58 rooms and villas, restaurants, bars, outdoor pool. Hotel rates: from $180.

Four Seasons Bali at Sayan
♥♥♥♥

Sayan, Gianyar, Ubud, Bali 80571. Tel: (361) 977577, Fax: (361) 977588. TYPE: Resort & Spa. LOCATION: Along the Ayung River 10 minutes to Ubud. DESCRIPTION: Elegant resort with fitness spa, sauna, cycling, trekking, rafting, kayaking. 46 rooms, restaurant, bar, swimming pool, tennis court. Hotel rates: from US375.

The Chedi Ubud
♥♥♥♥

Desa Melinggih Kelod Payangan, Ubud 80572. TYPE: Retreat & Spa. LOCATION: Amidst lush tropical foothills high above the Ayung river valley. SPA CLIENTELE: Women and men. DESCRIPTION: Picturesque Balinese style retreat with spa - The Spa at The Chedi - two 1,000 sq.ft. / 90 sq.m. deluxe spa villas for couples, open air spa with bathing pavilion, beauty treatments, mineral baths, body scrubs, herbal wraps, fitness center, jacuzzi, sauna. 60 rooms, 6 suites, restaurants, bar, open-air lobby. Hotel rates: from US$200.

UNGASAN
ᔨ **361**
✈ Ngurah Rai Airport (DPS) 25 km. / 16 mi.

Bali Cliff Resort
♥♥♥♥

Pura Batu Pageh, Ungasan, Bali 80361. Tel: (361) 771-992. Fax: (361) 771-993. TYPE: Resort & Spa. LOCATION: Southernmost tip of Bali overlooking the Indian Ocean. SPA CLIENTELE: Women and men. DESCRIPTION: First class resort hotel with fitness center, sauna, massages, gym, beauty salon. 175 rooms, 2 pools, restaurants,

Balinese art market. Hotel rates: from US$200.

JAVA ISLAND

YOGYAKARTA
ᔨ **274**
✈ Adi Sucipto Airport (AMI) 15 km. / 10 mi.

Hyatt Regency Yogyakarta
♥♥♥♥

Jl Palagan Tentara Pelajar, Yogyakarta 55581. Tel: (274) 869-123. Fax: (274) 869-588. TYPE: Resort & Spa. LOCATION: Situated amidst landscaped gardens with views of Mount Merapi & Seribu Mountain. SPA CLIENTELE: Women and men. DESCRIPTION: Secluded resort near Indonesian temples with full service spa offering health and beauty treatments, Javanese massage, aromatherapy, reflexology. 269 rooms, 9 suites, restaurants, lounges, freedom pool with waterfalls. Hotel rates: from US$150.

LOMBOK ISLAND

KELAMATAN PUJUT PRAYA
ᔨ **370**
✈ Mataram Int'l Airport (AMI) 60 km. / 38 mi.

Novotel Lombok Coralia
♥♥♥♥

Pujut Lombok Tengah, Nusa Tenggara Barat. USA/Canada reservations: (800) 257-5344 or (516) 944-5508. Fax: (516) 944-7540. TYPE: Beach Resort & Spa. LOCATION: On a beautiful coastal location on the southern shore of Lombok. SPA CLIENTELE: Women and men.

* Rooms: 85 deluxe rooms
* Bungalows: 23 Sasak bungalows; Villas: 4 Nyala villas
* Phone, CTV, A/C, minibar, hairdryer, safe deposit
* Restaurants, cafe, dining pavilion
* Reservations: required
* Credit Cards: VISA/AMEX/MC/DIS/EC

* Open: Year round; Rates: on request; TAC: 10%
* SPA on premises: **Mandara Spa**
* **Spa Facilities**: indoor treatment rooms, open air garden pavilions, fitness rooms, saunas, jacuzzi, massage rooms, beauty salon
* **Spa Programs**: beauty, pampering, fitness
* **Spa Treatments**: Mandara massages, Japanese Shiatsu, Thai and Balinese massages, stretching, acupressure, aromatherapy, facials with Indonesian herbs, spices and tropical fruits and vegetables.
* **Indications**: stress reduction, pampering

DESCRIPTION: Traditional Sasak village style resort with a unique architectural design creating a rustic but comfortable hotel aiming to reflect an authentic Lombok village. The Health Spa - **Mandara Spa** - features exotic Balinese style massages and beauty treatments.

MEDANA BEACH

⅂ 370

✈ Mataram Int'l Airport (AMI) 28 km. / 18 mi.

The Oberoi Lombok
♥♥♥♥♥

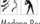

Medana Beach, West Lombok 83001. Tel: (370) 38444. Fax: (370) 32496. TYPE: Garden Resort & Spa. LOCATION: On Medana Beach on the northwest coast of Lombok Island. SPA CLIENTELE: Women and men. DESCRIPTION: Secluded resort in local style with Health Spa, treatment rooms, massages, herbal bath, steam shower, sauna, jacuzzi, beauty treatments, beauty salon. 50 Lombok style thatched-roofed 1-2BR villas and pavilions, swimming pool, poolside restaurant, beach side cafe, golf tours. Hotel rates: from US$255.

Photo: courtesy of **Mandara Spa**, Bali Indonesia

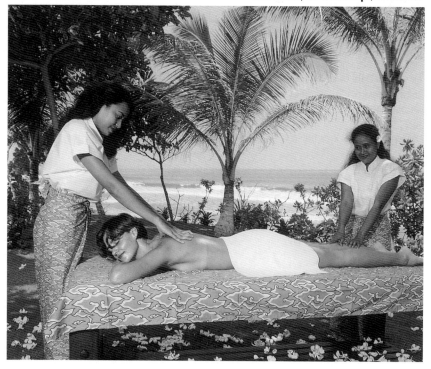

IRELAND

AREA: 27,136 sq. mi. (70,282 sq. km.)
POPULATION: 3,540,000
CAPITAL: Dublin
OFFICIAL LANGUAGE: English, Gaelic (Irish)
CURRENCY: Irish Pound (I£)
EXCHANGE RATE: 1 US$ = IR 0.68
TELEPHONE COUNTRY CODE: 353

ℹ️ Bord Fáilte (Irish Tourist Board)
Baggot St., Bridge, Dublin 2, Republic of Ireland
Tel: (+353-1) 602-4000. Fax: (+353-1) 602-4100

COOLAKAY
✈ 1
✈ Dublin Airport (DUB) 30 km. / 19 mi.

Powerscourt Springs Health Farm
❤❤❤

Coolakay, Enniskerry, Wicklow. Tel: (1) 2761000. Fax:
(1) 2761626. TYPE: Health Farm. LOCATION: In the
"Garden of Ireland" area 30 min. from Dublin. SPA CLIEN-
TELE: Women and men. DESCRIPTION: Health Farm set on
50 acres, surrounded by rivers and woodlands. The Spa
offers structured programs and it is dedicated to the needs
of those in search of rest, relaxation and rejuvenation.
Facilities include: swimming pool, sauna, steam room,
jacuzzi, sunbed, gym, beauty salon. Spa treatments: calorie counted gourmet meals, massages, reflexology, beauty

treatments, aerobics. Recreation: golf, horse riding, hill
walking and beaches nearby.

Claureen Health Farm
❤❤❤

Ennis, Clare. Tel: (65) 28969. Fax: (65) 42970. TYPE:
Health Farm. LOCATION: West of Ireland in an area known
for its unspoiled beauty. SPA CLIENTELE: Women and men.
DESCRIPTION: Health Farm with weight loss and holistic
programs. Spa facilities: sauna, gym, massage clinic, beauty salon. Spa treatments: massage, yoga, reflexology, aromatherapy.

CORK
✈ 21
✈ Cork Airport (ORK) 5 km. / 3 mi.

Thalassotherapy Centre
❤❤❤

c/o Rochestown Park Hotel, Rochestown Rd., Douglas,
Cork. Tel: (21) 894949. Fax: (21) 892178. TYPE:
Thalassotherapy Spa. LOCATION: in the first class
Rochestown Park Hotel on 7 acres of landscaped gardens,
10 mi. south of Cork. SPA CLIENTELE: Women and men.

* Hotel Rooms: 118 w/priv. bath.
* Suites: 5 w/jacuzzi
* Cottages: 8 self catering
* Phone, A/C, C/H, coffee tea making facilities
* Restaurant, business center, tennis court
* Open: Year round
* Hotel Rates: from I£45
* TAC: 10%
* Spa on premises: **Thalassotherapy Centre**
* **Spa Facilities**: sauna, steam room, whirlpool, gym,
  solarium, aerobics room, hydrotherapy pool and baths,
* **Spa Treatments**: thalassotherapy, hydrotherapy, sea-
  weed baths, massages, beauty treatments, aerobics
* **Spa Programs**: Anti-stress, beauty, fitness

DESCRIPTION: Thalassotherapy centre set in a wonderful

Roman style featuring a wide range of health, beauty and leisure treatments based on thalassotherapy, massages and exercises.

GALWAY
⟩ 91
✈ Galway AP

Galway Bay Health Farm
♥♥♥♥

Longhaunrone House, Oranmore, Co, Galway. Tel: (91) 790606. Fax: (91) 790837. TYPE: Health Farm. MANAGING DIRECTOR: Margaret McNulty. LOCATION: On a 50 acre deer farm overlooking Galway Bay. SPA CLIENTELE: Women and men. AGE RESTRICTION: must be 16 or older. SPECIAL RESTRICTIONS: Smoking not permitted.

* Rooms: 6. Suites: 6
* Phone, A/C, C/H, radio, clock, dining facilities
* Airport: Galway, free pick up
* Open: Year round
* Rates: from I£85
* TAC: 10%
* Spa on premises
* Year Established: 1994
* **Spa Facilities**: sauna, steam room, fully equipped gym, beauty salon, massage clinic, treatment room, lecture hall, tennis court, library
* **Spa Treatments**: reflexology, therapeutic massage, holistic massage, low impact aerobics, stretch classes, organized walks, aromatherapy, beauty treatments, yoga, low calorie balanced meals, organized walks and cycling, daily early morning swim in a 20 m indoor heated pool (3 min. drive away)
* **Spa Programs**: Weight loss, beauty, fitness, yoga, Structured daily program, Holistic program
* **Spa Packages**: 3-5 Day Programs, Non Resident Holistic Health Day, Week-End Program
* Email: lochan@iol.ie
* Web: www.galwaybayhealthfarm.ie

DESCRIPTION: Award winning Health Farm/Spa and Relaxation Center providing a kickstart to a healthy lifestyle through a balance of attitude, relaxation, exercise and eating plans. Elegant yet casual Health Farm in a beautiful Georgian Mansion offering a wide range of exercises and beauty treatments for relaxation, weight loss and pampering. The food is light and nutritious, low calorie, high protein and can be adjusted to different dietary requirements. Professional lectures are given on different health topics. The experience at Galway Bay Health Farm opens your mind to the benefits of good health, tones your body through exercise, fitness and relaxation and leaves the soul with a sense of peace and tranquility.

HORSELEAP
⟩ 506
✈ Dublin Airport (DUB)

Temple Country House & Spa
♥♥♥

Horseleap, Moate, Westmeath. Tel: (506) 35118. Fax: (506) 35118. TYPE: Country Spa. LOCATION: Just off N6 midway between Dublin and Galway. SPA CLIENTELE: Women and men. DESCRIPTION: 200 year old Farm House with a house spa that is personally supervised by the proprietors. The Spa Program includes; yoga, relaxation classes, reflexology, aromatherapy, hydrotherapy and beauty treatments. Spa facilities: sauna, steam room, hydrotherapy bath. Recreation: golf, horse riding, cycling tours.

KILLALOE
⟩ 61
✈ Shannon Airport (SNN)

Tinarana House
♥♥

Killaloe, Clare. Tel: (61) 376966. Fax: (61) 376773. TYPE: Health Spa. LOCATION: 6.4 km / 4 mi. from Killaloe once the ancient capital of Ireland. SPA CLIENTELE: Women and men. DESCRIPTION: Victorian mansion on 300 woodland acres offering spa treatments with a special emphasis on the Mayr Cure. Spa treatments: balneotherapy, hydrotherapy, fango therapy, aromatherapy, body massages, body wraps, colon treatments, procaine treatments, yoga, exercises. Recreation: horseback riding, golf, fishing, tennis, sailing.

MOORESFORT
ⵋ **62**
✈ Dublin Airport (DUB)

An Tearmann Beag
♥♥

Mooresfort, Kilross, Tipperary. Tel/Fax: (62) 55102. TYPE: Holistic & Retreat Centre. SPA DIRECTORS: Sally McCormack and Mary Condren. LOCATION: Heart of Irish countryside on 14 acre of land farmed organically. SPA CLIENTELE: Women and men. DESCRIPTION: Retreat centre looking out at the Galtee Mountains. Accommodations are in cottages and apartments as self-catering or full board. Spa treatments

include: aromatherapy, reflexology, holistic massage, allergy testing, energy bodywork, daily meditation.

WESTPORT
ⵋ **98**
✈ Connaught Regional AP, 48 km. / 30 mi.

Cloona Health Centre
♥♥♥

Westport, Mayo. Tel: (98) 25251. TYPE: Health Farm. LOCATION: 3 mi / 5 km from Westport, between Croagh and Clew Bay. SPA DIRECTORS: Emer and Dhara Kelly. SPA CLIENTELE: Women and men. DESCRIPTION: Founded 25 years ago the Cloona Health Center offers to opportunity to reflect, refresh and rejuvenate with holistic and structured programs. A healthy light, cleansing diet of fruit and organic vegetables will help you loose weight and feel good.

Photo courtesy of the **Galway Bay Health Farm**

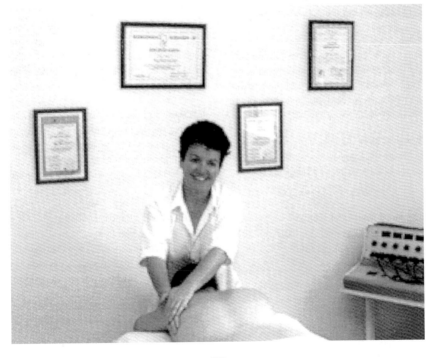

ISRAEL

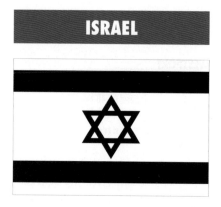

AREA: 7,847 sq. mi. (20,324 sq. km.)
POPULATION: 4,625,000
CAPITAL: Jerusalem
OFFICIAL LANGUAGES: Hebrew, Arabic
CURRENCY: Shekel (IS)
EXCHANGE RATE: 1 US$ = IS 4.20
TELEPHONE COUNTRY CODE: 972

Israeli health spas have been famous since biblical times. Today, the state of Israel considers the development and maintenance of the spa industry a top priority. The most famous Health Spa destination in Israel is the **Dead Sea**, the "Lowest Place on Earth". This is one of the world's most fascinating tourism destination. The Dead Sea region offers year-round health and beauty tourism combined with dramatic natural beauty and historical sites.

Most of the Health Spas in Israel have their own medical clinics or are located near clinics or hospitals. Excellent medical care by professionals is always readily available.

ℹ️ Israel Ministry of Tourism
800 Second Avenue, New York NY 10017
Tel: (212) 499-5652. Fax: (212) 499-5655

DEAD SEA SPAS
🍷 **7**
✈ Massada Airport, 20 km. / 13 mi.
Ben Gurion Airport (TLV); Atarot Airport (JRS)

Dead Sea area: A world famous Spa resort on the eastern shores of Yam HaMelah (the Salt Sea), at the lowest point on earth, 1,296 ft. / 393 m. below sea level. The Dead Sea, which is actually a landlocked saltwater lake, was already an important healing Spa in Biblical times. The notorious cities of Sodom and Gomorrah were said to have been located on its shores. The legend has it that King Herod the Great used the thermo-mineral water for cure and relaxation. The Dead Sea has a unique history that makes it one of Israel's most compelling tourist attractions.

The chemical composition of the Dead Sea water is a concentrated solution of chlorides of calcium, magnesium, sodium and potassium, with a high percentage of dissolved bromides. The combination of high mineral concentration (30%), high atmospheric pressure, dry heat, and non-polluted oxygen-rich air, makes the Dead Sea an excellent winter resort for natural therapy. Summers can be extremely hot with temperatures in the 100°F (38°c). But winters are comfortable with temperatures in the mid 70°sF (24°c). The low altitude filters out many of the sun's harmful rays, making possible safe sun treatments for skin ailments.

The high mineral concentration gives the Dead Sea a distinguished 'oily' character which keeps bathers afloat and leaves the skin smooth and moisturized. Dead Sea water must be kept away from the eyes or open wounds as this can be very painful.

Indications: Dead Sea treatments are recommended to reinvigorate the skin, treat psoriasis, asthma and certain respiratory problems. The therapeutic mud is used in the treatment of muscular, joint diseases and post-paralytic conditions, but the mud is also good for beauty and cosmetic applications.

Contraindications: acute skin inflammation, active tuberculosis, bleeding disorders, malignant growths, advanced renal and/or hepatic insufficiency, after effects of heart attack, heart failure, advanced peripheral arteriosclerosis, high blood pressure, psychosis, severe neurosis, epilepsy.

The Dead Sea offers balneological and climatological treatments at three locations: Ein Bokek, Hamme Zohar & Ein Gedi.

Ein Bokek is a Spa and tourist center on the shore of the Dead Sea with hot mineral (sulfur) springs, some 32 km. (20 mi.) southeast of Arad and 15 km. (9 mi.) south of Masada.

Hamme Zohar is a Hot springs Resort on the Dead Sea, 24 km. (15 mi.) southeast of Arad.

Ein Gedi is a charming desert oasis north of Masada, near Kibbutz Ein Gedi with lovely waterfalls and nature wildlife reserve. Visitors can relax by the Dead Sea, enjoy mud packs or dip in Ein Gedi's sulfur pools. Ein Gedi is located 28 km. (18 mi.) north of Ein Bokek.

The Dead Sea is located about one hour drive from Jerusalem through the Judean desert.

Caesar Premier Hotel Dead Sea
❤❤❤

Ein Bokek, Dead Sea 86980. Tel: (7) 668-9666. Fax: (7) 7652-0303. TYPE: Hotel & Spa. LOCATION: On the shores of the Dead Sea in Ein Bokek. SPA CLIENTELE: Women and men. DESCRIPTION: Spa hotel with mineral baths, mud treatments, massage, solarium, sauna & gym. 320 rooms, 20 suites, restaurants, indoor and outdoor salt water pools.

Carlton Galei Zohar Hotel
❤❤❤

Ein Bokek, Dead Sea 86930. Tel: (7) 658-4311. Fax: (7) 658-4503. TYPE: Spa Hotel. LOCATION: Dead Sea beach location. SPA CLIENTELE: Women and men, family oriented.

* Rooms: 250 w/private bath
* Phone, CTV, A/C
* Night Club, Bar & Video Room
* Conference Room: up to 350 seats
* Airport: Ben Gurion (Tel Aviv), 200 km. / 125 mi.
* Airport Transportation: bus, taxi
* Open: Year round
* Rates: from $120/day; TAC: 10%
* Spa on premises

* **Spa facilities**: Dermatologic & Rheumatic Clinic, health club, indoor / outdoor swimming pools
* **Spa Treatments**: see Dead Sea treatments
* Medical Supervision: medical clinic
* Treatments Approved: Ministry of Health

DESCRIPTION: Modern first class hotel near beach offering medically supervised Dead Sea treatments. Many hotel guests enjoy the spa benefits to the body and skin without medical treatments. Amenities: kosher kitchen, synagogue, dining rooms, game/card room, and parking.

Ein Gedi Resort Hotel & Spa
❤❤❤

Kibbutz Ein Gedi, Dead Sea 86980. Tel: (7) 659-4813, Fax: (7) 658-4544. Managing Director: Dov Litvinoff. Program Director: Moshe Shamir. TYPE: First class resort hotel & Spa. LOCATION: Dead Sea beach location. SPA CLIENTELE: Women and men. AGE RESTRICTIONS: Teenagers & children accepted.

* Rooms: 120 w/private bath
* CTV, A/C, C/H, phone
* Restaurant, bar
* Airport: Ben Gurion (Tel Aviv) 200 km. / 125 mi.
* Airport Transportation: bus, taxi
* Reservations: required for guest house
* Credit Cards: MC/VISA/AMEX/ACC/EC
* Open: Year round
* Rates: on request
* Name of Spa: **Ein Gedi Spa**
* Distance to SPA: 5 km. / 3 mi.
* Year Established: 1960
* **Spa Facilities**: Sulphur pools & showers, black mud, Dead Sea, fresh water pool
* **Spa Treatments**: see Dead Sea treatments. All treatments at the Ein Gedi SPA are self-applied
* **Spa Programs**: Light exercises in all pools, Night Programs, Bar-B-Que, Disco
* **Spa Packages**: Spa + lunch; Season Ticket (10 entries)
* **Indications**: Rheumatism and certain skin disorders
* **Contraindication**: persons with heart conditions; blood pressure problems or pregnant women are advised not

to enter sulphur pools
* Documentation from Physician: recommended
* Medical Supervision: 1 doctor; 3 RN
* Maximum number of guests: 2,000

DESCRIPTION: Resort hotel at the Ein Gedi Kibbutz, consisting of rustic air-conditioned cabins in a landscaped garden setting. Facilities: cafeteria, indoor and outdoor pools and a world famous Clinic specializing in climatological therapies. Regular shuttle takes the guests to the Ein Gedi Spa, an ultra modern facility with warm sulphur baths (38°c / 100°F), black mud pools, and sunbathing beach. The Spa has its own vegetarian restaurant which serves delicious low-cal and nutritious meals. Special activities for children are available during the high season. The hot springs of Ein Gedi Spa and the oxygen rich air, work wonders for relaxation, rejuvenation and rehabilitation.

Grand Nirvana on the Dead Sea Spa, Resort & Convention Center
❤❤❤❤

Mobile post Dead Sea 84960. Tel: (7) 6689444. Fax: (7) 6689400. TYPE: Deluxe Resort & Spa Hotel. MANAGER: Mr. Paul Milwidsky. LOCATION: 3.5 km. / 2 mi. south of Ein Bokek, on the shore of the Dead Sea. SPA CLIENTELE: Women and men. AGE RESTRICTION: Must be 16 years and older to access the spa.

* Rooms: 388 w/priv. bath, Suites:12, Apartments: 50
* Phone, CTV, minibar, hairdryer, safe, balcony, jacuzzi (in suites)
* Hotel Facilities: restaurant, bar, English pub, children's club, 2 lounges, mini golf, private beach, recreation beach, outdoor fresh water pool, rooms for disabled, spacy solarium on the hotel's roof
* Airport: Ben-Gurion (Tel Aviv), 175 km. / 109 mi.
* Airport Transportation: taxi, bus, rent a car
* Reservations: required
* Credit Cards: VISA/AMEX/MC/DIN/EC
* Open: Year round
* Hotel Rates: room from $145 including service charge

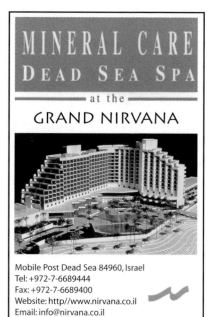

MINERAL CARE
DEAD SEA SPA
at the
GRAND NIRVANA

Mobile Post Dead Sea 84960, Israel
Tel: +972-7-6689444
Fax: +972-7-6689400
Website: http//www.nirvana.co.il
Email: info@nirvana.co.il

* TAC: 10%
* Spa on premises: open from 08:00 am - 23:00 pm
* Year Established: 1989, renovated 1998
* SPA Facilities: Health, Fitness & Beauty Center, stylish intimate health club with professional spa, indoor Dead Sea water pool (heated or chilled), dry & wet sauna, 2 jacuzzi pools, modern and fully equipped gym, Spa bar - beverages based on natural fruit juices, treatment rooms (35) for massages, special mud wraps rooms, individual mineral and oil baths, sulphur pool, beauty parlor
* Spa Programs: Beauty, pampering, Anti-Stress, Fitness, Medical
* Spa Treatments: hydrobaths, mineral & oil baths, seaweed, underwater massage, unique mud wraps, anti-cellulite, classic massages, shiatsu, reflexology, aromatherapy, beauty facials for women and men, hair and scalp treatments, all treatments based on highly professional Dead Sea and Mineral Care products
* Spa Packages: Beauty, rheumatology, anti-stress,

anti-cellulite packages available for 3-28 days
* **Indications**: Dead Sea Spas
* **Medical Supervision**: doctor on premises 24 hrs. a day
* **Email**: info@nirvana.co.il
* **Web**: www.nirvana.co.il

DESCRIPTION: Deluxe Spa Hotel on the shore of the Dead Sea with an easily accessible private beach with all beach facilities. The resort features a world class, intimate and highly professional Spa using first class cosmetic products of the "Mineral Care" line. The Nirvana's Spa offers pampering, beauty, anti-stress, rheumatology, and anti-cellulite treatments of the highest standards. The "Nirvana's way" offers for your leisure - entertainment every evening, pub, children's club, and mini golf. The Nirvana Hotel is where the High Society meets at the Dead Sea.

Hod Hotel
♥♥♥

Ein Bokek, Dead Sea 86930. Tel: (7) 584-644. Fax: (7) 584-381. TYPE: First class Spa hotel. LOCATION: Dead Sea beach location. MANAGING DIRECTOR: Mr. Udi Zicherman. SPA CLIENTELE: Women and men, family oriented.

* Rooms: 203 w/private bath
* Phone, CTV, A/C
* Restaurant, bar, disco
* Airport: Ben Gurion (Tel Aviv), 200 km. / 125 mi.
* Airport Transportation: bus, taxi
* Season: Year round
* Rates: from $160/day; TAC: 10%
* Spa on premises
* **Spa facilities**: Health Club, Clinic, Fitness room, Finnish sauna, jacuzzi, Dead Sea water pool, massage rooms
* **Spa Treatments**: massages, hot mud body pack
* Medical Supervision: medical clinic
* Treatments Approved: Ministry of Health

DESCRIPTION: Moderate first class spa hotel with air-conditioned rooms. The Health Spa features traditional treatments based on Dead Sea muds, seawater and other products. The health Club features the "Stauffer Concept" for weight loss and relaxation. Recreation: fashion shows, folk dancing, lectures on topics of health & beauty, bingo and casino evenings.

Hyatt Regency Dead Sea Resort & Spa
♥♥♥♥

Dead Sea Post, Ein Bokek. Hotel Tel: (7) 659-1234, Spa Tel: (7) 6591201. Fax: (7) 6591204. TYPE: Deluxe Resort Hotel & Spa. MANAGER: Mr. Gidon Laks. LOCATION: Western shore of the Dead Sea south of Kibbutz Ein Gedi. SPA CLIENTELE: Women, men. AGE RESTRICTION: must be 16 years or older.

* Rooms: 600, Suites: 38
* Phone, CTV, A/C, C/H, minibar, safe, balcony
* Jacuzzi, restaurant, bar, nightclub
* Reservations: required
* Open: Year round
* Rates: Hotel rooms from $180/day
  Spa entry: $8 (hotel guests) $25 (visitors)
  opening hours: 7:00am - 8:00pm
  Spa Treatments: $30 - $115 per treatment
* Spa on premises: **Mineralia**
* Year Established: 1996
* **Spa Facilities**: mineral & sulfur baths, skin treatment clinic, fresh water pools, sea water pools, jacuzzi, sauna, steam room, tennis, squash, gym
* **Spa Programs**: Beauty, Pampering, Relaxation
* **Spa Treatments**: hydrobaths, mineral baths, essential oils, seaweed, underwater massage, cellulite, mud and aromatherapy wraps, Swedish massage, Thai massage, Shiatsu, reflexology, so-jok, sports massage, aromatherapy, lymph drainage, facials, beauty treatments, hair treatments, skin treatments (based on Dead Sea and Mineralia products)
* **Indications**: See Dead Sea spas
* Medical Supervision: available on request
* Email: hyt_sale@inter.net.il

DESCRIPTION: Deluxe multistory Health Spa & resort. All rooms are tastefully decorated with sea or pool views. The Mineralia Health Spa offers a wide range of beauty, pampering, revitalizing and medical treatments in an elegant environment by highly qualified beauty and health professionals. The Hyatt Regency Dead Sea Resort & Spa is popular with spa afficionados from all over the world.

Radisson Moriah Gardens
Dead Sea
❤❤❤

🗿 ⚖ 🐎

Mobile post Dead Sea, Ein Bokek, Sodom 84960. Tel: (7) 658-4351. Fax: (7) 658-4383. TYPE: Spa Hotel. LOCATION: South end of the Dead Sea, 200 m. from the beach. SPA CLIENTELE: Women and men, family oriented.

* Rooms: 196 w/priv. bath. Suites: 10
* Phone (direct dial), A/C, CTV, video, radio
* Kosher restaurant, bar, cocktail lounge, night club
* Airport: Ben Gurion (Tel-Aviv), 200 km. (125 mi.)
* Airport Transportation: Bus, rent-a-Car
* Reservations: suggested
* Credit Cards: MC/VISA/AMEX/DC/EC
* Open: Year round
* Hotel Rates: from US$180; TAC: 10%
* Spa on premises
* **Spa Facilities**: Indoor and outdoor pools with Dead Sea water, jacuzzi, swimming pool, Beauty center, Health Club
* **Spa Programs**: 2 weeks spa program, Special Psoriasis Treatment, Beauty and Health Program
* **Spa Treatments**: bathing in Dead Sea mineral waters, Dead Sea mud treatments, psoriasis treatments
* **Indications**: skin diseases, psoriasis, atopic dermatitis, recovery after illnesses, neurological metabolic disorders, traumatic illnesses, allergies, bronchial, asthma; Dead Sea muds- rheumatism, post myelitic and post-paralytic illnesses, also good for relaxation
* **Contraindications**: see Dead Sea spas
* Treatments Approved: Ministry of Health

DESCRIPTION: Health Spa offering treatments based on Dead Sea products. Special treatments are available for psoriasis sufferers with natural ingredients including solarium. Family plan allows children up to the age of 18 to stay free with their parents.

Radisson Moriah Plaza
Dead Sea Hotel & Spa
❤❤❤

🗿 ⚖ 🐎 ❀

Hamme Zohar, M.P. 86910 Dead Sea. Tel: (07) 659-1591. Fax: (07) 658-4238.TYPE: Spa Hotel. LOCATION: Dead Sea beach location. SPA CLIENTELE:Women and men, family oriented.

* Rooms: 220 w/priv. bath. Suites: 5
* CTV, A/C, C/H, phone, minibar
* Restaurant, Bar, Nightclub, Kosher/Diet Cuisine
* Airport: Ben Gurion (Tel Aviv), 175 km. / 110 mi. nearby airstrip for local flights
* Airport Transportation: Bus, rent-a-car, taxi
* Reservation: required
* Credit Cards: MC/VISA/AMEX
* Open: Year Round
  High Season: 3/25 - 5/31& 9/19 - 11/30
* Hotel Rates: from US$200; TAC: 10%
* Spa on premises
* Year Established: 1973
* **Spa Facilities**: Health, Fitness & Beauty Center, air conditioned indoor pool containing heated Dead Sea water, 2 sulfur pools supplied with thermal water from the Zohar spring, 8 bath tubs for mineral, mud, carbon dioxide, air bubble and sulfur baths, with group recovery rooms, 2 tubs with private recovery rooms, a stretch and mineral whirlpool tub with weights and underwater massage, special small tubs for arm and leg treatment, Scotch shower, inhalation room, massage room, Fitness Room with "Universal" fitness equipment, dry Finnish Sauna, private bathing beach
* **Spa Programs**: Beauty, relaxation, medical
* **Spa Treatments**: Dead Sea water Hydrotherapy and Sulphur pools, private sulphur bath with mud pack, vapor inhalation of Dead Sea water and eucalyptus oil to clear respiratory passages and sinuses, massage, physiotherapy, fangotherapy (application of heated sea mud), low cal meals, solarium for the treatment of psoriasis; Beauty treatments include: massages, hydro-massage, facials, manicures & pedicures, aerobic

training, stress relaxation, body toning, dieting instructor, reflexology
* **Spa Package**: Beauty & Relaxation (7 nts) Rheumatic Package (14 nts)
* **Indications**: See Dead Sea spas
* **Contraindications**: See Dead Sea spas
* Medical Supervision: permanent medical team, 1 MD, 1 nurse
* Documentation from Physician: guests may be requested to bring their medical records plus relevant X-rays and prescriptions
* Treatments approved: Ministry of Health

DESCRIPTION: Spa hotel on the Dead Sea shore offering Spa programs and treatments under medical supervision in the modern spa on the hotel's ground floor. Guests can benefit from a wide range of medical treatments in the annexed medical clinic. Unique body pampering and beauty treatments are based on the world famous Dead Sea products & mud packs. This is a popular health Spa with many Israelis and Europeans. Recreation: tennis, bridge, movies, and sight-seeing.

EILAT

7

✈ Eilat Airport, 1 km. / 1/2 mi.

Eilat is Israel's southernmost port city on the Red Sea. It is the country's leading winter resort with Israelis and International tourism, especially from Scandinavia and Germany. Tourists arrive by the plane loads in the winter to soak the warm desert sun, enjoy the fine beaches, crystal clear sea water, and the modern hotels, restaurants and shopping centers. Summers are extremely hot with temperatures exceeding 110°F (45°c). Winters are pleasant with high temperatures in the 80°sF (28°c). Eilat is the point where the Israeli border meets Jordan (Aqaba) and Egypt (Taba).

Herods Sheraton Resort
❤❤❤❤❤

North Shore, Eilat. Tel: (7) 633-5256. Fax: (7) 633-

5253. TYPE: Resort Hotel & Spa. LOCATION: On the beachfront of Eilat's North Shore, bordered by the Red Sea and the New Lagoon. SPA CLIENTELE: Women and men.

* Rooms: 468 w/priv. bath and balcony all balconies provide shade and panoramic seaview
* Suites: 34 (including 1 Presidential Suite)
* No smoking rooms, rooms for the handicapped and the hearing impaired
* Phone, CTV, A/C, C/H, minibar, coffee maker safe deposit box
* Restaurant, Bar, Nightclub, Kosher/Diet Cuisine
* Airport: Eilat, bus, rent-a-car, taxi
* Reservation: required
* Credit Cards: MC/VISA/AMEX
* Open: Year Round High Season: winter
* Hotel Rates: from US$200
* TAC: 10%
* Spa on premises: **Herods Vitalis Spa**
* Year Established: 1999
* **Spa Facilities**: 2,500 sq. m. 27,500 sq. ft. spa facilities, thermal mineral salt pool, indoor and outdoor exercise pool, hydromassage waterfall, dry and wet saunas, treatment rooms indoors or out, skin care rooms (7), body treatment rooms (23), hydrojet massage rooms (3), massage rooms (10), Fitness center, pneumatic exercise equipment, aerobics studio, gym with panoramic windows overlooking the sea, beauty salon, Spa Restaurant
* **Spa Programs**: Beauty, pampering, relaxation, fitness
* **Spa Treatments**: thalassotherapy, hydromassage, massages, therapeutic body treatments, beauty treatments, fitness classes, spa cuisine
* **Spa Package**: Lifemasters - all inclusive 3,5 or 7 day programs, Open Spa package programs
* **Indications**: Anti-stress, pampering, fitness

DESCRIPTION: Elegant theme resort hotel and spa built on the shores of the Red Sea. The Herods Sheraton resort consists of three separate entities: Herods Palace, Herods Vitalis and Herods Forum. Herods Vitalis, health and lifestyle resort is dedicated to the promotion of well being and offer luxury thalassotherapy, beauty and fitness programs and treatments.

The Orchid Hotel & Resort
❤❤❤❤❤

South Beach, Eilat 81000. Tel: (7) 636-0360. Fax: (7) 637-5323. TYPE: Resort & Spa. LOCATION: On a hillside overlooking the Red Sea. SPA CLIENTELE: Women and men. DESCRIPTION: Distinctive Thai style resort hotel with Health Spa, gym, sauna, Thai massages, outdoor pools connected by waterfalls. 136 rooms. Thai restaurant, coffee shop, piano bar, poolside bar. Hotel rates: from $190/day.

HAIFA
🌙 **4**

✈ Haifa Airport, 20 km. / 13 mi.

Haifa, population 370,000, is the capital of the north. Beautifully situated on the slopes of Mt. Carmel overlooking the bay of Haifa, the city offers panoramic vistas, beautiful beaches and mild climate year round.

Carmel Forest Spa Resort
❤❤❤

Carmel Forest, Haifa. Tel: (4) 832-3111. Fax: (4) 832-3988. TYPE: Spa Hotel. LOCATION: On top of the Carmel mountain range, 20 min. from Haifa. SPA CLIENTELE: Women and men. DESCRIPTION: Spa hotel on landscaped forested grounds overlooking the sea. Spa facilities: sauna, jacuzzi, gym, beauty salon, swimming pools. spa treatments include: massages, facials and body treatments, fitness classes. No smoking policy. 97 rooms, restaurant with spa cuisine, Synagogue. Hotel rates: from US$240.

ROSH PINA
🌙 **6**

✈ Rosh Pina Airport

Rosh Pina, population 800, is a quaint little town founded in 1882. The region is known for its rolling verdant hills, picturesque villages and excellent climate.

Mizpe HaYamim
❤❤❤

Rosh Pina 12000. Tel: (6) 999666. Fax: (6) 999555. TYPE: Health Resort. LOCATION: Between Rosh Pina and Safed, 570 m / 1,880 ft. above sea level with views of Mt. Hermon, The Sea of Galilee and the Hula Valley. SPA CLIENTELE: Women and men.

* Rooms & Suites: 96 w/priv. bath
* Phone, CTV, A/C, C/H, minibar, coffee maker
* Restaurant: gourmet vegetarian cuisine
* Reservation: required
* Credit Cards: MC/VISA/AMEX
* Open: Year Round
* Hotel Rates: from US$160; TAC: 10%
* Spa on premises
* **Spa Facilities**: Vegeterian restaurant, swimming pool, sauna, jacuzzi, beauty salon, fitness center.
* **Spa Programs**: Beauty, fitness & diet
* **Spa Treatments**: Swedish massage, Thai massage, Chinese massage, aromatherapy, Feldenkrais, anti-cellulite, mud pack, facials, Shiatsu, reflexology, Indian massages, Reiki healing, thalassotherapy, body peeling, carniosacral balancing, massages, relaxation, physical exercise, water exercise, yoga, relaxation to music, aerobics, vegetarian cuisine

DESCRIPTION: Health Farm in the heart of the Galilee combining recreation and health activities with relaxation and comfort. The hotel offers nicely furnished rooms with period furniture, some with balcony. The spa offers a variety of health, slimming and beauty treatments administered by qualified professionals under medical supervision. Recreation: tennis, folk dances, horseback riding and walking tours.

TIBERIAS
🌙 **6**

✈ Haifa Airport 69 km. / 43 mi.

The **Sea of Galilee** Spas of **Tiberias** and **Hammat Gader** have been famous for the therapeutic value of their mineral springs since biblical times. Today, the spectacular development of the Tiberias Hot Springs turned the spa into a major internationally acclaimed balneological center and resort. Hammat Gader, a thermo mineral medical spa and recreation park, remains mostly a family oriented recreational facility built on the site of the ancient Roman baths.

Tiberias Hot Springs is a popular year-round resort town on the western shore of the Sea of Galilee in the north of Israel with health-restoring sulfur baths and hot water springs. The hot springs of Tiberias have been known for thousands of years for their therapeutic value. Herod Antipas founded the town of Tiberias around 18 AD in honor of the Emperor Tiberius, and the Romans built a genuine spa on the site.

The hot springs mineral content is similar to that at Aix-les-Bains in France, it contains 5,900 pico-Curies of radon per litre, and are classified as muriatic-calearious-sulfuric thermal waters. The mineral content is high, and the water is relatively hard which together with the high salinity renders it unsuitable for drinking. The Tiberias Hot Springs Health Center (Hamme-Teverya) is primarily a medical center and an International Spa Resort.

Indications: Under medical supervision people can get treatments for rheumatism, joint inflammation and muscular diseases, respiratory disturbances, gynecological complaints, and psychosomatic disorders.

Contraindication: for the spa treatments: cardiac insufficiency, coronary and vascular diseases, high blood pressure, and other chronic diseases. Some less strenuous treatments are available at the "recreation center" for healthy holiday makers for general health improvement and relaxation without medical supervision.

Tiberias is located 69 km. (43 mi.) east of Haifa, 132 km. (83 mi.) northeast of Tel Aviv.

Hammat Gader (El Hamma) hot springs, situated amidst the Golan and the Gilad mountains, is located about 20 km (13 mi.) southeast of Tiberias. Both spas can be reached by regular Egged bus service, or taxi Sherut (Service) from Haifa.

Holiday Inn Tiberias
❤❤❤

Habanim Street, Hamme Teverya, Tiberias 14100. Tel: (6) 679-2890. Fax: (6) 672-4443. TYPE: Spa hotel. LOCATION: On the Sea of Galilee in spacious wooded grounds. SPA CLIENTELE: Women and men. Family oriented.

* Rooms: 246 w/private bath. Suites: 14
* Phone, A/C, radio
* Restaurant, coffee shop, night club
* Gardens & private beach
* Airport: Haifa Airport, 69 km. (43 mi.)
* Airport Transportation: bus, taxi
* Open: Year round
* Credit Cards: AMEX/DC/VISA
* Rates: from $180/day
* TAC: 10%
* **Spa Facilities**: connected by bridge to the Hot springs Spa Center with pool and sauna nearby
* **Spa Program**: see Tiberias Hot Springs
* **Spa Treatments**: Treatments at Tiberias Hot Springs; at the hotel - ultrasound, solarium, physiotherapy & gymnasium.
* **Indications**: see Lake of Galilee Spas
* Medical Supervision: at Tiberias' Hot Springs
* Treatments Approved: Ministry of Health

DESCRIPTION: Contemporary lake front hotel with nice fully air-conditioned rooms. Kosher dining room overlooking the lake, wheelchair accessibility. Spa treatments at the Tiberias Hot Springs. Recreation: private beach, tennis courts, boating, fishing & swimming.

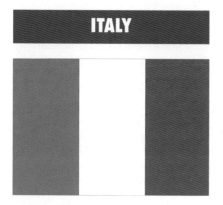

AREA: 116,303 sq. mi. (301,225 sq. km.)
POPULATION: 57,574,000
CAPITAL: Rome
OFFICIAL LANGUAGE: Italian
CURRENCY: Lira (Lit.)
EXCHANGE RATE: 1US$ = Lit. 1,684
TELEPHONE COUNTRY CODE: 39

Italy is famous for its spas and their mineral rich healing waters. Scientific research of balneology raised the traditional spa cure in Italy to impressive levels of contemporary medical care. Italian spas are located in different parts of Italy, and one can explore the cultural, geographical and historical heritage of their region.

ℹ️ ENIT - Ente Nazionale Italiano Per Il Turismo

Via Marghera 2, 00185 Roma, Italy
Tel: (+39-06) 49711. Fax: (+39-06) 4463379

ABANO TERME
🕽 049

✈️ Marco-Polo Tessera Airport (VCE)
32 mi. / 51 km. northeast of Abano

Abano is a small spa town near Padua, 25 miles (40 km) southwest of Venice. The town, surrounded by lovely parks, has interesting shops, galleries and fine restaurants. Abano is an important Thermal Spa and an internationally acclaimed medical center for treatments of specific physical problems.

Abano's principal treatment is based on Fango mud therapy. The thermal waters have a reputation for their healing powers thanks to their mineral content of sodium chloride, sodium sulfate, sodium bicarbonate, potassium chloride, lithium chloride, ammonium chloride, magnesium chloride, calcium, iodine, iron, alumina, and silica.

While taking a cure at Abano discover the beautiful city of Padua, rich with Roman origins and medieval history, and Venice with its romantic canals and glorious art treasures. Abano is accessible by car from either Venice or Padua.

Bristol Buja Spa
❤️❤️❤️❤️❤️

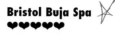

Via Monteortone, 2, Abano Terme 35031. Tel: (049) 866-9390, Fax: (049) 667-910. TYPE: Superior First Class Spa Hotel. LOCATION: Central location surrounded by park. SPA CLIENTELE: Women and men.

* Rooms: 152 w/private bath
* Suites: w/treatment sector
* Phone, A/C, CTV, minibar, balcony
* Restaurant, bar, TV rooms
* Wheelchair Accessible
* Airport: Venice, 25 mi. (40 km.), train, taxi
* Reservations: required
* Credit Cards: AMEX/VISA/DC/EC
* Open: year round (closed Nov. 19 - Dec. 17)
* Hotel Rates: from Lit. 260,000
* Spa on premises
* **Spa Facilities**: indoor/outdoor thermal pools, sun-terraces, natural grotto-sauna, gym, beauty center, SPA and mud treatment rooms on all floors
* **Spa Programs**: Thermal Cure (7 day) Beauty & Well Being (7 day)
* **Spa Treatments**: fango mud applications, thermal water showers, ozonized thermal baths, massages, underwater massages
* Medical Supervision: doctors, nurses, physiologist, dietitian, health senior

DESCRIPTION: Bristol Buja is a modern hotel offering comfortable rooms and pleasant atmosphere. The Spa program consists of a variety of health, beauty and fitness treatments based on mud applications and thermal baths. The Bristol Buja is a favorite hotel among many Spa enthusiasts.

Columbia Hotel
❤❤❤❤

Via Cornelio Augure 15, Abano Terme (Padova) 35031. Tel: (049) 866-9606. Fax: (049) 866-9430. TYPE: Spa hotel. LOCATION: 5 km. to Terme Euganee train station, 58 km to Venice's Marco Polo Airport. DESCRIPTION: Tourist class spa hotel with thermal treatments & cure facilities, connecting indoor & outdoor thermal pools, solarium, gym. Open March through November. 108 rooms, restaurant, bar, TV lounge, grotto garden & park. Hotel rates: from US$80.

Due Torri Morosini
❤❤❤❤

Via Pietro d'Abano 18, Abano Terme 35031. Tel: (049) 866-9277. Fax: (049) 866-9927. TYPE: Spa Hotel. LOCATION: Centrally located surrounded by a private park. SPA CLIENTELE: Women and men.

* Rooms: 80 w/private bath
* Phone, A/C, CTV, minibar, hair dryer
* Airport: Venice, 25 mi. (40 km.), taxi, train
* Reservations: suggested
* Credit Cards: VISA/AMEX/DC/EC
* Open: Year round
* Hotel Rates: from Lit. 120,000/day, rates are for room only, minimum stay 3 nights. SPA packages rates on request.
* SPA Facilities: Cure Department connected with guest rooms by lifts; two thermal swimming pools (one indoor), massage, inhalations, and therapy rooms, beauty salon
* Spa Programs: Medical, Beauty, Weight Loss
* Spa Treatments: mud applications, thermal baths, ozonized thermal baths, inhalations, vaginal irrigation, massages, under water massages, cosmetic and dermatology, diets

* **Indications**: arthritis, arthrose, gout, rheumatism, diseases from metabolism, after effects of fractures
* Medical Supervision: resident doctor, nurses and specialists

DESCRIPTION: A charming hotel decorated in a classic Italian style with old world ambience. The Spa is directly linked to the guest rooms via elevator and provides a variety of medical, beauty, and skin care treatments based on thermal waters and mud applications. Diet programs are available. Recreation: tennis, golf, and nightly entertainment.

Grand Hotel Trieste & Victoria
❤❤❤❤❤

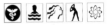

Via Pietro d'Abano 1, Abano Terme 35031. Tel: (049) 866-9101. Fax: (049) 866-9779. TYPE: Spa Hotel. LOCATION: Centrally located in a private park. SPA CLIENTELE: Women and men.

* Rooms: 94 w/private bath. Suites: 7
* Phone, A/C, CTV, mini bar
* Open air restaurant & bar
* Wheelchair Accessible
* Airport: Venice 60 km. / 38 mi.
* Train Station: Padova 12 km. / 8 mi.
* Airport/Train Transportation: taxi, bus
* Credit Cards: MC/VISA/AMEX/DC/EC
* Open: March - November
* Hotel Rates: from Lit. 160,000/day
* TAC: 10%
* Spa on premises
* Spa Facilities: indoor/outdoor thermal pools, sun-terraces, natural grotto-sauna, gym, cure cabins in private rooms, beauty salon
* Spa Programs: Health, beauty, relaxation, stress reduction, rejuvenation, weight loss, Physical Rehabilitation
* Spa Treatments: fango mud applications, thermal water showers, ozonized thermal baths, inhalations, massages, underwater massages, facial treatment, diet cuisine, exercises, rejuvenation treatments
* Indications: acute rheumatism, arthritis, metabolic disorders, neuralgia, fibrositis, gynecological

diseases, chronic congestion of the upper respiratory system, obesity, beauty and rejuvenation
* Contraindication: TBC
* Medical Supervision: 3 MD, 3 RN
* Treatments Approved: Italian Health Dept.

DESCRIPTION: A superior first class hotel combining tradition and elegance with contemporary comfort. The hotel offers a variety of one bedroom suites, some poolside, others with private treatment cabin for total privacy and comfort. Excellent beauty and rejuvenating center is available for therapeutic treatments with local mud and thermal water. Recreation: gala dinners, concerts, fashion show, tennis and golf privileges.

Metropole Terme
❤❤❤

Via F. Flacco 99, Abano Terme, Veneto 35031. Tel: (049) 861-9100. Fax: (049) 860-0935. TYPE: Spa Hotel. LOCATION: Walking distance from town center. SPA CLIENTELE: Women and men.

* Rooms: 115 w/priv. bath
* Phone, A/C, CTV, minibar, balcony, safe deposit
* Restaurant: diet menu
* Airport: Venice 55 km. / 35 mi.
* Train St'n: Terme Fuganef 5 km. / 3 mi.
* Airport/Train Transportation: taxi
* Credit Cards: MC/VISA/AMEX/DC
* Open: Year round
* Rates: from Lit. 170,000
* TAC: 10%
* Spa on premises
* **Spa Facilities**: thermal pools, sauna, fitness room, treatment department, solarium
* **Spa Treatments**: pressotherapy, facials, mud beauty wraps, baths, ozonized thermal baths, massage, inhalation, aerosoltherapy, mud applications, therapeutic exercises, shiatsu, Kinesitherapy (physical rehabilitation)
* **Indications**: arthritis, arthrosis, rheumatism, traumatic states, beauty and pampering
* Medical Supervision: 2 MD, 1 RN

DESCRIPTION: A modern 9-story Spa hotel with classic traditional decor. The Spa offers Thermal, Beauty & Cure programs.

President Hotel
❤❤❤❤❤

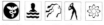

Via Montirone 31, Abano Terme I-35031. Tel: (049) 866-8288. Fax: (049) 667-909. TYPE: Modern Spa Hotel. LOCATION: Situated in its own park near town center. SPA CLIENTELE: Women and men.

* Rooms: 113 w/priv. bath, Suites: 7
* Phone, A/C, CTV, frigobar, hair dryer
* Restaurants, lounges
* Airport: Venice 55 km. / 35 mi.
* Nearest Train St'n: Terme Fuganef 5 km. / 3 mi.
* Airport/Train Transportation: taxi
* Reservations: required
* Credit Cards: MC/VISA/AMEX/DC
* Open: March - November
* Hotel Rates: from Lit. 165,000
* TAC: 10%
* **Spa Facilities**: thermal indoor and outdoor pools, sauna, treatment department
* **Spa Programs**: Beauty & Well Being
* **Spa Treatments**: mud baths, ozonized thermal baths, sports & toning massages, inhalation, aerosol-therapy, mud applications, therapeutic exercises, anti-cellulite, lymphatic drainage, aromatherapy
* **Indications**: arthritis, arthrosis, rheumatism cosmetics and anti-stress

DESCRIPTION: Large, elegantly classic Spa Hotel with interconnected indoor and outdoor pools. Beauty Club on premises. Golf nearby.

Quisisana Terme Hotel
❤❤❤

Viale delle Terma 67, Albano Terme (Padova) 35031. Tel: (049) 860-0099. Fax: (049) 860-0039. TYPE: Spa hotel. LOCATION: Near centre, 2 km to Abano Terme train station,, 50 km to Venice's Marco polo Airport. DESCRIP-

TION: Moderate first class Spa hotel with thermal treatments & cure facilities, gym, sauna, solarium. 82 rooms, 9 suites, 2 restaurants, 2 bars, entertainment, meeting facilities, tennis courts. Hotel rates: from Lit. 120,000.

La Residence Hotel
❤❤❤❤

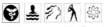

Via Monte Ceva 8, Abano Terme (Padova) 35031. Tel: (049) 866-9333. Fax: (049) 866-8396. TYPE: Thermal hotel. LOCATION: Just outside the town center. SPA CLIENTELE: Women and men. DESCRIPTION: Thermal hotel with beauty & fitness club, thermal swimming pool, sauna. 116 rooms, 6 suites, restaurant, lounge, tennis. Hotel rates: from Lit. 160,000.

Ritz Terme Hotel
❤❤❤❤

Via Monteortone 19, Abano Terme, Veneto 35031. Tel: (049) 866-9990. Fax: (049) 667549. TYPE: Spa Hotel. LOCATION: In a green valley surrounded by lawns and gardens. SPA CLIENTELE: Women and men.

* Rooms: 141 w/priv. bath. Suites: 12
* Phone, A/C, CTV, minibar, balcony, safe deposit
* American & garden bar, restaurants, nightclub
* Airport: Venice 55 km. / 35 mi.
* Train St'n: Terme Fuganef 5 km. / 3 mi.
* Airport/Train Transportation: taxi
* Credit Cards: MC/VISA/AMEX/DC
* Open: Year round
* Rates: from Lit. 170,000
* TAC: 10%
* Spa on premises
* **Spa Facilities**: thermal pools, sauna, gym treatment department, solarium
* **Spa Treatments**: pressotherapy, facials, mud beauty wraps, baths, ozonized thermal baths, massage, inhalation, aerosoltherapy, mud applications, therapeutic exercises, shiatsu, Kinesitherapy (physical rehabilitation)
* **Indications**: arthritis, arthrosis, rheumatism, traumatic states, beauty and pampering

* Medical Supervision: 2 MD, 1 RN

DESCRIPTION: Modern Spa hotel with classic traditional decor. The Spa offers Thermal, Beauty & Well Being Programs.

Smeraldo Terme Hotel
❤❤

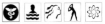

Via Flavio Busonera 174, Abano Terme (Padova) 35031. Tel: (049) 866-9555. Fax: (049) 866-9752. TYPE: Spa hotel. LOCATION: In a private park, 5 km. / 3 mi. to Euganaee train station. DESCRIPTION: Tourist class Spa hotel with thermal treatments, extensive cure facilities, connecting indoor & outdoor pools.130 rooms & suites. Restaurant, bar, TV lounge, tennis. Hotel rates: from Lit. 120,000.

Terme Patria
❤❤❤

Viale delle Terme 56, 35031 Abano Terme. Tel: (049) 861-7444. Fax: (049) 860-0635. TYPE: Spa Hotel. LOCATION: Central location in Spa area. SPA CLIENTELE: Women and men, family oriented.

* Rooms: 50 w/priv. bath
* Phone, A/C, CTV
* Restaurant: diet menu
* Airport: Venice 55 km. / 35 mi.
* Train St'n: Terme Fuganef 5 km. / 3 mi.
* Airport/Train Transportation: taxi
* Credit Cards: MC/VISA/AMEX/DC
* Open: Year round
* Rates: from Lit. 80,000; TAC: 10%
* Spa on premises
* **Spa Facilities**: thermal pools, sauna, fitness room, whirlpool, solarium
* **Spa Treatments**: pressotherapy, massotherapy, facials, fangotherapy, mud wraps and applications, baths, ozonized thermal baths, massage, inhalation, aerosoltherapy, therapeutic exercises, reflexology

DESCRIPTION: Small thermal hotel with indoor and outdoor

thermal pools featuring spa treatments and cures.

BELLAGIO
🕽 031
✈ Linate Int'l Airport (LIN)

Grand Hotel Villa Serbelloni
💗💗💗

Via Roma 1, Bellagio (Como) I-22021. Tel: (031) 950-216. Fax: (031) 951-529. TYPE: Palace hotel & Spa. LOCATION: On the shores of Lake Como, 35 km. to Como train station. DESCRIPTION: Deluxe Old World Palace hotel with health & beauty centre. Open April through October. 95 rooms, 3 suites, wheelchair access. Public room, dining room, bar, meting facilities, outdoor pool, 2 tennis courts, private beach. Hotel rates: from Lit. 60,000.

CAPRI ISLAND
🕽 081
✈ Capodichino Airport (NAP)

Capri, population 14,000, is the most famous, and most beautiful of all the Italian island. Located in the bay of Naples it is only 4 mi. / 6 km. long and 2 mi. / 3 km. wide. Capri is a favorite resort for the international jet-set, as well as artists, writers, honeymooners and hedonists in search of sun, sea, wine and great food. The **Blue Grotto** is the most famous tourist attraction on the island.

The island of Capri is linked to the mainland by a frequent ferryboat and hydrofoil service to and from Naples. The trip takes about 1 1/4 hour. In the summer there is regular hydrofoil service to Capri from Ischia, Amalfi and Salerno.

Hotel Palace - Capri Beauty Farm
💗💗💗💗💗

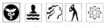

Via Capodimonte 2b, 80071 Anacapri, Island of Capri. Tel: (081) 837-3800. Fax: (081) 837-3191. TYPE: Deluxe Spa Hotel. GENERAL MANAGER: Dr. Tony Cacace. LOCATION: Set against Mount Solaro in Anacapri on the most

exclusive part of the Island of Capri. Panoramic views of the bay and Naples. SPA CLIENTELE: Men & Women.

* Rooms: 80 w/priv. bath, some with private pool. Plus 1 "Megaron" Suite
* Phone, CTV, A/C, C/H, minibar
* Restaurant, bar, piano bar
* Airport & Train Station: Naples
* Airport / Train Transportation: Limo (on request)
* Reservation: Required
* Credit Card: MC, VISA, AMEX, DC
* Season: From March - November
* Hotel Rates:
  Low season - Lit. 390,000 - Lit. 580,000 (double)
  Lit. 690.000 - 770.000, Suite Lit. 900.000
  (double with private pool)
  high season - Lit. 460,000 - Lit. 680,000 (double)
  Lit. 870.000 - 890.000 Suite 1,000.000
  (double with private pool)
* TAC: 10%
* Spa on premises: **Capri Beauty Farm**
* **Spa Facilities**: Heated swimming pool, gym, laboratory, electronic beauty equipment, Turkish baths, massage rooms, beauty salon, Kneipp basins,
* **Spa Programs**: Health, Fitness, beauty, weight loss
* **Spa Packages**: Beauty Program (7 day) Lit. 3,500,000 extra charges per person per week - single Lit.300,000; "Junior Suite" Lit. 500,000; double for single occupancy Lit. 700,000; w/private swimming pool Lit. 1,000,000. Complete Health and Beauty (7 day) Lit. 4,600,000; extra charges per person per week - single Lit. 300,000 "Junior Suite" Lit. 500,000 double for single occupancy Lit. 700,000 w/private swimming pool Lit. 1,000,000 The Programs are on a full board basis with dietetic food on a double occupancy basis.
* **Spa Treatments**: Medical examination, electrocardiogram, dermoaesthetic examination, body composition examination, hydromassage with marine algae and micronized seaweeds, massages, pressotherapy, muscular invigorating, electronic lymphodrainage, mud bath therapy, aromatherapy, ultrasound therapy, lasertherapy. Thermal treatments - inhalations, (aerosol), fango mud applications, thalassotherapy; Facial treatments - moisturizing, masque, with algae,

with collagen, biolifting. Peeling Body treatments; anti cellulitic, toning and specific for the breast. Aquatic gymnastics, gymnastics, ecological walks
* Length of Stay: 7 days required.
* Medical Supervision: 2 MD

DESCRIPTION: The Hotel Palace is a luxury hotel where good living goes hand in hand with the highest standards of service. It stands 300 m. / 990 ft. above sea level. All the rooms and suites have been designed with the ultimate comfort and discretion in mind. **Capri Beauty Farm** will purify your body and breathe new life into your spirit. Beauty treatments are specially designed for each individual to combat aging skin, acne, cellulite and other conditions. Guests are constantly looked over by a qualified team in an ultra-modern building equipped with state of the art equipment. Flexible personalized treatment programs have been conceived to satisfy the most diverse requirements.

Hotel Punta Tragara
❤❤❤❤

Via Tragara, 57, Capri I-80073. Tel: (081) 837-0844. Fax: (081) 837-7790. TYPE: Vila Hotel & Spa. LOCATION: On the island of Capri with a panoramic view of the sea. SPA CLIENTELE: Women and men.

* Rooms: 15 w/priv. bath. Suites: 30
* Phone, CTV, minibar, hair dryer, balcony
* Restaurant, taverna, piano bar, disco
* Nearest Port: Naples, 40 minutes by hydrofoil
* Open: April - October
* Hotel Rates: from Lit. 400,000
* Spa on Premises
* **Spa Facilities:** Saltwater pools, thermal baths, massage center, jacuzzi, solarium
* **Spa Treatments:** thalassotherapy, massages, thermal baths

DESCRIPTION: All suite hotel designed by Le Corbusier in 1925, overlooking the Mediterranean Sea. The Spa features thermal baths and thalassotherapy treatments. Popular with couples and honeymooners.

CASTROCARO TERME
☎ 0543

✈ Guglielmo Marconi Airport (BLQ)

Castrocaro Terme, population 7,000, is an historic spa town in Northern Italy, south of Bologna. Famed since ancient times for its curative waters, the spa offers healthy climactic environment for preventive treatments and rehabilitation. Castrocaro Terme is 10 km. (6 mi.) southwest of Forli, 70 km. (44 mi.) south of Bologna, and 342 km. (213 mi.) north of Rome.

The ultra modern spa facilities are fitted with state-of-the-art equipment, and use local natural mud and sulphurous and salsobromoiodic bearing waters for preventive, therapeutic and rehabilitative purposes.

Indications: rheumatism, arthritis, gynecological complaints, female sterility, respiratory diseases, digestive system complaints, and metabolism disorders.

Spa Treatments: thermal baths, irrigation, inhalations, oral balneotherapy, massotherapy, respiratory and rehabilitative physical exercises.

Grand Hotel Terme
❤❤❤

Via Roma, 2, 47011 Castrocaro Terme (FO). Tel: (0543) 767-114. Fax: (543) 768-135. TYPE: Hotel & Spa. LOCATION: In the beautiful Spa gardens. SPA CLIENTELE: Mixed.

* Rooms:100 w/priv. bath. Suites: 1
* Restaurants (2) special diet menu available
* Airport: Forli 10 km. / 6 mi.
* Train Station: Forli 8 km. / 5 mi.
* Airport/Train Transportation: taxi, rent a car
* Credit Cards: MC/VISA/AMEX/DC/DIS
* Open: May - October
* Rates: from Lit. 105,000 (full board); TAC: 8% Weight Loss (12 days) add Lit. 700,000
* **Spa Facilities:** All facilities at the nearby Terme di Castrocaro; In Hotel Thermal Cure Center
* **Spa Treatments:** see Spa; diet treatments in the hotel

* **Spa Package**: 12 day or more Weight Loss
* **Indications**: see introduction
* **Medical Supervision**: 5 MD, 30 RN (at the Spa)
* **Treatments Approved**: Medical Center

DESCRIPTION: A first class spa hotel with internal treatment facilities near the thermal center. Pleasant rooms, some with private balconies. Hotel guests can participate in all the spa treatments that are offered at the center. The hotel's own weight loss program requires a minimum of 12 night stay. Recreation: billiard, bowling, tennis, dancing and night club.

CHIANCIANO TERME
) 0578

✈ Peretola Airport (FLR) Florence
   70 mi. / 113 km. northwest

Chinciano Terme is a picturesque Etrusco Roman Spa town in the Province of Siena. Nestled on a verdant hillside it has magnificent views of the Tuscan countryside. The large spa with its thermal water, manicured parks, first class hotels and baths have made Chinciano Terme famous with spa aficionados worldwide.

Spa'deus
❤❤❤❤

😀 🏊 🏃 🚶

Via Le Piane 35, Chinciano Terme I-53042. Tel: (0578) 63232. Fax: (0578) 64329. TYPE: Spa Hotel. LOCATION: Nestled in the rolling hills of Tuscany. GENERAL MANAGER: Christina Newburgh. SPA CLIENTELE: Men & Women.

* Rooms: 50 w/priv. bath. Suites: 2
* Phone, CTV, frigobar
* Restaurant: special Spa diet menu
* Airport: Florence, 113 km. / 70 mi.
* Credit Cards: MC/VISA/AMEX/DC/DIS
* Open: Year round; TAC: 10%
* Spa on premises: **Centro Benessere**
* **Spa Facilities**: Sauna, solarium, gym indoor pool, Turkish bath, nature trails
* **Spa Treatments**: aromatherapy, thalassotherapy, nature walk, stretching, low impact aerobics, box

aerobics, circuit training, total body massage, herbal packs, non-surgical face-lift, ondapress- hydrotherapy, NIA (New Age Dance), Ai-Chi (aquatic gynmastic workout), fango, pressotherapy, Scottish showers, low impact step aerobics, organic facial treatments, chair exercise, abdominal and body toning, yoga, low cal gourmet vegetarian diet

* **Spa Packages**: Weight Loss, Fitness from
   Lit. 520,000 (day), Lit. 3,640,000 (7 day) to
   Lit. 620,000 (day), Lit. 4,340,000 (7 day)
   based on double room occupancy per person
   Lit. 600,000 (day), Lit 4,200,000 (7 day) to
   Lit. 700,000 (day); Lit. 4,900,000 (7 day)
   based on double room, single occupancy
* **Indications**: anti-stress, obesity, cosmetic improvement, pampering

DESCRIPTION: Spa'deus by Christina Newburgh is a modern California style Spa in the heart of the verdant hills of Northern Italy. Popular with celebrities it offers a unique environment where you can find complete harmony between yourself and nature. The Spa offers a variety of weight loss, fitness and beauty programs, tailored to the need of each individual. The weight loss program is based on a delicious local vegetarian cuisine which has been modified according to the low-fat and low-calorie dietary recommendations of the American Cancer Institute.

FIUGGI
) 0775

✈ Leonardo de Vinci Int'l AP (FCO) Rome
   90 km. / 56 mi.

Fiuggi has been a popular spa resort since the early 13th century. The famous Michelangelo was one of the many people who visited this spa to take advantage of its restorative powers. The beneficial effects of the thermal waters combined with fresh mountain air and beautiful scenery make this historic spa town, 38 miles (60 km.) southeast of Rome, a popular destination for many Italians. Fiuggi is an up and coming spa resort which is yet to be discovered by sophisticated international and North American travelers.

Indications: The oligo-mineral thermal water brings relief to some forms of kidney diseases and is excellent for relaxation.

Grand Hotel Palazzo della Fonte
❤❤❤❤❤

Via dei Vilini 7, Fiuggi I-03015. Tel: (0775) 5081. Fax: (0775) 506-752. TYPE: Deluxe Hotel & Spa. LOCATION: Scenic hilltop location. SPA CLIENTELE: Women and men.

* Rooms: 153 w/private bath
* Phone, CTV, A/C, hair dryer, safe deposit
* Restaurant, bar, lounge with terrace
* Airport: Fiumicino (Rome) 90 minutes
* Reservations: suggested
* Credit Cards: AMEX
* Open: May - October (closed Oct. 30 - Apr. 30)
* Hotel Rates: from Lit. 260,000/day (room only)
* Spa on premises
* **Spa Facilities**: Health & Beauty Center, out door pool, sauna
* **Spa Programs**: Beauty/Relaxation Week
* **Spa Treatments**: diet, extensive facial and scalp treatments, reflexogenic foot massage, thermal showers, in house specialty - hot phyto-plankton mud, applied over face and body to cleanse and reinvigorate the skin, massages, thermal water showers, fango facial masks, fango mud, aesthetic treatments
* **Indications**: stress reduction, relaxation
* **Medical Supervision**: physicians, estheticians

DESCRIPTION: Once home of the King of Italy, The Grand Hotel Palazzo della Fonte offers Health & Beauty programs with various massages and treatments.

Silva Hotel Splendid
❤❤❤

Corso Nuova Italia, 19, Fiuggi 03014. Tel: (0775) 55791. TYPE: Hotel & Spa. LOCATION: Centrally located. SPA CLIENTELE: Women and men.

* Rooms: 120 w/private bath
* A/C, Wheelchair Accessibility, Restaurant
* Airport: Fiumicino, Rome, 90 minutes
* Airport Transportation: paid Pick Up
* Reservations: suggested

* Credit Cards: AMEX
* Open: May - October (closed Oct. 30 - Apr. 30)
* Hotel Rates: from Lit. 160,000/day (room only)
* Spa on premises
* **Spa Facilities**: Health & Beauty Center, outdoor pool, sauna
* **Spa Programs**: Beauty/Relaxation Week
* **Spa Treatments**: diet, extensive facial and scalp treatments, reflexogenic foot massage, thermal showers, in house specialty - hot phyto-plankton mud, applied over face and body to cleanse and reinvigorate the skin, massages, thermal water showers, fango facial masks, fango mud, aesthetic treatments
* **Indications**: stress reduction, relaxation
* **Medical Supervision**: physicians, estheticians

DESCRIPTION: Health & Beauty Center with emphasis on beauty treatments based on natural products individually designed by professionals for each guest.Recreation: tennis and golf privileges nearby.

ISCHIA ISLAND
☏ 081

✈ Capodichino Airport (NAP)

Ischia is a charming island in the Tyrrhenian Sea off the coast of Naples. It is world famous for its excellent sulfurous hot springs that made it a fashionable spa resort already during the Roman period. The thermal spa claims to have beneficial effects on a wide range of ailments. Ischia is regaining popularity among the wealthy Italians and smart international travelers. To get to Ischia take a ferryboat, hydrofoil, or helicopter from Naples.

Indications: gout, retarded sexual development, or chronic rheumatism.

Continental Terme Hotel
❤❤

Via Michele Mazzella 74, Ischia Porto, Ischia (Napoli) I 80077. Tel: (081) 991-588. Fax: (081) 982-929. TYPE: Spa Hotel. LOCATION: Topical landscape setting 32 km. / 20 mi. to Naples by ferry. DESCRIPTION: 3-story tourist class hotel with thermal & cosmetic treatments, thermal pools, sauna, gym. Open April to October. 240 rooms, 4 suites, 2 restaurants, coffee shop, 2 bars, meeting facilities, business center, tennis. Hotel rates: from Lit. 190,000.

Grand Hotel Excelsior Belvedere
❤️❤️❤️

Via E. Gianturco 19, Ischia I-80077. Tel: (081) 991-522. Fax: (081) 984-100. TYPE: Spa Hotel. LOCATION: In a peaceful private pine grove, across from the beach. SPA CLIENTELE: Women and men. DESCRIPTION: 72 rooms, 3 Jr suites, adjacent Spa with thermal facilities, 5 thermo-mineral pools. Thermal and cosmetic treatments. Hotel Rates: from Lit. 300,000.

Grand Hotel Punta Molino Terme
❤️❤️❤️❤️

Lungomare C. Colombo 14, Ischia I-80077. Tel: (081) 991-544. Fax: (081) 991-562. TYPE: Spa Hotel. LOCATION: Set in pine woods, facing sea and private beach. SPA CLIENTELE: Women and men. DESCRIPTION: 88 rooms, 5 suites. 3 pools with thermal water, beauty and thermal treatments. Hotel Rates: from Lit. 310,000.

Jolly Hotel delle Terme
❤️❤️❤️❤️

Via A. De Luca, 42, 80070 Ischia. Tel: (081) 991-744. Fax: (081) 993-156. TYPE: Hotel & Spa. LOCATION: Centrally located, 200 yards from the Naples ferry terminal and close to the beach. CLIENTELE: Women and men, family oriented.

* Rooms: 208 w/priv. bath
* Suites: 1; Cottages & Apartments: 5
* Phone, CTV, A/C, minibar
* Restaurant & Piano Bar
* Reservations: 1 night deposit
* Credit Cards: MC/VISA/AMEX/DC/CB/EC
* Open: March - November
* Hotel Rates: from Lit. 175,000; TAC: 10%

* Spa on Premises: **Terme Jolly**
* **Spa Facilities**: Indoor private Spa, 50 treatment booths, gym, beauty salon
* **Spa Programs**: Medical, Diet/Fitness, Beauty
* **Spa Treatments**: physiotherapy, ionophoresis, Finnish sauna, radar-therapy, ultrasonics and connective tissue massage
* Medical Supervision: 5 MD, 15-20 RN
* Number of Customers per Doctor: 40
* Treatments Approved: Health Ministry

DESCRIPTION: The Jolly Hotel is a sophisticated Spa hotel set in one of the most beautiful part of Porto d'Ischia. The hotel features its own indoor Spa facilities for a variety of treatments under medical supervision. Direct lift service is provided to the thermal Spa area.

LACCO AMENO
🌙 **081**
✈️ Capodichino Airport (NAP) 25 mi. / 40 km.

Albergo Terme San Montano
❤️❤️❤️

Via Montevico, Ischia I-80077. Tel: (081) 994-033. Fax: (081) 980-242. TYPE: Spa Hotel. LOCATION: Set in pine woods, facing the sea and lovely views of Naples. SPA CLIENTELE: Women and men. DESCRIPTION: 67 rooms, 2 suites, thermal treatments, massage & beauty Center. Hotel Rates: from Lit. 260,000.

La Reginella Terme
❤️❤️❤️

Lacco Ameno, Ischia 80076. Tel: (081) 994-300. Fax: (081) 980-481. TYPE: Hotel & Spa. LOCATION: Seafront connected with thermal baths, opposite the elegant Regina Isabella hotel. SPA CLIENTELE: Women and men.

* Rooms: 52 w/priv. bath/shower. Suites: 2
* Phone, A/C, hair dryer, safe deposit
* Restaurant & piano bar
* Nearest Port: Ischia Harbor 7 km. (4 mi.) taxi

* Reservations: suggested
* Credit Cards: AMEX/DC
* Open: March 10 - October 31
* Hotel Rates: from Lit. 160,000/day; TAC: 10%
* **Spa Facilities**: Connected to thermal establishment, indoor/outdoor thermal pools, sauna, gym
* **Spa Treatments**: mineral water bathing, various medical type treatments

DESCRIPTION: La Reginella is a first class villa style resort. All rooms are comfortable and pleasantly appointed. It offers easy access to the attached Thermal Establishment for spa cures.

Regina Isabella Hotel
❤❤❤❤❤

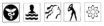

Piazza St. Restituta 3, Lacco Ameno, Ischia 80076. Tel: (081) 994-322. Fax: (081) 900-190. TYPE: Deluxe Spa Hotel. LOCATION: Scenic beach location adjacent to the Thermal Baths. SPA CLIENTELE: Women and men (many celebrities).

* Rooms: 134 w/private bath, All-Suite Annex
* Phone, A/C, private balcony
* Restaurants & terrace bars
* Port: Ischia Harbor, 7 km. (4 mi.), taxi
* Reservations: required
* Credit Cards: VISA/AMEX/EC/DC/ACC
* Open: April - October
* Hotel Rates: from Lit. 500,000 (room only)
* TAC: 10%
* **Spa Facilities**: connected to the Santa Restituta Thermal Spa, Health Spa, whirlpool baths, Beauty Salon, private beach, pools
* **Spa Treatments**: medical, fitness and beauty, therapeutic mud treatments, thermal water showers, underwater deep muscle massage, facial treatments, exercise sessions, lymphatic drainage body massage
* **Spa Programs**: Health & Beauty (7 day)
* Medical Supervision: available

DESCRIPTION: The ultimate in resort spa luxury on the island and long time favorite of celebrities and movie stars.

The Regina Isabella offers a complete range of spa treatments, many medically oriented. The food is excellent with a distinguished southern Italian flavor.

MERANO
✆ 0473

✈ Villafranca Airport, Verona
Kranebitten Airport (INN) Innsbruck (Austria)

Merano, population 31,000, is a quaint spa town in Northern Italy near the Swiss & Austrian borders. A lovely oasis of Mediterranean climate in Alpine environment where palm trees, oleander and laurel trees grow against the background of the snow covered mountains. The town is mostly Tyrol with medieval houses and a river flowing through the center. The beautiful landscape combined with spa cure and a variety of recreational activities make Merano the premier health resort in the South Tyrol. Merano is located 28 km. (18 mi.) from the Brennero highway exit "Bolzano-Sud"; 150 km. (94 mi.) by highway from the small airports of Verona or Innsbruck.

The thermal water have radioactive properties given by radon, a radium emanation that produces physical effects of a great benefit to the body. The radioactivity present in the air and ground assures positive effects even without actually taking the water, but a classic cure of 12 baths is the highlight of the spa treatment at Merano. Merano has various spa facilities for different cures: radon baths, mud baths, inhalations, sauna, massage, physiotherapy, thermal baths (indoor and outdoor swimming pools).

Indications: peripheral circulatory disorders, rheumatism and joint diseases, metabolic disorders, chronic disorders of the respiratory tract, geriatric complaints.

Palace Hotel
❤❤❤❤

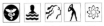

Via Cavour 2-4, 39012 Merano. Tel: (0473) 211-300, Fax: (0473) 234-181. TYPE: Health Resort & Congress Center. LOCATION: In an elegant residential area in the center of town on a large private park. SPA CLIENTELE: Women and men, family oriented.

* Rooms: 127 w/priv. bath. Suites: 7
* Phone, CTV, radio, frigobar, hair dryer, bidet
* Restaurant & grill room
* Airports: Munich/Milan, 350 km. (220 mi.)
* Airport Transportation: train, bus
* Reservations: required
* Credit Cards: VISA/AMEX/DC
* Open: March - November, Dec. 12 - Jan. 1
* Hotel Rates: from Lit. 185,000/day; TAC: 8%
* Spa on premises
* **Spa Facilities**: indoor and outdoor swimming pools, sauna, solarium, gymnasium, thermal cure department, beauty parlor
* **Spa Treatments**: mud baths, radon mineral baths, massages, exercise, medical consultation; slimming diet or fit menu, facials, medical relaxing baths, herb-packs, mineral drinking cure
* **Spa Packages**: Cure Package, Beauty & Fitness
* Medical Supervision: 1 MD

DESCRIPTION: An elegant hotel with extensive thermal spa facilities for medical cures and/or slimming and beauty treatments mainly for a female clientele. The hotel stresses mineral drinking cures, and a classic "Heirler" whey cure is available under the supervision of Doctor Anemüller.

MONTECATINI TERME
☎ 0572

✈ G. Galileo Airport, Pisa (PSA) 50 km. / 31 mi.

Montecatini Terme, one of the best and most elegant spas in Italy is located in the lovely Val di Nievole near Florence, Pisa and Viareggio. It is an internationally acclaimed spa with nine termes (spas) known for the treatment of liver diseases and affections of the digestive tract and metabolism. The numerous mineral springs are mainly enriched in chloride-sulfate and bicarbonate-sodium. The water temperature is between 24°c-34°c (75°F - 93°F) and are radioactive. *La Tettuccio* spring is the most active on the liver.

Spa Treatments & Indications: Carbonic baths for the treatment of hyper and hypo tensions; Sulfur baths (dermatosis); Iodine Salt Baths (rheumatic and lymphatic complaints); Oral Balneotherapy (paradentosis); Intestinal Irrigation (constipation); vaginal Irrigation (gynecological

affections); Inhalations (tonsillitis, laryngitis, bronchitis); tubotympanic insufflations (rhinogenous deafness); massotherapy (electric massage in water and under spray); Radioactive treatments (uricemia, gout, obesity); Electrical treatments; eudermal treatments (treatment of the skin - mud packs, filiform sprays tending to produce facial improvement e.g. in case of dermatosis, erythema, acne, seborrhea, affections of the scalp).

Contraindication: Ulcerative gastritis and duodenitis, acute abdominal complaints, serious cardiac affections, marked arteriosclerosis, acute and chronic nephrosis, active tuberculosis, malignant tumors. Due to the serious medical treatments offered it is necessary to consult a physician before starting the treatments.

Montecatini has recently started to offer a wide gamut of beauty treatments that include aesthetics and are directly linked to the thermal therapy. Only natural products and methods based on mineral waters, thermal muds, and massages are used in these treatments. Many celebrities including Sophia Loren, the late Princess Grace and others have come in the past for treatments at Montecatini Terme.

Cappelli - Croce Di Savoia
❤❤❤

Viale Bicchierai 139, 51016 Montecatini Terme. Tel: (0572) 71151. Fax: (0572) 71154 TYPE: Hotel & Spa. LOCATION: Centrally located near the thermal area. SPA CLIENTELE: Women and men.

* Rooms: 72 w/private bath
* Train Station: Montecatini Terme
* Airport: Pisa Airport, 50 km. (31 mi.)
* Airport Transportation: train, bus, taxi
* Credit Cards: MC/VISA/AMEX/DC
* Rates: from Lit. 110,000/day
* Distance to the Spa: 100 m. (100 yds.)
* **Spa Facilities**: Thermal baths nearby; heated swimming pool
* **Spa Treatments**: Mineral water baths, mud baths, weight lose program - special diet cooking, and all the treatments that are available at Montecatini Terme

* Medical Supervision: at the thermal facilities
* Indications: see above
* Contraindication: see above

DESCRIPTION: Quiet hotel near the thermal area with pleasant rooms and lovely garden area. Special diet meals are available upon demand.

Grand Hotel Croce di Malta
♥♥♥♥

Viale VI Novembre, 18, 51016 Montecatini Terme. Tel: (0572) 75871. Fax: (0572) 767-516. LOCATION: Quiet central area near the Thermal Park. CLIENTELE: Women and men, family oriented.

* Rooms: 106 w/priv. bath. Suites: 18
* Phone, CTV, A/C, C/H, minibar,
* Bar & garden restaurant with diet menu
* Airport: Pisa Airport, 50 km. (31 mi.)
* Airport Transportation: taxi
* Credit Cards: MC/VISA/AMEX/DC/EC
* Rates: from Lit. 160,000/day; TAC: 8.5%
* Distance to the Spa: 200m (200 yrds)
* **Spa Facilities**: Thermal baths nearby, heated heated swimming pool, sauna
* **Spa Treatments**: Mineral water baths, mud baths, and all the spa treatments that are available at Montecatini Terme.
* Medical Supervision: at the thermal facilities
* **Indications**: see above
* **Contraindication**: see above

DESCRIPTION: Elegant and inviting first class hotel in the middle of the thermal park and near all the cure establishments. Guests may choose to take rooms only or a full or half pension plan with meals. Special diet meals are available upon request. Conference Center facilities hold up to 150 people.

Grand Hotel e la Pace
♥♥♥♥♥

Vialle Della Torretta 1, Montecatini Terme 51016. Tel:

(0572) 75801. Fax: (0572) 78451. TYPE: Hotel & Spa. LOCATION: Near the thermal establishments. CLIENTELE: Women and men (many celebrities).

* Rooms: 106 w/priv. bath. Suites: 18
* Phone, CTV, A/C, C/H. minibar, safe deposit
* Restaurants & bar, landscaped garden
* Airport: Pisa Airport, 50 km. (31 mi.)
* Airport Transportation: taxi
* Reservations: requested
* Credit Cards: MC/AMEX/DC/EC
* Open: April 1 - October 31
* Hotel Rates: from Lit. 290,000/day
* TAC: 10%
* **Spa Facilities**: Complete Health Facilities including: sauna, massage rooms, gym, solarium, pool
* **Spa Treatments**: hydro (underwater) and manual massage, Swiss showers,diet, physiotherapy, health and beauty treatments - fango mud wraps, baths in Leopoldine spa, scalp & facial treatments
* **Spa Programs**: one or two weeks programs tailored to the individual's needs
* Medical Supervision: specialized doctors, dieticians, sports directors, physiotherapists
* **Indications**: see above
* **Contraindication**: see above

DESCRIPTION: Distinguished Palace style hotel, with special appeal to celebrities. Everything in the hotel indicates Old European Royal charm. The architecture is a classic European with extensive use of Italian marble and objets d'art. The hotel provides spa programs that emphasize natural health. Recreation: clay court tennis, golf.

Grand Hotel Tamerici E Principe
♥♥♥

Viale IV Novembre, I-55016 Montecatini Terme. Tel: (0572) 71041. Fax: (0572) 72992. TYPE: Hotel & Spa. LOCATION: In residential area near the thermal facilities. MANAGER: Tullio & Egenio Pancioli, owners. SPA CLIENTELE: Mixed

* Rooms: 157 w/priv. bath. Suites: available
* Phone, CTV, A/C, C/H, balcony

* Roof Garden, bar & cocktail terrace
* Airport: Pisa 45 km. / 28 mi.
* Train Station: Montecatini 2 km. / 1 mi.
* Airport/Train Transportation: taxi
* Credit Cards: MC/VISA/AMEX/DC/DIS/EC
* Open: March - November
* Hotel Rates: from Lit. 190,000/day; TAC: 10%
* Spa off Premises: 500 m/yards away
* **Spa Facilities**: heated swimming pool, covered swimming pool with hydromassage, Beauty Center, gym, sauna, solarium, massage room; Public thermal facilities nearby
* **Spa Programs**: fitness, beauty, diets

DESCRIPTION: Modern hotel near the thermal facilities. All rooms and apartments are furnished in elegant old style with sound-proof walls and two bathrooms. Recreation: swimming pool, solarium, golf.

Grand Hotel Vittoria
♥♥♥

Viale della Liberta 2-A, 51016 Montecatini Terme. Tel: (0572) 79271. Fax: (0572) 910-520. TYPE: Spa Hotel. LOCATION: Residential area near thermal facilities. SPA CLIENTELE: Women and men.

* Rooms: 84 w/priv. bath. Suites: 3
* Phone, minibar, C/H, some balconies
* Restaurant with summer garden, bar & lounge
* Airport: Pisa 45 km. / 28 mi.
* Train Station: Montecatini 2 km. / 1 mi.
* Airport/Train Transportation: taxi
* Reservations: required
* Credit Cards: MC/VISA/AMEX/DC
* Open: April 1 - October 31
* Rates: from Lit. 135,000/day
* Spa off Premises: 500 m/yards away
* **Spa Facilities**: Beauty Farm, pool, solarium

DESCRIPTION: Traditional hotel near the thermal facilities. The hotel does not have its own in house spa facilities but features in house Beauty Farm. Recreation: swimming pool, solarium, tennis.

MONTEGROTTO TERME
☊ 049

✈ Marco Polo Airport (VCE) 40 km. / 25 mi.

Health Spa in the Venice area close to Abamo Terme. Their thermal water have similar curative properties. Montegrotto means - "mountain of the sick". The town has ruins of a spa from the times of Julius Caeser.

Continental Hotel Terme
♥♥♥

Via Neroniana 16, Montegrotto Terme (Padova) I-35036. Tel: (049) 793-622. Fax: (049) 891-0683. TYPE: Spa Hotel. LOCATION: In quiet park 100 meters to train station. DESCRIPTION: HOTEL: 110 rooms, 40 suites, wheelchair access.Thermal & Beauty treatments, mud treatment, ozone bath, massage, sauna, gym. Dining room (Special diets on request), TV & bridge room, outdoor pool, 2 tennis courts. Hotel rates: from Lit. 121,000.

Hotel Esplanade Tergesteo
♥♥♥♥

Via Roma 54, Montegrotto Terme (Padova) I-35036. Tel: (049) 891-1777. Fax: (049) 891-0488. TYPE: Spa Hotel. LOCATION: In town center, 2 km to train station. DESCRIPTION: First class spa hotel with cure facilities, thermal & mud treatments, indoor/outdoor thermal pool, solarium. 124 rooms, 15 suites, nonsmoker rooms, wheelchair access. Restaurant, garden grill, 2 bars, lounge, meeting facilities, tennis, 18-hole golf course. Hotel rates: from Lit. 150,000.

International Hotel Bertha
♥♥♥♥

Largo Traiano 1, Montegrotto Terme (Padova) I-35036. Tel: (049) 891-1700. Fax: (049) 891-1771. TYPE: Spa Hotel. LOCATION: Park setting, 16 km. to Padua train station. DESCRIPTION: Superior first class Spa hotel with Cure facilities, thermal treatments, physiotherapy center, sauna, gym, termal swimming pool. 110 rooms, 16 suites, nonsmoker rooms, wheelchair access. 2 restaurants, 2 bars, meeting facilities, business center, 2 tennis courts. Hotel rates: from Lit. 120,000.

RIMINI
0541

 Miramare Airport

Il Grand Hotel
❤❤❤

Pizzale Fellini 2 Rimini (Forli) I-47037. Tel: (0541) 56000. Fax: 0541-568-66. TYPE: Hotel & Spa. LOCATION: In park on private beach.SPA CLIENTELE: Women and men. DESCRIPTION: First class hotel featuring beauty spa, with beauty treatments, massage, sauna. 163 rooms, 6 suites, wheelchair access. Restaurant, breakfast room, nightclub, bar, meeting facilities, 2 pools., water sports. Hotel rates: from Lit. 230,000.

ROME
06

Leonardo de Vinci Int'l (FCO) 10 km. / 16 mi.

Rome Cavalieri Hilton
❤❤❤❤

Via Alberto Cadiolo 101, Rome I-00136. Tel: (06) 35091. Fax: 06-3509-2241. TYPE: Deluxe Hotel & Spa. LOCATION: In a private park overlooking Rome and St. Peter's Cathedral, 10 minutes to the Vatican. DESCRIPTION: Stylish hotel with Spa and La Prairie of Switzerland beauty center, turkish bath, massage, exercise room, juice bar. 358 rooms, 16 suites. 2 restaurants, bar, lounge, meeting facilities, business center, indoor/outdoor pool, tennis. Hotel rates: from Lit. 480,000.

SALSOMAGGIORE
0524

Linate Int'l Airport (LIN) 90 km. / 56 mi.

Salsomaggiorre, located half way between Bologna and Milano, is an elegant spa town with a romantic charm of a bygone era. Its salty iodic water were first used to extract salt during the II century BC, but the therapeutic value of its 48 thermal wells were only later discovered in the 19th century. In 1839 a doctor named Lorenzo Berzieri experimented with the iodine water on a young girl suffering from acute osteitis and was amazed by the extraordinary effects of the water. In 1923 the "Terme Berzieri" was inaugurated and became the property of the Italian state.

Indications: The bromo-iodine-salt water of Salsomaggiore can be used for the treatment of the following diseases: rheumatic forms, gynecological forms, respiratory and otorhinolaryngological forms, certain dysmetabolic and dyshormonal processes, and pediatric illnesses.

Spa Treatments: bathing in natural iodine water, baths with oxygen, baths with hydromassage, inhalations, dry and wet atomization, nasal irrigation, balneotherapy of the mouth, vaginal irrigation, muds, paraffin therapy, massages, vacuum therapy, kinesitherapy.

The Thermal establishment offers medical assistance free of charge with most thermal cures. However, there is a charge for special services such as check upsor laboratory controls. All rates for medical services are displayed at the ticket offices of the different thermal departments. A special salt-iodine water swimming pool for preventive therapy is available with gymnasium, sauna, massage services for simple physio-therapeutic applications. Due to the particular nature of the spa and the wide variety of treatments offered, it is necessary to consult a physician to determine the type of treatments that are appropriate for those who wish to take the cure at Salsomaggiore spa.

Centrale Bagni Hotel
❤❤❤

Largo Roma 4, 43039 Salsomaggiore Terme. Tel: (524) 572-441. Fax: (524) 574-028. TYPE: Spa Hotel. LOCATION: In the center of Salsomaggiore Terme. SPA CLIENTELE: Women and men, family oriented.

* Rooms: 96 w/priv. bath. Suites: 5
* American bar & lounges, restaurant

* Nearest Airport: Milano Linate, 1 hour
* Airport Transportation: taxi
* Credit Cards: VISA/AMEX/DC
* Open: May - October
* Hotel Rates: from Lit. 160,000/day
* TAC: 10%
* Spa on premises
* **Spa Facilities**: Thermal establishment
* **Spa Treatments**: medical
* Medical Supervision
* Treatments approved: Medical assoc.

DESCRIPTION: First class hotel offering complete Spa treatments under medical supervision. Cocktail, banquet and meeting rooms for up to 190 people. Private garden for relaxation.

Grand Hotel Poro
♥♥♥♥

Viale Porro 10, I-43039 Salsomaggiore Terme. Tel: (0524) 578221. Fax: (524) 577-878. TYPE: Hotel & Spa. LOCATION: Centrally located. SPA CLIENTELE: Women and men.

* Rooms: 82 w/priv. bath
* SPA on premises: in the hotel
* Airport: Milano Airport, 90 km. (56 mi.)
* Airport Transportation: free pick up, limo
* Credit Cards: VISA/AMEX/DC
* Open: April - November
* Rates: from Lit. 190,000/day
* TAC: 10%
* **Spa Facilities**: Thermal establishment with private medical service, complete fitness center, swimming pool, sauna, solarium
* **Spa Treatments**: medical, beauty, diet, thermal
* Medical Supervision: 1 MD, 6 RN
* Treatments approved: Medical Assoc.

DESCRIPTION: Well furnished hotel with spa facilities for medical and beauty treatments. All rooms are fully air-conditioned with private thermal bath or shower and are decorated in period furniture. Diet meals are available.

SARDINIA ISLAND
⌖ 070

✈ Elmas Airport (CAG) 46 km. / 29 mi.

The second largest island in the Mediterranean, Sardinia offers beautiful beaches, crystal clear seawater and historical sites. The climate is mild, especially in the southern region which is protected from cold northern winds by a range of mountains. Average temperatures range from 15°c / 59°F in April to 30°c / 80°F in August. Casual, practical clothing is recommended.

Forte Village
♥♥♥♥♥

55195 km 39,600 Forte Village, Santa Margherita di Pula (Cagliari) Sardinia I-09010. Tel: (070) 921-516. Fax: (070) 921-246. TYPE: Resort Complex & Spa. SPA MANAGER: Ute Simon. LOCATION: On 55 wooded acres on the southern tip of Sardinia. SPA CLIENTELE: Women and men. AGE RESTRICTION: Children under 14 years of age are not admitted.

* Bungalows: 725 w/priv. bath
* Phone, CTV, A/C, C/H, minibar, safe deposit
* Restaurant, bar, nightclub
* Airport: Cagliari, taxi
* Credit Cards: MC/VISA/AMEX/DC
* Open: April - October
* Rates: from Lit. 190,000/day
* TAC: 10%
* Spa on premises: **Thermae Del Parco**
* Year Established: 1983
* **Spa Facilities**: Thermae complex, saunas, curative pools, sea-oil tubs, Turkish baths, massage rooms, fully equipped gym, Spa restaurant: dietetic cuisine
* **Spa Treatments**: thalassotherapy, mud treatments, massage, Shiatsu, osteopathy sessions, water gymnastics, lymph-drainage, loofba, aerobics, water aerobics, beauty collagen treatments, anti-cellulitis, sea-oil treatments
* **Spa Programs**: Anti-stress, nutrition, beauty, wellbeing, thalassotherapy, Cardiofitness

* **Spa Packages**: Thalassotherapy and Total Well Being Thalassotherapy and Beauty, Thalassotherapy and Stress; Thalassotherapy and Nutrition. All packages are for 6 nights. Prices start at Lit. 2,883,000
* Medical Supervision: 2 MD

DESCRIPTION: Magnificent beachfront village resort complex consisting of 5 hotels and bungalows on the loveliest beach in Sardinia. Accommodations include the elegant Hotel Castello (4-star), the exclusive Villa del Parco (5-star) and Le Dune (5 star). The 'Thermae del Parco' offers open air thalassotherapy pools, Turkish bath and gym and a wide range of beauty, pampering, and rejuvenation programs and treatments for body and soul.

SATURNIA
꒐ 0564

✈ Grosseto Airport,45 km. / 28 mi.

Saturnia is a tiny hilltop village in southern Tuscany, half way between Rome and Florence. Located in the province of Grosseto it is archeologically one of Italy's richest and most interesting region of prehistoric, Etruscan, and Roman epochs. Nearby Grosseto, the administrative capital of the Province, is a modern town with walls dating from the Medici period. East of Saturnia lies the town of Orvieto, one of the most interesting cities in Italy. The town is a beautifully mixture of Etruscan, medieval, and renaissance traditions.

Saturnia can be reached by train from Rome, Florence, Orvieto or Grosseto. By car you can reach Saturnia from the North via the Bologna-Florence-Siena motorway and then the road leading to Grosseto and Scansano. From the South via the Rome-Civitavecchia motorway, then up to Albinia and east to Manciano.

The thermal springs cascade into the valley below with unique therapeutic qualities, pouring from the volcano Saturnia. At the source of the thermal springs lies the peaceful and elegant **Terme di Saturnia**.

The thermal water gush out at a constant 37°c (98°F) and contain a vegeto-mineral thermal substances. Their healing effect is most notable in curing and revitalizing the skin.

Terme di Saturnia
♥♥♥♥

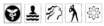

58050 Saturnia (Grosseto). Tel: (0564) 601061 or 601099. Fax: (0564) 601266. TYPE: Spa Hotel. LOCATION: In the valley below the village amidst country scenery and hot thermal springs. SPA CLIENTELE: Women and men.

* Rooms: 104 w/private bath
* Phone, CTV, A/C, C/H, frigobar
* Villa Montepaldi Restaurant
* Airport: Grosseto, 45 km. (28 mi.)
* Airport Transportation: Pick-up
* Reservations: suggested
* Credit Cards: AMEX/DC
* Open: Year round
* Rates: from Lit. 195,000 (optional half or full board)
* Spa on premises
* **Spa Facilities**: Complete Thermal Spa, Institute of Aesthetic Medicine, Benessere Club, gym, sauna, Spa swimming pool on top of the volcano spring at 37°c (98°F) water temperature year round, massage rooms, therapy rooms
* **Spa Programs**: Health, Fitness, Beauty
* **Spa Treatments**: medical, surgical, thermal, physiokinesitherapeutic and cosmetic, bathing in thermal water, mud applications, thalassotherapy, climatotherapy, hydrotherapy, massotherapy, Gerovital H3, Aslan method,diet
* Medical Supervision: doctors, nurses
* Treatments Approval: S.U. of Milan

DESCRIPTION: A large Spa hotel in a country setting. Accommodations are spacious and beautifully appointed. Adding to the sense of luxury is the superb restaurant - Villa Montepaldi with its Royal gourmet menus. Amidst all this luxury and peacefulness there is a world class Spa offering thermal, medical, aesthetic and Geriatric prevention treatments based on its thermal water and therapeutic mud. Terme di Saturnia is world famous for its unique range of skin care treatments.

SIRMIONE
꒐ 030

✈ Verona Villafranca Airport 35 km. / 22 mi.

Grand Hotel Terme
❤❤❤

😀 🏊 🐎 🚶 ❄

Viale Marconi 7, Sirmione/Lake Garda (Brescia) I-25019. Tel: (030) 916-568. Fax: (030) 916-568. TYPE: Spa Hotel. LOCATION: Lakefront garden setting near the Old Castle, 15 Km. / 10 mi. to Verona train station. DESCRIPTION: First class hotel with health and beauty spa, thermal & cosmetic treatments, sauna, gym, indoor & outdoor pool. Open April through October. 57 rooms, 1 suite, limited wheelchair access. Restaurant, bar, meeting room, 3 tennis courts, private beach, water sports. Hotel rates: from Lit. 280,000.

STRESA
🌙 0323

✈ Linate Airport (LIN)

Stresa is a picturesque medieval town and a fashionable resort in the beautiful Lake Region on the western shore of Lake Maggiore. The "Jewel City of Lake Maggiore" has fabulous vegetation, magnificent views, and mild climate year round. Stresa can be reached in about one hour from Milan via the Simplon Railway.

Centro Benessere di Stresa
❤❤❤❤❤

😀 🏊 🐎 🚶 ❄

c/o Grand Hotel Des Iles Borromees, Corso Umberto I, 67, Stresa 28049. Tel: (0323) 30431. Fax: (0323) 32405.

TYPE: Deluxe Resort & Spa. LOCATION: In a park overlooking Lake Maggiore. SPA CLIENTELE: Women and men.

* Rooms: 173 w/private bath. Suites: 15
* Phone, CTV, frigobar, C/H, A/C, balcony or terrace
* Restaurant & bar, snack bar, business center
* Airport: Malpensa 60 km. / 38 mi.
* Train Station: Stresa Stn 500 m./yds.
* Airport/Taxi Transportation: taxi
* Credit Cards: MC/VISA/AMEX/DC/EC/ACC
* Open: Year round
* Hotel Rates: from Lit. 360,000
* TAC: 10%
* Spa on premises
* **Spa Facilities**: Health & Beauty Center, Turkish bath, massage rooms, gym, sauna, indoor whirlpool
* **Spa Programs**: Health, fitness, beauty, weight loss, stress reduction, weekly program
* **Spa Treatments**: face & body treatments, herbal wraps, facials, gourmet diet menu, makeup lessons, mud packs, oil baths, hydrowave pressure massage in water enriched with marine algae, Shiatzu massage, body masque, total body peeling, aquatic exercises, jogging, aerobics
* Medical Supervision: 4 MD, cosmetologist, dietitians, exercise experts, medical screening

DESCRIPTION: Stresa Centro Benessere is an impressive spa with the latest in spa facilities. Located at the grand Hotel des Iles Barommées it offers exotic beauty treatments and professional diet and exercise programs for small groups of no more than 34 people. The luxurious accommodations and superb cuisine make this spa one of the best in Europe.

JAMAICA

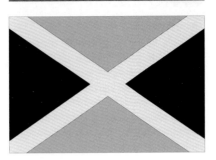

AREA: 4,411 sq. mi. (11,424 sq. km.)
POPULATION: 2,200,000
CAPITAL: Kingston
OFFICIAL LANGUAGE: English
CURRENCY: Jamaican Dollar (J$)
EXCHANGE RATE: 1US$ = J$ 35.95
INTERNATIONAL PHONE CODE: 876

Jamaica is an exciting Caribbean island with a pleasant climate, beautiful scenery, and a diversity of sports and recreation. Little is known that the North Coast mineral springs near Ocho Rios have curative power, and their location was selected as the site for Jamaica's premier International Spa.

 Jamaica Tourist Board
ICWI Bldg., 2 St. Lucia Ave. Kingston 5 Jamaica
Tel: (876) 929-9200. Fax: (876) 929-9375

IRISHTOWN

⟩ No area code
✈ Norman Manley Int'l Airport (KIN) 24 km. / 15 mi.

Strawberry Hill - Aveda Spa
♥♥♥♥

St. Andre, Irishtown. Tel: 944-8400. Fax: 944-8408. TYPE: Hotel & Holistic Spa. LOCATION: Nestled amidst 26 acres in the hills of the Blue Mountains. SPA CLIENTELE: Women & men. DESCRIPTION: Picturesque hotel dating

from the 1800's with holistic health studio specializing in preventive care, massages, nature walks. 18 cottages with mahogany plantation antiques some with full kitchen, phone, CD player, minifridge, restaurant, afternoon tea. Hotel rates: from US$250.

MONTEGO BAY

⟩ No area code
✈ Donald SangsterInt'l Airport (MBJ)
2 mi. / 3 km. east of Montego Bay

Half Moon Golf, Tennis & Beach Club
♥♥♥♥♥

P.O. Box 80, Montego Bay. Tel: (876) 953-2211. Fax: (876) 953-2731. Toll Free (800) 626-0592. TYPE: All Inclusive Resort & Spa. MANAGING DIRECTOR: Heinz

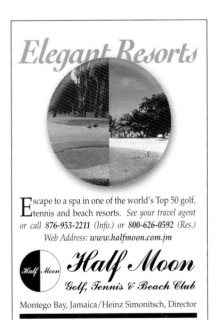

Simonitsch. LOCATION: On private beach, 7 mi. / 11 km. from Montego Bay town center. SPA CLIENTELE: Men, Women.

* Rooms: 418 w/priv. bath (rooms, suites & villas)
* Phone, CTV, Air-conditioning, minibar, jacuzzi, restaurants, bar, nightclub
* Reservations: deposit required
* Credit Cards: MC/VISA/AMEX
* Open: Year round
* Hotel Rates: from $130-$175/day (inclusive plan) per person; Spa Treatments: $25-$70 each
* TAC: 12%
* Spa on premises: **Body Works**
* Year Established: 1996
* **Spa Facilities**: Health & Fitness center, weight rooms, aerobic studio, massage rooms, sauna, jacuzzi, 4 tennis courts, pools, croquet & squash courts,
* **Spa Programs**: Pampering, Fitness
* **Spa Package**: Spa Plan (includes one Spa treatment per day plus all other health and fitness services)
* **Spa Treatments**: Swiss & Vichy showers, hydrotherapy, salt glo, natural Moor Mud, Sea Algae thalassotherapy, aromatherapy; body wraps and scrubs, facials, massage therapy, reflexology, aerobics, yoga, fitness classes
* **Medical Supervision**: medical diagnostic center
* **Email: hmoondat@infochan.com**
* **Web: www.halfmoon.com.jm**

DESCRIPTION: Elegant resort comprising of rooms, suites, cottages and villas on 400 acres of tropical gardens with 1 mile of private beach. The Spa and Fitness center - **Body Works** is a state of the art luxurious center with top notch massage therapists, fitness instructors and sports facilities.

Round Hill Hotel & Villas
❤❤❤❤❤

PO Box 64, Montego Bay, Tel: 956-7050. Fax: 956-7505. TYPE: Deluxe Resort. LOCATION: 8 mi. / 13 km. from Montego Bay on a peninsula. DESCRIPTION: Caribbean resort with fitness center, aerobics, massages. 110 rooms, 74 suites. Hotel rates: from US$270.

Royal Court Hotel & Natural Health Retreat
❤❤❤

PO Box 195, Montego Bay. Tel: 952-4531 or 4100. Fax: 952-4532. TYPE: Holistic Health Spa. LOCATION: Hilltop one mile from beach, overlooking Montego Bay. SPA CLIENTELE: Women and men. DESCRIPTION: Relaxing retreat with emphasis on mental and physical fitness. Health spa, swimming pool, gym, holistic health consultation, yoga, massages, workshops on healthy living, vegetarian cuisine, juice bar, disco. Hotel rates: from US$80.

NEGRIL

No area code

Negril Airport (NEG) 3 mi. / 5 km. north

Negril is a quiet beach resort on the western tip of the island with fine tourist facilities, Club resort complexes, nudist beach, and water sports: scuba diving, snorkeling, sailing, windsurfing, and water-skiing. Negril can be reached by car from Kingston via Hwy A2 west, or from Montego Bay, the second largest city in Jamaica about 30 miles (48 km.) east via Hwy A.

Sandals Negril Beach Resort & Spa
❤❤❤❤

PO Box 12, Negril. Tel: 957-5216. Fax: 957-5338. TYPE: Resort & Spa. LOCATION: Beachfront, 1.5 hrs. from hours from Sangster Airport. SPA CLIENTELE: Women and men. DESCRIPTION: All-inclusive couples only resort with full service European Spa. Hotel rates: from US$1,100 (2 nights).

Swept Away
❤❤❤

1400 longboat Rd., Long Bay, Negril. Tel: (809) 957-4040. TYPE: Resort Complex. LOCATION: On the Negril beach. SPA CLIENTELE: Men and women.

* Rooms: 134 verandah suites

* Restaurant, bar, piano lounge
* Airport: Montego Bay 30 mi. / 48 km.
* Hotel Rates: from US$570
* TAC: 10%
* Spa on premises
* **Spa Facilities**: Sports complex, gym, exercise lap pool, steam, sauna & massage rooms
* **Spa Treatments**: aerobics, yoga, massage

DESCRIPTION: 20 acres beach resort for couples with comprehensive fitness facilities.

OCHO RIOS

> No area code

✈ Ocho Rios Airport (OCJ) 11 mi. / 18 km. north

Ocho Rios, is a beach resort on the North Coast of Jamaica. The long stretch of beach from Negril to Ocho Rios has soft, powdery beaches, and a diversity of water sports and recreation. Of particular interest are the Dunn's River Falls and beach where clear mountain waters rush down a wooded gorge, and the mineral springs that are said to have curative effects for the treatment of rheumatism, arthritis, and certain skin problems.

Ocho Rios can be reached by car from Kingston via the main highway A1 north.

Charlie's Spa
❤❤❤❤❤

c/o Grand Lido Sans Souci, P.O. Box 103, Main St., Ocho Rios. Tel: 974-2353. Fax: (809) 974-2544. TYPE: Deluxe Resort & Spa. LOCATION: Beachfront on 12 acres of tropical hillside beach front, 2 miles (3 km.) east of Ocho Rios. SPA CLIENTELE: Women and men.

* Rooms: 12 w/priv. bath. Suites: 99
* Phone, CTV, A/C, minibar, balcony
* Nightly Entertainment, bar
* Airport: Montego Bay 65 mi. / 104 km.
* Airport Transportation: private car transfer
* Open: Year round
* Reservations: 3 night deposit required

* Credit Cards: MC/VISA/AMEX
* Hotel Rates: from US$420 (room only)
* TAC: 10% (on room only)
* Spa on premises
* **Spa Facilities**: fresh and mineral water swimming pools and Spa. Duplex pool & fitness pavilion, weight-training center, panoramic Jacuzzi, massage and therapy rooms
* **Spa Programs**: fitness, beauty and pampering; Diet & Weight Management
* **Spa Treatments**: bath in mineral water, low impact aerobics, massage and beauty therapies, aromatherapy, body scrub, weight-training sessions, fitness/lifestyle consultation, yoga, aquacize, gourmet spa diet meals (1,000 - 1,200 calories per day)
* **Indications**: relaxation, weight loss; mineral water are effective in the treatment of rheumatism, arthritis, and certain skin diseases
* Medical Supervision: local MD on call. resident health professionals, nutritionists, estheticians

DESCRIPTION: Charlie's Spa was created by Christine Cox from the Phoenix Fitness resort in Houston (TX), and it is named after Charlie, the giant green turtle, that has lived in the spa's mineral water-fed grotto. The elegant spa offers structured fitness, beauty and weight loss programs with professional counselling. Recreation: 4 tennis courts, private beach, snorkeling, waterskiing, sailing, windsurfing, deep-sea fishing, and scuba.

Elysium Spa & Salon
❤❤❤❤

c/o Ciboney Ocho Rios, 104 Main St., PO Box 728, Ocho Rios. Tel: 974-1027. Fax: 974-7148. TYPE: Spa & Beach Resort. LOCATION: On 45 acres of hills overlooking the sea. SPA CLIENTELE: Women and men. DESCRIPTION: Mediterranean style all inclusive beach resort with health club and spa, body scrubs, wraps, facials, waxing, relexology, aerobics studio, exercise & weight studio, sauna, steamrooms, massage, manicure, pedicure, jogging trail, walking course. 63 rooms, 18 junior suites, 199 one-bedroom villa suites, 7 two-bedroom villas, 4 three-bedroom villas. 4 restaurants, 2 cafes, 7 bars, conference facilities, 2 pools, 6 tennis courts, squash courts, "Hot Slot" gaming room, water sports, beach. Hotel rates: from US$690 (3 nights).

Enchanted Garden
❤❤❤

🏊 🚶 ❋

St. Ann, PO Box 284, Ocho Rios. Tel: 974-1400, Fax: 974-5823. TYPE: Resort & Spa. LOCATION: On 20 acres of landscaped gardens near Dunns River Falls. SPA CLIENTELE: Women and men. DESCRIPTION: All inclusive beach resort with fully equipped health spa, natural pools with waterfalls, jacuzzi, seaquarium, swim up bar. 113 rooms and suites, 5 restaurants, 4 bars, nightclub. Hotel rates: from US$180.

Grand Lido Sans Souci
❤❤❤❤❤

🏊 🚶

St. Ann, PO Box 103, Ocho Rios. Tel: 974-2353. Fax: 974-2544.TYPE: Resort & Spa. LOCATION: Beachfront in tropical gardens, 5 mi. / 9 km. from downtown. SPA CLIENTELE: Women and men. DESCRIPTION: All inclusive deluxe beachfront resort with health spa. Spa treatments include: facials, body scrubs, reflexology, massage, manicures, pedicures, aerobics, yoga, mineral springs. Hotel rates: from US$460.

Sandals Dunn's River
Golf Resort & Spa
❤❤❤❤❤

🏊 🚶

PO Box 51, Ocho Rios. Tel: 972-1610. Fax: 972-1611. TYPE: Resort & Spa. LOCATION: Beachfront. SPA CLIENTELE: Women and men. DESCRIPTION: All inclusive couples-only resort with a full service European Spa. 256 rooms, 6 bars, 4 restaurants, outdoor pools, tennis, golf, water sports. Hotel rates: from US$1160 (2 nights).

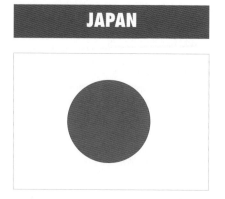

JAPAN

AREA: 145,730 sq. mi. (377,441 sq. km.)
POPULATION: 117,100,000
CAPITAL: Tokyo
OFFICIAL LANGUAGE: Japanese
CURRENCY: Yen (¥)
CURRENCY EXCHANGE: 1US$ = ¥ 120
TELEPHONE COUNTRY CODE: 81

Japan is a chain of volcanic islands with twenty thousands hot springs called Onsen in Japanese. The spa tradition in Japan goes back to A.D. 552 when Buddhism was first introduced. Some hot springs developed facilities similar to the fashionable 19th century great European spas, but they are still very intimate, traditional and Japanese in essence.

In Japan you can find a wide range of medicinal spas with healing waters, exotic spas with fantastic 'jungle baths', and large public baths. However, although Japan offers hundreds of hot springs resort areas with multiple type of hot bathes, banquet halls and massage rooms, unfortunately none of them target on the international market.

ℹ️ **Japan Nat'l Tourist Organization**
One Rockefeller Plaza, Suite 1250,
New York, NY 10020
Tel: (212) 757-5640. Fax: (212) 307-6754

ATAMI
ﾑ **557**

✈️ Atami Airport, 4 km. / 2.5 mi.

Atami is a popular sea-side hot-spring resort about 100 km. (63 mi.) southwest of Tokyo overlooking the Sagami Bay with the snow covered Mt. Fuji in the backdrop. Atami "hot sea" in Japanese, is a favorite spa destination close to the capital. Here you can discover hundreds of mineral springs and some of the best bathing facilities in Japan. The waters are simple thermal with salt and calcium sulfate. Taking the water may help calm the nerves, irritated skin, and invigorate blood circulation.

Atami can be reached from Tokyo by Shinkansen (bullet train) in less than one hour, or use the private Odakyu Line from Shinjuku (Tokyo) and change to the Tokaido Main Line at Odawara.

New Fujyia Hotel
❤❤❤

1-16 Ginzacho, Atami, Shizuoka Pref. 413. Tel: (557) 81-0111. Fax: (557) 81-8052. TYPE: Hotel & Spa. LOCATION: Centrally located, few blocks inland. SPA CLIENTELE: Men and women, family oriented.

* Rooms: 316, Japanese & Western style rooms w/private bath
* Suites: 5 w/cooking facilities
* CTV, A/C, C/H
* Restaurants, Night Club & Bar
* Airport: Atami Airport, 2-1/2 mi. / 4 km.
* Airport Transportation: bus, taxi
* Credit Cards: AMEX/DC
* Hotel Rates: from ¥8,000
* TAC: 10%
  Rates include two meals and free use of Spa
* Spa on premises
* **Spa Facilities**: Health Club, indoor thermal pool, outdoor Hot Spring Spa, public bath
* **Spa Treatments**: bathing in hot mineral water, massage, sauna

DESCRIPTION: Popular resort hotel with staff that is trained to deal with foreigners. The main activity is bathing in hot mineral water at the outdoor hot-spring spa. Recreation: Nightclub, entertainment and fine dining.

BEPPU SPA
☏ **977**
✈ Oita Airport (OIT) 25 mi. / 40 km. southeast

Beppu, population 134,000, is a world famous spa region with more than 3000 thermally active hot springs. Located in Oita Prefecture on the northeastern coast of Kyushu it can be easily accessed via the bullet train from Tokyo.

The hot springs are rich in iron (over 10 mg of Fe^{2+} or Fe^{3+}) and other minerals. They have a beneficial effect on the body and the skin, and contribute to a general feeling of well being. When imbibed: the water helps in blood production. In Beppu you will discover a great number of spa facilities and treatments ranging from hot springs bathing to hot sand bath, mud bath, and steam bath.

indications: rheumatism, neurologia, menopause, sterility and anemia.

Suginoi Hotel
❤❤❤

Kankaiji, Beppu 874. Tel: (977) 24-1141. Fax: (977) 21-0010. TYPE: Spa Hotel. LOCATION: On a wooded hill with breathtaking views of the town and the harbor below. SPA CLIENTELE: Women and men, Family oriented. Popular with Japanese and foreign visitors.

* Rooms: 586; 80 (Western style) Suites: 32
* Japanese Restaurant & Bars
* Phone, CTV, A/C
* Airport: Oita Airport, 1 hour, bus, taxi
* Reservations: suggested
* Credit Cards: MC/VISA/AMEX/DC
* Hotel Rates: from ¥15,500
* TAC: 10%
  Rates include 2 meals and use of thermal bath
* Spa on premises
* **Spa Facilities**: Large dome-covered mineral water Public Baths set amidst a tropical garden; Two separate baths for men and women; swimming pool,
* SPA Treatments: bathing in hot mineral water

DESCRIPTION: Large Hotel offering a variety of accommodations with the majority in traditional Japanese style. Very popular with Japanese and many foreign tourists who come here to enjoy the exotic large public mineral bath. Try the Dream Bath or Flower Bath. For about ¥2,000 (free for hotel guests) you can indulge in a fantasy spa experience with hundreds of other people (same sex bathing). Another extraordinary experience for spa enthusiasts is the Hoyoland complex of open-air communal baths.

FUKUOKA CITY
92
✈ Fukuoka Airport (FUK), 10 km. / 6 mi.

Grand Hyatt Fukuoka
❤❤❤❤

1-2-82 Sumiyoshi, Hakata-ku Fukuoka City 812, Fukuoka Prefecture. Tel: (92) 282-1234. Fax: (92) 282-2817. TYPE: Hotel & Spa. LOCATION: Downtown Fukuoka, 1.6 km. to Hakata train station. SPA CLIENTELE: Women and men. DESCRIPTION: Resort hotel with a fitness center and spa. 356 rooms, 14 suites, nonsmoker rooms, 10 restaurants, 2 bars, lounge, meeting facilities.

HAKODATE
138
✈ Hakodate Airport 35 mi. / 56 km.

Hakodate-Onuma Prince Hotel
❤❤❤

148 Nishi-Onuma-Onsen, Nanae-cho, Kameda-gun 041-13, Hokkaido Prefecture. Tel: (138) 67-1111. Fax: (138) 67-3660. TYPE: Resort & Spa. LOCATION: Wooded area near Hakodate-Onuma Nanae Ski area, 5 km. to train station. SPA CLIENTELE: Women and men. DESCRIPTION: First class resort with Hot Spring baths, sauna. 418 rooms 4 suites, nonsmoker rooms, 3 restaurants, bar & lounge, banquet hall, indoor pool 16 tennis courts, 45 holes of golf, Mahjong room. Hotel rates: from ¥ 15,000.

Hakodate Yunokawa Wakamatsu
❤❤❤

1-2-27 Yunokawa-cho, Hakodate 041-0932, Hikkaido Prefecture. Tel: (138) 5902171. Fax: (138) 59-3316. TYPE: Ryokan hotel & Spa. LOCATION: Overlooking the Tsugaru Straits, 15 minutest to Hakodate train station. SPA CLIENTELE: Women and men. DESCRIPTION: Traditional Japanese Inn with Yunokawa Spa hot springs.

HAKONE
460
✈ Haneda Airport, Tokyo (HND) 40 mi. / 64 km.

Hakone Yumoto group of hot springs is located about 50 miles (80 km.) southwest of Tokyo. It is a favorite weekend get away for Tokyo residents. The hot springs are located in a National Park called Fuji-Hakone-Izu and provide a peaceful setting of magic mountains, blue lakes and views of Mt. Fuji.

The spring water composition is simple thermal with sodium chloride. Bathing in the water provides a sense of well being and relief to almost any kind of ailments. The most famous public bath in Hakone is Senninburo where thousands of people can take the water at the same time.

Fujiya Hotel
❤❤❤❤

359 Miyanoshita, Hakone, Kanagawa Pref. 250-04. Tel: (460) 22211. Fax: (460) 22210. TYPE: Mountain Resort & Spa. LOCATION: In the Fuji-Hakone National Park. SPA CLIENTELE: Women and men.

* Rooms: 145 (western type) w/private bath
* Suites: 8
* Phone, C/H, Dining Room, Tea Lounge
* Japanese Gardens
* Train Station: Odawara, 7.5 mi. / 12 km.
* Credit Cards: MC/VISA/DC/AMEX
* Rates: from ¥16,000/day; TAC: 10%
* Spa on premises
* **Spa Facilities**: hot spring baths, outdoor

swimming pool, indoor thermal pool
* **Spa Treatments**: bathe in thermal waters

DESCRIPTION: An International hotel, one of the oldest and the most revered in Hakone. The architecture is traditionally Japanese, with buildings shaped like a pagoda or a Japanese temple. The public garden is serene with waterfalls and ponds. Accommodations are in western style rooms, with excellent service. English is spoken. The hotel offers thermal baths with hot spring for pleasure and relaxation.

Ichinoyu
❤❤❤

90 Tonosawa, Hakone-machi, Kanagawa-pref. 250-03. Tel: (460) 5-5333/5334. Fax: (460) 5-5335. TYPE: Ryokan & Spa. LOCATION: A riverside location, five minutes walk from the Yumoto Station Odakyu Line. SPA CLIENTELE: Women and men.

* Rooms: 22; 10 w/private bath
* Airport: Haneda (80 km. / 50 mi.)
* Train Station: Odawara (8 km. / 5 mi.)
* Train Station Transportation: bus, taxi
* Reservations: required, no deposit
* Credit Cards: VISA/AMEX/MC/DC
* Open: Year round
* Rates: from ¥26,000/day; prices include room, 2 meals, tax and service charge
* TAC: 13-16%
* Spa on premises: **Tonosawa Spa**
* **Spa Facilities**: wooden bathtubs, communal tubs fed by natural mineral spring waters

DESCRIPTION: A romantic 350 years old Ryokan with charming Japanese style rooms and spa facilities. A great experience in an old fashioned Japanese spa tradition.

IBUSUKI
⟩ **933**
✈ Kagoshima Airport (KOJ) 49 mi. / 78 km.

Ibusuki Spa is a famous hot-spring honeymoon type resort in southern Kyushu's eastern Satsuma Peninsula. It is locat-

ed some 45 km. (28 mi.) south of Kagoshima city. The Spa owes its popularity in part to the lovely white seashore and lush tropical vegetation which surrounds it. Sand bathing, also known as natural sauna, is an experience unique to Ibusuki. The best place for hot black sand bathing is at the **Surigahama Public Beach**, located within a walking distance of the main station. In addition to the famous hot sand bathing, there are hot salty springs (185°F - 85°c) which are alkali saline.

How to get there: Fly from Tokyo to Kagoshima (1hr. 40 min.) JAL, ANA & JAS have 8 daily flights to Kagoshima. From Kagoshima Airport 1 hr. 50 min. by bus.

Indications: Bathing in the hot springs has a beneficial effect in cases of gastroenteric disorders, nervous conditions, and female disorders. The climate is relatively mild in the winter with average temperatures in January between 28°F low - 64°F high (-2°c - 18°c); summer temperatures vary between 66°F low - 95°F high in July (19°c - 35°c).

Ibusuki Iwasaki Hotel
❤❤❤

3755 Juni-cho, Ibusuki City 891-04, Kagoshima - Prefecture. Tel: (993) 22-2131. Fax: (993) 24-3215. TYPE: Resort & Spa. LOCATION: Centrally located near the main train station. SPA CLIENTELE: Women and men, family oriented.

* Rooms: 428; 362 western type. Suites: 9
* Phone, CTV, A/C, minibar, private balcony
* Dining room, bar, night club
* Seafood 'Jungle' Restaurant
* Airport: Kagoshima AP, 75 km. / 47 mi.
* Airport Transportation: bus, taxi
* Train Station: Ibusuki Station, 3 km. (2 mi.)
* Train Station Transportation: taxi, bus
* Reservations: suggested
* Credit Cards: MC/VISA/AMEX/DC
* Open: Year round
* Rates: from ¥15,000 (room only); TAC: 10% Sand bath: ¥1,500
* Spa on premises: distance 100 m. / yards

* **Spa Facilities**: Jungle bath - separate and co-ed thermal bathing, indoor and outdoor exotic hot-sand bath
* **Spa Treatments**: springs & hot-sand baths
* **Indications**: hot springs - gastroenetric problems, neuralgia, female disorders. Hot sand bath - rheumatism, muscular aches, improving blood circulation
* **Treatments Approved**: Kagoshima Pref. Government hygienic laboratory

DESCRIPTION: A modern Western-style self-contained resort & spa complex built along the beach of the scenic Kinko-bay. The resort features an immense hot-springs 'Jungle Bath' and indoor and outdoor hot-sand bathing facilities. It was designed as a tropical paradise for Japanese tourists and honeymooners. Recreation: tennis, golf, and nightly entertainment.

Ibusuki Park Hotel Hakusuikan
♥♥♥

Tarahama-kaigon, Ibusuki City. Tel: (993) 23131. TYPE: Hotel & Spa. LOCATION: Centrally located near the main train station. SPA CLIENTELE: Family oriented.

* Rooms: 237; 50 Western style
* Beer Garden (summer only)
* Train Station: Ibusuki Station, 6 min., taxi
* Reservations: suggested
* Open: Year round
* Room Rates: from ¥14,000/day. Rates include accommodations, free use of spa facilities, two meals.
* **Spa Facilities**: Indoor hot-sand bath, outdoor hot-spring for men and women, 3 pools
* **Spa Treatments**: mineral, hot-sand baths
* **Indications**: gastroenteric troubles, neuralgia, female disorders

DESCRIPTION: A pleasant first class hotel with a variety of accommodations ranging from typical Japanese to contemporary Western. Excellent mineral water and hot-sands baths facilities.

MATSUYAMA CITY
✈ 89

✈ Matsuyama Airport (MYJ) 5 mi. / 8 km. southwest

Matsuyama city, population 450,000, is the largest town in Shikoku the smallest island in Japan. The island is beautiful with rugged mountains, mild climate and many historical sites including Buddhist temples.

Spa lovers in search of exotic spas will enjoy visiting the famous **Dógo Onsen**, the oldest hot-spring spa in Japan (3,000 years old). The main attraction here is Shinrokaku, a public bathhouse complex accommodating up to 2,000 people. The spa water is alkaline and odorless with softening effect on the skin. Inhalation of steam helps in clearing of the bronchial tubes.

Matsuyama is accessible from Hiroshima, Osaka, Beppu and Kobe by hydrofoil or ferry. From Tokyo by air in about 2 hours.

Indications: diabetes, gout, drug addiction, gallstones, bronchial problems.

Funaya Hotel
♥♥♥

1-33, Dogo Yunomachi, Matsuyama, Ehime. Tel: (899) 47-0278. TYPE: Hotel & Spa. LOCATION: At the hot spring resort east of Matsuyama. SPA CLIENTELE: Family oriented.

* Rooms: 43, 22 w/private bath, 3 Suites
* Japanese Garden
* Restaurant: Japanese Cuisine
* Airport: Matsuyama Airport, 7 mi. / 11 km.
* Airport Transportation: taxi, limo
* Credit Cards: MC/VISA/AMEX/DC
* Open: Year round
* Hotel Rates: from ¥25,000/day
* Spa on premises
* **Spa Facilities**: hot spring, mineral baths, indoor & outdoor, public bathhouses nearby
* **Spa Treatments**: bathing in hot alkaline mineral water
* **Indications**: see above

DESCRIPTION: Ryokan with Japanese style rooms in a beautiful Japanese Garden setting. Price include two Japanese meals a day.

MISASA SPA
⟩ 858
✈ Okyama Airport

Hotel Mansuiro
♥♥♥♥

5 Yamada, Misasa-machi, Tohaku-gun 682-0122, Tottori Prefecture. Tel: (858) 43-0511. Fax: (858) 43-2616. TYPE: Ryokan hotel & Spa. LOCATION: On the banks of the Misasa River in Misasa Spa, 20 minutes to Kurayoshi station. DESCRIPTION: Traditional hotel in Misasa Spa known for the rejuvenating radium content of its hot springs. 77 rooms, restaurant, coffee shop. Hotel rates: from ¥23,000.

NAHA CITY
⟩ 98
✈ Okinawa / Naha Airport (OKA) 2 mi. / 3 km.

Loisir Hotel Okinawa
♥♥♥♥

3-2-1 Nishi, Naha City 900, Okinawa Prefecture. Tel: (98) 868-2222. Fax: (98) 860-2000. TYPE: Hotel & Spa. LOCATION: Harbor front area, 5 km. to Naha Airport. DESCRIPTION: Attractive hotel with Spa, massage, sauna, indoor pool. 416 Western & Japanese rooms, 3 suites, wheelchair access. Chinese, French, & Japanese restaurants, coffee shop, sushi bar, 2 bars, meeting facilities, outdoor pool. Hotel rates: from ¥19,000.

Renaissance Okinawa Resort
♥♥♥♥

3425-2 Yamada, Onnason, Kunigami-gun, Okinawa Prefecture, Tel: (98) 965-0707. Fax: (98) 965-5011. TYPE: Resort Hotel & Spa. LOCATION: In Okinawa State Park, 40 km. to Naha Int'l Airport. SPA CLIENTELE: Women and men. DESCRIPTION: Elegant beachfront resort hotel with Spa, indoor & outdoor pools, Hot Spring bath. 262 Western rooms, 20 Japanese rooms, 9 suites, nonsmoker rooms, wheelchair access. 6 restaurants, coffee shop, bar, lounge, disco meeting facilities, private beach, marine sports club. Hotel rates: from ¥30,000.

NARUKO
⟩ 229
✈ Sendai Airport

Naruko is a medicinal hot-springs resort in northern Honshu. The thermal water contain sulfur, or sodium chloride and has a unique skin softening effect. Naruko is accessible by the Rikuuto Line to the Naruko Station, the hot-springs are nearby within walking distance.

Indications: The thermal water can be recommended for treatment of symptoms of nervous tension, indigestion, and stiff joints.

Yusaya Country Inn
♥♥

84 -Yumoto, Narugo, Miyagi Pref., 989-68. Tel: (229) 83-2565. Fax: (229) 83-2566. TYPE: Hot Springs Inn. LOCATION: Northern part of Japan, 2-1/2 hours from Tokyo via the new express train. Sendai, the nearest large city is one hour drive south. SPA CLIENTELE: Family oriented.

* Rooms: 14, Ryokan Japanese Style
* Airport: Sendai Airport, 1 hour drive
* Credit Cards: MC/DC
* Season: Year round
* Hotel Rates: from ¥13,000; TAC: 10%
* Spa on premises
* **Spa Facilities:** indoor thermal baths
* **Spa Treatments:** beauty, medical, thermal mineral water containing skin softening sulfur or sodium chloride
* **Indications:** skin treatment, nervous tension, indigestion, stiff joints
* **Contraindications:** general contraindication for thermal bathing treatments

DESCRIPTION: Two-story building made of cypress and cider wood. The interior decoration is in traditional Japanese country style. Excellent food and banquet facilities.

NOBORIBETSU

) 143

✈ Okadama Airport, Saporo (OKD) 40 mi. / 64 km.

Noboribetsu, population 52,000, is one of Japan's best hot springs resorts just south of Sapporo in the northern island of Hokkaido.

There are 11 hot springs in the Spa with temperatures ranging between 113°F and 197°F (45°c - 92°c). The thermal waters represent almost any available thermal combinations that exist in Japan. The major mineral content includes: sulfur, salt, iron, sodium hydrogen-carbonate, sodium sulfate, and acid-aluminum sulfate. Some springs are radioactive, others are simple thermal or mineral free hot water. Several hospitals and research centers in Noboribetsu Onsen use the hot springs and offer balneological facilities and treatments.

Indications: motor disturbances, diabetes, rheumatism, arthritis, eczema, and chronic digestive problems.

Noboribetsu Spa is more than a place for a cure, the town is alive with fine restaurants, shops and nightlife. Noboribetsu Spa is located about 15 minutes bus drive from the town center.

Daiichi Takimotokan
❤❤❤

55 Noboribetsu Onsen, Noboribetsu City 059-05. Tel: (143) 842111. TYPE: Ryokan & Spa. LOCATION: Noboribetsu Onsen. SPA CLIENTELE: Family oriented.

* Rooms: 340, 8 western style w/beds
* Ceiling Fan, TV with paid video, fridge
* Japanese Garden
* Restaurant: Japanese Cuisine
* Airport: Sapporo, 60 mi. (96 km.)
* Airport Transportation: taxi, limo

* Open: Year round
* Hotel Rates: from ¥14,000/day
* Spa on premises
* **Spa Facilities**: hot spring pools, mineral bath, indoor and outdoor facilities, public bath houses nearby
* **Spa Treatments**: hot mineral rich water
* **Indications**: see above

DESCRIPTION: The best known Ryokan in the Spa first opened 126 years ago. Most rooms are Japanese style with tatami.

Noboribetsu Grand Hotel
❤❤❤

Noboribetsu Onsen, Noboribetsu City 059-05. Tel: (143) 842101. Fax: (143) 842543. TYPE: Hotel & Spa. LOCATION: Hilltop above the bus terminal. SPA CLIENTELE: Men and women, family oriented.

* Rooms: 259, Japanese or western style
* Restaurant, rock garden, games room
* Airport: Sapporo, 60 mi. (96 km.)
* Airport Transportation: bus, taxi
* Reservations: suggested
* Open: Year round
* Hotel Rates: from ¥15,000/day
* Spa on premises
* **Spa Facilities**: Elegant Public Bath with thermal water, indoor/outdoor sections for men, indoor for women, saunas for men and women, public bathhouses nearby
* **Spa Treatments**: bathe in thermal water, massages
* **Indications**: see above

DESCRIPTION: A large hotel complex with rooms in Japanese or Western style, most with private bath. The hotel features thermal pools and a public bathhouse.

Kanko Hotel Takinoya
❤❤❤❤❤

162 Noboribetsu-Onsen. Noboribetsu, Hokkaido. Tel: (143) 84-2222. TYPE: Deluxe Ryokan. LOCATION: Hill and River side in the center of town, 5 min. walk to Hell Valley

and Bear Ranch. SPA CLIENTELE: Family Oriented.

* Rooms: 72; 50 w/private bath. Suites: 4
* Japanese Garden, banquet facilities
* Train Station: Noboribetsu, 8 km. (5 mi.) taxi, bus
* Reservations: 10% deposit required
* Credit Cards: MC/VISA/AMEX/DC
* Hotel Rates: from ¥ 15,000; TAC: 10%
* Spa on premises
* **Spa Facilities**: Outdoor public hot spring baths; indoor thermal baths
* **Spa Treatments**: bathing in hot mineral water
* **Indications**: see Noboribetsu spa
* **Medical Supervision**: none

DESCRIPTION: A Japanese Hot Spring resort with invigorating thermal pools. The accommodations are traditional Japanese. A place to enjoy the serenity of the Orient.

OSAKA CITY

 6

✈ Osaka Int'l Airport (OSA) 10 mi. / 16 km.
Kansai Int'l Airport (KIX) 31 mi. / 50 km.

Imperial Hotel Osaka
♥♥♥♥♥

8-50 Tenmabashi 1-Chome, Kita-ku, Osaka 530-0042, Osaka Prefecture. Tel: (6) 881-1111. Fax: (6) 881-4111. TYPE: Hotel & Spa. LOCATION: Downtown adjacent to parklands overlooking the Okawa river. 10 minutes to train station, 55 minutes to Kansai Int'l Airport. DESCRIPTION: Deluxe hotel with full service spa, beauty treatments, fully equipped health club with gym, sauna, massages, jacuzzi, aerobics. 373 rooms, 17 suites, nonsmoker rooms. 12 restaurants, bars, lounges, meeting facilities, business center, 3 tennis courts, indoor pool. Hotel rates: from ¥22,000

Hotel Nikko Kansai Airport
♥♥♥♥

1 Kita, Senshu-Kutu, Izumisano City 549-0001, Osaka Prefecture, Tel: (724) 55-1111. Fax: (724) 55-1155.

TYPE: Hotel & Spa. LOCATION: At Kansa Int'l Airport connected to airport passenger terminal & train station. DESCRIPTION: Resort style airport hotel with fully equipped spa and large 15 meter / 50 ft. pool. 562 rooms, 14 suites, nonsmoker rooms, wheelchair access. Restaurants, bars, karaoke bar, lounge, shops. Hotel rates: from ¥22,000.

The Ritz-Carlton Osaka
♥♥♥♥♥

2-5-25 Umeda, Kita-ku, Osaka, Osaka Prefecture. Tel: (6) 343-7000. Fax: (6) 343-7001. TYPE: Hotel & Spa. LOCATION: Osaka's Umeda business & shopping district, across from Osaka train station, 40 km. to Kansai Int'l Airport. SPA CLIENTELE: Women and men. DESCRIPTION: Elegant hotel with complete spa & fitness club, indoor pool workout studio, Japanese baths, sauna, indoor & outdoor jacuzzis, massage rooms. 264 Western rooms, 2 Japanese rooms, 26 suites, nonsmoker rooms, wheelchair access. 5 restaurants, bar, lounge, entertainment, meeting facilities, business center. Hotel rates: from ¥28,000.

SENDAI

) 22

✈ Sendai Airport 35 mi. / 56 km.

Hotel Zuiho
♥♥♥♥

26-1 Akiu-cho Yumoto, Taihauku-ku, Sendai 989-33, Miyagi Perfecture. Tel: (22) 397-1111. Fax: (22) 397-1131. TYPE: Resort hotel & Spa. LOCATION: Natural cliff side setting. SPA CLIENTELE: Women and men. DESCRIPTION: Pleasant resort hotel with spa facilities, large public baths, mist baths, waterfall like showers, open air baths, fitness center. 105 rooms, 13 suites, nonsmoker rooms, wheelchair access. 2 restaurants, 2 bars, meeting facilities, 2 pools, 2 tennis courts, Japanese gardens. Hotel rates: from ¥25,000.

SHIMA SPA

) 279

✈ Haneda Int'l Airport (HND)
Narita Int'l Airport (NRT) 156 mi. / 250 km.

Shima Hot Spring is a picturesque Japanese Spa in the northeastern Gumma Prefecture (north of Tokyo). The Spa is located along Shima River and it is surrounded by green forests and rolling hills. The hot springs have medicinal value. The water composition includes sodium, calcium-chloride, and sulfate thermal waters at temperatures between 54°c - 75°c (130°F - 167°F).

How to get there: take the Joetsu Line from Ueno Station in Tokyo to Shibukawa. From there take the Agatsuma Line to Nakanojo (JR) and from there continue by bus or taxi to the hot spring.

Indications: Rheumatism, neuralgia, and gastroenteric diseases.

Sekizenkan
♥♥♥

ko-4236, Shima, Nakanojo-machi, Agatsuma-gun, Gumma-ken, 377-06. Tel: (279) 64-2101. Fax: (279) 64-2369. LOCATION: In Joshinetsu Highland National Park. SPA CLIENTELE: Women and men, family oriented. SPECIAL RESTRICTIONS: Japanese only spoken. Foreign guests need Japanese speaking guide.

* Rooms: 83; 20 w/priv. bath
* Suites: 350 (no cooking facilities)
* Distance to Hot Springs: 50 m. (150 ft.)
* Airport: Narita (Tokyo), 250 km. / 156 mi.
* Train Station: Nakanojo (JR), 15 km. / 10 mi.
* Train Station Transportation: bus, taxi
* Reservations: must speak Japanese
* Credit Cards: MC/DC/JCM
* Open: Year round
* Rates: from ¥20,000; TAC: 15%-20%
* **Spa Facilities**: thermal pools, outdoor hot springs
* **Spa Treatments**: thermal medicinal baths, drinking medicinal water

DESCRIPTION: The ryokan Sekizenkan consists of three wooden buildings from different periods (built in 1691, 1936 and 1986). The accommodations are in traditional Japanese style. The spa consists of a large European-style

bath, and small thermal pools both indoor and outdoor for bathing and recreation.

SHIRABU SPA

238

✈ Yamagata Airport

Shirabu Spa is a rustic hot-spring resort in the mountains of northern Honshu few miles south of Yonezawa City in southeastern Yamagata Prefecture.

The mineral water of Shiabu Onsen is enriched with hydrogen sulphide and calcium sulfate and has a rather strong smell. Water treatments are beneficial for those who suffer from gastrointestinal disorders. The town's scenic location makes it an ideal location for health tourism.

How to get there: take the Ou Main Line to Yonezawa Station and from there continue with bus service to Shirabu Onsen and get off one station before the bus reaches the terminal.

Nakaya Ryokan
♥♥♥

1534 Ohaza Seki, Yonezawa-shi, Yamagata Pref. Tel: (238) 55-2111, 55-2121. TYPE: Ryokan & Spa. LOCATION: Central location. SPA CLIENTELE: Family oriented.

* Rooms: Japanese style
* Japanese Garden
* Train Station: Yonezawa, 50 min.
* Train Station Transportation: bus
* Open: Year round
* Rates: from ¥15,000/day
* Spa on premises
* **Spa Facilities**: Thermal waterfall bath, 3 mineral water spouts (cold, warm & hot)
* **Spa Treatments**: thermal water bathing
* **Indications**: stomach complaints, obesity, general well being

DESCRIPTION: One of the three original thatch roofed ryokan

connected to each other and sharing the hot sulfur springs that pour from the mountains into their pools. The accommodations are in a traditional Japanese style. The main attraction besides the hot-springs is the excellent 14-course dinner and the delicious breakfast. Meals are included.

TOCHIOMATA
🕿 **238**

✈ Haneda Int'l Airport (HND)
  Narita Int'l Airport (NRT)

Tochiomata Hot Springs is a medicinal spring located south of Niigata City (Niigata Prefecture) some 120 mi. (190 km.) northwest of Tokyo. This is a traditional Japanese hot spring resort going back to the eighth century which offers an inexpensive spa holiday centered around bathing.

The water which are radio active are not extremely hot. Their temperature is around 102°F (39°c) which permits lengthy bathing with no discomfort.

Indications: insomnia, neuralgia, skin irritations, rheumatism, and the water have a reputation to be effective in cases of infertility.

How to get there: take the Joetsu Shinkansen (bullet train) from Ueno Station in Tokyo to Urasa Station, from there proceed by bus, about 1 hour drive.

Hogando
♥♥

Tochiomata, Yunotani-mura, Kita Uonuma-gun, Niigata 946. Tel: (2579) 5-2216. TYPE: Ryokan & Spa. MANAGER: Mrs. Tomoko Hoshi. LOCATION: In a mountainous region south of Niigata. SPA CLIENTELE: Mixed.

* Rooms: 15 w/shared bath only
* Season: Year round
* Rates: from ¥10,000 with two meals
* Spa on premises
* **Spa Facilities**: indoor facilities, hot springs, 5 different type of baths, fitness room

* **Indications**: see general indications for Tochiomata Hot Springs

DESCRIPTION: Old Japanese Ryokan. All rooms have tatami mats, TV, but without private bath or cooking facilities. Breakfast and dinners are included in the price of the room, lunch can be served at additional cost.

TOKYO
🕿 **3**

✈ Haneda Int'l Airport (HND) 11 mi. / 18 km.
  Narita Int'l Airport (NRT) 41 mi. / 66 km.

Four Seasons at Chinzan-So
♥♥♥♥♥

10-8 Sekiguchi, 2-chome, Bunkyo-ku, Tokyo 112, Tokyo Perfecture. Tel: (3) 3943-2222. Fax: (3) 3943-2300. TYPE: Deluxe Hotel & Spa. LOCATION: In city center of historic Chinzan-So Gardens, 19 km to Haneda Int'l Airport & 60 km to Narita Int'l Airport. DESCRIPTION: Deluxe hotel combining Japanese and western design with mineral spring baths, health club, sauna, gym, indoor pool. 234 rooms, 49 suites, nonsmoker rooms, wheelchair access. 4 restaurants, 2 bars, meeting facilities, business center. Hotel rates: from ¥36,000.

Hotel Nikko Tokyo
♥♥♥♥♥

1-9-1 Daiba, Minato-Ku, Tokyo 135-8625, Tokyo Perfecture. Tel: (3) 5500-5500. Fax: (3) 5500-2525. TYPE: Hotel & Spa. LOCATION: Mid-city overlooking Tokyo Bay, direct access to Daiba station, 15 minutes to Haneda Airport. DESCRIPTION: Stylish waterfront hotel featuring a spa with indoor pool, indoor & outdoor jacuzzis, steam room, sauna, tanning beds, exercise studio, fitness classes, massage, aromatherapy, facial & body treatments. 453 rooms & suites, nonsmoker rooms, wheelchair access. 6 restaurants, 2 bars, nightclub, meeting facilities, business center. Hotel rates: from ¥27,000.

YUNOHIRA
⟩ 977
✈ Oita Airport

Yunohira - Onsen is a famous spa and a National Registered Health resort near Beppu on the island of Kyushu. The spa is famous for its potable mineral water which contains sodium chloride and is served in most of the local hotels or Ryokans.

Indications: drinking the water brings relief from indigestion, heartburn, constipation and other gastroenteric disorders. The hot springs water are recommended for bathing.

Shimizu-Ryokan
❤❤

♨

Yonohira Yofuin-cho, Oita-Gun, Oita-Pref 879-53. Tel: (0977) 86-2111. TYPE: Hotel - Ryokan. MANAGER: Soji Shimizu, GM. LOCATION: On the Kagono River near the Handa Highlands in Central Oita Pref. near Beppu. SPA CLIENTELE: Men, Women.

* Rooms: 13
* Japanese Garden
* Train Station: Yunohira Station
* Train Station Transportation: free pick up
* Season: Year round
* Rates: from ¥11,000/day
* TAC: 10%
* Distance to the Spa: 50 m (50 yards)
* **Spa Facilities**: Hot springs cave bath
* **Spa Treatments**: drinking cure of bottled mineral water, bathing in hot spring
* Treatments Approved: doctors in Kyushu University

DESCRIPTION: A Traditional Japanese style spa hotel (Ryokan), with a tatami floor and Japanese type bedrooms only. The Spa facility consists of a big cave-like bath made of rocks where guests can take a bath, relax and refresh themselves. The atmosphere is calm and serene and the innkeepers pledge a warm welcome to foreign visitors. The autumn changing of the season is one of the most beautiful times of the year to stay in Yunohira.

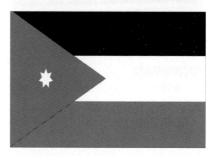

JORDAN

AREA: 35,000 sq. mi. (90,650 sq. km.)
POPULATION: 2,779,000
CAPITAL: Amman
OFFICIAL LANGUAGE: Arabic
CURRENCY: Jordanian Dinar (JD)
EXCHANGE RATE: 1US$ = JD 0.70
INTERNATIONAL PHONE CODE: 962

ℹ Jordan Tourism Board
P.O. Box 830688, Amman 11183 Jordan
Tel: (+962) 6-6477951. Fax: (+962) 6-647915

AMAN
⟩ 6
✈ Queen Alia Int'l Airport (AMN)

Hotel Intercontinental Jordan
❤❤❤❤

🐎 🏃

Queen Zair St. Tel: (6) 641361. Fax: (6) 645217. TYPE: Hotel & Spa. LOCATION: Hilltop in diplomatic and residential area. SPA CLIENTELE: Women and men. DESCRIPTION: Deluxe tower hotel with health spa, gym, sauna, jacuzzi, indoor heated lap pool, rooftop sundeck. 400 rooms, 34 suites, restaurants, nightclub, cocktail lounge. Hotel rates: from US$210.

HAMMAMAT MA'IN
⟩ 8

✈ Queen Alia Int'l Airport (AMN) 40 km. / 25 mi.

Hammamat Ma'in is a popular thermal spa town with its own 4-star hotel one hour drive from downtown Aman.

Ashtar Ma'in Hotel
♥♥♥♥

Hammamat Ma'in. Tel: (8) 545500. Fax: (8) 545550. TYPE: Spa Hotel. LOCATION: Zarqa Ma'in, 10 km. / 6 mi. east of the Dead Sea. SPA CLIENTELE: Women & men. DESCRIPTION: Four-star hotel at the natural mineral sources and waterfall of Zerqa Ma'in with swimming pool and Turkish bath.

SALT LAND VILLAGE (Dead Sea)
⌐ 9

✈ Queen Alia Int'l Airport (AMN) 40 km. / 25 mi.

The Dead Sea area is located at the northern end of the Great Rift Valley. This is the lowest point on earth at 400 m. / 1,320 ft. under sea level.

Dead Sea Spa Hotel
♥♥♥

Salt Land Village. Tel: (9) 802028 or (6) 601554. Fax: (6) 688100. TYPE: Spa Hotel. LOCATION: Seafront 10 km. / 6 mi. from hot water springs. SPA CLIENTELE: Women & men. DESCRIPTION: Hotel and bungalows with outdoor fresh water pool and skin clinic. Closed: January 16 - March 1. 96 rooms, 6 suites, restaurant, coffee shop, limited room service. Hotel rates: from US$170.

LATVIA

AREA: 24,595 sq. mi. (63,700 sq. km.)
POPULATION: 2,681,000
CAPITAL: Riga
OFFICIAL LANGUAGE: Latvian, Russian, Polish
CURRENCY: Latvian Lats (LVL)
EXCHANGE RATE: 1US$ = LVL 0.57
INTERNATIONAL PHONE CODE: 371

JURMALA
⌐ 2

✈ Riga Airport (RIX) 30 km. / 19 mi.

Baltija Hotel
♥♥♥

11 Dzintaru Prospect, Jurmala LV-2015. Tel: (2) 762151. Fax: (7) 892746. TYPE: Hotel & Spa. LOCATION: 15 minutes from Riga Int'l Airport, 25 min. to downtown Riga. SPA CLIENTELE: Women and men. DESCRIPTION: Hotel featuring Health Spa with spa medical treatments, mineral water pool, gym, steam bath, turkish bath, solarium, and massages. 150 rooms, 7 suites. Restaurant, bar, 3 lunges, meeting facilities. Hotel rates: from US$50.

Majori Spa
♥♥♥

7 Trigonu St., Majori. Tel: (2) 764242. Fax: (2) 762457. TYPE: Spa Complex with Hotel. LOCATION: Downtown

majori near the sea. SPA CLIENTELE: Women and men. DESCRIPTION: Health Spa complex in wood cottages and historic buildings, swimming pool with mineral water, gym, steam bath, sauna, Turkish bath, solarium, massages, medical treatments, mini golf, tennis nearby. 276 units with private bath, refrigerator, minibar, phone, room service, bar, banquet facilities. Hotel rates: on request.

Rigas Licis Hotel
❤❤❤

51 Dubultu Prospect, Jurmala LV-2015. Tel: (2) 761180, Fax: (2) 761166. TYPE: Hotel & Spa. LOCATION: Garden setting, beach access, 3 km. to city center, 20 km. to Riga Airport. DESCRIPTION: First class hotel with full health & spa facilities, beauty treatments, dental & medical services. 49 rooms, 28 suites, nonsmoker rooms. Restaurant, bar, lounge entertainment, meeting & banquet facilities, 3 tennis courts, indoor pool. Hotel rates: from US$60.

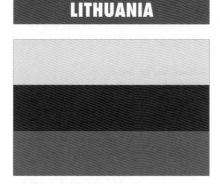

LITHUANIA

AREA: 25,174 sq. mi. (65,200 sq. km.)
POPULATION: 3,690,000
CAPITAL: Vilnius (Vilna)
OFFICIAL LANGUAGE: Lithuanian, Russian, Polish
CURRENCY: Lithuanian Litas (LTL)
EXCHANGE RATE: 1US$ = LTL 4.00
INTERNATIONAL PHONE CODE: 370

DRUSKININKAI
✈ Vilnius Airport (VNO) 82 mi. / 130 km.

Druskininkai Spa is a famous spa town 60 km. / 38 mi. east of the Polish border and 130 km. / 82 mi. west of Vilnius. The spa is nestled among beautiful landscapes and pine forest on the banks of the river Nemunas. The spa offers medical treatments, mineral springs and unique climate conditions. Druskininkai has its own treatment and diagnosis facilities.

Spa "Egle"
❤❤❤

Druskinininkai Spa. Reservations through Poland: Tel: (+48-58) 3412761. Fax: (+48-58) 39124554. TYPE: Hotel & Spa. LOCATION: Large pine forest by the river Gruta. SPA CLIENTELE: Women and men.

* Rooms: 500 w/priv. bath.
* Apartments: available
* Restaurant: traditional and international cuisine

* Coffee shop, bar, newsstand, post office
* Airport: Vilnius
* Airport/Train Transportation: transfers or car rental
* Reservations: required
* Open: Year round
* SPA on premises
* **Spa Facilities**: outpatient polyclinic, thermal swimming pool, sauna, beauty parlor
* **Spa Programs**: medical, beauty, relaxation
* **Spa Treatments**: climatism, hydrotherapy, muds
* **Spa Packages**: 14 days with full board
* **Indications**: digestive tract disorders, metabolic disorders, circulatory and respiratory disorders, locomotive disorders, rheumatic conditions, nervous system disorders
* Medical Supervision: medical staff
* Email: holidays@holidays.com.pl

DESCRIPTION: Large Health Spa complex offering climatic, thermal and specialized medical services.

LUXEMBOURG

AREA: 999 sq. mi. (2,587 sq. km.)
POPULATION: 378,000
CAPITAL: Luxembourg
OFFICIAL LANGUAGE: Luxembourgeois, French, German
CURRENCY: Luxembourg Franc (LF), Euro
EXCHANGE RATE: 1US$ = LF 34.50
INTERNATIONAL PHONE CODE: 352

🛈 Luxembourg Nat'l Tourist Office

17 Beekman Place, New York NY 10022
Tel: (212) 935-8888 . Fax: (212) 935-5896

MONDORF-LES-BAINS

> No area code

✈ Findel Int'l Airport (LUX)

The Thermal Spa of Mondorf-Les-Bains, population 3000, is located in the Moselle Valley near Luxembourg City. The resort was established in 1842 after the discovery of the highly mineralized sulphurous springs with hydrotherapeutic benefits at a temperature of 24°c (75°F).

The modern spa center, attended by 5000 visitors each year mainly from Luxembourg and neighboring countries, offers three weeks cure programs for various medical conditions, weight loss and fitness.

For entertainment the Casino 2000 is located in a park like setting in the heart of Mondorf-les-Bains with gaming rooms, restaurants, and international shows.

Mondorf Le Domaine Thermal
❤❤❤❤

Avenue des Bains, L-5610 Mondorf-les-Bains. Tel: 6612121. Fax: 661593. TYPE: Spa Hotel. LOCATION: 20 km. / 13 mi. from downtown Luxembourg City and train station. SPA CLIENTELE: Women and men.

* Rooms: 113 w/priv. bath. Suites: 29
* Phone, CTV, minibar, hairdryer, balcony
* Restaurant, piano bar, garden, terrace
* Airport: Luxembourg 30 min. taxi
* Train Station: Luxembourg 20 min. taxi
* Reservations: required
* Credit Cards: VISA/AMEX/MC/DIS/EC
* Open: Year round
* Hotel rates: from LF 3,470; TAC: 10%
* Spa on premises
* **Spa Facilities**: "Domaine Thermal" cure complex, sauna, gym, massage rooms, two thermal indoor and outdoor pools, Club Fitness Center, Gallo Roman and Turkish Baths, Finnish sauna, Japanese baths (ladies only), Tyrolean steam bath, Spa Leisure floor with whirlpools, salt baths, solarium, carbo-gas baths, multi-jet baths, fitness trails, aerobics, beauty institute
* **Spa Programs**: medical, beauty, fitness, weight loss, 50+ programs, anti back-pain, slimness
* **Spa Treatments**: hydrotherapy, fangotherapy, physio-therapy, massages, baths, medical showers, inhalation, mineral mud packs,
* **Indications**: rheumatism, respiratory insufficiencies, hepatitis, obesity, hypercholesterol, back pain, articular problems, liver and gall bladder complaints
* Medical Supervision: complete medical center
* Treatments Approval: health insurance organization at Thionville (Belgian, French & German coverage)

DESCRIPTION: First class spa hotel with complete thermal establishment and cure center in the "green heart of Europe". The spa features a wide range of treatments and services for medical conditions, beauty, or relaxation. The hotel connected to the Thermal establishment is an elegant 4-star hotel with comfortable rooms and faultless and dis-creet service. Recreation: casino, tennis, minigolf, fishing, horseback riding.

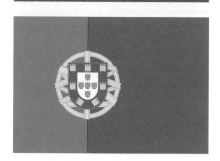

MACAU

AREA: 6 sq. mi. (16 sq. km.)
POPULATION: 238,400
CAPITAL: Macau
OFFICIAL LANGUAGE: Chinese / Portuguese
CURRENCY: Pataca or Hong Kong Dollar
EXCHANGE RATES: 1 US$ = P 7.99
TELEPHONE COUNTRY CODE: 853

Macau is a Portuguese territory 40 mi. / 65 km. west of Hong Kong and it is connected to China via a narrow strip of land. Macau was founded in 1557 by the Portuguese and it is the oldest European settlement in Asia. Macau offers old Portuguese charm, a relaxed pace of life with a relatively Mediterranean flavor. Macau is known for its gambling casinos, fine restaurants, and quaint shops. Macau is slated to become part of China in 1999.

TAIPA ISLAND
No area code
Macau Int'l Airport

Hyatt Regency Macau
❤❤❤❤

P.O. Box 3008, 2 Estrada, Almirante, Taipa Island, Macau. Tel: 831-234. Fax: 830-195. TYPE: Superior First Class Resort & Spa. LOCATION: On Beautiful Taipa Island south of Hong Kong overlooking the South China Sea. SPA CLIEN-TELE: Women and men. AGE RESTRICTIONS: No children under 12 years in Spa.

* Rooms: 307, Suites: 19 all with private bath
* Phone, CTV, A/C, C/H, minibar, jacuzzi
* Restaurant, bar, casino
* Airport: Macau Int'l, Free shuttle
* Credit Cards: MC, VISA, AMEX, JBC
* Open: Year round
* Hotel Rates: from US$150
* Spa on premises
* **Spa Facilities**: Health Club, hot tub, cold plunge, sauna, steam room, solarium, whirlpool, fitness center, relaxation lounge, beauty salon
* **Spa Programs**: Relaxation, beauty, fitness
* **Spa Packages**: on request
* **Spa Treatments**: massages, back scrub (men only), manicure, pedicure, foot massage (men only), fitness
* Medical Supervision: 1MD, 1 RN

DESCRIPTION: The Hyatt Regency Macau is a deluxe Portuguese villa style resort on Taipa Island. Guest rooms and villas have a pleasing decor and soft color schemes. A complete Fitness Center and Spa facilities are at your service to stay in shape, loose weight or indulge in beauty and pampering treatments. Recreation: casino, squash, tennis.

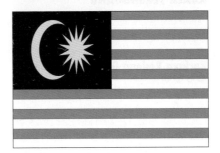

MALAYSIA

AREA: 128,308 sq. mi. (332,318 sq. km.)
POPULATION: 17,377,000
CAPITAL: Kuala Lumpur
OFFICIAL LANGUAGES: Malay, Chinese, English
CURRENCY: ringgit (R)
EXCHANGE RATE: 1US$ = R 3.80
INTERNATIONAL PHONE CODE: 60

🛈 **Malaysia Tourism Board**
27th Fl. Menara Dato Onn, Putra World Trade Center
45 Jalan Tun Ismail. Kuala Lumpur, Malaysia
Tel: (+60-3) 293-5188 . Fax: (+60-3) 293-5884

JOHOR BAHRU
🌙 **7**
✈ Sultan Ismail Airport, 18 mi. / 28 km.

Hyatt Regency
❤❤❤❤

Jalan Sungai Chat, PO Box 222, Johor Bahru 80720. Tel: (7) 222-1234. Fax: (7) 223-2718. TYPE: Hotel & Spa. LOCATION: Overlooking the Straits of Johor, 45 min. to Singapore via causeway. SPA CLIENTELE: Women and men. DESCRIPTION: Modern hotel with recreational spa facilities, various spa treatments, gym, sauna, jacuzzi. 390 rooms, 10 suites, Regency Club, nonsmoker rooms, wheelchair access. 4 restaurants, lounge, fun pub, meeting facilities, business center, 2 tennis courts, outdoor pool. Hotel rates:

from R 350.

KUALA TERENGGANU

 9

✈ Sultan Mahmud Airport, 19 mi. / 30 km.

Berjaya Redang Golf & Spa Resort
❤❤❤❤

Pulau Redang, PO Box 126, Kuala Terengganu 20928. Tel: (9) 697-111. Fax: (9) 697-1199. TYPE: Resort & Spa. LOCATION: Secluded island resort overlooking the South China Sea. SPA CLIENTELE: Women and men. DESCRIPTION: First class resort hotel with spa, beauty treatments, sauna, gym.100 rooms & suites. Restaurants, lounge, bar, meeting facilities, outdoor pool, games room, 9-hole golf course, water sports. Hotel rates: from R 250.

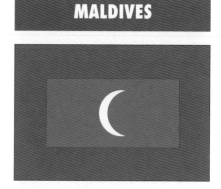

MALDIVES

AREA: 115 sq. mi. (298 sq. km.)
POPULATION: 206,000
CAPITAL: Male
OFFICIAL LANGUAGES: Divehi
CURRENCY: Maldivian rufiyaa (MR)
EXCHANGE RATE: 1US$ = MR 11.77
INTERNATIONAL PHONE CODE: 960

MALE

⌇ No area code

✈ Male International Airport (MLE), 1.2 mi. / 2 km.

Banyan Tree Maldives
❤❤❤❤

Vabbinfaru Island, North Male Atoll. Tel: 443-147. Fax: 443-843. TYPE: Resort & Spa. LOCATION: Beachfront in the middle of the North Male Atoll, 8 km. / 5 mi. or 20 minutes by speedboat to Male Int'l Airport. DESCRIPTION: Exclusive beachfront resort with Spa Pavilion, beauty treatments and exotic massage. 487 villa units, 1 presidential villa unit. 2 restaurants, bar, TV room, water sports, diving school. Hotel rates: from US$280.

Kuda Huraa Reef Resort
❤❤❤❤

North Male Atoll. Tel: 444888. Fax: 441188. TYPE: Tropical 1996 villa resort. LOCATION: A North Male Atoll island 16 km. / 10 mi. to Male Int'l Airport. SPA CLIEN-TELE: Women and men. DESCRIPTION: Tropical villa resort with a complete health and beauty spa, Herbal aromatherapy, facials, massages. Health Club with sauna, whirlpool, and gym. 106 villa rooms and villa suites. Restaurant, cafe,, bar lounge entertainment, dive center, beach, water sports shop. Hotel rates: from US$250.

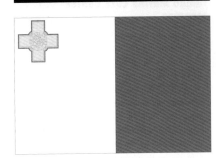

MALTA

AREA: 122 sq. mi. (316 sq. km.)
POPULATION: 360,000
CAPITAL: Valleta
OFFICIAL LANGUAGE: Maltese, English,
CURRENCY: Maltese Lire (M£)
EXCHANGE RATE: 1 US$= M£ 0.39
TELEPHONE COUNTRY CODE: 356

Malta consists of three inhabited islands: The Island of Malta which is the largest, the island of Gozo, and the tiny island of Comino (between Malta & Gozo) popular with international divers. Connection between Malta Island and the other islands is via an efficient ferry service and helicopter flights. Malta is located 93 km. / 58 mi. south of Italy, and 230 km. / 145 mi. north of North Africa.

CLIMATE: Summers are hot and dry with temperatures in the high 80's; winters are mild and comfortable with little rainfall; average temperatures of 14°c / 57°F and 6 hours of sunshine daily.

Malta National Tourist Office
Empire State Building, 350 Fifth Avenue,
Suite 4412 New York NY 10118 (USA)
Tel: (212) 695-9520. Fax: (212) 695-8229

GOZO ISLAND

SAN LAWRENZ
No area code

Luqa Airport (MLA)

Thalgo Marine Cure Center
♥♥♥♥

c/o San Lawrenz Leisure Resort, Triq Il-Rokon, San Lawrenz GRB 104. Tel: 680167, 685021. Fax: 680010. TYPE: Resort Hotel & Spa. LOCATION: Just outside the cream-colored village of San Lawrenz overlooking Dwejra Valley. SPA CLIENTELE: Women and men, all ages. DESCRIPTION: Thalgo Thalassotherapy center offering a wide range of marine algae and baths in addition to herbal and fresh water treatments.

MALTA ISLAND

ST. JULIANS
⌐ No area code
✈ Luqa Airport (MLA) 6 mi. / 10 km. SW

The Apollo Club
♥♥♥♥

c/o San Georg Corinthia Hotel, St. George's Bay, St. Jullians. Tel: 374114. Fax: 374039. TYPE: Hotel & Spa. LOCATION: On a secluded promontory at St. George's Bay, on the outskirts of St. Julians. SPA CLIENTELE: Women and men, all ages. DESCRIPTION: Marine treatment, beauty and fitness centre offering thalassotherapy, fitness and beauty programs. The spa is located at the 250 rooms, 5-star San Georg Corinthia Hotel.

Westin Dragonara Resort
♥♥♥♥

Dragonara Rd., St. Julians, STJ 02. Tel: 381000. Fax: 381347. TYPE: Hotel & Spa. LOCATION: On its own peninsula with stunning seaviews. SPA CLIENTELE: Women and men, all ages. DESCRIPTION: Beauty & Fitness center at the 5-star, 311 rooms Westin Dragonara Resort.

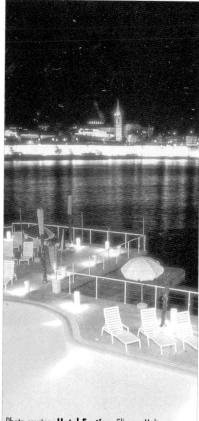

Photo courtesy **Hotel Fortina**, Sliema Malta

SLIEMA
⌐ No area code
✈ Luqa Airport (MLA) 6 mi. / 10 km. SW

Spa Méditerranée Thalassotherapie
♥♥♥♥

c/o Hotel Fortina, Tigné Seafront, Sliema SLM 15. Tel: 342-976 or 343-380 (ext:149). Fax: 339-388. TYPE: Hotel & Spa. LOCATION: Right on the waterfront in a quiet but central area in Sliema. SPA CLIENTELE: Mixed, all ages.

* Accommodations: **Hotel Fortina******
  deluxe 4-star hotel with 220 rooms and suites
* Phone, A/C, minibar, priv. bath
* Restaurants (3), bars (3)
* Reservations: deposit required
* Credit Cards: MC, VISA, AMEX, DISC
* Open: Year round
* Rates: (accommodations only) from: M£37-M£64
* TAC: 10%
* Spa on premises: **Spa Mediterranée Thalassotherapie**
* Year Established: 1996
* **Spa facilities:** Treatment rooms, Thalasso therapy pool, gym, mineral bath, sauna, Beauty Salon.
* **Spa Programs:** Anti Stress, Well Being & Physiotherapy, Anti-Cellulite, Anti-Arthritic / Anti Rheumatism. Get Fit & Firm, Post Natal. 1,5,6 or 12 days programs
* **Spa Packages:** (and Hotel Packages) full use of gym, 2 thalassotherapy treatments per day, aerobics, step and acqua aerobics supervised by trained personnel
* **Spa Treatments:** facials and beauty treatments, algotherapy, seawater therapy, acquaciser (underwater treadmill), bain d'algues, jet showers, massage, skin tonic, body fat testing, pressotherapy, aerobics
* **Cost of Treatments:** (for hotel residents)aprox. M£15 per person per day. Non residents may use the facilities
* **Email:** info@hotelfortina.com
* **Web:** http://www.hotelfortina.com

DESCRIPTION: Spa Mediterrannée is located in the elegant 4-star all inclusive Hotel Fortina, along the Sliema waterfront. The spa focuses on a variety of programs including "Anti-Stress, Well-Being and Physiotherapy" treatments. A unique system has been developed where the sea water is used is three times stronger in salt and mineral elements, giving you three times the benefits than any other centre in the world. A highly qualified team of physiotherapists and international body of beauty therapists will assure you enjoy a variety of unique spa treatments.

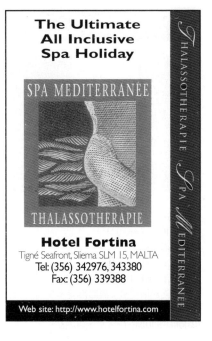

SAN ANTON

No area code

Luqa Airport (MLA) 6 mi. / 10 km. SW

Athenaum Spa
❤❤❤❤

c/o Hotel Corinthia Palace, De Paule Avenue, San Anton. Tel: 440-301. Fax: 465-713. TYPE: Hotel & Spa. LOCATION: close to the Presidential Palace and the San Anton Botanical Gardens, right in the center of the island. SPA CLIENTELE: Mixed, all ages. DESCRIPTION: Centre for vitality, beauty and well-being. 50 therapies include: beauty programs, relaxation, sports therapy, mud baths, oxygen treatment, specialized nutrition and meditation.

MEXICO

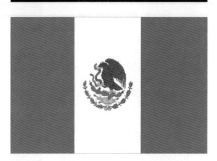

AREA: 761,601 sq. mi. (1,972,546 sq. km.)
POPULATION: 67,400,000
CAPITAL: Mexico City
OFFICIAL LANGUAGE: Spanish
CURRENCY: Mexican peso (MEX$)
EXCHANGE RATE: US$1 = MEX$10
COUNTRY CODE: 52
NATIONAL HOLIDAY: Cinco de mayo, May 5

Mexico the southernmost country in North America offers exciting tourist attractions, lovely beaches, high mountains historic towns and archeological sites. Ever since the Aztecs first built a health resort in the hills southwest of Mexico City, visitors arrive in Mexico seeking opportunities for renewal, rejuvenation and relaxation in the popular balnearios of Mexico.

ⓘ Secretaria du Turismo
Mexican Ministry of Tourism
Presidente Masaryk #172, 11587 Mexico D.F.
Tel: (+52-5) 211-0099

CABO SAN LUCAS
☽ 114
✈ Los Cabos Airport (SJD) 10 mi. / 16 km.

Villa Del Palmar Resort & Spa
♥♥♥

Km 0.5 Camino Viejo a San Jose, Cabo San Lucas (Baja California Sur), 23410. Tel: (114) 32694. Fax: (114) 32664. TYPE: Hotel & Spa. LOCATION: In private enclave on Medano Beach. SPA CLIENTELE: Women and men. DESCRIPTION: Beach resort condo complex with European style spa, aerobic room, weight room, whirlpool, sauna, steam room, beauty salon, massage cabins. 132 condo units 1-3BR, restaurant, bar, minimarket, deli. Hotel rates: from US$140.

Casa del Mar
♥♥♥♥

Km 19.5 Carretera, Cabo San Lucas (Baja California Sur) 23400. Tel: (114) 40030. Fax: (114) 40034. TYPE: Inn & Spa. LOCATION: 5 mi. / 9 km. north of Cabo San Lucas against the Sea of Cortés.

* Rooms: 32 w/priv. bath
* Phone, CTV, A/C, C/H, minibar
* Restaurant, bar, lounge, games room
* Airport: Cabo San Lucas 8 mi. / 13 km.
* Reservations: deposit required
* Open: Year round
* Hotel Rates: from US$290
* TAC: 10%
* Spa on premises
* **Spa Facilities**: health & beauty spa, fitness room, 6 swimming pools, jacuzzis,
* **Spa Programs**: beauty, pampering, fitness
* **Spa Treatments**: massages, beauty and skin care treatments, aromatherapy, fango packs, herbal wraps, yoga, cardiovascular equipment

DESCRIPTION: Elegant intimate colonial style Inn with full health and beauty spa facilities and treatments. Recreation: tennis, golf, horseback riding, racquetball, water sports.

Melia Cabo Real
Beach & Golf Resort
♥♥♥♥

Carretera Cabo San Lucas km 19.5, San Jose del Cabo

(Baja California Sur) 23400. Tel: (114) 40000. Fax: (114) 40101. TYPE: Golf Resort & Spa. LOCATION: Between San José del Cabo and Cabo San Lucas on the best beach in this area. SPA CLIENTELE: Women and men.

* Rooms: 300 w/priv. bath. Suites: 14
* Phone, CTV, A/C, C/H, minibar
* Restaurant, bar, lounge, poolside bar
* Airport: Cabo San Lucas 10 mi. / 15 km.
* Reservations: deposit required
* Open: Year round
* Hotel Rates: from US$220
* TAC: 10%
* Spa on premises
* **Spa Facilities**: health & beauty spa, fitness center, sauna, steam room, jacuzzis, fully equipped gym
* **Spa Programs**: beauty, pampering, fitness
* **Spa Treatments**: massages, beauty and skin care treatments, aromatherapy, fango packs, herbal wraps, yoga, cardiovascular equipment, reflexology, T'ai chi

DESCRIPTION: Beach resort hotel with complete health and fitness spa facilities. Home of the Senior Slam. Recreation: golf, sport fishing, tennis, bicycling and water sports.

CANCUN
⟩ 98
✈ Cancun Int'l Airport (CUN) 10 mi. / 16 km.

Calinda Beach & Spa Cancun
❤❤❤❤

Blvd Kukulcan Section C lote 1, Zona Hotelera, Cancun (Quitana Roo) 77500. Tel: (98) 831600. Fax: (98) 831416. TYPE: Resort & Spa. LOCATION: Beachfront, 5 min. from downtown, overlooking the Caribbean. SPA CLIENTELE: Women and men.

* Rooms: 470 w/priv. bath.
* Phone, CTV, A/C, C/H, minibar, in room safe
* Restaurants, bar, lounge, beach bar
* Airport: Cancun 9 mi. / 14 km.
* Reservations: deposit required
* Open: Year round

* Hotel Rates: from US$100
* TAC: 10%
* Spa on premises
* **Spa Facilities**: health & beauty spa, fitness center, sauna, steam room, jacuzzis, fully equipped gym, jogging trails
* **Spa Programs**: beauty, pampering, fitness
* **Spa Treatments**: massages, beauty and skin care treatments, aromatherapy, fango packs, herbal wraps, yoga, cardiovascular equipment

DESCRIPTION: Pyramid shaped all inclusive resort with full service health and fitness spa. The fitness center features aerobics classes, and conditioning workouts. The beauty spa has a wide range of beauty and pampering services. Recreation: golf, tennis, water sports, swimming, basketball, horseback riding.

Casa Turquesa
❤❤❤❤❤

Blvd. Kukulkan km 13.5, Zona Hotelera, Cancun (Quitana Roo) 77500. Tel: (98) 852924. Fax: (98) 852922. TYPE: Resort & Spa. LOCATION: Beachfront in beautiful landscaped gardens 8 mi. / 13 km. from downtown. SPA CLIENTELE: Women and men.

* Suites: 33
* Phones (3), CTV, VCR, A/C, C/H, compact disc player, minibar, in-room safe, hair dryer, balcony, jacuzzi
* Airport: Cancun 9 mi. / 14 km.
* Reservations: deposit required
* Open: Year round
* Hotel Rates: from US$275
* TAC: 10%
* Spa on premises
* **Spa Facilities**: health & beauty spa, fitness center, sauna, steam room, jacuzzis, fully equipped gym,
* **Spa Programs**: beauty, pampering, fitness
* **Spa Treatments**: massages, beauty and skin care treatments, aromatherapy, fango packs, herbal wraps

DESCRIPTION: Luxurious all-suite hotel with intimate health spa featuring an abundance of beauty and pampering services. Recreation: golf, tennis, watersports, horseback riding, excursions to archeological sites.

Fiesta Americana Condesa Cancún
❤❤❤❤❤

Blvd. Kukulkan Km 16.5, PO Box 5478, Cancun (Quitana Roo) 77500. Tel: (98) 851000. Fax: (98) 851800. TYPE: Resort & Spa. LOCATION: Beachfront opposite Convention Center close to Plaza Caracol. SPA CLIENTELE: Women and men.

* Rooms: 502 w/priv. bath. Suites: 26
* Phone, CTV, A/C, C/H, minibar, hair dryer
* Restaurants (4), bars (3), games room
* Airport: Cancun 10 mi ./ 16 km., taxi
* Reservations: deposit required
* Credit Cards: MC/VISA/AMEX/CB/DC
* Open: Year round
* Hotel Rates: from US$155
* TAC: 10%
* Spa on premises
* **Spa Facilities**: Health & Beauty Spa, Fitness center, weight & cardio equipment
* **Spa Programs**: Beauty, wellness and fitness
* **Spa Treatments**: massages, loofah scrubs, seaweed wraps, aromatherapy, facials, aerobics, yoga

DESCRIPTION: All-suite oceanfront resort overlooking the Caribbean. The resort features modern spa, one of the island's best, with a wide range of beauty, skin care and renewal services. Recreation: golf, tennis, watersports, fishing.

Melia Cancun Resort & Spa
❤❤❤❤❤

Blvd. Kukulcan km 16.5, Zona Hotelera, Cancun 77500. Tel: (98) 851114. Fax: (98) 851963.TYPE: Resort & Spa. LOCATION: Beachfront location 15 km. / 10 mi. from downtown. SPA CLIENTELE: Women and men.

* Rooms: 450 w/priv. bath. Suites: 37
* Phone, CTV, A/C, C/H, minibar, hair dryer

* Wheelchair accessible
* Restaurants (5), bars (4), meeting facilities
* Airport: Cancun 10 mi. / 16 km., taxi
* Reservations: deposit required
* Credit Cards: MC/VISA/AMEX/CB/DC
* Open: Year round
* Hotel Rates: from US$180
* TAC: 10%
* Spa on premises
* **Spa Facilities**: Health & Beauty Spa, Fitness center, weight & cardio equipment
* **Spa Programs**: Beauty, wellness and fitness
* **Spa Treatments**: massages, loofah scrubs, seaweed wraps, aromatherapy, facials, aerobics

DESCRIPTION: Elegant resort hotel on one of the best beaches in Cancun. The full-service health and beauty spa offers a variety of soothing and pampering treatments in the spa or open-air cabanas. Recreation: golf, tennis, water sports, sport fishing, horseback riding.

CIHUATLAN
🛬 335

 Gustavo Diaz Ordaz AP (PVR) 190 km. / 120 mi.

Hotel Bel-Air Costa Careyes
❤❤❤❤

Km 53.5 Carr. Barra de Navidad, Puerto Vallarta, Cihuatlan (Jalisco) 48970. Tel: (335) 10000. Fax: (335) 10100. LOCATION: In the secluded Costa Careyes overlooking the Pacific coast, 2 hrs. south of Puerto Vallarta. SPA CLIENTELE: Women and men.

* Rooms: 41 w/priv. bath. Suites: 10
* Phone, CTV, A/C, C/H, minibar, hair dryer
* Restaurant, bistro, cinema
* Airport: Puerto Vallarta, 2 hrs.
* Reservations: deposit required
* Credit Cards: MC/VISA/AMEX/CB/DC
* Open: Year round
* Hotel Rates: from US$155
* TAC: 10%
* Spa on premises

* **Spa Facilities**: European Spa, Fitness center, weight & cardio equipment
* **Spa Programs**: Beauty, wellness and fitness
* **Spa Treatments**: massages, loofah scrubs, seaweed wraps, aromatherapy, facials, aerobics, yoga

DESCRIPTION: Luxurious intimate hotel nestled between the emerald jungle and the ocean. The resort features a large full service 3,500 sq. ft. / 318 sq. m. European spa and a beautiful serpentine pool winding through lush gardens. Recreation: golf, tennis, sport fishing, nature tours.

CUAUTLA
⟩ 735
✈ Benito Juarez Int'l Airport (MEX) 60 mi. / 96 km.

Hotel Hacienda Cocoyoc
♥♥♥♥

Carreter Cuernasvaca-Cuautla km 32.5, Cocoyoc (Morelos) 62736. Tel: (735) 62211. Fax: (735) 62155. (Mailing Address: PO Box 300, Cuautla, Morelos 62740). TYPE: Resort & Spa. LOCATION: Central Mexico, one hour drive from Mexico City. SPA CLIENTELE: Women and men.

* Rooms: 300 w/priv. bath
* Suites: 24 each with private pool
* Restaurants (4), disco, games room
* Swimming pool & children wading pool
* Airport: Mexico City, 1 hour
* Reservations: deposit required
* Credit Cards: MC/VISA/AMEX/CB/DC
* Open: Year round
* Rates: from US$140; TAC: 10%
* Spa on premises: **Spa Coyoc**
* **Spa Facilities**: Health & beauty Spa, fitness center, sauna, steam room, Swiss showers, jacuzzi
* **Spa Programs**: beauty, wellness and fitness
* **Spa Treatments**: mud baths, body treatments, massages, facials, hydrotherapy, Evian shower, aerobics, yoga, jogging

DESCRIPTION: Highly regarded colonial style resort in tropi-

cal gardens with full service European spa. The Spa Cocoyoc offers lavish beauty and pampering treatments including exfoliating loofah scrub, body sculpting seaweed wraps and several relaxing massages. Recreation: golf, tennis, horseback riding, archeological tours.

CUERNAVACA
⟩ 73
✈ Benito Juarez Int'l Airport (CVJ) 55 mi. / 90 km.

Hosteria las Quintas
♥♥♥♥

Av. Diaz Ordaz 9, PO Box 427, Cuernavaca (Morelos) 62120. Tel: (73) 174000. Fax: (73) 174155. LOCATION: An inner-city oasis in Cuernavaca " the land of eternal spring" a short journey from Mexico City. SPA CLIENTELE: Women and men.

* Rooms: 8 w/priv. bath. Suites: 52
* Phone, CTV, covered terrace, jacuzzi, fireplace (some)
* Restaurant, cocktail lounge, meeting facilities
* Swimming pools (2)
* Airport: Mexico City, 1 hour
* Reservations: deposit required
* Credit Cards: MC/VISA/AMEX/CB/DC
* Open: Year round
* Rates: from US$100
* TAC: 10%
* Spa on premises
* **Spa Facilities**: Health & beauty Spa, fitness center, fully equipped gym, sauna, steam room, jacuzzi
* **Spa Programs**: beauty, wellness and fitness
* **Spa Treatments**: massages, facials, body wraps, loofah scrubs, hydrotherapy, aromatherapy, thalassotherapy, fangotherapy, yoga, aerobics
* **Spa Packages**: Supreme Pampering (4 nts)

DESCRIPTION: Charming atmospheric Hacienda-style hotel on lovely tropical grounds, 7 blocks from downtown. The hotel features a full service European style spa with services focusing on fitness, health and pampering. Recreation: golf, tennis, water sports, horseback riding, archeological sites.

Mission del Sol Resort & Spa

♥♥♥

Av. Gral. Diego Diaz Gonzalez 31, Cuernavaca (Morelos) 62440. Tel: (73) 210999. Fax: (73) 211195. TYPE: Resort & Spa. LOCATION: 15 minutes from downtown on tropical gardens. SPA CLIENTELE: Women and men.

* Rooms: 50 w/priv. bath; Suites: 10
* Restaurant: gourmet organic cuisine
* Airport: Mexico City, taxi, car rental
* Reservations: deposit required
* Credit Cards: MC/VISA/AMEX/DC/CB
* Open: Year round
* Rates: from US$120
* TAC: 8%
* Spa on premises
* **Spa Facilities**: Health & Fitness spa, fitness room, fully equipped gym, sauna, steam room, jacuzzi
* **Spa Programs**: beauty, wellness and fitness
* **Spa Treatments**: seaweed therapy, electro-quartz, acupuncture, hydrotherapy, yoga, meditation, massage, workshops on stress management, health & nutrition

DESCRIPTION: Appealing hotel with Moorish architecture featuring full service health and fitness spa.

GUADALAJARA

⟩ 3

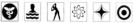 Miguel Hidalgo Airport (GDL)

Guadalajara, population 2,500,000, is the capital of the Jalisco state. It is located in 1,650 m. (5,450 ft.) altitude, 696 km. (435 mi.) northwest of Mexico City. The climate is sunny and comfortable year round. Mid-June through August is the tropical rain season with evening storms. November through February are cold and rainy. Rio Caliente spa is located 18 miles (29 mi.) from Guadalajara in what used to be an ancient Indian healing and spiritual center. Trips are organized to Guadalajara for shopping and sightseeing.

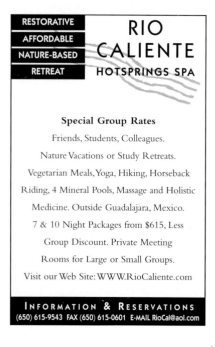
Rio Caliente
Hot Springs Spa

♥♥♥

Information and Reservations: c/o PO Box 897, Millbrae, CA 94030 (USA). Tel: (650) 615-9543. Fax: (650) 615-0601. MANAGING DIRECTOR: Caroline Durston. PROGRAM DIRECTORS: Lou Catching & Viviana Dean. TYPE: Hot Springs Spa Resort. LOCATION: Remote Pine Forest near Guadalajara (Jalisco). SPA CLIENTELE: Men, Women. GENDER & AGE RESTRICTIONS: Must be 15 years or older. MEDICAL RESTRICTIONS: must be able to climb, and feel well at 5,000 ft./ 1500 m. OTHER RESTRICTIONS: Arrival no later than 10pm.

* Rooms: 50 w/priv. bath; Suites: 2, Cottages: 2
* Restaurant: gourmet vegetarian meals
* Airport: Guadalajara 25 mi. (40 km.), taxi
* Reservations: US$250 per person deposit
* No Credit Cards

* Open: Year round
* Rates: from US$105 sgl; US$88 dbl /day; rates are per person including room, meals, activities, & tips. Tax is 15% (to be added); TAC: 8%
* Spa on premises
* Year Established: 1962
* **Spa Facilities**: 4 mineral hot pools, natural volcanic steam room, yoga and massage rooms, gym, conference center, therapy rooms
* **Spa Programs**: Preventive Health & Anti-Aging (7-10 day); The Tune-Up (7-10 day); Memory & Brain Booster (10 day min.); Allergy Relief & Immune System Builder (10 day)
* **Spa Treatments**: thermal baths, natural steam, vegetarian diet, beauty treatments, mud-wraps, acupuncture, massages, skin lifting, homeopathics, Iridology, electromagnetic field therapy, cupping, natural therapy, human growth hormone, cell therapy, DHEA, chelation therapy, bio-oxidine therapy, collagen & fibroblast injections, pool exercise, yoga, tai chi
* **Medical Supervision**: American Doctor 30 minutes away and a good hospital; the administrative staff are experienced in First-Aid techniques; carry stock of remedies for minor ailments as recommended by US physician
* Maximum Number of Guests: 75
* Number of clients per doctor: 10 per day
* **Email: RioCal@aol.com**
* **Web: www.riocaliente.com**

DESCRIPTION: An affordable Spa and holistic retreat near Guadalajara offering beauty services and preventive health and anti-aging treatments. The accommodations are simple but tastefully decorated in local style. Buffet style meals consist of locally grown fresh fruit, grains, vegetables and cheeses. Special low calorie vegetarian meals are prepared for weight loss. Spring water are tapped to supply mineral water to the bedrooms, they are purified and safe to drink. Two walled pools are available for clothing optional soaking, or sunbathing. Recreation: hiking, swimming, horseback riding, social events, excursions.

ISLA MUJERES
98
Isla Mujeres Airport, Cancun Int'l AP (CUN)

Isla Mujeres, "The Island of Women" is a dazzling strip of a Caribbean island with powder-fine sand beaches about 5 mi. / 8 km. off the coast of Cancun. The island offers many hotels, restaurants, bars and cater to tourists from all over the world.

Puerto Isla Mujeres Resort & Yacht Club
❤❤❤❤

Blvd. Kukulcan, km 45, Isla Mujeres 77500, Quintana Roo. Tel: (98) 833208. Fax: (98) 831228. TYPE: Resort & Spa. LOCATION: Beachfront in Isla Mujeres. SPA CLIENTELE: Women and men.

* Suites & Villas: 26
* Phone, CTV, VCR, A/C, hair dryer
* Computer/fax hook up
* Restaurants (2), bar, meeting room, full service marina
* Outdoor pool, private beach
* Airport: Cancun 18 mi. / 29 km.
* Airport transfers: available on request
* Reservations: deposit required
* Open: Year round
* Hotel Rates: from US$160
* TAC: 10%
* Spa on premises
* **Spa Facilities**: Health & Beauty spa, fitness room
* **Spa Programs**: Beauty, wellnes & fitness
* **Spa Treatments**: aromatherapy, massages, salt glow, body wraps, seaweed body mask, thalassotherapy, cellulite firming, tea tree spritzer

DESCRIPTION: Mexican Caribbean style Marina hotel with intimate spa offering privacy and peaceful ambiance. A wide range of beauty and pampering treatments are offered by highly trained staff. Recreation: water sports, swimming, marina.

IXTAPAN
527
Benito Juarez Int'l AP (MEX) 70 mi. / 112 km.

Ixtapan, population 13,700, is a famous medicinal hot

springs resort known for its radio-active mineral waters, some 70 miles (112 km) southwest of Mexico City. The municipal spa is located right at the town center. Ixtapan de la Sal can be reached from Mexico City via car or bus on road 55 going to Taxco. The driving time is about 2 hours.

Hotel Spa Ixtapan
❤❤❤❤

Blvd. Arturo San Ramon s/n, Ixtapan 51900. Tel: (527) 143-0304. Fax: (527) 1430304. TYPE: Resort & Spa. MANAGING DIRECTOR: Felipe Tapia. PROGRAMS DIRECTOR: Alyssia. LOCATION: Secluded resort built around hot springs at 6,000ft. altitude (1,800m). SPA CLIENTELE: Women and men, children accepted. SPECIAL RESTRICTIONS: The spa is not wheelchair accessible.

* Rooms: 250 w/private bath. Villas: 50
* Night club, disco, meeting facilities
* Airport: Mexico City, 70 mi. (112 km.)
* Airport transfers: available on request
* Reservations: full payment by check or CC
* Open: Year round
* Hotel Rates: from US$133; TAC: 10%
* Spa on premises
* Year Established: 1920
* **Spa Facilities**: Thermal (105°F - 40°c) mineral springs, Roman private baths, Spa Beauty & Health Clinic, Men's Health Club, 20 private thermal water pools, swimming pool, jacuzzis, 500 ft / 150 m Alpine water slide
* **Spa Programs**: Health & Beauty; Health & Fitness Diet Spa, Relax, & Sport programs
* **Spa Treatments**: aquatic exercises, mineral bath, aerobics, mud wraps, herbal wraps, reflexology, loofa bath, hair treatment, complete beauty salon service, yoga, acupuncture, Swedish massage, Shiatsu, sport massage, facials
* **Spa Packages**: Diet from US$1,095; Relax from US$985; Sport from US$975, Relax from US$985
* Length of stay Required: 4-7 day for Spa packages
* Medical Supervision: 1 MD

DESCRIPTION: Spa resort complex with rooms, suites and villas on a beautifully landscaped 45 acres of exotic tropical garden. The resort is popular with Spa aficionados who come 'to take the water' and indulge in luxurious spa treatments for both men and women. The spa emphasizes beauty, weight loss, fitness and relaxation. The ambience is laidback without vigorous morning aerobics or spa routines. Recreation: 9 hole golf-course, horseback riding, bowling and billiard, movies, and a folkloric ballet group.

LAKE TEQUESQUITENGO
⌇ 73

✈ Benito Juarez Int'l AP (CVJ) 60 mi. / 96 km.

Villa Bejar Hotel & Grand Spa
❤❤❤

Lake Tequesquitengo, Cerro dela Estrell No. 3, Campestre Churubusco 0420. Tel: (73) 470620. Fax: (73) 470269. TYPE: Resort & Spa. LOCATION: On Lake Tesquesquitengo just 15 min. from Cuernavaca. SPA CLIENTELE: Women and men.

* Suites: 45 w/priv. bath
* Restaurants, disco boat
* Airport: Mexico City, 60 mi. (96 km.)
* Airport transfers: available on request
* Reservations: full payment by check or CC
* Open: Year round
* Rates: from US$1000/week; TAC: 10%
* Spa on premises
* **Spa Facilities**: Health Spa, Beauty Salon, weight and cardio equipment, state-of-the-art gym
* **Spa Programs**: beauty, wellness and fitness
* **Spa Treatments**: massage, facials, herbal wraps, loofa scrubs, yoga, aerobics.

DESCRIPTION: Lakeside health resort in one of Mexico's wealthiest outpost of luxury. The area is known for its pure mountain air and scenic location. The Grand Spa is a full service health and beauty spa with highly trained staff members. Recreation: tennis, 18-hole golf, water sports. Excursions can be arranged to Mexico's richest historical landmarks: The thousand waterfalls of Grenada, The Pyramids of Tepoztlan or Xochicalco.

MAZATLAN
🌙 69

✈ Rafael Buelna Int'l AP (MZT) 15 mi. / 24 km.

El Cid Mega Resort
❤❤❤❤

Av. Camaron Sabalo. PO Box 813, Mazatlan (Sinaloa) 82110. Tel: (69) 133333. Fax: (69) 141311. TYPE: Mega Resort & Spa. LOCATION: Set on 720 beachfront acres. SPA CLIENTELE: Women and men.

* Rooms: 1,320 w/priv. bath
* Phone, CTV, A/C, C/H, minibar, purified water
* Restaurants (14), bars (14), nightclub
* Private marina, golf courses, tennis courts (14)
* Airport: 12 mi. / 19 km., taxi
* Reservations: required
* Credit Cards: VISA/AMEX/MC
* Open: Year round
* Hotel Rates: from US$115
* Spa on premises
* **Spa Facilities:** Full service spa and fitness center, beauty salon, gym, saunas, steam room, jacuzzi
* **Spa Programs:** beauty, wellnes and fitness
* **Spa Treatments:** aromatherapy, body scrubs, facials, massage therapies, aerobics, yoga, T'ai Chi

DESCRIPTION: El Cid is Mexico's largest self-contained resort comprising of four hotels, thousands of newly decorated guest rooms, and magnificent sports and health facilities. The full spa center features virtually every treatment or therapy. Recreation: golf, tennis, swimming, water sports, sport fishing, and horseback riding.

MEXICO CITY
🌙 5

✈ Benito Juarez Int'l AP (MEX) 4 mi / 6.5 km

Hotel Marquis Reforma & Spa
❤❤❤❤❤

Paseo de la Reforma 465, Colonia Cuauhtemoc, Mexico City 06500. Tel: (5) 211-3600. Fax: (5) 211-5561. TYPE: Hotel & Spa. LOCATION: Downtown, 5 min. walk from the "Pink Zone", Chapuletepec Park, shops and restaurants. SPA CLIENTELE: Women and men. DESCRIPTION: Deluxe Art-Deco highrise hotel with complete health club and beauty salon featuring gym, massage, whirlpool, solarium, steam room, jacuzzi and juice/fresh fruit bar. 208 rooms, 84 suites, restaurant, coffee shop, bar and business center. Hotel rates: from US$235.

PLAYA DEL CARMEN
🌙 98

✈ Playa del Carmen AP (PCM) 3 mi. / 5 km.

El Dorado Resort & Spa
❤❤❤❤

PO Box 512, Km 95 Tulum-Cancun Hwy, Kantenah, Playa Del Carmen, Quintana Roo. Tel: (98) 843242. TYPE: Resort & Spa. LOCATION: Secluded paradise amidst 280 coconut palm-dotted acres on the Caribbean beach. SPA CLIENTELE: Women and men.

* Suites: 135 ocean view JR suites
* Phone, CTV, minibar, A/C
* Restaurants, bars, nightclub, game room
* Airport: Playa del Carmen, shuttle transfers
* Reservations: required
* Credit Cards: VISA/AMEX/MC
* Open: Year round
* Hotel Rates: from US$110
* Spa on premises
* **Spa Facilities:** health spa and fitness center, gym, sauna, steam room, beauty salon
* **Spa Programs:** beauty, wellness and fitness
  3 nights minimum stay
* **Spa Treatments:** beauty and body treatments, fitness center, gym with weight and cardio equipment

DESCRIPTION: Secluded beach resort with health and beauty spa adjacent to a sparkling pool. Recreation: golf, tennis, swimming, sport fishing, excursions to Mayan ruins. Evening turtle watch during May - August. Half day tours to

Tulum and Xel-ha.

PUERTO VALLARTA
✈ 322
✈ Gustavo Diaz Ordaz AP (PVR) 4 mi. / 6.5 km.

Puerto Vallarta, population 70,000, is a cosmopolitan beach resort on the Pacific coast of Mexico. It gained world fame after the shooting of the classic Hollywood film "Night of the Iguana". The town is divided by the River Cuale. The expensive hotels, resorts, the airport and the port are located north of the river.

La Jolla de Mismaloya Resort & Spa
♥♥♥♥

Km 11.5 Zona Hotelera Sur, Puerto Vallarta (Jalisco) 48300. Tel: (322) 80853. Fax: (322) 80660. TYPE: Resort & Spa. LOCATION: On Mismaloya Bay. SPA CLIENTELE: Women and men. DESCRIPTION: All-suite resort hotel with health and fitness spa facilities. 303 1-2BR suites, presidential suites, restaurants, lounges, swimming pools, swim-up bar. Hotel rates: from US$150.

Paradise Village
Beach Resort & Spa
♥♥♥♥♥

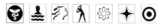

Paseo de los Cocoteros 001, Nuevo Vallarta, Nayarit. Tel: (322) 66727. Toll Free (800) 995-5714. Fax: (322) 66726. TYPE: Deluxe Beach Resort & Spa. HOTEL MANAGER: Ricardo Orozco. SPA DIRECTOR: Diana Mestre. LOCATION: Banderas Bay in Nayarit, north of Puerto Vallarta. SPA CLIENTELE: Men, Women. AGE RESTRICTION: Children not accepted in spa. Kids club for children.

* Suites: 175; Apartments: 484 (1-3 BR apts)
* Phone, CTV, minibar, cooking facilities, A/C
* Restaurant, bar, nightclub, casino
* Airport: Puerto Vallarta, 20 min.
* Airport/Train Transportation: taxi
* Reservations: required
* Credit Cards: VISA/AMEX/MC

* Open: Year round
* Rates: Winter (high season) Dec. 19- Apr. 11 from US$200/day; Summer (off season) Apr. 12 - Dec. 18 from US$150/day
* Spa on premises
* Year Established: 1995
* Spa Package: 3 day Escape package and 7 day Total Renewal package. (available only through wholesalers, Spa Finders and Spa Traveler agency) Tax: 15%
* Name of Spa: Spa Palenque
* Spa Facilities: 22,500 sq. ft. (2,045 sq. m.) deluxe Mayan style building facing our marina; Mayal Beach Spa station; Palenque healthy snack bar; lap pool, Shel-ha body shop; service areas for men and women, hydrotherapy center, gym and aerobic rooms, extensive cardiovascular equipment, Paramount and Life Fitness weight equipment, whirlpool, saunas, steam, pressure showers, beauty salon
* Spa Programs: Hydrotherapy, Fitness, Beauty
* Spa Treatments: aerobics, free weight, meditation, yoga, manicures, pedicures, back massage, aromatherapy, acupressure shiatsu, anti-cellulite lymphatic drainage, reflexology, alpha massage, holistic relaxation, facials, back cleansing, salt body rub, seaweed mask, vichy shower, slimming treatment silk body with paraffin, electro-Acuscope anti pain & stress therapy, hydromassage, herbal wraps, thermal clay treatments, sea fango massage, botanical body wrap, deluxe mayan wrap, computerized body composition analysis, computerized fitness evaluation, Iris diagnosis, Orthogen 200 energy analyzing system,
* Indications: beauty, pampering, anti-stress, fitness, and general well being.
* Email: spa@paradisevillage.com
* Web: www.paradisevillage.com

DESCRIPTION: Paradise Village Beach Resort & Spa is a delightful beachfront holiday complex with spacious suites and apartments in distinctive Mayan style architecture. All suites and apartments offer breathtaking views. The Paradise Village Spa was created in the image of the world's great resort spas and it is the only one of its kind in Mexico. The Spa offers European-style hydrotherapy, body treatments, holistic massages, and fitness instructions. The

Spa staff includes 55 highly trained employees to meet the needs of the most sophisticated clientele. Recreation: watersports, 18 hole golf course, nightlife and shopping in nearby Puerto Vallarta.

Qualton Club & Spa Vallarta
❤❤❤❤❤

🐎 🚶 ◉

Ave. Francisco Medina Ascencio km 2.5, PO Box 308, Puerto Vallarta (Jalisco) 48300. Tel: (322) 44446. Fax: (322) 44447. TYPE: Spa Hotel. SPA MANAGER: Silvia Medina Velasco. LOCATION: Ocean front overlooking Banderas Bay. SPA CLIENTELE: Women and men. AGE RESTRICTION: Must be 16 years or older.

* Rooms: 218 w/priv. bath
* Suites: 4 2BR suites with jacuzzi
* Phone, CTV, A/C, ocean view balcony
* Restaurants (2), bars (3), Theme dinners
* Airport: Puerto Vallarta, 10 min. taxi
* Reservations: required
* Credit Cards: VISA/AMEX/MC
* Open: Year round
* Hotel Rates: from US$175
* Spa on premises: **Qualton Club & Spa Vallarta**
* Year Established: 1990
* **Spa Facilities**: Full service health & beauty spa, state-of-the-art gym with a 22 station strength and condition circuit
* **Spa Programs**: Beauty, wellness, fitness, weight loss
* **Spa Treatments**: massages, herbal wraps, reflexology, aromatherapy, lymphatic drainage, salt and loofah exfoliation, thermal clay, seaweed wrap, anti-cellulite therapies, facials, non surgical face lift, loofah scrubs, herbal wraps, yoga, step and aqua aerobics, exercise classes, eucalyptus inhalation, guided outdoor walks
* **Spa Packages**: Basic (US$91); Beauty (US$106); Natural (US$123); Relax (US$145); Detoxification (US$140); Slimming (US$162).
* **Indications**: beauty, pampering, anti-stress, fitness, and general well being.

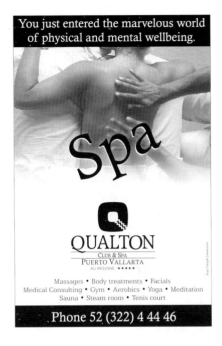

* Email: qualton@npvnet.com.mx drios@qualton.com
* Web: www.qualton.com

DESCRIPTION: Elegant ocean-front All-inclusive resort hotel with full service spa, where guests can enjoy the latest in beauty, well being and relaxation treatments by highly qualified and trained staff. Recreation: golf, tennis, water sports, adventure excursions and horseback riding.

Velas Vallarta Grand Suites Resort
❤❤❤❤

🐎 🚶

Paseo de la Marina, Puerto Vallarta (Jalisco). Tel: (322) 10091. Fax: (322) 10755. TYPE: Hotel/Time-Share & Spa. LOCATION: In the Marina Vallarta development adjacent to 18 hole golf course. SPA CLIENTELE: Women and men. DESCRIPTION: Beachfront resort hotel and time share with full service health and fitness spa. 361 suites, restaurants, bars, business center. Hotel rates: from US$180.

ROSARITO
⟩ 661

✈ General Abelardo Rodrigues AP (TIJ)
Linbergh Field Int'l AP (SAN) 40 mi. / 64 km.

Rosarito Beach Hotel & Spa
❤❤❤

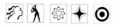

Blvd. Benito Juarez 31, Rosarito (Baja California Norte) 22710, (mail: PO Box 430145 San Diego, CA 92143), Tel: (661) 20111 or 21106. Fax: (661) 21176 or 211-25. TYPE: Resort & Spa. LOCATION: On tropical gardens, 18 mi. / 29 km. from Tijuana. SPA CLIENTELE: Women and men. DESCRIPTION: Hacienda style resort with health spa, swimming pools, tennis, racquetball, basketball. 280 rooms, 90 efficiency suites. Restaurants, bars, business center. Hotel rates: from US$110.

SAN MIGUEL DE ALLENDE
⟩ 415

✈ Leon Guanajuato AP

La Puertercita Boutique'otel & Spa
❤❤❤❤

Santo Domingo 75, San Miguel de Allende (Guanajuato) 37740. Tel: (415) 25011. Fax: (415) 25505. TYPE: Hotel & Spa. LOCATION: On the edge of San Miguel de Allende. DESCRIPTION: Charming boutique hotel with a full service health spa, massage, whirlpool, gym, exercise equipment. 24 rooms, 6 suites w/garden bath, jacuzzi and fireplace, bar and wine cellar, games room, bike excursions. Hotel rates: from US$120.

TECATE
⟩ 6

✈ Linbergh Field Int'l AP (SAN) 40 mi. / 64 km.

Rancho La Puerta
❤❤❤❤

km 5 Caretera Fed., Tecate, Baja California. Tel: USA (760) 744-4222. Fax: (760) 744-5007. Mexico Tel: (6) 654-1155. Fax: (6) 654-1108. TYPE: Health & Fitness Resort. LOCATION: In Baja California, 3 mi. / 5 km. west of Tecate. SPA CLIENTELE: Women and men. 3 couple's only weeks in March and October. SPECIAL RESTRICTIONS: Smoking not permitted.

* Cottages: 83 w/private bath
* Fireplace, garden patio
* Mexican restaurant, organic vegetable garden
* Airport: San Diego 40 mi. (64 km.)
* Reservations: deposit required
* Rates: from $1,200/week
* TAC: 10%
* Spa on premises
* **Spa Facilities**: Women's Health Center, Men's Therapy Center, aerobic gyms, weight & cardio gym, pools, hot whirlpools, saunas, beauty salon, mountain hiking trails
* **Spa Programs**: Full-day health program, Weekly Spa Program, Couple's Only Weeks, Fitness Instructors Training Week
* **Spa Treatments**: Vegetarian diet (800 - 1000 calories/day), massages, herbal wraps, facials, exercises, aerobics, calisthenics, sports, beauty and skin care, meditation, yoga, T'ai Chi, meditation, self defense
* **Special Restrictions**: guests who weigh 35% above norm, have difficulty walking, or seeing, or those with serious health problems are not admitted

DESCRIPTION: Mexican colonial style health retreat on 150 acres of landscaped grounds at the foot of the 'sacred' Mt. Kuchumaa. The accommodations vary from cozy Rancheras to cottages and villas. The Spa program emphasizes beauty, wellness and fitness through exercise, natural vegetarian cuisine, and sports. The beauty salon offers luxurious treatments. Recreation: tennis, hiking, and swimming.

VALLE DE BRAVO
⟩ 726

✈ Benito Juarez Int'l AP (MEX) 80 mi. / 130 km.

Avandaro Golf & Spa Resort
❤❤❤❤

Vega del Rio s/n Fracc. Avandaro, Valle de Bravo (Mexico) 51200. Tel: (726) 60366. Fax: (726) 60122. TYPE: Golf Resort Hotel & Spa. LOCATION: At 6,300 ft. / 1,910 m. high in the Sierra Madre Mountains. SPA CLIENTELE: Women and men.

* Suites: 100 junior and master
* Phone, CTV, minibar, fireplace, balcony
* Restaurants (2), bars (2)
* Olympic size swimming pool (heated, outdoor)
* Airport: Mexico City, 80 mi. (130 km.)
* Reservations: deposit required
* Hotel Rates: from $120
* TAC: 10%
* Spa on premises
* **Spa Facilities**: Full service spa, gym, whirlpools, saunas, beauty salon, massage rooms
* **Spa Programs**: Beauty, wellness and fitness
* **Spa Treatments**: massages, anti-cellulite, facials, loofah scrubs, herbal wraps, yoga, aerobics, low calorie spa cuisine

DESCRIPTION: Superior first class golf resort hotel with a full service European spa. The resort is located in a charming area known as "Little Switzerland". Recreation: golf, tennis, hiking, water sports, horseback riding.

MONACO

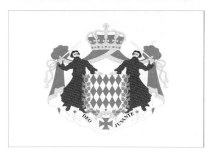

AREA: 482 acres
POPULATION: 30,000
CAPITAL: Monaco Ville
OFFICIAL LANGUAGE: French
CURRENCY: Monégasque Franc, FF or Euro
EXCHANGE RATES: 1US$ = 5.60 FF
TELEPHONE COUNTRY CODE: 377

Monaco is one of the smallest states in Europe. The tiny principality occupies a one-square mile tucked in a scenic area of Southern France on the famous French Riviera. Monte Carlo, the main city, is located in a panoramic setting overlooking the blue Mediterranean bay. Monaco, a mixture of old world charm and modern technology is synonymous with all that is luxurious and glittering in the world of travel.

The climate is mild and pleasant year round. It is similar to the climate of Southern California. Winters are mild with temperatures in the 60"sF (16°c). Summers are warm, sunny and dry with temperatures in the 80°sF (28°c).

His majesty Prince Rainier III has requested to design a "Sea water thermal baths of Monte Carlo". The establishment recaptures the glamour of the old Thermal Baths of Monte Carlo which were inaugurated at the turn-of-the-century and soon became one of the most famous sea water therapy center in Europe. The new **Les Thermes Marins** de Monte Carlo is one of the most fashionable Thalassotherapy centers in the world.

The principality attracts wealthy tourists to its world class casinos, fashionable marina, car races and festivals. Although Monaco is a sovereign State it is politically linked to France. There are no customs formalities crossing the border with France and French Franc is a legal tender.

ⓘ Monaco Gvmt Tourist Office

Direction du Tourisme et des Congès
2a blvd. des Moulins, Monte-Carlo MC 98030
Tel: (+377) 9216-6166

MONTE CARLO

☽ 6

✈ Côte d'Azur Airport (NCE) France
15 mi. / 24 km. Southwest

Les Thermes Marins
❤❤❤❤❤

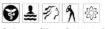

2, Avenue d'Ostende, Monte Carlo MC 98000. Tel: 9216-3636. Fax: 9216-6913. TYPE: Thalassotherapy Center. LOCATION: Monte Carlo facing the most beautiful rock of Europe with panoramic views of the Mediterranean Sea. SPA CLIENTELE: Women and men.

* Accommodations: at the superior deluxe **Hotel de Paris** & the deluxe **Hotel Hermitage**. Both hotels are directly linked to the Thermal Institute.
* Rooms & suites: 550 all with private bath
* Phone, CTV, A/C, C/H, minibar, jacuzzi

* Restaurants, bars, casinos
* Airport: Côte d'Azur Airport 15 mi. / 24 km.
* Train station: Monte Carlo
* Credit Cards: MC, VISA, AMEX,
* Open: Year round
* Hotel Rates: from FF 1,100
* Spa on premises
* **Spa Facilities**: Les Thermes Marins, 4 levels of treatment areas, seawater pools (2), jet showers (4) application cabins (4), balneotherapy cabins (8) diffusing shower cabins (2); massage cabins (8), cardiofitness studio, gym, aqua gym, sophrology room, aerosol and pressotherapy rooms, saunas (2), hammam (2), ultraviolet rooms (2), Beauty Salon
* **Spa Programs**: Anti-Stress, Weight Loss Anti-Cellulite, Menopause, Young Mothers, Beauty Cruises, Fitness, Well Being, Medical & Tobacco Withdrawal programs
* **Spa Treatments**: Thalassotherapy, under-water showers, shower-jets, seaweed applications, body wraps, hydromassage, balneotherapy, massages, manual therapy, facials, beauty and pampering

DESCRIPTION: Les Thermes Marines is a 6,600 sq. m. / 72,600 sq. ft. luxurious temple of well being. It features an indoor salt water pool and therapy facilities in a sumptuous decor of pink marble, light woods and clear glass. The thalasotherapy center offers unique programs and treatments based on seawater and techniques used in the world's most distinguished spas. Recreation: PGA championship 18-hole golf course at the Monte Carlo Golf Club, and clay courts at the Monte Carlo Tennis Club.

NETHERLANDS

AREA: 15,892 sq. mi. (41,160 sq. km.)
POPULATION: 14,910,000
CAPITAL: The Hague
OFFICIAL LANGUAGES: Dutch
CURRENCY: Dutch Florin (Dfl)
EXCHANGE RATE: 1US$ = Dfl 1.90
COUNTRY TELEPHONE CODE: 31

🛈 **Nederlands Bureau voor Tourism**
Postbus 458, 2260 MG Leidschendam, The Netherlands
Tel: (+31-70) 3705705. Fax: (+31-70) 3201654

BAD VALKENBURG a/d GEUL
☏ **4406**
✈ Maastricht Airport (MST) 10 mi. / 15 km.

Thermae 2000
♥♥♥♥

Cauberg 25, PO Box 198, NL-6300 AD Bad Valkenburg
a/d Geul. Tel: (4406) 16050. Fax: (4406) 14777.
TYPE: Spa Resort. LOCATION: In the Limburg Hills near
Maastricht. MANAGING DIRECTOR: Dhr. Verschuur. SPA
CLIENTELE: Women and men. Teenagers accepted. SPECIAL
RESTRICTION: Children up to the age of six have no admission to Thermae 2000.

* Hotel: **Thermaetel**
* Rooms: 51 w/priv. bath. Suites: 9

* Phone, CTV, minibar, terrace, spa facilities
* Wheelchair Accessible
* Restaurant, bar, meeting facilities
* Reservations: deposit required
* Credit Cards: MC/VISA/DC/AMEX/EC
* Airport: Mastricht, 15 km. / 10 mi., taxi
* Train Station: Valkenburg, taxi
* Open: Year round
* Hotel Rates: from Dfl 385; TAC: 8%
* Spa on premises: **Thermae 2000**
* Year Established: 1989
* **Spa Facilities**: Thermal springs, sauna park, Turkish
  bath, solarium, gym, hydrogym, beauty salon,
  Thalgo Thalasso, whirlpools, fitness rooms,
  indoor and outdoor pools, Spa shops
* **Spa Programs**: Health, Beauty, Anti-stress, Fitness
* **Spa Treatments**: hydrotherapy, thalassotherapy,
  baleotherapy, massage, body mud-pack, herbal bath,
  "Cleopatra" wrapping, floating bath, hydro-jet
  massage, cosmetic treatments, yoga, meditation
* **Indications**: Beauty, wellness and fitness
* Maximum Number of Guests: 120 (hotel); 1000 spa
* Medical Supervision: no

DESCRIPTION: Elegant health resort complex nestled in the
verdant hills with panoramic views of the South Limburg
countryside. Accommodations available at the **Thermaetel**,
a modern 4-star hotel with comfortable rooms and suites all
equipped with their own terrace and spa facilities. The hotel
is directly linked to **Thermae 2000**, a large Thermal/
Thalasso spa center based on the 40,000 year old curative
waters with revitalizing and stimulating effects. As a part of
your stay at the Thermaetel a visit to Thermae 2000 is
included where you can select a wide range of health, well-
being and beauty treatments by highly professional staff.

BERGAMBACHT
☏ **182**
✈ Rotterdam Airport (RTM)

Hotel de Arendshoeve
♥♥♥♥

Molenlaan 14, Bergambacht NL-2661 LB. Tel: (182)

351000. Fax: (182) 351155. TYPE: Hotel & Spa. LOCA-TION: Set in a rose garden 15 min. from Rotterdam. SPA CLIENTELE: Women and men. DESCRIPTION: Hotel with Vithalgo Health Spa, fitness center, sauna, jacuzzi, solarium. Hotel rates: from Dfl 215.

HOUTHEM/ST. GERLACH
) 4406
✈ Maastricht Airport (MST)

Château L'Ermitage
♥♥♥♥

Meerssenderweg 30-34, 6301 PJ Houthem/St.-Gerlach. Tel: (4406) 41594. Fax: (4406) 41150. TYPE: Resort Hotel & Medical Cosmetic Centre. LOCATION: In natural setting on a hillside with scenic views of the Geul Valley, just outside of the rural village of Houthem/St. Gerlach. DIREC-TOR: E. Geurts van Kessel. SPA CLIENTELE: Women and men.

* Rooms: 60 w/priv. bath
* Phone, CTV, minibar, patio or balcony
* Wheelchair Accessible
* Restaurant (spa cuisine), intimate bar
* Reservations: deposit required before arrival
* Credit Cards: MC/VISA/DC/AMEX/EC
* Open: Year round
* Rates: from Dfl 2,125 (6 days)
* TAC: 8%
* Spa on premises
* **Spa Facilities**: Beauty center, medical cosmetic center, luxurious bathing complex, indoor thermal swimming pool, sauna, hammam, massage department, Kneipp bath, Scottish showers,fitness room, solarium
* **Spa Programs**: Beauty, Ozon-Therapy, Anti Cellulite, Lasertherapie-lifting, Micro Pigmantation, Aslan Therapy,
* **Spa Treatments**: collagen, face packs, phytotherapy, biotherapy, serum therapy, homeopathy, oxygen therapy, ozone-therapy, massages, kneipp therapy, therapeutic baths, hydrotherapy, autogene training, light therapy, colon hydrotherapy
* **Indications**: skin problems, acne, cardiac complaints,

circulation disorders, arteriosclerosis, disorders in the motor system, rheumatism, arthrosis, arthritis, metabolic problems, diabetes, female complaints, disorders of the immune system, allergies, general symptoms of exhaustion, sleeping problems, depression, headaches and migraines, memory loss
* Medical Supervision: medical clinic
* Treatments Approved: Deutche Aslan Gesellschaft

DESCRIPTION: The elegant Château L'Ermitage is a romantic estate in a peaceful setting near Maastricht. The location is one of the most beautiful places in the Netherlands. The Medical Cosmetic Center offers a variety of beauty, cosmetic and anti-aging treatments by highly qualified professional staff. The list of people that participated in the programs includes many well known celebrities.

NIEUWESCHANS
) 597
✈ Elde Airport, Groningen

Nieuweschans, population 2,000, is a small old fort-town, in a rural setting, some 47 km. / 30 mi. east of Groningen on the German border.

The Kuurcentrum is a modern health complex with state-of-the-art facilities that include: solariums, beauty salon, massage and treatment rooms, indoor thermal pool, and a spa restaurant. The Health Center specializes in dermatology, in particular in the treatment of psoriasis by the method of balneo-fototherapy (combination of thermal baths and ultraviolet light).

The thermal waters are rich in iron, iodine, calcium and sulfate and gush forth from a depth of 630 m (2,079 ft) at a constant temperature of 36°c (97°F). Water treatments are excellent for general well being and beauty.

Golden Tulip Fontana Spahotel
♥♥♥

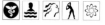

Weg naar de Bron 7, 9693 GA Nieuweschans. Tel: (597) 527777. Fax: (597) 528585. TYPE: Spa Hotel. LOCA-TION: Northern Holland on the German border, about 25

mi. (40 km.) east of Groningen. SPA CLIENTELE: Women and men. SPECIAL RESTRICTIONS: No pets allowed.

* Rooms: 67 w/priv. bath
* Phone, CTV, minibar, patio or balcony
* Wheelchair Accessible
* Restaurant, bar, meeting facilities
* Reservations: deposit 2 wks before arrival
* Credit Cards: MC/VISA/DC/AMEX/EC
* Open: Year round
* Hotel Rates: from Dfl 130
* TAC: 8%
* Spa on premises
* **Spa Facilities**: open air thermal baths, indoor swimming pool, whirlpool, solarium, fitness center, beauty salon
* **Spa Programs**: Thermal & Health 1 - 14 days
* **Spa Treatments**: balneotherapy, balneofototherapy, massage, beauty, thalassotherapy, reflexology, treatment of psoriasis
* **Indications**: skin problems, psoriasis, stress
* **Contraindications**: epilepsy, open wounds, heart operation less than 6 wks, blood pressure medication
* Medical Supervision: 3 MD, 3 RN
* Treatments Approved: Academic Hospital Groningen

DESCRIPTION: Modern hotel situated in the heart of Nieuweschans with a modern international Spa center based on 36°c (97°F) warm thermal bath with paramedical and medical treatments. The establishment is famous for thalassotherapy and treatment of psoriasis. Recreation: tennis, horseback riding and water sports.

OOTMARSUM
✈ 541

✈ Twente Airport, Enschede

Hotel de Wiemsel
♥♥♥♥

Winhofflaan 2, Ootmarsum NL-7631 HX. Tel: (541) 292-155. Fax: (541) 293-295. TYPE: Hotel & Spa. LOCATION: In wooded setting 10 km. / 6 mi. from Oldenzaal. SPA

CLIENTELE: Women and men.

* Rooms: 49 w/priv. bath
* Phone, CTV, minibar, kitchenette
* Wheelchair Accessible
* Restaurant, lounge, bar, meeting facilities
* Reservations: deposit required
* Credit Cards: MC/VISA/DC/AMEX/EC
* Open: Year round
* Hotel Rates: from Dfl 260
* TAC: 8%
* Spa on premises
* **Spa Facilities**: Beauty salon, sauna, solarium, indoor and outdoor swimming pool
* **Spa Programs**: Beauty, wellness and fitness
* **Spa Treatments**: hydro-gymnastics, massage, beauty treatments in the Beauty Farm

DESCRIPTION: Country retreat with Beauty Farm.

SCHEVNINGEN
✈ 70

✈ Rotterdam Airport (RTM) 13 mi. / 20 km. Schipol Int'l AP (AMS) 28 mi. / 45 km.

Kuur Thermen Vitalizee
♥♥♥♥

Strandweg 13F, 2586 JK Scheveningen. Tel: (70) 4166500. Fax: (70) 4166501. TYPE: Thermal Spa. LOCATION: Heart of Scheveningen near the beach with an unspoiled view of the sea. SPA CLIENTELE: Women and men. SPECIAL RESTRICTION: No swimwear allowed in the Thermen.

* Hotel: can be arranged with the Spa
* Open: Year round , 10:30am - 24:00
* **Spa Facilities**: thermal baths, sauna, cold plunge, steambaths, whirlpools (2), Dead Sea "floating" baths, relaxation room, treatment rooms (30), pool, gym
* **Spa Treatments**: Thalassotherapy, hydrotherapy, balneotherapy, quick bronza, aqua-jet, massage, seawater massage, Vichy massage, underwater

massage, hydromassage bath, algotherapy, facials, skin treatments (Helena Rubinstein, Thalgo), collagen masks, herbal baths,
* **Spa Programs**: Beauty, wellness, medical thalasso, stop smoking
* **Spa Packages**: range from several hours to a couple of days. Inquire direct.
* **Indications**: beauty, pampering, stress, fatigue, cellulite, menopause complaints, smoking

DESCRIPTION: A modern thermal center complex with extensive facilities offering a large array of beauty, wellness and well being treatments by highly trained staff. Enjoy Beauty & Healthy day packages or longer thalasso cures for medical purposes. Hotel accommodations nearby can be arranged directly with the spa.

VENLO
⟩ 77
✈ Düsseldorf Int'l Airport (DUS), Germany

Venlo, population 62,000, is a resort town on the German-Dutch border in southern Holland.

De Bovenste Molen Hotel
❤❤❤❤

🏇 🚶

Bovenste Molenweg 12, Venlo NL-5912 TV. Tel: (77) 359-1414. Fax: (77) 354-8257. TYPE: Hotel & Spa. LOCATION: By a lake in 80 acres of forest at the German border.

SPA CLIENTELE: Women and men.

* Rooms: 83 w/priv. bath. Suites: 8
* Phone, CTV, whirlpool, minibar, balcony
* Restaurant, cafe, bar
* Open: Year round
* Hotel Rates: from Dfl 230
* Spa on premises
* **Spa Facilities**: Beauty farm, health club, sauna, jacuzzi,solarium, gym with exercise equipment
* **Spa Programs**: Beauty, wellness, fitness

DESCRIPTION: Country hotel with beauty farm and golf clinic. Recreation: tennis, golf, archery.

ZANDVOORT
⟩ 23
✈ Amsterdam Schipol Airport (AMS), 25 mi. / 40 km.

Golden Tulip Zandvoort Hotel
❤❤❤❤

🏇 🚶

Burgemeester v Alphenstraat 63, Zandvoort NL-2041 KG. Tel: (23) 571-3234. Fax: (23) 571-9094. TYPE: Resort & Spa. LOCATION: On the North Sea beach, near Circuit Park Zandvoort. SPA CLIENTELE: Women and men. DESCRIPTION: Resort hotel complex with Beauty Center, sauna, Turkish bath, solarium, whirlpool. 211 rooms, 19 suites. Restaurant, bar, brasserie. 10 min. to golf course. Hotel rates: from Dfl 240.

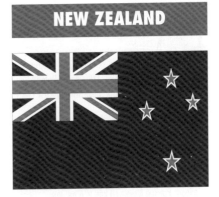

NEW ZEALAND

AREA: 103,736 sq. mi. (268,676 sq. km.)
POPULATION: 3,389,000
CAPITAL: Wellington
OFFICIAL LANGUAGES: English, Maori
CURRENCY: New Zealand Dollar (NZ$)
EXCHANGE RATE: 1 US$ = NZ$ 1.79
COUNTRY TELEPHONE CODE: 64

Health Spas are a rarity in New Zealand with only the Millbrook Resort (near Queenstown) having one with international standards. Rotorua has Geothermal area with abundance of hot pools/springs. Many people visit Rotorua to soak in the thermal pools for relaxation and recreation.

ℹ️ New Zealand Tourism Board
501 Santa Monica Blvd.m #300, Santa Monica CA 90401
Tel: (310) 395-7480. Fax: (310) 395-5453

HANMER SPRINGS
🌙 **3**
✈️ Christchurch Int'l AP (CHC), 90 mi. / 140 km.

Hanmer is an Alpine village and a super winter playground. It is a scenic alpine and thermal resort of the South Island. When the springs were discovered the hot water rose to the surface under artesian pressure. Today the thermal water are pumped to the thermal pools for therapeutic purposes.

Alpine Spa Lodge
❤️❤️❤️

1-11 Harrogate St., Hanmer Springs. Tel/Fax: (3) 315-7311. TYPE: Alpine Lodge & Spa. LOCATION: Directly opposite Thermal pools complex near town centre, restaurants and shopping. SPA CLIENTELE: Women and men.

* Rooms: 20 w/priv. bath
* Tower block suites w/spa baths
* Phone, CTV, cooking facilities
* Airport: Christchurch
* Credit Cards: MC/VISA/AMEX/DC/CB/EC
* Open: Year round
* Hotel Rates: on request
* Opposite Thermal Pools Complex
* **Spa Facilities**: see Hanmer Springs Thermal Reserve
* **Spa Treatments**: see Hanmer Springs Thermal Reserve

DESCRIPTION: Chalet style Alpine lodge near thermal pools. Recreation: bungy jumping, jet boating, river rafting, helicopter flights.

Hanmer Springs Thermal Reserve
❤️❤️❤️

Amuri Rd., PO Box 30, Hanmer Springs. Tel: (3) 315-7511. Fax: (3) 315-7511. TYPE: Hot Springs Spa. LOCATION: In famous hot springs area. SPA CLIENTELE: Women and men. DESCRIPTION: Spa complex with seven thermal pools, freshwater swimming pool, Finnish sauna and steam room w/shower, plunge pool and dressing area. A therapeutic massage, gym, aqua therapy and beauty treatments are also available. **Indications**: orthopedic conditions such as bone fractures and soft tissue injuries.

MOTUEKA
🌙 **3**
✈️ Nelson Airport, 60 mi. / 90 km.

Kimi Ora Health Resort
❤️❤️❤️

Kaiteriteri Beach, Motueka. Tel: (3) 527-8027. Fax: (3) 527-8134. TYPE: Health Resort. LOCATION: One hour from Nelson. SPA CLIENTELE: Women and men. DESCRIPTION:

Kimi Ora offers a healthy, peaceful, smoke free environment and a healthy vegetarian cuisine. Spa Facilities: gym, sauna, pool, beauty salon. Treatments: naturopathy, yoga, aerobics, meditation, medical baths, facials, massages. Accommod-ations in comfortable chalets. Accommodations: Hammer Springs Lodge - Tel: (3) 315-7021. Fax: (3) 315-7071.

QUEENSTOWN

↘ 3

✈ Frankton Airport (ZQN) 10 mi. / 15 km.

Millbrook Resort
❤❤❤❤

Malagans Rd. Arrowtown. Mailing address: Private bag, Queenstown. Tel: (3) 441-7015. Fax: (3) 441-7016. TYPE: Resort & Spa. LOCATION: Set in a lovely surroundings with striking mountain views. SPA CLIENTELE: Women and men. DESCRIPTION: Health & Fitness resort with sauna, solarium, massage, indoor lap pool. 56 rooms, villas, restaurants, bars, 18 hole golf, tennis courts, jogging tracks. Hotel rates: from NZ$260.

ROTORUA

↘ 7

✈ Rotorua Airport (ROT) 5.5 mi. / 9 km. East

Rotorua, population 48,000, is a popular hot-springs resort town on the shores of Lake Rotorua. The town is famous for its thermal activity consisting of mud pools, sulfur free flowing hot springs and geysers of all sizes and shapes. Visitors can discover some of New Zealand's best-known Maori settlements in the area. Located 158 mi / 254 km southeast of Auckland it can be reached from Auckland via coach or air.

Indications: Rotorua spa gained international recognition since the late 19th century as a treatment center for arthritis with the cure based on natural thermal and therapeutic spa packs.

Millenium Rotorua
❤❤❤❤

Corner Eruera & Hinemaru Sts. PO Box 1044. Rotorua. Tel: (7) 347-1234. (7) 348-1234. TYPE: Resort Hotel & Spa. LOCATION: Near the shores of Lake Rototua. SPA CLIENTELE: Women and men.

* Rooms: 227 w/private bath. Suites: 2
* Phone, CTV, minibar, refrigerator
* Rooms for non-smokers
* Restaurants (2), bars (2)
* Airport: Rotorua Airport 10 km. / 6 mi. taxi
* Credit Cards: MC/VISA/AMEX/DC/CB/EC
* Open: Year round
* Hotel Rates: from NZ$250/day
* TAC: 10%
* Spa on premises
* **Spa Facilities**: Near thermal baths, spa pools, sauna, steam room, plunge pool, gym
* **Spa Treatments**: bathing in mineral water, steam & massages, fitness & aerobics
* **Indications**: arthritis, skin care, anti-stress

DESCRIPTION: Attractive resort hotel. Conveniently located to thermal baths with view of Lake Rotorua.

Moose Lodge
❤❤❤❤

State Hwy 30. RD 4, Lake Rotoiti. Tel: (7) 362-7823. Fax: (7) 362-7677. TYPE: Sporting Lodge & Spa. LOCATION: Just outside Rotorua City Limits. SPA CLIENTELE: Women and men.

* Rooms: 20 w/priv. bath
* Suites: 4 w/priv. spa bath
* Restaurant, lounge, billiard room
* Airport: Rotorua Airport 11 km. / 6 mi.
* Airport Transportation: free transfer
* Credit Cards: MC/VISA/AMEX/DC/CB/EC
* Open: Year round
* Hotel Rates: from NZ$375/day
* TAC: 10%

* Spa on premises
* **Spa Facilities:** hot mineral spa, gym
* **Spa Treatments:** bathing in mineral water, steam & massages, fitness & aerobics
* **Indications:** anti-stress

DESCRIPTION: An elegant lakefront sporting lodge with hot mineral spa. Recreation: trout fishing, hunting, boating, water sports.

Polynesian Spa
❤❤❤❤

Hinemoa St., PO Box 40, Rotorua. Tel: (7) 348-1328. Fax: (7) 348-9486. TYPE: Thermal Spa. LOCATION: Rotorua thermal area. SPA CLIENTELE: Women and men. SPA DIRECTOR: Mr. Martin Lobb. DESCRIPTION: The complex has 33 mineral pools, 10 public pools, 17 luxury private pools. The Radium and Priest Hot Springs are famous for the relief of aches and pains, arthritis, rheumatism and travel weariness. Also offers Aix massage done under jets of hot water. The Polynesia Spa is New Zealand's leading thermal bathing attraction.

Regal Geyserland Hotel
❤❤❤❤

Fenton Street, P.O. Box 800, Rotorua. Tel: (7) 348-2039. (7) 348-2033. TYPE: Resort & Spa. LOCATION: Overlooking Whakarewarewa Thermal Reserve, 1 mi. (1.6 km) from city center. SPA CLIENTELE: Family oriented.

* Rooms: 69 w/private bath. Suites: 4
* Phone, CTV, minibar, in-room safe
* Restaurant, bar, meeting room
* Airport: Rotorua 6 mi / 9 km
* Airport Transportation: free pick up
* Reservations: 1 night deposit req'd
* Credit Cards: MC/VISA/AMEX/DC

* Open: Year round
* Hotel Rates: from NZ$115
* TAC: 10%
* **Spa Facilities:** Health center, heated pool, indoor thermal spout pool, saunas, gym
* **Spa Treatments:** Bathing in mineral water, sauna, massage, diet and fitness

DESCRIPTION: Resort-style Motor Hotel overlooking one of the best thermal reserves in Rotorua. The main attraction are the hot springs and thermal pools at the hotel. Recreation: golf course nearby, lake fishing and boating.

Sheraton Rotorua Hotel
❤❤❤❤

Fenton Street, P.O. Box 983, Rotorua. Tel: (7) 349-5200. Fax: (7) 349-5201. TYPE: Resort & Spa. LOCATION: Overlooking Whakarewarewa Thermal Reserve, 1 mi. (1.6 km.) from city center. SPA CLIENTELE: Family oriented.

* Rooms: 130 w/private bath
* Suites: 8 w/spa bath & balcony
* Phone, CTV, minibar, refrigerator, balcony
* Restaurants, bars, lounge, entertainment
* Airport: Rotorua, 10 km. / 6 mi.
* Reservations: 1 night deposit req'd
* Credit Cards: MC/VISA/AMEX/DC
* Open: Year round
* Hotel Rates: from NZ$250/day
* TAC: 10%
* Spa on premises
* **Spa Facilities:** heated indoors and outdoors thermal pools, gym, sauna
* **Spa Treatments:** Bathing in mineral water, sauna, massage, diet and fitness

DESCRIPTION: Victorian style hotel offering thermal balneotherapy pools and health club facilities.

PALAU (REPUBLIC OF)

POLAND

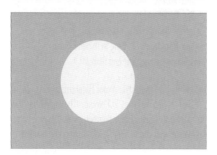

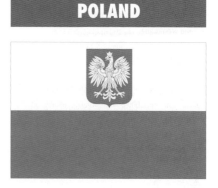

AREA: 177 sq. mi. (458 sq. km.)
POPULATION: 15,122
CAPITAL: Koror
OFFICIAL LANGUAGES: English, Palauan
CURRENCY: US$
INTERNATIONAL PHONE CODE: 680

Palau is an island destination in the Western Pacific, known for some of the world's finest diving and fishing.

KOROR

🤙 No area code

✈ Koror Airai Int'l (ROR)

Outrigger Palasia Hotel Palau
♥♥♥♥

P.O. Box 125, Koror, Republic of Palau 96940. (680) 488-8888. Fax: (680) 488-8800. TYPE: Resort Hotel & Spa. LOCATION: On the island of Koror overlooking the famous Rock Islands. SPA CLIENTELE: Women and men. DESCRIPTION: Elegant resort hotel with health spa, fitness facilities, swimming pool. 165 rooms w/priv. bath, shops, restaurants (4), banquet facilities. Hotel rates: from US$182.

AREA: 120,725 sq. mi. (312,678 sq. km.)
POPULATION: 35,800,000
CAPITAL: Warsaw
OFFICIAL LANGUAGE: Polish
CURRENCY: Zloty (Z)
EXCHANGE RATE: 1 US$ = Z 3.45
TELEPHONE COUNTRY CODE: 48

Polish health resorts are located in different regions of the country. They offer numerous mineral water springs of various physiochemical components, therapeutic muds, and climatology centers. The most popular spas are located in the south, in the Carpathian and Sudeten Mountains and along the Baltic Coast. The spas operate more like sanatoriums and are medically oriented with their own diagnostic laboratories and medical care.

ⓘ Sport & Tourism Administration
00-916 Warszawa, ul. Swietokrzyska 12, Poland
Tel: (22) 8264515. Fax: (22) 6945161.

USA
Polish National Tourist Office
275 Madison Ave., Suite 1711, New York NY 10016.
Tel: (212) 338-9412. Fax: (212) 338-9283.

BUSKO
🤙 **496**

✈ Balice Int'l Airport (KRK) Cracow

Busko, population 11,200, lies 60 miles (100 km.) northeast of Crakow in the broad, picturesque Niecka Nidzianska valley between the Gory Swietokrzyskie and the Wyzyna Krakowsko-Czestochowska mountains. The curative qualities of the spa's mineral waters were known as far back as the times of the Piast and Jagiello dynasty. Busko dates as a health resort from the beginning of the 19th century. Buildings for the first baths, erected in 1836, were designed in the classical style by the famous architect Marconi, and being modernized, are still in use. The Marconi health station and related health resort buildings are located on a 124 acre (50 hectare) park. The therapeutic cures at Busko are provided by the sodium chloride, iodide and bromide waters; sodium chloride and sulfide waters; the table water "Buskowianka"; and therapeutic mud.

While taking a cure at Busko one can enjoy open-air concerts at the spa park, and evening dancing at the spa's modern style restaurant and coffeehouse. The entertainment hall contains a cinema and rooms for various cultural and artistic events. Excursions are available to the nearby mountains and places of historical interest such as Checiny with its old castle; Oblrgorek the home of the polish writer Henryk Sienkiewicz; and the historical towns Wislica, Pinczow and Szydlow.

Marconi
❤❤❤

P.P. Uzdrowisko Busko-Solec, ul. gen F. Rzewuskiego 2, 28-100 Busko. Reservations: Orbis Tel: (22) 273673. Fax: (22) 271123. TYPE: Health Resort. LOCATION: In the middle of a 124 acre park. SPA CLIENTELE: Women and men.

* Rooms: singles & double w/private bath
  singles & doubles without private bath
* Restaurant, bar
* Airport: Cracow, 60 mi. / 100 km.
* Transportation: train or bus to Busko
* Reservations: required
* Open: Year round
* Rates: on request
* Treatment duration: minimum 10 - 21days
* Spa on premises: **Marconi Health Station**

* **Spa Facilities**: Indoor swimming pool, baths, latest balneotherapeutic equipment, gymnasium, laboratories, varied sports facilities
* **Spa Programs**: Rejuvenation, relaxation, general fitness, beauty and medical
* **Spa Treatments**: Therapeutic baths, hydrotherapy, lavages, electrotherapy, thermotherapy, light therapy, inhalation, mud packs, physiotherapy, drinking water
* **Indications**: circulatory system diseases, gynecological problems, nervous system disorders, rheumatic diseases, skin diseases, traumatic & orthopedic conditions
* **Medical Supervision**: Qualified doctors, nurses, physiotherapists, dieticians
* Treatment Approval: Medical Academies and International Federation of Thermalism and Climatism FITEC

DESCRIPTION: Sports and exercise are an important part of the Busko treatment. The resort has an outdoor swimming pool, sport stadium with soccer (football) field, smaller fields and other game courts .

CIECHOCINEK
✈ Bydgoszcz 40 mi. / 67 km.

Ciechocinek is the largest brine and mud health resort in Poland. It is situated in the Kujawy region of central Poland. The spa is located in the picturesque Vistula River valley 110 mi. / 180 km. northwest of warsaw and 40 mi. / 67 km. southeast of Bydgoszcz. The resort is mostly known for its thermal brine, mild climate and effective treatments. The first baths were built in 1849, then enlarged and modernized over the years. Since world war II and especially in the 1960's the health resort has been expanded to include new health stations and modern treatment facilities.

The mild climate with little rain fall is strongly influenced by the salt graduation towers; during graduation ozone is produced and released into the air which becomes saturated with the salty iodine enriched humidity. The air quality resembles sea air and has similar therapeutic qualities. The graduation towers turns the spa park into a natural saline inhalatorium. The thermal springs contain sodium chloride, iodides and bromides at temperatures averaging 80°F - 95°F (27°c - 35°c).

The spa's own drinking water "Krystynka" contain 0.36% sodium chloride. The major indications for therapeutic treatments include: orthopedic and traumatic disorders, rheumatic, circulatory, respiratory and nervous system diseases.

Ciechocinek is accessible by train or bus service from Warsaw, Lodz, or Poznan.

Dom Zdrojowy
♥♥♥

P.P. Uzdrowisko, ul. Kosciuszki 10, 87-720 Ciechocinek, Poland. Reservations: Orbis Tel: (22) 273673. Fax: (22) 271123. TYPE: Health resort. LOCATION: In the center of town in the spa park. SPA CLIENTELE: Women and men.

* Rooms: singles & doubles w/private bath
* Restaurant, bar
* Airport: Bydgoszcz 40 mi. / 67 km.
* Transportation: train & bus service to and from Warsaw and Bydgoszcz
* Season: Year round
* Rates: on request
* Treatment duration: minimum 10-21 days
* Spa on premises
* **Spa Facilities**: swimming pools, baths, balneo-therapeutic equipment, gymnasium, diagnostic and analytic laboratories, sports facilities
* **Spa Programs**: Medical, relaxation, general fitness, and weight loss
* **Spa Treatments**: Therapeutic water baths, mud baths, inhalation therapy, hydrotherapy, lavages, gynecological irrigations, mud packs, electrotherapy, light therapy, thermotherapy, massage, physical therapy, drinking cures
* **Indications**: circulatory system diseases, nervous system disorders, respiratory tract diseases, rheumatic diseases, traumatic & orthopedic conditions
* Medical Supervision: doctors, nurses, physio-therapists, dieticians
* Treatment Approval: Medical Academies and International Federation of Thermalism and Climatism FITEC

DESCRIPTION: A spa hotel sanatorium with a wide range of accommodations from suites to simple rooms without private bath. The hotel has its own medical center and offers a complete medically spa package including full board, lodging and medical treatments.

CIEPLICE ZDROJ
✈ 22

✈ Wroclaw, 80 mi. / 133 km.

Cieplice Zdroj, one of the oldest health resorts in Poland is located in the Jelenia Gora Basin, 3 miles (5 km.) from the town of Jelenia Gora (population 56,000). The Karkonosze, Izerskie, Kaczawskie and Janowickie Mountains surround the basin, have an important tempering influence on the climate and create a magnificent panoramic scenery. Cieplice can be reached by direct bus and train lines from Warsaw, Szcezecin or Poznan.

The town's springs were discovered in 1175; and the first thermal bath was erected in 1403. In the 17th century it gained popularity as a health resort throughout Europe. Cieplice was rebuilt after World War II and plans call for the enlargement and further expansion of the resort facilities. The spa's thermal waters are slightly mineralized and include fluoride. The spa produces its own mineral table water known as the "Marysienka".

Indications: orthopedic and traumatic disorders, rheumatic, nervous system, urinary tract and kidney diseases.

Dom Zdrojowy
♥♥♥

Zespol Uzdrowisk Jeleniogorskich, ul. Mireckiego 4, 58-560 Cieplice Zdroj. Reservations: Orbis Tel: (22) 273673. Fax: (22) 271123. TYPE: Health resort. LOCATION: In the spa park. SPA CLIENTELE: Men, Women.

* Rooms: suites w/private bath
  singles & doubles without private bath
* Restaurant, coffee house, library
* Airport: Wroclaw, 80 mi. / 133 km.
* Transportation: train & bus

* Open: Year round
* Rates: on request
* Treatment duration: minimum 10-21days
* **Spa Facilities**: swimming pools, baths, latest balneotherapeutic equipment, gymnasium, diagnostic & analytic laboratories, sports facilities
* **Spa Programs**: Medical, relaxation, well being
* **Spa Treatments**: Therapeutic water baths, mud baths, hydrotherapy, electrotherapy, light therapy, thermotherapy, inhalation therapy, irrigations, gynecologic packs, massages, physical therapy, drinking cures
* **Indications**: nervous system disorders, rheumatic diseases, traumatic and orthopedic conditions, urinary tract diseases
* Medical Supervision: doctors, nurses, dieticians, physiotherapists
* Treatment Approval: Medical Academies and International Federation of Thermalism and Climatism FITEC

DESCRIPTION: Modern hotel offering a variety of accommodations in different styles. The hotel features its own medical facilities and offers mainly a medical spa package that includes full board, lodging and treatments.

INOWROCLAW
⟩ 536

✈ Okecie Airport (WAW)

Inowroclaw, population 80,000, is located in the West Kujawy region of northern Poland, about 220 km. / 140 mi. northwest of Warsaw. The area is connected with many historical sites linked to the early days of the Polish State. The climate is typical for lowlands with mild winters and pleasant summers.

Inowroclaw Health Resort
♥♥

P.P. Uzdrowisko Inowroclaw, ul. Solankowa 77, Inowroclaw 88-100. (536) 740-11, Fax: (536) 740-16. TYPE: Health Resort. LOCATION: In a large park in the southwestern part of the city. SPA CLIENTELE: Women and men. MED-

ICAL RESTRICTIONS: Not accepted after cardiac infraction.

* Rooms: 20 with private bath
* Phone, CTV, C/H, minibar
* Airport: Warsaw
* Airport Transportation: Taxi, limo, bus
* Open: Year round
* Hotel Rates: from US$60 / per day
* Spa on premises
* Name of Spa: **P.P. Uzdrowisko Inowroclaw**
* Year Established: 1875
* **Spa Facilities**: Sports and recreation center, outpatient clinic, mud therapy department, natural physiotherapy department, war veterans sanatorium, patient service department
* **Spa Treatments**: Saline, gas-bubble and carbonic acid baths, peat wrappings, poultices, inhalation, paradontopathies, gymnastics, therapeutic and rehabilitation pools
* **Indications**: Rheumatic troubles, osteoarticular system diseases, circulatory system and peripheral vessels diseases, digestive tract diseases, obesity and other metabolic disorders, diabetes, upper respiratory tract and genital tract diseases; women's infertility, functional liver disturbances after virus hepatitis and fatty liver
* Length of Stay Required: 14 - 24 days
* Medical Supervision: 17 MDs, 100 RNs
* Treatments Approved By: Balneoclimatic Institute

DESCRIPTION: The Inowroclaw Health Resort is a large complex with six separate buildings. The resort has a long term partnership with research centers and specializes in medical treatments. Patients are given treatment directly after operations, myocardial or cerebral infractions. Great importance is given to therapeutic gymnastics under supervision of professional kinesitherapeutists. The resort meets all the requirements of post hospital rehabilitation.

KOLOBRZEG
⟩ 965

✈ Koszalin, 28 mi. / 46 km.

Kolobrzeg, population 25,000, is a commercial fishing port and a seaside resort with saline bathing at the mouth of the

Parseta River, 28 miles (46 km.) from Koszalin. The district of the Kolobrzeg Spa is located in the northern part of the city along the seacoast. The whole health resort is managed by the "Uzdrowisko Kolobrzeg" State enterprise which run the clinics and sanatoriums. Tel: (965) 22441. Fax: (965) 22516.

The cures at Kolobrzeg consist of therapeutic sea water baths, therapeutic mud treatments, sea water aerosol inhalations, and drinking cures of table waters containing sodium chloride, bromide and iodide.

Indications: diabetes, circulatory, respiratory and rheumatic diseases.

Mewa V & Muszelka
❤❤❤

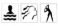

ul. Jana Kasprowicza 3, P.P. Uzdrowisko Kolobrzeg, 78100 Kolobrzeg. Tel: (965) 2516. TYPE: Health resort hotel. LOCATION: in the Spa Park along the Baltic Sea. SPA CLIENTELE: Women and men.

* Rooms: singles & doubles w/priv. bath singles & double without priv. bath suites w/ priv. bath
* Restaurants, cafes, cinemas
* SPA on premises
* Airport: Koszalin, 28 mi. / 46 km.
* Transportation: train & bus
* Reservations: required
* Season: Year round
* Rates: from US$50/day
* Treatment duration: minimum 10-21days
* **Spa Facilities**: swimming pools, baths, balneotherapeutic equipment, sauna, gym, diagnostic and analytic laboratories, sports facilities
* **Spa Programs**: Medical, relaxation, fitness,
* **Spa Treatments**: therapeutic water baths, massages, mud packs & baths, inhalations, electrotherapy, light therapy, thermotherapy, lavages, physiotherapy
* **Indications**: circulatory system diseases, diabetes, respiratory tract & rheumatic diseases
* Medical Supervision: doctors, nurses,

dieticians, physiotherapists
* Treatment Approval: Medical Academies

DESCRIPTION: Hotel and sanatorium with a wide range of accommodations. The hotel features thalassotherapy spa treatments based on sea water and sea products. Medical supervision and treatments included in their packages.

KRYNICA
ℷ 135
✈ Balice Int'l Airport (KRK) Cracow

Krynica, population 10,200, is Poland's most fashionable spa known as the "Pearl of Polish Health Resorts". Situated in the Kryniczanka River valley it is an important winter sports resort. The secluded south facing valley is protected from the freezing north wind by high wooded slopes and makes Krynica one of the warmest places in the area. The spa's mineral rich springs are carbonic acid, alkaline acidulous, containing iodides. Krynica can be reached by train or bus from Warsaw and other main cities.

Indications: diabetes, circulatory, digestive and urinary diseases, women infertility.

Nowy Dom Zdrojowy
❤❤❤

Nowotarski - Allee 7, 33380 Krynica. Tel: (135) 2815. TYPE: Spa Hotel. LOCATION: On mountain slope with a winter garden. SPA CLIENTELE: Women and men.

* Rooms and suites w/ private bath
* Restaurant, coffee shop, cinema
* Airport: Cracow, 80 mi. / 133 km.
* Transportation: train or bus from Cracow
* Reservations: required
* Open: Year round
* Rates: from $70/day
* Treatment duration: minimum 10-21days
* Spa on premises
* **Spa Facilities**: swimming pools, baths, latest balneotherapeutic equipment, gym, diagnostic and analytic laboratories, sports facilities

* **Spa Programs**: Medical, relaxation, fitness
* **Spa Treatments**: therapeutic water & gas baths, inhalation therapy, light therapy, electrotherapy, thermotherapy, physical therapy, mud treatment, drinking cures
* **Indications**: circulatory system diseases, diabetes, digestive tract diseases, heart & liver diseases, urinary tract diseases
* **Medical Supervision**: doctors, nurses, physiotherapists, dieticians
* **Treatment Approval**: Medical Academies and International Federation of Thermalism and Climatism FITEC

DESCRIPTION: A modern spa hotel with a variety of accommodations. The spa features thermal springs, therapeutic muds and gazes for medical and recreational purposes. Spa packages include medical supervision and treatments.

KUDOWA
ɔ 135

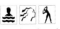 Strachowica Airport (WRO) Wroclaw

Kudowa, one of the oldest European health resorts, is situated in southwest Poland in the deep, sheltered Klodzko valley. Kudowa gained its popularity as one of the best known spas in Europe when the railroad was built in 1901. The therapeutic waters of Kudowa are carbonic acid containing sodium and calcium hydrocarbonates, ferruginous, arsenic and radioactive. Kudowa can be reached by train and bus services from Warsaw, Wroclaw, Szczecin, and Lublin.

Indications: circulatory system diseases, and diseases of the thyroid.

Zameczek
❤❤❤

Zespol Uzdrowisk Klodzkich, ul. Zdrojowa 43, 57-350 Kudowa-Zdroj. Reservations: Orbis - Tel: (22) 273673. Fax: (22) 271123. TYPE: Health resort. LOCATION: near the Spa Park. SPA CLIENTELE: Women and men.

* Rooms: singles & doubles w/priv. bath, singles

& double w/o private bath suites w/priv. bath
* Restaurant, bar
* Airport: Wroclaw, 60 mi. / 100 km.
* Transportation: train or bus
* Open: Year round
* Rates: from US$60/day
* Treatment duration: minimum 10-21days
* Spa on premises
* **Spa Facilities**: balneotherapeutic equipment, baths, gym, diagnostic & analytic labs
* **Spa Programs**: Medical, relaxation, fitness
* **Spa Treatments**: therapeutic water & gas baths, massages, hydrotherapy, electrotherapy, light therapy thermotherapy, physical therapy, inhalation therapy
* **Indications**: circulatory system diseases, diabetes, digestive tract diseases, heart diseases, liver diseases, urinary tract diseases
* **Medical Supervision**: doctors, nurses, physiotherapists, dieticians
* **Treatment Approval**: Medical Academies

DESCRIPTION: This spa is medically oriented. Spa packages include accommodations, full board, medical supervision and treatments.

POLANICA
 Strachowica Airport (WRO) Wroclaw

Polanica, is a thermal and climatic resort 72 miles (120 km.) south of Wroclaw near the Czech border. The resort is surrounded by a lovely park, decorative shrubs and flower gardens. The therapeutic waters, climate and scenery contributes to Polanica's success as a health resort. The cures at Polanica consist of carbonic acid waters containing hydrocarbonate; therapeutic water "Wielka Pieniawa"; and table water "Staropolanka". Polanica can be reached by train or bus service from Wroclaw, Warsaw, Lublin and Szczecin.

Indications: circulatory and digestive system diseases.

Wielka Pieniawa
❤❤❤

Zespol Uzdrowisk Klodzkich, ul. Zdrojowa 37, 57-320

Polanica. Reservations: Orbis - Tel: (22) 273673. Fax: (22) 271123. TYPE: Health resort. LOCATION: in a lovely park. SPA CLIENTELE: Women and men.

* Rooms: w/shared or priv. bath, suites
* Restaurants, coffee house, cinema
* Airport: Wroclaw, 72 mi. / 120 km.
* Transportation: train or bus
* Open: Year round
* Rates: from $70/day
* Treatment duration: minimum 10-21days
* **Spa Facilities**: pool, balneotherapeutic equipment, gym, drinking cure room, diagnostic and analytic laboratories, sports facilities
* **Spa Programs**: Medical, relaxation, fitness
* **Spa Treatments**: therapeutic water baths, massages, hydrotherapy, electrotherapy, light therapy, thermotherapy, physical therapy, inhalation therapy, drinking water treatment
* **Indications**: circulatory and digestive diseases
* Medical Supervision: doctors, nurses
* Treatment Approval: Medical Academies

DESCRIPTION: Health spa with a variety of accommodations. The spa is medically oriented. The drinking room is in the spa's park. Recreation: tennis courts, swimming pool with a beach and spring board, sports field and jogging trail for exercises.

POLCZYN
⌐ 22

✈ Koszalin 36 miles (60 km.)

Polczyn, population 8,000, is located in the Koszalin Province 36 miles (60 km) from the Baltic Sea and 36 miles from Koszalin. The climate is continental and typical to the plains. The summer is comparatively warm and the air is clear and pollution free. The health resort with the kursaal or spa buildings is located in a separate part of the town amidst a large park. In 1964 salt brine of therapeutic value was found and is now used for treatment purposes. The cure elements consist of mineral waters rich in sodi-

um chloride, bromide and iodide, therapeutic mud and the mineral table water "Polczynianka".

Indications: gynecological, rheumatic, and nervous system diseases, orthopedic and traumatic troubles, disease of the digestive system, heart troubles, anemia.

Irena
❤❤❤

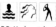

P.P. Uzdrowisko Polczyn, ul. K. Marksa 6, 78-320 Polczyn. Reservations: Orbis - Tel: (22) 273673. Fax: (22) 271123. TYPE: Health resort. LOCATION: in the spa park. SPA CLIENTELE: Women and men.

* Rooms: w/private or shared bath, suites
* Restaurant, coffee shop, library, game room
* Nearest Airport: Koszalin 36 miles (60 km)
* Transportation: train & bus
* Reservations: required
* Open: Year round
* Rates: from US$60/day
* Treatment duration: minimum 10-21days
* Spa on premises
* **Spa Facilities**: balneotherapeutic equipment, gym, laboratories, baths
* **Spa Programs**: Medical, relaxation, fitness,
* **Spa Treatments**: therapeutic water & gas baths, massages, mud packs & baths, electrotherapy, light therapy, thermotherapy, hydrotherapy, physical therapy, inhalation, lavages, drinking water treatments
* **Indications**: gynecological problems, nervous system disorders, traumatic & orthopedic conditions, rheumatic diseases,
* Medical Supervision: doctors, nurses, physiotherapists, dieticians
* Treatment Approval: Medical Academies

DESCRIPTION: Spa hotel with a variety of accommodations. The Spa is medically oriented. Good results are observed in the treatment of gynecological diseases, particularly sterility. Spa packages include full board, lodging, medical supervision and treatments.

PORTUGAL

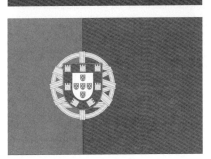

AREA: 35,549 sq. mi. (92,072 sq. km.)
POPULATION: 10,470,000
CAPITAL: Lisbon
OFFICIAL LANGUAGE: Portuguese
CURRENCY: Portuguese Escudo (ESC$)
EXCHANGE RATE: 1 US$ = ESC$171
TELEPHONE COUNTRY CODE: 351

Portugal is one of the oldest nations in Europe. The country offers beautiful historic sites, sunny weather, sandy beaches and gambling casinos. Portugal has a long tradition of thermal cure that can be traced back to the times of the Romans. Today there are many spa towns all over Portugal. However most spas in Portugal are thermal water resorts aimed at an older market group and offer a very limited type of services. The only true international world-class spa in Portugal is The **Vilalara Thalasso** Spa resort in the fashionable Algarve.

ℹ Direcção-Geral do Turismo
Av. António Augusto de Aguiar, 86 -1050
Apartado 1929 -1004 Lisboa Codex
Tel: (+351-1) 357-5086. Fax: (+351-1) 315-0308

USA
Portuguse National Tourist Office
590 Fifth Ave., 4th Fl., New York NY 10036-4704
tel: (212) 354-4403/4. Fax: (212) 764-6137
Web: www.Portugal.org

ALGARVE
⟩ 82
✈ Faro Airport (FAO) 27 mi. / 43 km.

Vilalara Thalasso
❤❤❤❤

8365 Armação de Pêra, Algarve. Tel: (82) 310-7000. Fax: (82) 314-956. TYPE: Health Resort & Thalassotherapy Center. LOCATION: Beachfront on a cliff in the heart of the Algarve. GENERAL MANAGER: Mr. Wilfried Royer. SPA CLIENTELE: Women and men.

* Suites: 100 luxury suites
* Apartments: 9 self-contained phone, satellite CTV, safe, priv. terrace, A/C
* Restaurants (3), bars/lounges (5)
* Reservations: required
* Open: Year round
* Rates: from 21,000$00 (room only)
* Spa on premises: **Thalassotherapy Center**
* Year established: 1990
* **Spa Packages**: Thalassotherapy from 37,000$00 per person per day; individual treatments from 3,000$00
* **Spa Facilities**: Thalassotherapy Center, relaxation rooms, bar/restaurant, water jet pools, dynamic pool, bathing area, therapy rooms, gym, massage rooms, saunas,Turkish baths, Pediluve, Maniluve
* **Spa Programs**: Beauty, Thalassotherapy, Anti Tobacco cure, Osteopathic treatment, Anti-cellulitis cure
* **Spa Treatments**: massage, pressotherapy, aerosol, algotherapy, acupuncture, shiatsu, beauty treatments (algotherm, la Prairie)
* **Indications**: Anti-stress, physical fitness, smoking cessation, respiratory difficulties, nervous system problems, circulation problem, digestive problems, rheumatic pain, contraction and muscular strain, back pain, headaches, muscular injuries, convalescence
* Medical Supervision: doctors, nurses, physiotherapists, dieticians
* **Web**: www.vilalara.com

DESCRIPTION: Luxury resort hotel in a magnificent beachfront garden location. The Thalassotherapy Center, one of the finest in Europe, offers a wide variety of treatments for beauty, pampering, stress relief and certain medical conditions. Treatments are totally natural based on seawater and its derivatives such as mud, algaes and seaweed. All treatments are under strict medical supervision and can be designed and adapted to your individual need. The "Dietetico" restaurant feature gourmet dishes high in taste but low in calorie. Recreation: tennis, golf, watersports. Member: *"Small Luxury Hotels of the world"*

TERMAS DE CURIA
ˀ 31
✈ Petros Rubras Int'l Airport (OPO), Porto

Aquae Curiva was the name given by the Romans to the thermal springs they discovered and explored during their occupation of the Iberian Peninsula. From the word Curiva came the name of the town Curia, which is one of the oldest and most famous spas in Portugal. The waters at Curia contain mainly sulfates, calcium and magnesium.

The Curia Spa offers a combination of Spa tradition with the comfort of modern technology. The spa specializes in hydrotherapy and thermal cure treatments for a wide range of medical problems under qualified medical staff. However, the spa welcomes international holiday makers to enjoy relaxing and pampering services at the spa for a stress free vacation.

Hotels das termas - Curia is located 8 km. / 5 mi. from the EN1 Mealhada Highway exit, 94 km. / 59 mi. south of Porto and 245 km. / 153 mi. north of Lisbon.

Indications: metabolism, endocrinopathy (particularly gout), calculus and kidney infections, hypertension, rheumatism, and muscular-skeletal illnesses.

Grande Hotel da Curia
♥♥♥

Parque de Curia, 3780 Anadia. Tel: (31) 512720, Fax:

(31) 515317. TYPE: Spa Resort. LOCATION: In the quiet environment of a luxurious park, 1-1/2 hrs. from Lisbon. SPA CLIENTELE: Women and men. MEDICAL RESTRICTIONS: Previous medical appointment obligatory.

* Rooms: 84 with private bath. Suites: 3
* Phone, CTV, A/C, C/H, minibar
* Restaurant, bar, conference rooms (3)
* Airport: Porto - 70 km. / 44 mi.
* Train Station: Curia
* Airport/Train Transportation: Taxi, limo, bus
* Reservations: Required
* Credit Cards: MC, VISA, AMEX
* Season: Year round
* Hotel Rates: from ESC$ 11,000
* Spa: Annex to Hotel Das Termas
* **Spa Facilities**: Health & Fitness Center; sauna, indoor / outdoor pools, gym, beauty salon
* **Spa Treatments**: Massage, electrotherapy; ultrasonic vibrations, short wave and microwave treatments, ultra-violet & infrared rays, diadynamic currents. Treatments for the metabolism, endocrinopathy (particularly gout), calculus & kidney infections, hypertension, rheumatism and muscular-skeletal illnesses; oral water ingestion, bathing (with underwater douche or air bubble), douches (jet or shower) circular and lumbar, automatic hydromassage
* **Spa Packages**: All include 3 treatments per day, medical consulting. 4-14 nights No packages in high season
* **Indications**: see Spa indications
* **Length of Stay Required**: 12 - 14 days
* **Medical Supervision**: 5 MDs
* **Treatments Approved By**: Health Ministry

DESCRIPTION: First class attractive hotel in the grandiose architectural style of the early 20th century. Set on the grounds of a quiet and beautiful park. All rooms and suites are air-conditioned with private bath. The hotel is adjacent to the thermal spa institute and all the spa treatments are available to the guests at the hotel. The Hotel das Thermas offers the ideal setting for a relaxing holiday or a business meeting. Recreation: swimming, tennis, squash, jogging trails, sightseeing.

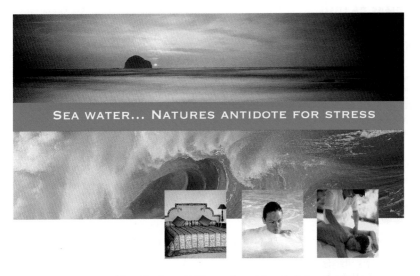

SEA WATER... NATURES ANTIDOTE FOR STRESS

The concept of "small is beautiful", together with secluded park - like gardens, a private bay and a tranquil atmosphere, provide guests of the hotel

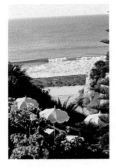

and spa resort of Vilalara with the perfect environment for relaxation.

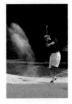

Personal attention and efficient service are the hallmarks of Vilalara's philosophy to provide complete privacy and the highest standards of hospitality. Among the excellent facilities, a choice of low calorie cuisine and the finest gourmet are available.

THALASSOTHERAPY

Vilalara is also home to one of the finest Thalassotherapy Centres in Europe, offering the age-old use of seawater and its natural derivatives such as seaweed and mud, to cleanse, detoxify and deep heal the muscles of the body - all under expert supervision and strict medical guidance. Those who seek both relaxation and the revitalising, invigorating benefits of these totally natural treatments, will find the hotel and spa resort of Vilalara an incomparable destination point on the magic Algarve coast. A true antidote to stress for mind, body and soul.

VILALARA

THALASSO

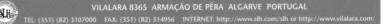

VILALARA 8365 ARMAÇÃO DE PÊRA ALGARVE PORTUGAL

TEL: (351) (82) 3107000   FAX: (351) (82) 314956   INTERNET: http://www.slh.com/slh or http://www.vilalara.com/

TERMAS DE LUSO
⌐ 31

✈ Petros Rubras Int'l Airport (OPO), Porto

Thermas de Luso is a small Spa town in northern Portugal. It is situated on a hill above a valley with a park and lake. Nearby is Buçaco with its centuries old forest. The nearest beaches are located in Mira and Figueira da Foz. The Spa's water composition is subsaline with silicates.

Indications: respiratory system, kidneys/urinary system, rheumatism, and muscular-skeletal ailments.

Grand Hotel de Luso
❤❤❤

Rua dos Banhos, Thermas de Luso P-3050. Tel: (31) 930450. Fax: (31) 930350. TYPE: Resort & Spa Hotel. LOCATION: In a private park in the center of town, a few yards from the spa baths. 171 rooms, 2 suites w/priv. bath, restaurant, pool, jacuzzi, sauna, gym, tennis, squash. Rates: from ESC$ 8,400.

VIDALGO
⌐ 76

✈ Petros Rubras Int'l Airport (OPO), Porto

The Spa of Vidalgo is located in Northern Portugal, 503 km / 314 mi. from Lisbon and 135 km / 85 mi. from Porto. The thermal and climatic Spa is nestled in a verdant area 300 m / 990 ft. above sea level. The thermal water characteristics are: hypothermal, hypersaline, and mesosaline, containing carbonates, carbon dioxide, sodium bi carbonate, low fluoride content, with acid reaction although their function is strongly alkaline. Means of cure: water ingestion, baths, enteroclysis, physiotherapy, intramuscular injec-

tions of mineral water, sauna. **Spa Season**: June 1 - October 15.

Indications: Dyspepsia, hepato-biliary dysfunctions, allergic states, metabolic disturbances, asthma, migraines.

Vidalgo Palace Hotel
❤❤❤❤

Parque, Vidalgo P-5425. Tel: (76) 356/7/8, Fax: (76) 97359. TYPE: Spa Resort. LOCATION: In the quiet environment of a luxurious park with thermal waters. SPA CLIENTELE: Women and men.

* Rooms: 81 with private bath. Suites: 9
* Phone, CTV, A/C, C/H, minibar
* Restaurants (2), bar, conference room
* Airport: Porto - 135 km. / 80 mi.
* Reservations: Required
* Credit Cards: MC, VISA, AMEX
* Open: Year round
* Hotel Rates: from ESC$ 11,000
* Spa: adjacent to Thermal Spa
* **Spa Facilities**: Health & Fitness Center; sauna, indoor / outdoor pools, gym, beauty salon, solarium
* **Spa Treatments**: balneotherapy, hydrotherapy, medical treatments, inhalations, water drinking, physiotherapy
* **Indications**: see Spa indications
* Length of Stay Required: 12 - 14 days
* Medical Supervision: 5 MDs
* Treatments Approved By: Health Ministry

DESCRIPTION: Classic old-world Palace Hotel (1910) in the Spa park with convenient access to the thermal facilities. Recreation: tennis, golf, fishing, clay pigeon shooting, entertainment.

PUERTO RICO

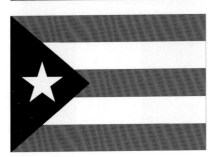

AREA: 3,515 sq. mi. (9,104 sq. km.)
POPULATION: 3,522,037
CAPITAL: San Juan
OFFICIAL LANGUAGES: Spanish, English
CURRENCY: US$
INTERNATIONAL PHONE CODE: 1

Puerto Rico, the shining star of the Caribbean, has a status of American Commonwealth. Located some 1,000 mi. / 1,600 km. southeast of the tip of Florida it is a major air and sea hub of the Caribbean islands. The climate is tropical and stable year round at 76° F (25°c) with cooling trade winds. Puerto Rico offers great beaches, casinos, rain forests, and 500 years of history.

DORADO

) **787**
✈ Luis Munoz Marin Int'l AP (SJU)

Hyatt Regency Dorado Beach & Cerromar Beach
♥♥♥♥♥

Road 693, Dorado PR 00646. Tel: 796-1234. Fax: 796-4647. TYPE: Resort & Spa. LOCATION: Oceanfront on the northern coast, 22 mi / 35 km from San Juan. SPA CLIENTELE: Women and men. DESCRIPTION: Deluxe beach resort hotel with Full health club and spa. Hotel rates: from US$185.

LOS CROABAS

) **787**
✈ Luis Munoz Marin Int'l AP (SJU)

El Conquistador Resort & Country Club
♥♥♥♥♥

1000 El Conquistador Ave., Las Croabas, PR 00738. Tel: 863-1000. Fax: 8634-3280. TYPE: Resort & Spa. LOCATION: Beachfront perched on a cliff overlooking the Caribbean Sea. SPA CLIENTELE: Women and men. DESCRIPTION: Beachfront resort hotel with full service health spa. Hotel rates: from US$345.

RIO MAR

) **787**
✈ Luis Munoz Marin Int'l AP (SJU)

The Westin Rio Mar Beach Resort & Country Club
♥♥♥♥♥

6000 Rio Mar Blvd, PO Box 2006, Rio Mar. Tel: 888-6000. Fax: 888-6600. TYPE: Resort Hotel, Country Club & Spa. LOCATION: Along the northeastern coast. SPA CLIENTELE: Women and men. DESCRIPTION: Beach resort with a spa and casino. Hotel rates: from US$205.

SAN JUAN

) **787**
✈ Luis Munoz Marin Int'l AP (SJU) 9 mi. / 14 km.
Isla Grand Airport (SIG) 4.5 mi. / 7 km.

Caribe Hilton
♥♥♥♥

PO Box 1872, San Juan, PR 00902. Tel: 721-0303. Fax: 725-8849. TYPE: Hotel & Spa. LOCATION: Oceanfront on a secluded beach. SPA CLIENTELE: Women and men. DESCRIPTION: Highrise resort hotel with full service spa.

Hotel rates: from US$195.

Ritz-Carlton San Juan Hotel & Casino
❤❤❤❤

6961 State Rd., 187, Isla Verde, Carolina, PR 00979. Tel: 253-1700. Fax: 253-0700. LOCATION: Beachfront in San Juan's Isla Verde area. SPA CLIENTELE: Women and men. DESCRIPTION: Deluxe resort hotel with full service spa,11 treatment rooms, health club, pool & water sports, casino. 414 rooms & suites. Hotel rates: from US$300

San Juan Grand Beach Resort & Casino
❤❤❤❤❤

Isla Verde Road 187, Isla Verde, PO Box 6676, Santurce, PR 00914.Tel: 791-6100. Fax: 791-8525. TYPE: Resort Casino Hotel & Spa. LOCATION: Beachfront of 5 tropical acres with 3 mi / 5 km of white sand. SPA CLIENTELE: Women and men. DESCRIPTION: Impressive resort hotel with a full service health spa. Hotel rates: from US$225.

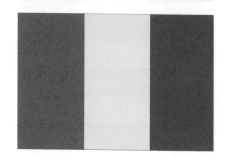

ROMANIA

AREA: 91,699 sq. mi. (237,500 sq. km.)
POPULATION: 23,250,000
CAPITAL: Bucharest
OFFICIAL LANGUAGE: Romanian
CURRENCY: Lei (ROL)
EXCHANGE RATE: 1US$ = ROL 630
TELEPHONE COUNTRY CODE: 40

Romania has over 160 health spas in different parts of the country which are known for their mineral springs, mud baths, and beautiful natural surroundings. Most of the Romanian spas specialize in medical treatments. Romanian spas offer Geriatric treatments based on Gerovital H3 and Aslavital products developed by the late Dr. Ana Aslan to combat aging and premature aging diseases.

ℹ️ Romania Ministry of Tourism
17 Apolodor St., 70663 Bucharest V, Romania
Fax: (+40-1) 3120481

USA
Romanian Nat'l Tourist Office
14 East 38th St., 12th Fl. New York NY 10016
Tel: (212) 545-8484. Fax: (212) 251-0429

BAILE FELIX
🌙 **59**
✈️ Otopeni Int'l AP (OTP) Bucharest

Baile Felix, the largest health resort in Romania lies 8 km.

(3 mi.) from Oradea in northwestern Romania, near the border with Hungary. Its elevated location 459 ft. (140 m.) above sea level, accounts for the resort's microclimate which is mild with only a slight temperature variations. The average temperature is 50°F (10°c) with a January mean temperature of 30°F (-1°c) and August mean temperature of 69°F (20°c). The spa's slightly radioactive waters and therapeutic mud are recommended for afflictions of the locomotory apparatus, nervous and digestive ailments. Baile Felix is a year round health resort.

Baile Felix Spa
♥♥♥

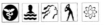

Baile Felix R-3733. TYPE: Health Spa. Accommodations: **Nufarul Hotel** (78 rooms & suites) Tel: (59) 261142, Fax: (59) 136532. **Thermal Hotel** Tel: (59) 261215, Fax: (59) 133231. **Poienita Hotel** Tel: (59) 261172. SPA CLIENTELE: Women and men.

* Rooms: 600 plus w/priv. bath (various hotels)
* Airport: Oradea, 5 miles (8 km.), bus or trams
* Train: local station
* Hotel Rates: from US$40/day
* Spa Water Composition: Bicarbonated, oligometallic thermal mineral waters rich in sodium, sulfate, calcium, silicium; slightly radioactive; temperature from 68°F -118°F (20°c - 48°c)
* **Spa Facilities**: Indoor and outdoor pools, thermal pools, tub, mud baths, inhalation rooms, massage rooms, gym, consulting rooms
* **Spa Programs**: Revitalization,rejuvenation, relaxation, general fitness, beauty and medical
* **Spa Treatments**: Hot mineral baths, mixed peat-bog and fissile sapropelic hot mud wraps, kinetotherapy, vertebral traction, electrotherapy, hydrotherapy, paraffin wraps, gynecological therapy, inhalation and aerosols, rehabilitation and medical gymnastics
* **Indications**: Inflammatory, degenerative and abarticular rheumatic diseases, post-traumatic afflictions, central and peripheral nervous system afflictions and associated metabolic, nutrition, endocrine and gynecological
* Medical Supervision: Medical section for muscular

articular tests & functional explorations, clinical laboratories and radiology section
* Treatment Approval: Romanian govn't.
* Treatment Duration: varies 14-21 days
* Special Geriatric Treatments: Gerovital H3, Aslavital, special Pell-amar, Ulcosivanil and Boicil Forte.

DESCRIPTION: Modern highrise Hotels & Spa overlooking Baile Felix offering balneary cure. Accommodations facilities 6,320 beds in two and three star hotels, with restaurants and therapy centers, fully integrated into the hotel-thermal treatment system.

BAILE HERCULANE
 ⟩ 55
✈ Otopeni Int'l AP (OTP) Bucharest

Baile Herculane is an historic spa in the southwest of Romania on the banks of the Cerna River. The Spa stretches to the foot of the Domogled massif at an altitude of 524 ft. (1,100 m.) above sea level amidst a famous nature reserve. Although the spa is in a mountainous zone it enjoys a fine Mediterranean like climate. The average annual temperature is 49°F (9°c) with a January mean of 30°F (-1°c) and a July mean of 72°F (22°c). The surrounding forests shield the resort from strong winds. Winters are mild with little snow, and the summers are cool.

Baile Herculane Spa
♥♥♥

Baile Herculane R-1600. TYPE: Health Spa. Accommodations: **Roman Hotel** (182 rooms) Tel: (55) 560390, **Minerva Hotel** Tel: (55) 560767; **Diana Hotel**, Baile Herculane R-1600, Tel (55) 5607030. SPA CLIENTELE: Women and men.

* Rooms: 500 w/priv. bath
* Train Station: local station 3 mi. / 5 km., bus
* Hotel rates: from US$40
* Spa Water Composition: Oligometallic thermal mineral waters rich in sulfate, calcium, magnesium; temperature 106°F -140°F (41°c - 60°c)
* **Spa Facilities**: Indoor and outdoor swimming pools,

thermal pools, tub, mud baths, inhalation rooms, massage rooms, gymnasium, consulting rooms, sauna
* **Spa Programs**: Rehabilitation, revitalization, relaxation, general fitness, beauty and medical
* **Spa Treatments**: Hot mineral baths, kinetotherapy, electro and hydrotherapy, gynecological therapy, inhalations, aerosols, ultrasound, acupuncture, massage, apiphytotherapy, balneary therapy, gymnastics, massage, Asian therapy, reducing cures, cosmetic sessions.
* **Indications**: locomotor apparatus and peripheral nervous system diseases, posttraumatic locomotor sequels, myosites, tendinites, chronic synosites and associated diseases, gynecological, upper respiratory, digestive, chemical poisoning,diabetes, eye diseases
* **Medical Supervision**: Medical rehabilitation radiology, stomatology, and laboratory
* **Treatments Approved**: Romanian govn't.
* **Treatment Duration**: 14-21 days
* **Special Geriatric Treatments**: Gerovital H3, Aslavital, special Pell amar, and Boicil forte

DESCRIPTION: Modern highrise Hotels & Spa overlooking the town and the mountains. Accommodations facilities 1,100 beds in 2 and 3 stars hotels, and 2,700 beds in villas of the 1-4 stars levels. All hotels are linked by passageways to the medical services; they also include restaurants and coffee houses.

BUCHAREST

➔ 1

✈ Otopeni Int'l Airport (OTP) 11 mi. / 18 km. North
Baneasa Airport (BBU) 5-1/2 mi. / 9 km. North

Bucharest, population 2,000,000, is the political, economic and cultural capital of Romania. It is situated on a forest plain just 37 miles (61 km) from the Danube River and 80 miles (130 km) from the Carapthian Mountains. The city shows a certain French influence dating from the early 1930's and manifested by the broad boulevards, outdoor cafes and restaurants. Even the replica of the Arcul de Triumf is there to remind you of Paris. Other attractions include large parks, lakes and monuments.

In 1952 the first geriatric institute in the world was established in Bucharest and five years later "Gerovital H3" was medically approved for treatments. The drug was developed by the late Professor Dr. Ana Aslan after a long and painstaking scientific experiments. Few years later a new biotophic product - Aslavital was developed.

Flora Hotel
♥♥♥♥

🐵 ♨ 🏇 🏃 ❀

1 Blvd. Poligrafiei, Bucharest 71556. Tel: (1) 222-3900. Fax: (1) 312-8344. TYPE: Geriatric Cure Hotel & Spa. LOCATION: In the northern outskirts lakes and parks district of Bucharest near Herastrau Park. SPA CLIENTELE: Women and men (mature clientele).

* Rooms: 155 w/private bath
* Suites w/air-conditioning
* Phone, radio, TV, refrigerators
* Restaurant (special diets), lounge, brasserie, bar
* Airport: Bucharest, 12 mi. / 19 km., taxi, bus
* Open: year round
* Hotel Rates: from US$115 (room only)
* Spa on premises: **Flora Geriatric Cure**
* **Spa Facilities**: consulting rooms, laboratories, swimming pool, gym, sauna, solariums, balneo-physiotherapy centre, cosmetic centre
* **Spa Programs**: Rejuvenation, revitalization, relaxation, stress reduction, general fitness, beauty, Geriatric Programs
* **Spa Treatments**: Electrotherapy, hydrotherapy, rehabilitation exercises, massage, baths, medical gymnastics & cosmetics, Gerovital H3, Aslavital
* **Indications**: Physical and intellectual asthenia, aging of skin, hair & nails, articulation diseases of rheumatic origin atherosclerosis, arterial hypertension, angina pectoris infection sequels, Parkinson's disease,neuritis, arthroses, spondyloses, osteopareses, psoriasis, bronchial asthma, gastroduodenal ulcer, hormonal disturbances
* **Medical Supervision**: medical personnel with knowledge of foreign languages

DESCRIPTION: The hotel has a semi-circular shape, on three floors with a patio and two elevators. The Spa program is medically oriented and geared towards the treatment of geriatric problems. Recreation: golf, tennis courts, and bowling facilities nearby.

Otopeni Clinical Centre
❤❤❤

Bucharest. Fax: (1) 3120481. TYPE: Clinical Centre. LOCATION: 10 miles / 16 km north of Bucharest on main hwy (DN 1). SPA CLIENTELE: Women and men.

* Rooms: 120 w/priv. bath and balconies
* Doubles and suites for 300 guest
* Phone, radio, TV
* Restaurant (special diets), shops, handicraft kiosk
* Beauty parlor, barber shop
* Airport: Bucharest 1 km. / 1/2 mi.
* Airport Transportation: taxi, bus
* Open: year round
* Rates: from US$115, Special Geriatric
  treatment from US$660/2 weeks.
* Spa on premises
* **Spa Facilities**: consulting rooms, laboratories, x-ray, pool, gym, pharmacy, emergency ward
* **Spa Programs**: Rejuvenation, revitalization, relaxation, stress reduction, general fitness, Geriatric Programs
* **Spa Treatments**: Electrotherapy, hydrotherapy, rehabilitation exercises, massage, baths, medical gymnastics, medical cosmetics, Gerovital H3, Aslavital
* **Indications**: Physical and intellectual asthenia, aging of the skin, hair and nails, articulation diseases of rheumatic origin atherosclerosis, arterial hypertension, angina pectoris infection sequels, Parkinson's disease, neuritis, arthroses, spondyloses, osteopareses, psoriasis, bronchial asthma, gastroduodenal ulcer, hormonal disturbances
* Medical Supervision: medical personnel with knowledge of foreign languages

DESCRIPTION: Renovated ancient palace hotel built in a large park area featuring a medical program specializing in geriatric treatments. Daily bus service assures transport to and from Bucharest center.

COASTAL SPAS: Eforie Nord / Mangalia / Neptun
☾ 41
✈ Constantsa Airport

Coastal spas are a string of black sea resorts south of Constanta which are known as the "Mythology Belt" of the sea coast "miracle" cures. The Coastal spas can be accessed from Constantsa by regular bus service or taxi. The resorts have sandy shores on one side and easy access to a chain of fresh water lakes on the other. Lake Techirghiol is the main source of the effective sapropedic mud, and is highly recommended for the treatment of rheumatic ailments.

A number of centers in the area offer thermal treatment facilities. The best known are **Eforie Nord**, **Neptun**, and **Mangalia**. Eforie Nord is the northernmost of the three, sitting between Lake Techirghiol and the Black sea. Neptun is relatively a new resort among others whose development begun in 1960 and are all named after planets. Mangalia is the southernmost coastal resort built right on the site of the Greek city of Callatis. The average annual mean temperature is 52°F (11°c) . It is around 70°F (21°c) in the Summer with high humidity.

The natural cure factors of the spas consist of the climate, the therapeutic waters (mesothermal waters, Black Sea water, salt water), the sapropelic mud, and the beach sand. The mesothermal waters are sulfurous, bicarbonated, sodic and hypotonic. The sea water temperature in the Summer is between 75°F - 8°2F (24°c - 28°c). Lake Techirghiol's water contains predominantly sodium chloride, but it is also rich in sodium, bromide, magnesium, and potassium. The lake's sapropelic mud is rich in organic mineral substances, humic acids, estrogenes, regenerating enzymes, vitamins (C, E, B2, B12), and biostimulators. The peat mud and sand are used externally for hot wraps and baths.

Indications: locomotor afflictions related to inflammatory, degenerative and abarticular rheumatism, orthopedic afflictions, peripheral nervous disorders, skin diseases, gynecological diseases and metabolic disturbances. Aerosol treatments are applied for asthmatic bronchitis, rhinites and sinusitis. Internal cure is applied for some digestive and renal afflictions.

Doina Cure Hotel
♥♥♥

Neptun-Olimp 8720. Tel: (41) 731818. TYPE: Spa Hotel. LOCATION: Overlooking the sea. SPA CLIENTELE: Family oriented.

* Rooms: 330 doubles w/private bath
* Phone, C/H, A/C, TV in rooms
* Restaurant, bar, disco
* Swimming pool, sport grounds
* Airport: Constantsa 12 mi. / 20 km, taxi, bus
* Train: Local station
* Open: Year round
* Hotel Rates: from US$70/day
* Spa on premises
* **Spa Facilities**: Indoor pool, thermal pools, tubs, inhalation rooms, mud baths, massage rooms, gym,sauna, consulting rooms
* **Spa Programs**: Revitalization, rejuvenation, relaxation,fitness, medical, Geriatric Programs
* **Spa Treatments**: Thermal baths, sea water baths, underwater douche, mud therapy, electrotherapy, hydrotherapy, rehabilitation and medical gymnastics
* **Special Geriatric Treatments**: Gerovital H3, Aslavital, Pell Amar, and Boicil Forte
* Treatment Duration: 14-21 days
* Medical Supervision: medical personnel with knowledge of foreign languages
* Treatments Approved: Romanian govn't.

DESCRIPTION: Six story deluxe hotel with in house treatment facilities in a small park overlooking the Black Sea. The Doina Hotel is part of the Neptun balveary complex. Recreation: swimming, volleyball, tennis, minigolf, bowling, water sports, cabaret programs.

Eforie Nord Spa
♥♥

Tudor Valdimirescu Blvd., Eforie Nord 8712. **Meduza Hotel** Tel: (41) 742770 or 742772, Fax: (41) 742980. **Delfinu Hotel**, Tel: 41-742630 or 742632. **Steaua de**

Mare Hotel, Tel: 41-742480 or 742482.TYPE: Balneary Tourist Complex. LOCATION: connected to the Delfinul, Medzua, and Steaua de Mare Hotels by a heated lobby walkway. SPA CLIENTELE: Women and men.

* Rooms: 1,200 (various hotels)
* Airport: Constanta 7 mi. / 12 km.
* Airport Transportation: taxi, bus
* Train: local station
* Spa Facilities: Indoor swimming pool, thermal pools, tubs, mud baths, inhalation & massage rooms, gymnasium, sauna, 20 consulting rooms
* **Spa Programs**: Revitalization, rejuvenation, relaxation, general fitness, beauty, medical, Geriatric
* **Spa Treatments**: Hot mineral baths, hot sea water, mixed peat-bog and fissile sapropelic hot mud wraps, kinetotherapy, electro and hydrotherapy, gynecological therapy, inhalation and aerosols, vertebral elongation, rehabilitation, medical gymnastics.
* **Special Geriatric treatments**: Gerovital H3, Asiavital, Pellamar, Boicil Forte
* Medical Supervision: medical personnel with knowledge of foreign languages
* Treatments Approved: Romanian govn't.
* Treatment Duration: 14-21 days

DESCRIPTION: This resort offers hotel rooms and villas in 1-3 star level mostly in the balneary-tourist complex formed by the "Delfinul", Meduza" and Steaua de Mare" hotels (2 stars) which are directly linked to the cure center. Recreation: minigolf, summer theatre, electronic games, billiard, disco, water slides and water sports.

Europa Hotel
♥♥♥

20 Republicii Blvd, Eforie Nord, Romania 8712. Tel: (41) 742990. TYPE: Spa Hotel. LOCATION: 390 feet (100 meters) from the beach. SPA CLIENTELE: Family oriented.

* Rooms: 242 w/private bath and balconies
* Phone, TV, swimming pool
* Restaurant, brasserie, bar

* Tourist shops, hairdresser's Salon
* Currency exchange, tourist office
* Central heating, elevators, parking
* Spa off premises: Cure Sanatorium
* Open: Year round
* Hotel Rates: from US$55

DESCRIPTION: Highrise hotel in a small park overlooking the Black Sea. Spa treatments are available at the Cure Sanatorium. Many leisure activities available nearby.

Mangalia Cure Hotel
♥♥♥

Mangalia 8712. Tel: (41) 751968. TYPE: Balneary Hotel. LOCATION: In a small park overlooking the Black Sea. SPA CLIENTELE: Family oriented.

* Rooms: 293 w/private bath
* Phone, TV in rooms
* Restaurant, bar, disco
* Central heating, elevators, parking
* Swimming pool, sauna, sport grounds
* Airport: Constanta 21 mi. / 36 km.
* Airport Transportation: taxi, bus
* Train: Local station
* Open: Year round
* Hotel Rates: from US $57/day
* Spa on premises
* **Spa Facilities**: Indoor pool, thermal pools, tubs, inhalation rooms, mud baths, massage rooms, gymnasium, sauna, consulting rooms
* **Spa Programs**: Revitalization, rejuvenation, relaxation, fitness, medical, Geriatric Programs
* **Spa Treatments**: Sulfurous mesothermal baths, carbon dioxide baths, sea water baths, underwater douche, mud therapy, kinetotherapy, electrotherpay, hydrotherapy, gynecological therapy, inhalation and aerosols, vertebral elongation, pneumotherapy, rehabilitation and medical gymnastics
* Treatment Duration: 14-21 days
* Medical Supervision: medical personnel with knowledge of foreign languages
* Treatments Approved: Romanian govn't.

DESCRIPTION: A highrise cure hotel with its own in house medical treatment facilities in the Balneary complex which has an integrated therapy centre. Recreation: indoor pool, horseback riding, tennis, minigolf, water sports.

COVASNA
1

✈ Bacau Airport 93 mi. / 150 km.

Located in central Romania at the foot of the western Vrancea mountains, Covasna Spa "The watering place of the 1,000 health springs" is the most popular spa for the cure of the heart and circulatory diseases. The climate is cool and refreshing with a yearly average temperature of 8°c / 48°F.

Indications: digestive tract diseases - chronic hypo and hyperacid gastritis, ulcerous diseases; diseases of the bile, bladder and ducts - stabilized chronic hepatitis; affections of the kidney and urinary ducts; degenerative affections of old age; nutrition diseases - gout, diabetes, obesity; affections of the locomotor apparatus, rheumatism, sexual neuroses, different types of sexual impotence.

Covasna Spa
♥♥♥

Covasna. Reservation - Fax: (1) 3122594. TYPE: Spa Complex. LOCATION: Intramountain location north of Bucarest. SPA CLIENTELE: Women and men.

* Rooms: 600 w/private bath (various hotels)
* Phone, CTV, C/H
* Restaurant, bars, coffee shops, elevators, parking, reading room, conference hall
* Airport: Bucharest, Train: Local station
* Spa on premises
* Open: Year round
* Hotel Rates: from US$70
* **Spa Facilities**: thermal pools, tubs, inhalation rooms, mud baths, massage rooms, fitness center, sauna, consulting rooms, beauty center

* **Spa Programs**: Revitalization, rejuvenation, relaxation, general fitness, medical
* **Spa Treatments**: Thermal baths, salt water baths, underwater douche, sapropelic mud therapy, heliotherapy, kinetotherapy, electrotherapy, hydrotherapy, paraffin wraps, rehabilitation and medical gymnastics
* **Indications**: see Covasna Spa
* **Medical Supervision**: medical personnel with knowledge of foreign languages
* **Treatments Approved**: Romanian govn't.

DESCRIPTION: Modern Spa complex with hotels and villas from 1 to 4 stars. The hotels include therapy sections and restaurants.

SINAIA
⟩ 44
✈ Otopeni Int'l Airport (OTP) 78 mi. / 125 km.

The resort of Sinaia, the "Pearl of the Carpathians" is located 125 km / 78 mi. north of Bucharest. It combines mountain resort, winter sports and climatic health spa. Located on the River Prahova Valley, at the foot of the Bucegi mountains at 800 m / 2,640 ft. it has a cool 6°c / 43°F yearly average temperature. Sinaia Spa offers bioclimate, pure air rich in UV radiation, and thermal sulphurous, bicarbonated, oligomineral water.

Indications: asthenic neurosis, endocrine affections, occupational diseases, rheumatismal diseases, affections of the digestive tract and of the annex glands, physical asthenia, stress.

Mara Hotel
❤❤❤❤

Sinaia R-2180. Reservation - Fax: (1) 312-0481. TYPE: Spa Complex. LOCATION: Overlooking the lake. SPA CLIENTELE: Popular with women.

* Rooms: 150 w/private bath

* Phone, CTV, C/H
* Restaurant, bars, coffee shops, elevators, parking, reading room, conference hall
* Airport: Bucharest, Train: Local station
* Spa on premises
* Open: Year round
* Hotel Rates: from US$70
* **Spa Facilities**: thermal pools, tubs, inhalation rooms, mud baths, massage rooms, fitness center, sauna, consulting rooms, beauty center
* **Spa Programs**: Revitalization, rejuvenation, relaxation, general fitness, medical
* **Spa Treatments**: Thermal baths, salt water baths, underwater douche, sapropelic mud therapy, heliotherapy, kinetotherapy, electrotherapy, hydrotherapy, paraffin wraps, rehabilitation and medical gymnastics
* **Indications**: see Sinaia Spa
* **Medical Supervision**: medical personnel with knowledge of foreign languages
* **Treatments Approved**: Romanian govn't.

DESCRIPTION: Modern 4-star spa hotel complex with swimming pool, tennis, squash, casino and shopping. Recreation: skiing (winter), fishing, hiking, alpinism (summer).

SOVATA
⟩ 65
✈ Tirgu Mures Airport

Sovata lies in the central Transylvanian Plateau at an altitude of 1740 ft. (530 m.) above sea level. It has won its fame thanks to the exceptional therapeutic properties of the salt water of its heliothermal lakes. The concentrated sodium chloride waters of the five lakes Urus, Alunis, Negru, Rosu and Verde are the main cure source of the spa. Sovata has a dry subalpine climate with clean air. Winters are mild; summers cool; and autumns prolonged. The annual average temperature is 48°F (9°c). The January mean temperature is 25°F (-4°c); the July mean is 65°F (18°c).

Indications: Gynecological, rheumatic and peripheral nervous diseases, secondary sterility, diseases of the locomotor apparatus, arthrosis.

Sovata Spa
❤❤❤

Sovata Hotel (164 rooms), Str Trandafirilor 85, Sovata Spa R-3295. Tel: (65) 578151, Fax: (65) 578335. Bradet Hotel (90 rooms), Str Trandafirilor, Spa Complex, Sovata R-3295, Tel: (65) 578311. Alunis Hotel (130 rooms) Tel: (65) 678801. TYPE: Spa Complex. LOCATION: Overlooking the lake. SPA CLIENTELE: Popular with women.

* Rooms: 500 w/private bath (various hotels)
* Phone, CTV, C/H
* Restaurant, bars, coffee shops, elevators, parking, reading room, conference hall
* Airport: Tirgu Mures 37 mi. / 61 km., bus or train
* Train: Local station
* Spa on premises
* Open: Year round
* Hotel Rates: from US$70
* Spa Facilities: thermal pools, tubs, inhalation rooms, mud baths, massage rooms, gym, sauna, consulting rooms, laboratories
* Spa Programs: Revitalization, rejuvenation, relaxation, general fitness, medical
* Spa Treatments: Thermal baths, salt water baths, underwater douche, sapropelic mud therapy, heliotherapy, kinetotherapy, electrotherapy, hydrotherapy, paraffin wraps, rehabilitation and medical gymnastics
* Geriatric Treatments: Gerovital H3, Aslavital, Pell Amar and Boicil Forte
* Indications: Degenerative, inflammatory and abarticular rheumatism, posttraumic and peripheral nervous system afflictions, gynecological disorders, endocrine and cardiovascular disorders, varicose ulcerous, acrocyanosis, Raynaud's disease
* Medical Supervision: medical personnel with knowledge of foreign languages
* Treatments Approved: Romanian govn't.

DESCRIPTION: All hotels are linked by interconnected by lobby walkways to the balneo cure establishment of the Sovata Spa. Recreation: swimming. casino, electronic games, ski facilities.

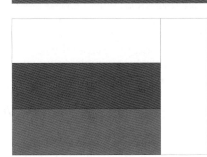

RUSSIA

AREA: 6,592,812 sq. mi. (17,075,400 sq. km.)
POPULATION: 147,500,000
CAPITAL: Moscow
OFFICIAL LANGUAGE: Russian
CURRENCY: Rubel
EXCHANGE RATE: 1 US$ = R 17.45
COUNTRY TELEPHONE CODE: 7

MOSCOW
☎ 095
✈ Domodedovo Airport (DME) 25 mi. / 40 km.
Sheremetyevo Airport (SVO) 18 mi. / 29 km.
Vnukovo Airport (VKO) 18 mi. / 29 km.

Aerostar Hotel
❤❤❤❤

37 Leningradsy Prospekt, Korpus 9, Moscow 125167. Tel: (502) 213-9000. Fax: (502) 213-9001. TYPE: Hotel with Health Club. LOCATION: Centrally located across from Petrovsky Palace and Dynamo Stadium. SPA CLIENTELE: Women and men. DESCRIPTION: Elegant hotel with full health club, gym, sauna, massage, exercise equipment and aerobics. 413 rooms, 8 suites, restaurants, bars. Hotel rates: from US$235.

Hotel Metropole Moscow
❤❤❤❤❤

1/4 Teatrainy Proezd, Moscow 103012. Tel: (501)927-6000. Fax: (501) 927-6010. TYPE: Hotel with Health Club. LOCATION: Centrally located in downtown Moscow, just a few minutes walk to the Red Square, Kremlin and Bolshoi Theatre. SPA CLIENTELE: Women and men. DESCRIPTION: Elegant Landmark Hotel built at the turn of the century (1903) with beautifully appointed Fitness Center, well-equipped gym, saunas, massage, indoor swimming pool. 403 rooms, 70 suites, restaurants, bars, lounges, night club, casino. Hotel rates: from US$310.

SOCHI
⌐ 862
✈ Sochi Airport, 17 mi. / 27 km.

Sochi is the largest and most popular Russian Black Sea resort. It owes its popularity to the proximity of the medicinal springs, some 8 mi / 13 km from the city center. Sochi has a pleasant subtropical climate. The average temperature in January and February is 43°F (6°c). The summer heat (85°F/29°c) is tempered by sea breezes. The summer season starts in mid-June and lasts through mid-October. The most pleasant season is Autumn when the humidity falls; there are long hours of sunshine and the mountain winds are warm.

The first baths were built in the early 1900's, but no real medical supervision was available until the 1950's when new installations were built for treatment. The wells yield several million gallons a day of thermal water and contain 27 different elements. Sulfureted hydrogen, chlorides and sodium in various concentrations provide the treatments.

Indications: treatments of muscle, bone and joint diseases, nervous and cardio-vascular systems, women's gynecological disorders and skin afflictions, bronchial, lung and nervous complaints.

Dagomys Tourist Complex
♥♥♥

7 Leningradskaya St., Sochi 354224. Tel: (862) 232-1600. TYPE: Resort Complex & Spa. LOCATION: Between the Sea and Intourist's motor route "The Great Caucasian

Ring" 12 miles (20 km) from the city center. SPA CLIENTELE: Men, Women.

* Rooms: 1,361 w/priv. bath. Suites: 97
* Restaurants: 7, Coffee Shops, Bars
* Spa on premises: Polyclinic
* Spa Water Composition: Sulfuretted hydrogen, chlorides and sodium
* Airport: Sochi 26 mi. / 43 km.
* Train Station: Sochi 11 mi. / 18 km.
* Open: Year round
* Hotel Rates: from US$90/day
* Treatment duration: 24 days
* Spa Facilities: Thermal pools, inhalation, massage & diagnostic rooms, sun terrace, 3 salt water swimming pools, sports facilities
* Spa Programs: Rejuvenation, relaxation, general fitness, beauty and medical
* Spa Treatments: Injections underwater & general massage, sunbathing, remedial exercise, sea radon, iodine-bromine & coniferous baths, remedial inhalation, gynecological washing, poultices
* Indications: Cardiovascular, nervous, gynecological, locomotive and skin disorders
* Medical Supervision: Over 70 Medical Services including biological analysis, x-ray, functional diagnostics, hydropathy, therapeutics, stonatology, gynecology, surgery, and optometry
* Translation Services: during treatment and doctor examination
* Treatment Approval: Polyclinic

DESCRIPTION: A modern complex on 60 acres (24 hectares) with access to the sea by one of six lifts or a stairway. It consist of the 115 room Meridian Motel built in 1980, the 230 room Olymiyskaya Hotel built in 1981, the 1013 room Dagomys Hotel built in 1982 and the the newly opened Polyclinic treatment center. A large forest park borders the complex on the east.

Kamelia Hotel
♥♥♥

Kurortny Prospekt 89, Sochi 354032. Tel: (862) 299-

0398. TYPE: Resort Hotel & Spa. LOCATION: In a large park near the beach 3 miles (4 km) from the city center. SPA CLIENTELE: Men, Women.

* Rooms: 184 w/priv. bath. Suites: 31 two room
* Restaurants, coffee shops, bars
* Airport: Sochi 19 mi. / 31 km.
* Seaport: Sochi 3 mi. / 5 km.
* Train Station: Sochi 3 mi. / 5 km.
* Transportation: Intourist car, bus, taxi,
* Season: Year round
* Rates: from US$90/day
* Treatment duration: 24 days
* Spa off premises: Polyclinic No. 1
* Spa Water Composition: Sulfuretted hydrogen, chlorides and sodium
* **Spa Facilities:** Thermal pools, inhalation, massage & diagnostic rooms, sauna bath, 3 salt water swimming pools, sports facilities
* **Spa Programs:** Rejuvenation, relaxation, general fitness, beauty and medical
* **Spa Treatments:** Injections underwater & general massage, sunbathing, remedial exercise, sea radon, iodine-bromine and coniferous baths, remedial inhalation, gynecological washing, poultices
* **Indications:** Cardiovascular, nervous, gynecological, locomotive and skin disorders
* Medical Supervision: Over 70 Medical services including biological analysis, x-ray, functional diagnostics, hydropathy, therapeutics, stonatology, gynecology, surgery, and optometry
* Translation Services: during treatment and doctor examination
* Treatment Approval: Polyclinic

DESCRIPTION: Two multistory hotels in a large park near the beach with medical treatment rooms, sauna and massage. Spa treatments are at the nearby Polyclinic No. 1.

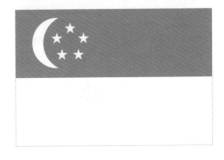

AREA: 226 sq. mi. (585 sq. km.)
POPULATION: 2,704,000
CAPITAL: Singapore
OFFICIAL LANGUAGES: Chinese, Malay, Tamil, English
CURRENCY: Singapore dollar (S$)
EXCHANGE RATE: 1 US$ = S$ 1.65
COUNTRY TELEPHONE CODE: 65

SINGAPORE

꒐ No area code
✈ Changi Int'l Airport (SIN) 11 mi. / 18 km.

Clark Hatch Life Spa
♥♥♥♥♥

c/o Pan Pacific Hotel, 7 Raffles Bolvd, #04-00, Singapore City 939595. Hotel Tel: 336-8111, Fax: 339-1861. Spa Tel: 334-5139, Fax: 333-4586. TYPE: Hotel & Spa. LOCATION: 5 minutes to financial district & 10 minutes to Orchard Street. DESCRIPTION: Deluxe hotel with full service spa & fitness center, gym, sauna, massage. 784 rooms & suites, nonsmoker rooms. Restaurants (5), coffee shop, lounge, meeting facilities, business center, tennis courts (2), outdoor pool. Hotel rates: from S$300.

Lifestyle Spa & Fitness Centre
♥♥♥♥

c/o Merchant Court Hotel, 20 Merchant Road, Singapore

City 058281. Hotel Tel: 337-2288, Fax: 334-0606. Spa Tel: 438-7080, Fax: 438-7090. TYPE: Hotel & Spa. LOCATION: Near the Singapore River, within walking distance of China town and Festival Village. DESCRIPTION: Contemporary hotel with full service Health Spa & Fitness Center. 476 rooms 7 suites, nonsmoker rooms, wheelchair access. 3 food & beverage outlets, meeting facilities, business center, pool. Hotel rates: from S$260.

Ritz Carlton Millenia Singapore
♥♥♥♥♥

7 Raffles Ave., Singapore City 039799. Tel: 337-888. Fax: 338-0001. TYPE: Hotel & Spa. LOCATION: On 7 acres in the heart of the Marina Centre. SPA CLIENTELE: Women and men. DESCRIPTION: Impressive high-rise deluxe hotel with Fitness Center, gym, sauna, massage, steam room, aerobics, jacuzzi, outdoor pool, tennis. 608 rooms, 80 suites, Summer Pavilion, Greenhouse Restaurant, lobby lounge, ballroom, business center. Hotel rates: from S$430.

Sheraton Towers Singapore
♥♥♥♥♥

39 Scotts Rd., Singapore City 22830. Tel: 737-6888. Fax: 737-1072. TYPE: Hotel & Spa. LOCATION: Central, 10 min. walk to Orchard Road main shopping district. SPA CLIENTELE: Women and men. DESCRIPTION: Deluxe hotel with Health Club, gym, fitness trainer, aerobics, physical therapist on site, indoor pool, sauna, massages. 411 rooms, 22 suites, restaurants, atrium bar. Hotel rates: from S$370.

St Gregory Javanna Spa
♥♥♥♥

c/o Hotel Plaza, 7500A Beach Road #03-00, Singapore City 199591. Hotel Tel: 298-0011, Fax: 296-3600. Spa Tel: 290-8028, Fax: 290-8063. TYPE: Hotel & Spa. LOCATION: Edge of business district, 20 km. / 13 mi. to airport. DESCRIPTION: Crescent shaped moderate first class hotel with full service spa, gym, steam bath, squash court. 350 rooms & suites. Restaurant, cafe, lounge, Karaoke, business center, outdoor pool. Hotel rates: from S$230.

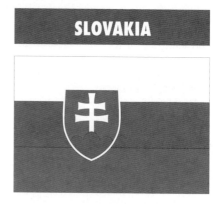

SLOVAKIA

AREA: 18,928 sq. mi. (48,455 sq. km.)
POPULATION: 5,000,000
CAPITAL: Bratislava
OFFICIAL LANGUAGE: Slovak
CURRENCY: Slovak Crown (Sk)
EXCHANGE RATE: 1US$ = Sk 36.55
COUNTRY TELEPHONE CODE: 421

The history of Slovak Spas dates back to Roman times when they were discovered by Marcus Aurelius and his legions. The health restoring mineral springs attract thousands of spa goers from all over the world. Most of the Spas are concentrated in the northern and western regions of the Slovak Republic along the River Vah. Teplice is the oldest of the Slovak Spas. All of the Spa programs include medical supervision and treatments.

ⓘ Tetra Travel
212 E. 51st St., New York NY 10022. USA Tel: (212) 466-0533. Fax: (212) 486-1456

BARDEJOV
✈ Kosice Airport

Bardejov, population 17,400, is a mineral springs Spa in northeastern Slovakia near the Polish border. It is located in a colorful valley setting on the southern slopes of the Carpatian mountains. It enjoys a mild climate, with an annual average temperature of 13°c (55°F). The natural curative mineral waters and climatic conditions make this

Spa an excellent health resort.

Spa treatments are based on the curative agents that are found in the mineral water of some 8 mineral springs. The strong alkaline-hydrocarbonic water contain: sodium, chloride,·with traces of lithium, zinc, cobalt etc., which is administered for therapeutic purposes in the forms of drinking cures, inhalations, and mineral baths. Modern balneotherapy provides a variety of treatments and facilities, including a covered mineral pool, two beaches for rehabilitation and recreation. Special diets and regular daily spa programs are also part of the complex treatment offered at the spa.

There is a museum of folk architecture on the spa premises, and nearby you can visit an interesting wooden Orthodox church dating from the 18th century. There are many old Gothic style villages that are worth a visit in the region. Bardejov Spa can be reached by air-travel to Kosice or Poprad airport, and then by bus to the Spa. You may also take the train to Presov, and then by bus to the Spa.

Indications: disorders of the digestive system, ulcers, liver diseases, as well as diseases of the pancreas and intestines. The Spa also treats diabetes, and illnesses of metabolic disturbances. Patients are accommodated at the sanatorium Ozón (see description below) which is directly connected with the balneotherapeutic center.

Bardejovské Kúpele - Ozón
♥♥♥

Bardejovské Kúpele 08631. Tel: 2824. TYPE: Hotel & Spa.
LOCATION: Central location near thermal establishments.
CLIENTELE: Women and men.

* Rooms: 234 w/priv. bath. Apartments: 3
* Airport: Kosice, or Poprad, 80 km. / 50 mi.
* Airport Transportation: taxi, bus
* Reservations: payment before arrival
* Credit Cards: MC/VISA/AMEX/DC
* Open: Year round
* Rates: from US$130/day; TAC: 10%; rates include accommodations, medical examination and selective Spa treatments. There is extra charge for Gerovital

treatment, Oxygen-therapy and acupuncture
* Spa on premises
* **Spa facilities**: hot springs, thermal baths, massage and therapy rooms, linked to balneotherapy center, covered pool in the balneotherapy unit, two beaches
* **Spa Programs**: medical, weight reduction, rehabilitation
* **Spa Treatments**: mineral water drinking cure, inhalations, mineral baths, hydrotherapy, massages, electrotherapy, remedial exercises, paraffin applications, intestinal douches, diet, gerovital H3, oxygen-therapy, acupuncture
* **Indications**: see Spa indications
* Medical Supervision: 8 MD, 24 nurses
* Treatments Approved: Institute of Human Bioclimatology, Bratislava

DESCRIPTION: A modern sanatorium offering a complete Spa therapy based on mineral water under medical supervision. Prices include: inpatient spa care, medical examinations and treatments, balneotherapeutic services including prescribed drugs, diets, treatments of minor ailments, and all medical examinations. Gerovital H3 treatments are available at additional charge.

PIESTANY SPA
↘ **838**
✈ Ivanka Airport (BTS) 50 mi. / 80 km.

Piestany is the largest spa town in Slovakia. It is a reputable Spa for rheumatic patients in the Vah River Valley in West Slovakia 50 mi. / 80 km. northeast of Bratislava. Nature has been particularly kind to Piestany with a sunny position, pleasant climate, rare thermal springs and curative mud.

The Piestany springs are gypseous-sulfide thermal containing 1,500 mg of mineral substances in solution per 1 liter of water, and free gases, the most important of which is hydrogen (mono) sulfide. The springs gush out from a depth of 2,000 m. (6,560 ft.) at the rate of 3.5 million liters daily. The therapeutic use of its mineral waters and mud for relief of rheumatism and other disorders goes back to very early times and is well documented in the town's Balneological Museum.

Piestany has its own airport with direct flights to Prague, and is connected with Bratislava and Vienna by an express motor coach. Bus service brings patients and visitors to and from its express train station. The Spa is also accessible by car via route E 16.

Balnea Esplanade
♥♥♥

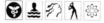

Pavlova Street, 92101 Piestany. Tel: (838) 724210. TYPE: Spa Hotel. LOCATION: On the Spa Island. SPA CLIENTELE: Women and men.

* Rooms: 512 w/private bath
* Restaurant & bar
* Airport: Piestany 2 km. / 1.5 mi., free pick up, bus
* Credit Cards: MC/VISA/AMEX/DC
* Open: Year round
* Rates: from US$110. including accommodations, selective Spa treatments & medical supervision
* TAC: 10%
* Spa on premises
* Spa Facilities: hot springs, indoor swimming pool, balneotherapeutic equipment, sauna, solarium, gym, consulting rooms, varied sports facilities
* Spa Programs: Rejuvenation, relaxation, general fitness, beauty and medical
* Spa Treatments: Peloid mud packs and mud baths, complex water procedures, dry and wet massage, paraffin, electrotherapy, ultrasound, physical therapy, Gerovital H3. There is extra charge for Gerovital treatment, Oxygen therapy, and acupuncture
* Indications: Progressive arthritis, ankylosing spondylitis (Bechterev's disease), coxarthroses in all stages, arthrosis of joints, rheumatism, gout, arthrosis, locomotor disorders
* Medical Supervision: 22 MD, 60 nurses
* Treatment Approved: Research Institute for Rheumatological Diseases, Piestany

DESCRIPTION: One of the four interconnected hotels comprising the Balnea Center. Hotel guests and patients can make use of all the treatment centers practically under one roof. This modern hotel includes a dining room, coffee shop, and a Nightclub.

Balnea Grand-Splendid
♥♥♥

Pavlova Street, 92101 Piestany. Tel: (838) 724210. TYPE: Spa Hotel. LOCATION: On the Spa Island. SPA CLIENTELE: Women and men.

* Rooms: 400 w/priv. bath. Apartments: 10
* Blue Lounge, coffee shop, nightclub
* Airport: Piestany, 15 min., free pick up, bus
* Reservations: deposit prepaid
* Credit Cards: MC/VISA/AMEX/DC
* Open: Year round
* Rates: from $110 including accommodations, meals, selected Spa treatments, medical supervision. Gerovital treatments, acupuncture (additional cost)
* TAC: 10%
* Spa on premises
* Spa Facilities: hot springs, outdoor swimming pool; directly connected to the new Balnea Treatment Center; balneotherapeutic facilities, consulting rooms,
* Spa Programs: medical, diet, & Beauty
* Spa Treatments: hydrotherapy, electrotherapy, kinesitherapy, skin and mud treatments, physical exercises, massages, whirlbaths, pearl baths, Scotch showers, under water massage, contrast baths, Magnetic-Field Therapy, Gerovital therapy
* Medical Supervision: 12 MD, 36 Nurses
* Treatments Approved: Research Institute for Rheumatological Diseases

DESCRIPTION: A modern Spa connected to the new Balnea Treatment Center offering quality accommodations, good service and easy access to all the Spa facilities and programs. Rates are all inclusive but some treatments are offered on à la carte basis.

Minotel Magnolia
♥♥♥♥

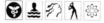

Ul. Nalepkova 1, 92101 Piestany. Tel: (838) 726251.

Fax: (838) 721149. TYPE: Spa Hotel. LOCATION: On the Spa Island. SPA CLIENTELE: Women and men.

* Rooms: 122 w/private bath. Suites: 7
* Restaurant, bar, lounge
* Airport: Piestany, 15 min. free pick up, bus
* Credit Cards: MC/VISA/AMEX/DC
* Open: Year round
* Rates: from $90 including accommodations, meals, selected treatments, medical supervision. Gerovital treatments, acupuncture (extra charge)
* TAC: 10%
* Spa Facilities: hot springs, outdoor swimming pool; directly connected to the new Balnea Treatment Center; balneotherapeutic facilities, consulting rooms, laboratories
* Spa Programs: medical, diet, & beauty
* Spa Treatments: hydrotherapy, electrotherapy, kinesitherapy, skin and mud treatments, physical exercises, massages, whirlbaths, pearl baths, Scotch showers, under water massage, contrast baths, Magnetic-Field Therapy, Gerovital therapy
* Medical Supervision: 12 MD, 36 Nurses
* Treatments Approved: Research Institute for Rheumatological Diseases

DESCRIPTION: A modern 9-story Spa hotel connected to the new Balnea Treatment Center offering quality accommodations, good service and easy access to all the Spa facilities and programs. Rates are all inclusive but some treatments are offered on à la carte basis. Recreation: skiing, horseback riding.

Thermia Palace
❤❤❤

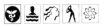

Pavlovova Street, Piestany 92101. TYPE: Hotel & Sanatorium. LOCATION: In the town's park like spa island of Kupelny Ostrovr. SPA CLIENTELE: Women and men.

* Rooms: 190 w/shared bath. Apartments: 6
* Restaurant & bar
* Airport: Piestany 2 km. / 1.5 mi., bus
* Credit Cards: MC/VISA/AMEX/DC

* Open: Year round
* Rates: from $90/day with treatment
* Treatment Duration: 13-20 days
* TAC: 10%
* Spa on premises
* Spa Facilities: indoor swimming pool, latest balneotherapeutic equipment, sauna, solarium, gym
* Spa Programs: Rejuvenation, relaxation, fitness, beauty and medical
* Spa Treatments: Peloid mud packs and mud baths, massages, paraffin, electrotherapy, ultra sound, physical therapy, Gerovital H3 (available at additional cost)
* Indications: Progressive arthritis, ankylosing, spondylitis (Bechterev's disease), coxarthroses in all stages, arthrosis of joints, rheumatism, gout, arthrosis, locomotor disorders
* Medical Supervision: 9 MD, 27 Nurses
* Treatment Approval: Research Center for Rheumatological Diseases, Piestany

DESCRIPTION: The oldest of the four interconnected cure hotels comprising the Balnea Center on the Spa Island. Built in 1913 in the late 19 century decorative style, it is a favorite of many foreign guests and patients due to its turn of the century charm and ambience. Thermia Palace is directly connected to the IRMA balneotherapeutical establishments. The major draw back is that the rooms do not have private bath and WC.

STRBSKE PLESO
🕿 969

✈ Poprad Airport

Srbske Pleso is a reputable climatic Spa located in the scenic High Tatras mountain range. The Spa enjoys a high mountain climate (8,528 ft. altitude / 2,600 m.), and six months of snow. The Tatra Mountains region may be reached by air via the Poprad airport, or through the railway station Poprad-Tatry which is connected with the Spa by an electric tramway.

The Tatra Mountains region is a protected nature reservation known as the Tatran National Park, with wild life, mountain lakes, and unique valleys. The local high-mountain climate saturated with solar radiation with ultraviolet rays, few days without sunshine, low atmospheric pressure, and a low relative humidity are the Spa's main assets with beneficial influence in the treatment of chronic diseases indicated for climatic treatments.

Indications: nonspecific affections of the respiratory tract, bronchial asthma, allergic rhinitis, and hay fever. As acclimatization during the treatment takes place in stages with some negative effects during the third week, an appropriately longer period of at least 4 weeks is recommended.

Helios
❤❤❤

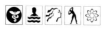

Strbske Pleso, 05985. Tel: (969) 92131. TYPE: Modern Sanatorium for Asthmatics. LOCATION: Mountain location at high altitude. SPA CLIENTELE: Women and men, children & Adolescents (3-15 years).

* Rooms: 234 w/private bath. Apartments: 3
* Night Club
* Airport: Poprad, 60 km / 38 mi. taxi, train
* Reservations: prepayment required
* Credit Cards: MC/VISA/AMEX/DC
* Open: Year round
* Rates: from $110 including accommodations, inpatient spa care, meals, medical examination, cure treatments, and treatments of minor ailments; TAC: 10%
* **Spa Facilities**: Up-to-date modern diagnostic and therapeutic facilities, indoor swimming pool,inhalation and treatment rooms
* **Spa Programs**: Climatic & medical therapy (Bronchial asthma & Allergic Colds)
* **Spa Treatments**: climatic treatments, open air exercises, inhalations, hydrotherapy, massages, water procedures and diet
* **Indications**: Bronchial asthma, allergic colds, hay fever
* **Medical Supervision**: 10 MD, 30 Nurses
* **Treatment Approval**: Institute of Human Bioclimatology, Bratislava

DESCRIPTION: The Helios offer quality accommodations and Spa specializing in climatic and medical cure of bronchial asthma and allergic colds under strict medical supervision.

A special department has been designated to take care of young patients ages of 3 and 15. Recreation: swimming, mountain climbing, skiing, tourism.

TRENCIANSKE TEPLICE
✈ Piestany Airport

Trencianske is one of the oldest and most frequently visited spas in the Slovak Republic. Situated in Western Slovakia surrounded by wooded hills, it is commonly known as "The Carpathian Pearl". It owes its fame to the fact that three of its five mineral springs spout directly into basins situated above them; patients can actually bath in the springs themselves. The water temperature is an ideal 104°F (40°c); heating, cooling and pumping are not required. The main therapy is from hot sulfate waters containing hydrogen sulfide and from the therapeutic sulfur mud used for the tub baths and pool baths. The Spa offers geriatric program based on the application of Gerovital, and a special program has been prepared for rheumatic patients suffering from Diabetes.

The amenities of Trencianske Teplice are enhanced by summer festivals, promenade concerts in the park, and daily social events. Since 1937, a series of concerts, called "Hudobne Leto" (Musical Summer) have been held with international participation each year. Trencianske Teplice can be reached by flights to Piestany airport. Airport transportation can be arranged with the Spa.

Indications: locomotor apparatus disorders, degenerative rheumatic diseases, chronic inflammatory forms of rheumatism, muscular rheumatism, chronic neurology, spinal disorders, and post-accidental states.

Krym Hotel
❤❤❤

Trencianske Teplice, 914 51. Tel: 2321. TYPE: Hotel & Spa. LOCATION: In the center of town near the train station and the Spa treatment facilities. SPA CLIENTELE: Women and men.

* Rooms: 254 w/priv. bath. Apartments: 3

* Terrace balconies for sunbathing
* Phone, CTV available, radio,
* Restaurants, bar, cafe, recreation room
* Library, lounge, social room, night club
* Airport: Piestany, 36 mi. / 60 km., taxi
* Reservations: Prepayment required
* Credit Cards: MC/VISA/AMEX/DC
* Open: Year round
* Rates: from $180 including accommodations, meals, selective treatments and medical supervision
* TAC: 10%
* **Spa Facilities**: indoor swimming pool, latest balneotherapeutic equipment, sauna, solarium, gymnasium, consulting rooms, sports facilities
* **Spa Programs**: Rejuvenation, relaxation, fitness, diet, beauty, medical
* **Spa Treatments**: mineral baths, mud baths, pool baths, hydrotherapy, classic & segmental massage, water massage, electrotherapy, remedial exercise, sauna, diet, Gerovital H3
* **Indications**: Chronic Polyarthritis, Artrosis, Spondylosis, post traumatic & operative conditions of locomotor disorders; Neuritis, Plexitis, Rasiculitis, Sciatica, Lumbosciatica, Cerviobrachial Synd. or Neurological ailment; Atheriocletosis, high cholesterol Geriatric problems
* Medical Supervision: 8 MD, 24 nurses
* Treatment Approval: Research Institute for Rheumatological Diseases, Piestany

DESCRIPTION: This Health Spa is the flagship of the contemporary Slovak Spa industry. Public spaces are tastefully decorated and guest rooms are beautifully furnished. The Spa emphasizes natural hot springs therapy, and is suitable for relaxation and recreation. All the treatments are administered at the hotel.

Pax Hotel
♥♥♥

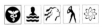

Trencianske Teplice, 914 51. Tel: 2321. TYPE: Hotel & Spa. LOCATION: In the center of town near the SPA treatment facilities and the Hammam. SPA CLIENTELE: Women and men.

* Rooms: 267 w/priv. bath. Apartments: 1
* Terrace balconies for sunbathing
* Radio, phone, TV available
* Restaurant, bar, cafe, recreation room
* Airport: Piestany, 36 mi. / 60 km., taxi
* Reservations: Prepayment required
* Credit Cards: MC/VISA/AMEX/DC
* Open: Year round
* Rates: from $180 including accommodations, meals, selective treatments and medical supervision, Gerovital treatments (extra charge)
* TAC: 10%
* Spa on premises
* **Spa Facilities**: Thermal pool & mud dept., consulting rooms, gymnasium, sauna, solarium, connected to SINA balneotherapy complex
* **Spa Programs**: Rejuvenation, relaxation, fitness, diet, beauty, medical
* **Spa Treatments**: mineral baths, mud baths, pool baths, hydrotherapy, classic & segmental massage, water massage, electrotherapy, remedial exercise, sauna, diet, Gerovital H3
* **Indications**: Chronic polyarthritis, artrosis, spondylosis, post traumatic & operative conditions of locomotor disorders; neuritis, plexitis, rasiculitis, sciatica, lumbosciatica, cerviobrachial synd. or neurological ailment; atheriocletosis, high cholesterol geriatric problems
* Medical Supervision: 8 MD, 24 nurses
* Treatment Approval: Research Institute for Rheumatological Diseases, Piestany

DESCRIPTION: Pax is a modern Spa complex offering quality accommodations in the vicinity of the balneotherapeutic facilities and sulfurous baths. The hotel offers a complete medical Spa program based on hot springs and mud therapy. It is directly connected with the SINA complex for a convenient in hotel cure. Non medical Spa programs are available for relaxation, regeneration, beauty and recreation.

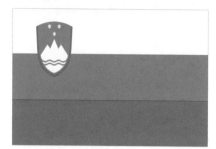

SLOVENIA

AREA: 7,814 sq. mi. (20,251 sq. km.)
POPULATION: 2,100,000
CAPITAL: Ljubljana
OFFICIAL LANGUAGE: Slovenian
CURRENCY: Slovenian Tolar (Slt)
EXCHANGE RATE: 1 US$ = Slt 161
COUNTRY TELEPHONE CODE: 386

Slovenia boasts more than 300 mineral, thermal and radio-active springs in over 100 spas. Their spas are traditionally linked to the Romans who were the first to discover the great healing powers of Slovenia's thermal spas.

The health resorts are well developed and equipped with teams of qualified experts and medical specialists. The spas are easily accessible and connected to the major towns by a good communication system. Whether you prefer a sunny Mediterranean resort or a cool mountain setting, Slovenian spas are an excellent choice.

ⓘ Slovenian Tourist Board

WTC, Dunajska 156, 1000 Ljubljana, Slovenia
Tel: (+386-61) 189-1840. Fax: (+386-61) 1891841

ATOMSKE TOPLICE
⌐ 63
✈ Pleso Airport (ZAG) Croatia 44 mi. / 70 km.

Atomske Toplice Thermal health resort is located at an altitude of 220 m. / 726 ft. surrounded by forested hills. The

spa is built around thermal water with magnesium, calcium, hydrogen carbonate content at 30°c - 37°c (86°F - 99°F) which is pumped from a depth of 500 m. / 1,650 ft.

Atomske Toplice Health Resort
♥♥♥

Zdraviliska c. 24, SI-3254 Podcetrtek. Tel: (63) 829000. Fax: (63) 829-024. TYPE: Health Resort. LOCATION: Eastern Slovenia near the Croatia border. SPA CLIENTELE: Women and men.

* Rooms: 149 w/priv. bath. Apts: 136
* Restaurants, bar
* Airport: Zagreb, Croatia, bus
* Credit Cards: MC/VISA/AMEX/DC
* Open: Year round
* Rates: from US$100; TAC: 10%
* Spa on premises
* **Spa Facilities**: thermal swimming pool complex, Turkish and Finnish saunas, cold waterpools, solarium, fitness hall, athletic grounds, laboratories
* **Spa Programs**: medical, fitness
* **Spa Treatments**: balneotherapy, hydrotherapy, mechanotherapy, electrotherapy, lasertherapy, acupuncture, alternative medicine
* **Indications**: skin diseases (psoriasis, eczema), rheumatic diseases, diseases of the locomotor system, convalescence after surgery or injuries, arterial circulation disorders, stress
* **Medical Supervision**: medical clinic

DESCRIPTION: Alpine chalet style health resort nestled amidst forested hills. The health resort features natural remedy based on thermal water and special therapies of the alternative medicine. Recreation: tennis, minigolf, cycling, deer hunting and fishing.

CATEZ
⌐ 608
✈ Pleso Airport (ZAG) Croatia 22 mi. / 35 km.

Catez Spa is located in eastern Slovenia near the Croatian border, about 35 km. / 22 mi. from Zagreb and 100 km.

/ 63 mi. from Ljubliana. The spa lies at an altitude of 142 m. / 469 ft. surrounded by forests. The climate is sub-alpine with mild winters and moderately warm winters. The accratohyperthermal springs with temperatures ranging from 41°c - 62°c (106°F - 144°F) provide natural remedy.

Indications: inflammatory rheumatoide diseases, degenerative and extra-articular rheumatism, convalescence after injuries and surgical treatments of the locomotor system, after oncological treatment, nervous diseases and obesity.

Terme Hotel
♥♥♥

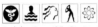

Topliska Cesta 35, Brezice SI-8250. Tel: (608) 57000. Fax: (608) 62721. TYPE: Spa Hotel Complex. LOCATION: On the bank of Sava River. SPA CLIENTELE: Women,men.

* Rooms: 149 w/private bath
* Restaurant & bar
* Airport: Zagreb, Croatia, bus
* Credit Cards: MC/VISA/AMEX/DC
* Open: Year round
* Rates: from US$100
* TAC: 10%
* Spa on premises
* **Spa Facilities**: indoor/outdoor thermal pools (9), gym, sauna, solarium, whirlpools, Catez Spa facilities
* **Spa Programs**: Rejuvenation, relaxation, general fitness, beauty and medical
* **Spa Treatments**: balneotherapy, thermotherapy, kinesitherapy, fango, massage, dietetics, beauty cures, slimming courses, acupuncture,
* **Indications**: see Catez Spa

DESCRIPTION: Terme hotel is one of several hotels in the spa holiday village with direct access to the Catez Thermal Spa. Recreation: cycling, boating, tennis, table-tennis, basketball and sandball.

MORAVSKE TOPLICE
⌐ 69
✈ Thalerhof AP (GRZ) Graz, Austria 60 mi. / 96 km.

Moravske Toplice is a health resort in northeastern Slovenia, in the border area with Austria and Hungary.

Moravske Toplice Spa
♥♥♥

Kranjceva 12, Moravske Toplice SL-69221 Martjanci. Tel: (69) 12280. Fax: (69) 48607. TYPE: Spa Resort Complex. LOCATION: Center of town. SPA CLIENTELE: Women and men.

* Accommodations: Ajda Hotel (4-star), Thermal Hotel (3-Star)
* **Spa Facilities**: Thermal Institute, fitness studio indoor/outdoor thermal pools (7), fitness trail
* **Spa Treatments**: hydrotherapy, balneotherapy physical therapy, medicamentosis, diets
* **Indications**: rheumatism, convalescence after injuries, chronic lung and skin diseases

DESCRIPTION: Spa complex with hotel facilities featuring natural remedy provided by natural medicinal water of the fossil mineral hyperthermal group. Recreation: tennis, basketball, handball.

PORTOROZ
⌐ 66
✈ Brnik Airport (LJU) 81 mi. / 130 km.

Portoroz or "the port of roses" is a well known seaside natural health resort in the northern part of the Adriatic, close to the Italian border. It is 2 mi. (3 km.) from Piran, the ancient Roman village with its romantic pastel colors, cobblestone streets and busy market places; 11 mi. (18 km.) from Koper.

Portoroz has been known as a health resort since 1890 when the mud from salt beds was first used for therapeutic purpose. The medical mud combined with sea water is noted for its thermal properties and is used to prepare peloid packs and baths. It contains iodine, chloride, bromine, magnesium, sodium and potassium.

Indications: various rheumatic ailments, post-traumatic

conditions, paraplegia, paresis, neuritis, allergic diseases of the skin, and the respiratory organs, conditions following surgery of the nervous system, nervous tension, fatigue, burns, and insomnia.

Grand Hotel Palace
❤❤❤❤

Obala 45, Portoroz SL-66320. Tel: (66) 747041. Fax: (66) 747188. TYPE: Hotel & Spa Complex. LOCATION: In the center of town surrounded by gardens. SPA CLIENTELE: Women and men.

* Rooms: 206 most w/priv. bath
* Suites: 7
* Phone, CTV, A/C, C/H, minibar
* Restaurants, bars, casino and tennis nearby
* Airport: Ljubliana AP
* Credit Cards: ACC/AMEX/DC/EC/MC/VISA
* Open: Year round
* Rates: from $70/day
* Treatment duration: 2 weeks
* Spa on premises: **Thalassotherapia**
* **Spa Facilities**: Indoor and outdoor swimming pools, latest balneotherapeutic equipment, sauna, gym, consulting rooms, varied sports facilities
* **Spa Programs**: Medical, relaxation, general fitness, anti-stress, beauty
* **Spa Treatments**: Sea water baths, peloid packs and baths, massages, electrotherapy, kinesitherapy, ionophoresis, acupuncture, magneto-therapy, laser therapy, inhalation, special diets
* **Indications**: Rheumatic ailments, posttraumatic conditions, paraplegia, paresis, neuritis, skin allergies, respiratory allergies, nervous tension, fatigue, burns, insomnia, cellulitis
* Medical Supervision: Examinations and laboratory tests
* Treatments Approved: Government

DESCRIPTION: First class Spa hotel in the center of town. Treatment and medical care is provided by the staff of the Terme Thalassotherapia affiliated with the Palace Hotel. Recreation: water sports, tennis, mini-golf.

Strunjan Health Resort
❤❤❤

Zdravilisce Strunjan, Portoroz SL-66320. Tel: (66) 78-882. Fax: (66) 78-618. TYPE: Hotel & Spa Complex. LOCATION: On the calm side of Strunjan Bay surrounded by gardens. SPA CLIENTELE: Women and men.

* Rooms: 160 most w/priv. bath
* Restaurants, bars, casino and tennis nearby
* Airport: Ljubliana AP 120 km. / 75 mi.
* Open: Year round
* Rates: on request
* Spa on premises
* **Spa Facilities**: Health Spa, indoor and outdoor pools with sea water, medical and therapy facilities
* **Spa Programs**: health-preventive program, medical, rehabilitation, beauty& fitness programs
* Spa Treatments: thalassotherapy, balneotherapy, fangotherapy, hydrotherapy, electrotherapy, kinesitherapy, mechanotherapy, beauty and pampering treatments, aerobics, exercise
* **Indications**: diseases of the lungs and the respiratory tract, rheumatic diseases, convalescence after injuries and surgical treatments of the locomotor system, nervous and skin diseases, general well being, anti-stress, beauty and pampering
* **Contraindications**: decompensated states of the vital organs, mental disorders and acute infectious diseases

DESCRIPTION: The Strunjan Health Resort offers natural remedy supported by mild Mediterranean climate and natural remedies based on sea water and sea mud. Recreation: tennis courts, mini golf and valley ball. Variety of events and excursions are organized for the guests including various programs for children.

RADENCI
🌙 69

✈ Pleso Airport (ZAG) Croatia 96 mi. / 160 km.

Radenci lies in the northeastern plain near the meeting point of the borders of Slovenia, Austria and Hungary, 27 mi. / 45 km. from Maribor and 96 mi. / 160 km. from

Zagreb (Croatia). It is a natural health resort and the source of one of the most popular mineral waters in Europe, known by the sign of "Three Red Hearts" of Radenska.

The springs produce mineral water with a temperature between 54°F (12°c) and 61°F (16°c) containing mostly sodium, calcium and potassium. They have a high content of free carbon dioxide and are pleasant to the taste.

Indications: angina pectoris, symptoms of arteriosclerosis, high blood pressure, heart and blood vessels diseases, kidney diseases, obesity, and neurological diseases. The spa is equipped with indoor and outdoor pools, therapy rooms, special baths, saunas and a solarium. All the treatments are medically supervised.

Radenci Health Resort
♥♥♥

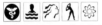

Radenci SI-9502. Tel: (69) 331-66594. Fax: (69) 331-66604. TYPE: Hotel & Spa. LOCATION: Situated in a beautiful Spa park. SPA CLIENTELE: Women and women.

* Rooms: 214 beds, w/priv. bath
* Phone, CTV, A/C, C/H,
* Restaurant, cocktail lounge, coffee bar with music
* Tennis, horseback ridding, bowling
* Airport: Zagreb (Croatia), 96 mi. / 160 km.
* Season: Year round
* Rates: from $829/week
* Spa on premises
* **Spa Facilities**: indoor swimming pool, latest balneotherapeutic equipment, sauna, solarium, gymnasium, consulting rooms, sports facilities
* **Spa Programs**: Rejuvenation, vitalcure, relaxation, general fitness, anti-stress, diet, beauty and medical
* **Spa Treatments**: Ozone, mineral baths, inhalation, massages, electrotherapy, kinesitherapy, skin brushing, thermotherapy, drinking cure
* **Indications**: Angina pectoris, symptoms of arteriosclerosis, cardiovascular, kidney and urinary tract diseases, rheumatism, obesity, paradentosis, neurogetative dystnia, neurological diseases
* Medical Supervision: Examinations and

laboratory tests
* Treatments Approved: Government

DESCRIPTION: Modern resort complex nestled in parks and promenades offering natural remedy based on thermomineral water rich in carbon dioxide. The Spa specializes in the treatment of heart and circulatory diseases.

ROGASKA SLATINA
↘ 63

✈ Pleso Airport (ZAG) Croatia 50 mi. / 80 km.

Rogaska Slatina is one of the most beautifully laid-out hotel/spa complexes in Slovenia. It is located 20 mi. / 33 km. from Celje and 28 mi. / 47 km. from Maribor in a scenic valley surrounded by mountains.

The springs have been known since the 12th century, and later were documented in a 16th century book describing their therapeutic use and praising them as unique in Europe.

The Rogaska Slatina mineral waters bear the well known labels "Donat", "Tempel", and "Styria". The first two are known in Europe as palatable mineral waters. The waters at their source have a temperature of 49°F (9°c) to 52°F (11°c) and are heated for therapeutic purposes to temperatures prescribed by the treating doctors. The waters contain magnesium, sodium, hydrocarbonate and sulfate. Magnesium is the dominate constituent of the "Donat" water, which makes it suitable for the treatment of many digestive disorders.

Rogaska Health Resort
♥♥♥♥

Rogaska Slatina, SL-63250. Tel: (63) 811-4000. Fax: (63) 811-6427. TYPE: Health Resort Complex. LOCATION: At an altitude of 228 m / 752 ft., among forest covered hills. SPA CLIENTELE: Women and men.

* Rooms: 416 w/private bath & telephone
* Restaurant, coffee shop, bar, nightclub
* Sports Hall, Meeting rooms, parking
* Nearest Airport: Zagreb, 96 miles (160 km.)

* Airport Transportation: limo, bus
* Rates: from $1959/21 day treatment
* **Spa Facilities**: Indoor thermal swimming pool, latest balneotherapeutic equipment, sauna, solarium, gym, consulting rooms, varied sports facilities
* **Spa Programs**: Rejuvenation, relaxation, general fitness, diet, beauty and medical
* **Spa Treatments**: mineral baths, massage, electrotherapy, mechanotherapy, thermotherapy, kinesitherapy, hydrotherapy, "Drinking Cure"
* **Indications**: Stomach, liver, bile and internal diseases, metabolism disorders, obesity, catarrh of the bile ducts and urinary tract, obesity, managerial illnesses, and psychosomatic diseases
* Medical Supervision: Examinations and laboratory tests
* Treatments Approved: Government

DESCRIPTION: The Rogaska Health Resort comprises of first class hotels connected by an underground corridor and together form a horseshoe shaped complex around the centralized Spa and Mineral Water establishment. The hotels and the Spa are completely modern with the most up to date equipment for treatments. Recreation: tennis, golf, hunting, cycling, hiking.

SMARJESKE TOPLICE
⌐ 68
✈ Brnik Airport (LJU) 56 mi. / 90 km.

Smarjeske Toplice lies in the valley of the Toplice stream, covered with many vineyards and evergreen forests, at an altitude of 554 ft. (169 m). This central Slovenian region, known locally as Dolenjska is located 7 mi. / 12 km. from Novo Mesto and it is within 2 mi. / 3 km. of the Zabreb-Ljublijana highway.

The history of the springs dates back to the 16th century. The thermal water at an average temperature of 90°F (32°c) has a high content of calcium and magnesium with trace of sodium, potassium, sulfate and chlorine. Carbon dioxide gas is particularly prominent.

Indications: the spa can be recommended for the treatment of the following disorders - rheumatism, psychoso-

matic disorders, blood pressure disorders, vegetative-hormone disturbance, and after-effect of injury to the locomotor system.

Smarjeske Tolpice Health Resort
❤❤❤

Smarjeske Toplice SI-8220. Tel: (68) 73230. Fax: (68) 73107. TYPE: Health Resort. LOCATION: Nestled in the hills of the Toplice valley. SPA CLIENTELE: Women and men.

* Rooms: 93 w/private bath
* Restaurant & bar, sports facilities, parking
* Airport: Ljubliana, limo, bus
* Open: Year round
* Rates: from $819/ 7 days
* Spa on premises
* **Spa Facilities**: 2 Indoor and 3 outdoor thermal swimming pools, latest balneotherapeutic equipment sauna, solarium, gymnasium, consulting rooms, varied sports facilities
* **Spa Programs**: Medical, relaxation, fitness, diet and beauty
* **Spa Treatments**: Mineral baths, massage, electrotherapy, mechanotherapy, thermotherapy, kinesitherapy, hydrotherapy
* **Indications**: degenerative rheumatism, psychosomatic disorders, blood pressure disorders, vegetative hormone disturbances, post-locomotor system injury
* Medical Supervision: Examinations and laboratory tests
* Treatments Approved: Government

DESCRIPTION: The Smarjeske Toplice Health resort is modern and contains complete health facilities with up-to-date balneotherapeutic equipment. It is only a short drive from Novo Mesto and is nestled in the hills for peaceful relaxation. The health resort features programs of natural remedies provided by hypothermal water. Fango, the mild subalpine climate and the rich ionization of the air add to the therapeutic effects. Recreation: table tennis, minigolf, football, basketball, fitness trail, mountain biking. Horse riding and boating nearby.

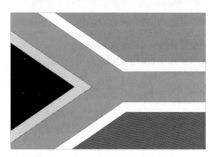

SOUTH AFRICA

AREA: 455,318 sq. mi. (1,179,274 sq. km.)
POPULATION: 34,492,000
CAPITALS: Cape Town, Pretoria
OFFICIAL LANGUAGES: Afrikaans, English
CURRENCY: Rand (R)
CURRENCY EXCHANGE: 1US$ = $ 5.80
COUNTRY TELEPHONE CODE: 27

 South African Tourism Board
500 Fifth Ave., New York NY 10110-0002 USA
Tel: (212) 730-2929. Fax: (212) 764-1980

BADPLAAS
ʔ **17**

Aventura Baadplas
❤❤❤

P.O. Box 15, Baadplaas 1190. Tel: (17) 844-1020. Fax: (17) 844-13991. TYPE: Hydro Spa. LOCATION: In Mpumalanga. SPA CLIENTELE: Women and men. DESCRIPTION: Hydro Spa with hotel accommodations, swimming pools, featuring a variety of soothing spa treatments.

CAPE TOWN
ʔ **21**

 D.F. Cape Town Int'l Airport (CPT) 14 mi. / 22 km.

Avalon Springs Hotel
❤❤❤❤

Uitvlugt St., Montagu, Western Cape 6720. Tel: (234) 41150, Fax: (234) 41906. TYPE: Hot Springs resort. LOCATION: 3 km from the town center. DESCRIPTION: Hotel, Timeshare & Spa. Health spa treatments, hot spring pools (5) of various temperatures, 2 indoor, 3 outdoor, gym, sauna. Restaurant (3) including Da Vinci's, bar, conference facilities, shops, tennis courts.

The Lord Charles Hotel
❤❤❤❤

Faure & Stellenbosch Roads, Somereset West, Cape Town (mail: PO Box 5151, Helderberg 7135). Tel: (21) 855-1040. Fax: (21) 855-4066. TYPE: Hotel & Spa. LOCATION: Near the Winelands, 5 km. / 3 mi. to the beach, 25 km. to the airport. DESCRIPTION: First class attractive hotel with health Spa. 188 rooms, 8 suites,, nonsmoker rooms, wheelchair access. Restaurant, coffee shop, bar, meeting facilities, 3 tennis courts, volleyball, outdoor pool. Hotel rates: from R 650.

The Table Bay Hotel
at the Waterfront
❤❤❤❤

Prince Alfred Breakwater, PO Box 50369 Cape Town 8002. Tel: (21) 405-5000. Fax: (21) 406-5767. TYPE: Hotel & Spa. LOCATION: On the Victoria & Albert waterfront 5 minutes to downtown, 20 minutes to airport. DESCRIPTION: Victorian style casino resort hotel with full service spa, gym, and beauty salon. 312 rooms, 18 suites, nonsmoker rooms, wheelchair access. Restaurants (3), bars (2), lounge, meeting facilities, business center, outdoor pool, shops. Hotel rates: from US$280.

PRETORIA / ERASMIA
ʔ **12**

 Wonderboem Airport (PRY)

Erasmia is a small community at the southern outskirts of

Pretoria and about 50 km. (31 mi.) north of Johannesburg. Hoogland Health Hydro Spa lies up in the Skurweberg Mountains near Hennops River. The rich natural surroundings allow guests to relax in a peaceful environment while taking spa cures and treatments. Both Pretoria and Johannesburg are nearby for the nightlife and excitement of large cosmopolitan cities.

Hoogland Health Hydro
❤❤❤

P.O. Box 34210, Erasmia 0023, South Africa. Tel: (12) 370-3322. Fax: (12) 370-3325. TYPE: Health Resort Complex. MANAGER: Mr. & Mrs. Pretorius. LOCATION: On a 1000 landscaped acres, within a 50 km. / 31 mi. range of Pretoria and Johannesburg. SPA CLIENTELE: Women and men. SPECIAL RESTRICTION: No children under 15.

* Rooms: 50 w/private bath
* Spa on premises
* Airport: Pretoria 70 km. / 44 mi.
* Credit Cards: VISA/MC/DC
* Open: Year round
* Rates: from US$110/day
* TAC: 10%
* **Spa Facilities**: Steam cabinets, sitz baths, sauna, Turkish bath, 9 fully equipped massage / beauty salons, swimming pool, nature trails
* **Spa Programs**: Health, Beauty and Fitness, Cleansing Fruit Diet
* **Spa Treatments**: massages, beauty, exercises, single fruit cleansing diet, nature walks, sitz baths
* Medical Supervision: 2 MD, 4 RN
* Number of Customers per Dr.: 25

DESCRIPTION: Hydro therapy and revitalization center for weight loss, fitness or daily stress. One week program is recommended. The cleansing diet is restricted to one type of fruit only, selected according to the season, and the degree of acidity in your system. Daily routine consists of early morning walk or exercises, massages, steam baths and sauna and underwater massage. Daily lectures on health and fitness subjects are available.

JOHANNESBURG
☽ 11
✈ Johannesburg Int'l AP (GCJ) 14 mi. / 22 km.

Park Hyatt Johannesburg & Peak Health Club
❤❤❤❤

191 Oxford Road, Rosebank. P.O. Box 1536, Saxonwold 2132. Tel: (11) 280-1234, Fax: (11) 280-1238. TYPE: Hotel & Spa. LOCATION: In suburban Rosebank, 7 mi. / 11 km. to city center, 15 mi. / 24 km. to airport. DESCRIPTION: Fashionable deluxe hotel in contemporary, ethnic architecture. The hotel offers complete Health Spa, saunas, steam rooms. The Peak Health Club specializes in hydrotherapy, beauty and fitness treatments providing antidote to the challenges of modern life. 219 rooms, 15 suites, nonsmoker rooms, wheelchair access. Restaurant, bar, entertainment, meeting facilities, business center, pool. Hotel rates: From R 1,000

STELLENBOSCH
☽ 21
✈ Capetown International AP (CPT)

Stellenbosch, population 30,000, is a beautiful university town on the famous South African Wine Route. The town is located 56 km. / 35 mi. east of Cape Town. Cape Town is a cosmopolitan port town with great beaches, museums, galleries, lively nightlife and lovely parks.

High Rustenberg Hydro
❤❤❤❤

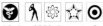

P.O. Box 2052, Dennesig, Stellenbosch, 7601. Tel: (21) 883-8600. Fax: (21) 886-5163. USA / Canada reservations: (800) 257-5344. TYPE: Health Spa. LOCATION: At the base of Simons Mountain, 5 km. / 3 mi. from Stellenbosch in the picturesque wineland area. SPA CLIENTELE: Women and men. SPECIAL RESTRICTIONS: No children under 18 years. MEDICAL RESTRICTIONS: Must be ambient, no wheelchairs.

* Rooms: 60 with private bath
* Phone, CTV, A/C, jacuzzi
* Airport: Cape Town Airport, 40 km. / 25 mi.
* Train St'n: Stellenbosch, 5 km. / 3 mi.
* Airport/Train Transportation: Bus
* Reservations: R 500 deposit required
* Credit Cards: MC/VISA
* Open: Year round
* Hotel Rates: from US$140
* TAC: 10%
* Spa on Premises
* **Spa Facilities**: Indoor (heated) and outdoor swimming pools, gym, auditorium, skin & body care clinic, sauna, massage and therapy rooms
* **Spa Programs**: Natural Healing (Naturopathy), diets, stress management, revitalization
* **Spa Treatments**: hydrotherapy, sauna, steam Kneipp therapy, yoga, progressive relaxation classes, water aerobics, aquatic classes, light exercise, lectures on diet, life-style and natural healing, electrotherapy, sitz bath, circulation treatment. Optional Extras; Clarins, Jeanne Gatineau & Rene Guinot beauty treatments, aromatherapy, cellulite & bust treatments, Shiatsu-acupressure massage, reflexology, seaweed treatments and various facial treatments
* Medical Supervision: 1 MD, 7 RN
* Number of customers per doctor: 20

DESCRIPTION: South Africa's largest and best known holistic health center with international reputation. The facilities are of a high standard. The natural healing resort emphasizes cleansing the system by means of fasting, raw natural foods, exercise, relaxation, plenty of sunshine, fresh air and positive mental attitudes. The 7 day programs include accommodations, meals, treatments (see Spa Treatments) and start on Sunday or Wednesday.

VAAL SPA

⤳ 534

✈ Johannesburg Int'l AP (GCJ)

Aventura Vaal Spa
♥♥♥

PO Box 19, Christiana 2680. Tel: (534) 2244. Fax: (534) 2354. TYPE: Hydro Spa. LOCATION: On the banks of the Vaal River between the Cape and the Gauteng. SPA CLIENTELE: Women and men. DESCRIPTION: Popular family getaway with natural mineral baths and well stocked game preserve. Accommodations are in thatched chalets and caravans. Facilities include: swimming pools, bubble-pools, bubble jet baths, and private baths with mineral water.

WARMBATHS

⤳ 14

✈ Johannesburg Int'l AP (GCJ) 90 mi. / 145 km.

Warmbaths, population 8,500, is a modern internationally acclaimed Spa with an African bushveld atmosphere. The resort is located 1.5 hrs. drive north of Joannesburg amidst an exciting combination of recreational facilities and exotic wildlife.

Aventura Spa
♥♥♥

PO Box 75, Warmbaths 0480. Tel: (14) 736-2200. Fax: (14) 736-4712. TYPE: Hydro Spa. LOCATION: In Gauteng north of Pretoria and Johannesburg. SPA CLIENTELE: Women and men. DESCRIPTION: Fashionable Hydro Spa modeled after the Baden Baden Spa in Germany with hotel accommodations and luxury chalets. The Hydro Spa features hydrotherapy, massage, and saunas. Recreation: water sports, squash, tennis, fishing, mountain biking.

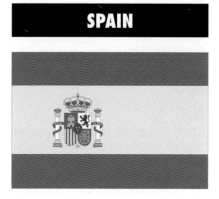

SPAIN

AREA: 194,881 sq. mi. (504,742 sq. km.)
POPULATION: 37,430,000
CAPITAL: Madrid
OFFICIAL LANGUAGES: Spanish, Catalan,
Basque, Galician, Valencian
CURRENCY: peseta (Pts.)
EXCHANGE RATE: 1US$ = Pts 142
COUNTRY TELEPHONE CODE: 34

Spain has more than 90 Spas in different locations around the country. Depending on the location some spas are open year round, others operate only seasonally. The Spas vary in style and size from traditional to modern resort complexes. Luxury spas offer European pampering and revitalizing programs. Their amenities include golf courses, and gambling casinos.

❶ Tourist office of Spain
666 5th Ave., New York NY 10022. USA
Tel: (212) 265-8822. Fax: (212) 265-8864

ARCHENA
〉 968
✈ Alicante Airport (ALC) 62 mi. / 100 km.

Archena, population 7,200, is located in the Costa Blanca Area; the southeastern province of Murcia along the banks of the Segura river. The climate and landscape are typical Mediterranean with fragrant pine, eucalyptus, palm, orange, and lemon trees everywhere giving their fresh and

stimulating aromas.

The average yearly temperature at the spa is 18°c (65°F) with hot summers and cool and windy winters. The spa mineral waters are hot at 52°c (125°F), and have a chloridized-iodine-bromine-sulfurous properties with regenerative power. The Archena spa is located 26 km. (16 mi.) northwest of Murcia, the province's capital, and 376 km. (235 mi.) southeast of Madrid.

The spa facilities at the Thermal Centre of Rheumatology & Functional Rehabilitation include: thermal pools, fitness area, massage and applications rooms, private cabinets, inhalation rooms. A variety of treatments are available under medical supervision and include: slimming massages, mud applications for anti-rheumatic purposes and beauty treatments, rehabilitation, massage under shower. For the spa treatment to be efficient a minimum stay period of 15 days is recommended.

Indications: Spa treatment can be effective in the cure of the following conditions: rehabilitation, rheumatism, respiratory affections, and obesity.

Hotel Termas
❤❤❤❤

Carretera del Balneario, s/n, Archena (Murcia) E-30600. Tel: (968) 670100. Fax: (968) 671002. MANAGING DIRECTOR: D. Nicasio Perez Menzel. TYPE: Spa Hotel. LOCATION: Convenient Spa location, 24 km. / 15 mi. to Murcia. SPA CLIENTELE: Women and men, children accepted. MEDICAL RESTRICTIONS: Heart problems.

* Rooms: 71 w/private bath. Suites: 6
* Phone, CTV, A/C, C/H, minibar
* Restaurant, bar
* Airport: Alicante Airport, taxi
* Reservations: required
* Open: Year round
* Hotel Rates: from pts. 8,700; TAC: 10%
* Spa on premises: **Balneario de Archena**
* Year Established: 1898
* **Spa Facilities**: Extensive spa facilities at the Thermal

Centre of Rheumatology and Functional Rehabilitation beauty salon, sauna (at the hotel)
* **Spa Treatments**: massages muds, thermal bath, jacuzzi, hydromassage
* Indications: rheumatism, respiratory and skin ailments
* Length of Stay Required: 15 days
* Medical Supervision: 2 MD
* Documentation required from Doctor
* Treatments Approved: Health Ministry
* Email: informacion@balneario-archena-sa.es

DESCRIPTION: Spanish style moderately elegant spa hotel with amenities and comfort that will satisfy international travelers who seek a new spa experience in a warm and friendly Mediterranean setting. The spa provides specialized treatments at the medical center, but can also be considered for relaxation, beauty and weight loss.

BARCELONA
) 93
 Barcelona Int'l Airport (BCN)

Princesa Sofia
Inter-continental Barcelona
❤❤❤❤❤

Plaza Pio XII 4, 08028 Barcelona. Tel: (93) 330-7111. Fax: (93) 330-7621. TYPE: Hotel & Spa. LOCATION: Barcelona's new Financial Centre. SPA CLIENTELE: Women and men. DESCRIPTION: Sleek high-rise convention hotel with Balneotherapy Centre, beauty parlours, gym, sauna, massage, aerobics, solarium, indoor and outdoor pools. 505 rooms, 23 suites, restaurants, coffee shop, bar, piano lounge. Hotel rates: from Pts 19,000.

CADIZ
) 956
 Jerez Airport 40 mi. / 64 km.

Iberostar Royal Andalus Golf Hotel
❤❤❤❤

Urb Novo Sancti Petri, Chiclana da la Frontera E-11130

(Cadiz). Tel: (956) 494109. Fax (956) 494490. TYPE: Hotel & Spa. LOCATION: On the Atlantic ocean beach, 24 km. / 15 mi. to Cadiz. DESCRIPTION: Glamorous first class hotel with complete health & beauty Spa, massage, body treatments, sauna, gym. 219 rooms, 44 suites. Restaurants (2), bars (3), entertainment, meeting rooms, business center, indoor & outdoor pools, 27-holes golf, tennis courts. Hotel rates: from Pts 13,000.

CALDES de MALAVELLA
) 972
 Barcelona Airport (BCN) 50 mi. / 80 km.

Vichy Catalan
❤❤❤

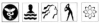

Avendia Doctor Furest 32, Caldes de Malavella E-17455 (Girona). Tel: (972) 470000. Fax: (972) 472299. TYPE: Spa Hotel. LOCATION: Girona area 80 km. / 50 mi. from Barcelona. SPA CLIENTELE: Women and men.

* Rooms: 80 w/private bath
* Airport: Barcelona Airport, 80 km. / 50 mi., train, taxi
* Open: Year round
* Hotel Rates: from pts. 13,700
* TAC: 8%
* Spa on premises
* **Spa Facilities**: thermal baths, bubble baths, shower massage (Vittel system), jet showers, Finnish sauna, thermal vapour sauna, inhalations, gym, solarium, beauty and aesthetics department
* **Spa Treatments**: hydrotherapy, mud baths, showers, massages, physiotherapy, beauty
* **Indications**: rheumatism, muscular stiffness, arthritis, obesity, respiratory and digestive complaints, stress
* Medical Supervision: medical clinic
* Treatments Approved: Health Ministry

DESCRIPTION: Arabesque style spa hotel built in 1891 by Dr. Furest. The spa has been improved and modernized to offer up to date spa facilities and treatments. Recreation: tennis, excursions, biking (rent-a-bike at the hotel).

FUENGIROLA
🌙 95
✈ Malaga Airport (AGP) 19 mi. / 30 km.

Fuengirola, population 26,000, is a charming resort in the Costa Del Sol near Malaga. The Costa Del Sol is a gentle riviera with a warm Mediterranean climate, fine beaches, romantic villages, and wonderful cuisine. Of special interest is the unique Andalusian folklore with flamenco songs and dances reflecting the happy character of its people. The pleasant climate make Fuengirola an ideal location for a Thalassotherapy cure at the **Hotel Babylos Andaluz** (see description below).

Hotel Byblos Andaluz
❤❤❤❤❤

Mijas Golf, Apt. 138, Fuengirola, (Malaga). Tel: (95) 246-0250/ (95) 247-3050. Fax: (95) 247-6783. TYPE: Deluxe Resort Hotel & Thalassotherapy Center. LOCATION: On the Costa Del Sol near the ancient Andalusian village of Mijas. SPA CLIENTELE: Women & men, teenagers accepted.

* Rooms: 105; and 39 luxurious suites
* Air-conditioning, color TV, mini-bar
* Restaurants: French haute cuisine, Andalusian cuisine, health-food, Bar
* Airport: Malaga Airport 12 mi. (19 km.)
* Airport Transportation: taxi, limo
* Reservations: required
* Credit Cards: VISA/AMEX/DC/EC
* Open: Year round
* Spa on premises: **Thalassotherapy Louison Bobet**
* Year Established: 1986
* **Spa Facilities**: Thalassotherapy Center Louison Bobet and Beauty Center "La Prairie", swimming pools (3), superb thermal baths, ultra-modern installations, gym, saunas, massage and treatment rooms
* **Spa Package Rates:** from Pts 213,000 (7 nights) including accommodations, diet or buffet breakfast luncheons or dinners, fruit basket in room on arrival
* **SPA Packages:** Classic Cure; Tonic Cure; Super Tonic Cure, Detoxication/Anti-Stress; 3 day Beauty Special

* **SPA Programs**: Health, Medical , Weight Loss
* **Spa Treatments**: massages, jet showers, submarine showers, bubbling bath, marine ultrasonic, submarine jets, pool exercises, algotherapy, thalassotherapy, gourmet low cal menu
* **Indications**: Rheumatic illnesses, post traumatic sequels, problems deriving from stress, loss of weight, cellulitis, relaxation, body pampering, fitness
* Maximum number of guests: 120
* Medical Supervision: doctors, specialists
* Email: bybbs@spa.es

DESCRIPTION: The Hotel Byblos Andaluz is a romantic luxury hotel built in local architecture with Roman, Arabic, Andalusian and rustic decor. Accommodations consist mostly of deluxe suites and mini-suites with views of the golf course or the town of Mijas. The Hotel offers a unique Thalassotherapy Center with a variety of health, medical, and stress reduction programs. All the treatments at the center are under a complete medical supervision by specialists in their particular fields. Recreation: golf, tennis, gourmet dining (diet available), sightseeing, and entertainment. Member: *The Leading Hotels of the World.*

ISLA DE LA TOJA
🌙 95
✈ Vigo Airport 40 mi. / 65 km.

Isla de la Toja, is a small island in the Atlantic Ocean, off the coast of Pontevedra in Galicia. Known to the locals as the 'Island of Health', it has thermal springs with curative powers, romantic beaches, and wooded areas.

The island, located 60 km. (38 mi.) from Vigo and 150 km. (94 mi.) from La Coruña, is ideal for peaceful relaxation, artistic inspiration and pleasant excursions.

The mineral waters are hot, contain sodium-chloride and are mildly radioactive at temperatures varying from 37°c - 60°c (98°F - 140°F).

Indications: Spa cure is effective in cases of rheumatism, rehabilitation, skin and lymph gland infections.

Gran Hotel de la Toja
❤❤❤❤

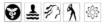

Isla de la Toja 36991, Pontevedra. Tel: (986) 730025. Fax: (86) 731201. TYPE: Resort Hotel & Spa. LOCATION: A beautiful beach location surrounded by woods and gardens. SPA CLIENTELE: Women and men.

* Rooms: 198 w/private bath. Suites: 4
* Phone, CTV, in-room safe, minibar, hair dryer
* Restaurants, gaming rooms, casino
* Airport: Santiago 85 km. / 53 mi.
* Reservations: suggested
* Credit Cards: MC/VISA/AMEX/ DC
* Open: Year round
* Hotel Rates: from Pts 12,000; TAC: 10%
* Spa on premises
* **Spa Facilities**: hyperthermal baths, inhalation rooms, gym, sauna, thermal water swimming pool
* **Spa Treatments**: thermal baths, mud and bubble baths, inhalations, showers, massages, physiotherapy; sauna, massage and gymnasium at the hotel
* **Indications**: skin diseases, articulation problems and breathing tracts, treatment of stress
* Medical Supervision: 1 MD, 2 RN
* Treatments Approved: Nat'l Assoc. of Thermal Baths

DESCRIPTION: Superior first class Old World Spa & Casino hotel built in 1903 and renovated in 1993. One of Spain's most distinguished Spa hotels. Classic construction and decor provide welcoming atmosphere in the style of Grand Hotels. Modern spa facilities, gambling casino and exquisite cuisine are few of the things that will make your spa vacation at this hotel a most delightful experience. Recreation: tennis, golf, swimming, excursions, Casino games, nightly entertainment.

MALLORCA ISLAND
☞ **971**
✈ Palma de Mallorca Int'l Airport (PMI)

Arabella Golf Hotel
❤❤❤❤❤

Carrer Vinagrella s/n, Son Vida, Palma de Mallorca E-07013. Tel: (971) 799999. Fax: (971) 799997. TYPE: Hotel & Spa. LOCATION: Son Vida residential area. SPA CLIENTELE: Women and men. DESCRIPTION: Sophisticated deluxe hotel in a classic Spanish country house with Beauty Farm. 93 rooms, restaurants, swimming pools, sauna, tennis. Hotel rates: from Pts 17,450.

Riu Palace Bonanza Playa Hotel
❤❤❤❤

Carreter de Illetas s/n, Illeta E-07015 (Mallorca). Tel: (971) 401112. Fax: (971) 405615. TYPE: Hotel & Spa. LOCATION: 7 km. to city center, 15 km. / 10 mi. to Airport. DESCRIPTION: First class waterfront resort hotel with Beauty & Therapeutic center, gym, sauna, jacuzzi. 279 rooms, 15 suites, nonsmoker rooms, wheelchair access. Restaurant, bars (2), meeting facilities, pools (2), tennis courts (2), water sports. Hotel rates: from Pts 11,500.

Hotel Son Vida
❤❤❤❤❤

Urb Son Vida, Palma de Mallorca E-07015. Tel: (971) 790000. Fax: (971) 790017. TYPE: Hotel & Spa. LOCATION: On a 1400 acre private estate overlooking Palma. SPA CLIENTELE: Women and men. DESCRIPTION: Deluxe hotel with Beauty Farm, Turkish bath, gym, sauna, jacuzzi. 171 rooms, 12 suites, restaurants (2), tea room, bar, indoor and outdoor pools, 18 hole golf course, tennis. Hotel rates: from Pts 19,150.

MARBELLA
☞ **95**
✈ Malaga Airport (AGP) 28 mi. / 45 km.

Marbella, population 54,000, is a year round seaside resort town on the famous Costa del Sol southwest of Malaga. Sheltered by the Sierra Blanca its climate is mild and pleasant. The major beaches are long with fine clean sand. The town is picturesque with well preserved historic remains such as the ancient citadel and the ruins of the moorish fortress. Many water sports, boating and yachting are available. Málaga, the capital of the Costa del Sol is 40 km. (25 mi.) northeast along the coast. Marbella is accessible by car from Málaga.

Incosol Spa & Resort
❤❤❤❤

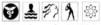

Golf Rio Real, Marbella, (Málaga), Costa del Sol. Tel: (95) 282-8500. Fax: (95) 282-3178. TYPE: Resort Hotel & Spa. LOCATION: In the Rio Real Valley, near the beach. SPA CLIENTELE: Women and men.

* Rooms: 197 w/private bath. Suites: 63
* Air-conditioning, telephone, color TV
* Restaurant: El Jardin & Bars
* Airport: Málaga 28 mi. (45 km.)
* Airport Transportation: taxi, rent-a-car
* Credit Cards: MC/VISA/DC/EC
* Spa on premises
* Open: Year round
* Hotel Rates: from Pts 14,000; TAC: 10%
* Spa Facilities: heated pools, gym, saunas, massage rooms, Beauty Salon, medical clinic, laboratory and a coronary-care unit
* Spa Treatments: diet and obesity treatments, massages, slimming and toning-up, Kneipp shower, laser therapy, acupuncture, physical exercises, facials, collagen and Clarins fresh cell facials, physiotherapy, hydrotherapy, mud baths, electrotherapy, ventilotherapy, Kinesitherapy, geriatrics cell therapy
* Spa Packages: Health & Beauty Package (7 nts) Geriatric Health Package available
* Indications: obesity, beauty, geriatric rehabilitation
* Medical Supervision: medical center

DESCRIPTION: Resort and spa in a fashionable Costa del Sol setting. The 9-story hotel is located on top of the renowned Los Monteros Estate, surrounded by gardens with views of the Mediterranean Sea and the mountains. The spa emphasizes scientifically oriented treatments of obesity and geriatric rehabilitation. Spa treatments are also available for relaxation, beauty treatments and fitness. Recreation: tennis, golf, squash.

PUENTE VIESGO
⟩ 942
✈ Prayas Airport 18 mi. / 28 km.

Puente Viesgo is a thermal resort with mineral/medicinal waters near Santander (Cantabria). The water are chlorated, sodic-bicarbonated, calcic at 34.6°c (94°F).

Gran Hotel Puente Viesgo
❤❤❤❤

B. La Iglesia s/n, 39670 Puente Viesgo (Cantabria). Tel: (942) 598061. Fax: (942) 598261. TYPE: Spa Hotel. LOCATION: On the banks of the Pas River near the Del Castillo Peak. SPA CLIENTELE: Women and men.

* Rooms: 98 w/priv. bath
* Phone, CTV, in-room safe
* Restaurants, cafeteria, private park
* Airport: Santander, 28 km. / 18 mi., taxi, bus
* Open: Year round
* Hotel rates: from Pts 15,000
* Spa on premises
* Spa Facilities: bath tubs, bubble baths, hydromassage baths, saunas, gym, open air swimming pool
* Spa Treatments: thermal baths, mud and bubble baths, showers, massages, physiotherapy, sauna, inhalations, ultra-violet rays
* Indications: cardiovascular illnesses, locomotive apparatus, arthrosis, rheuma, sinusitis, bronchitis, rhinitis, varices and circulation.
* Contraindications: accute infections
* Medical Supervision: 1 MD, 2 RN
* Treatments Approved: Nat'l Assoc. of Thermal Baths

DESCRIPTION: First class spa hotel with thermal treatment facilities.

TARRAGONA
⟩ 977
✈ Reus Airport (10 km. / 6 mi.)
  Barcelona Airport (BCN) 65 km. / 40 mi.

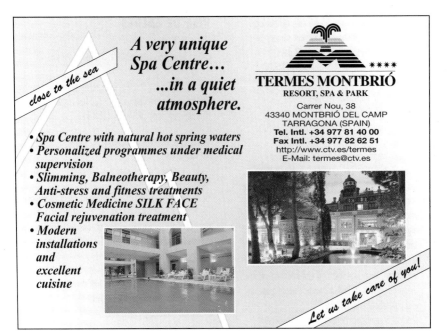

Tarragona is a beautiful city in the popular Costa Daurada southwest of Barcelona. During ancient times it was the favorite city of many Roman emperors who left giant architectural footprints in and around the city. Montbrio del Camp is located 15 km. / 10 mi. from Tarragona.

Hotel Termes Montbrio
❤❤❤

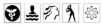

Carrer Nou 38, Montbrio del Camp - Tarragona. Tel: (0034-977) 81400. Fax: (0034-977) 826251. TYPE: Deluxe Hotel & Thermal Center. LOCATION: Costa Daurada region, about 15 km. / 10 mi. from Tarragona. SPA CLIENTELE: Women and men.

* Rooms: 140 w/private bath. Suites: 4 w/jacuzzi
* Telephone, CTV, minibar, hairdryer
* Restaurants (2): "**Le Sequoia**" gourmet international cuisine; "**l'Horta Florida**" French & Mediterranean

* Airports: Barcelona, Reus
* Train Station: Reus, Cambrils
* Airport/Train Transportation: taxi
* Reservations: required
* Credit Cards: VISA/AMEX/MC/DIS/EC
* Open: Year round
* Rates: see Spa Package rates
* TAC: 10% (travel agents) (to 20% tour operators)
* Spa on premises: **Termes Montbrió**
* **Spa Facilities**: Thermal pool, Sauna, Turkish bath, Scottish shower, hydrotherapy baths, massage therapy & relaxation rooms, beauty salon
* **Spa Programs**: Revitalization, Anti Stress, Anti Rheumatism, Weight Loss & Beauty, Fitness, Cosmetic Medicine
* **Spa Treatments**: Aquagym, aerobic, stretching, sauna & Turkish bath, Scottish shower, hydromassage, hydrotherapy with carbon dioxide, algae & mud packs, foot & hand shower, massages, manual lymphatic drainage, shiatsu, foot reflexology, antalgic ultra sounds, anti-cellulitis ultrasounds, pressure therapy,

electrolifting, thermoslim, body toner, Asthmology, Thymus therapy, plastic and cosmetic surgery
* **Spa Package Rates**: Short Break (2 days) Pts 38,000; Beauty & Relaxation Pts 89,500; Facial & Body Beauty (5 days) Pts 196,400; Anti-Stress (7 days) Pts 185,000; Slimming (7 days) Pts 218,800; Thymus Therapy (7 days) Pts 237,900; Balneotherapy (7 days) Pts 180,200; Thermal Water Treatment for Upper Respiratory Tract (7 days) Pts 166,800; Duo Form (2 days) Pts 49,500; Fitness (3 days) Pts 77,100; Silk Face (facial Rejuvenation - 11 days) Pts 795,000. Prices are per person per day, single supplements and high season supplements apply
* **Indications**: Anti-stress, loss of vitality, fatigue, premature aging, depression, artrial hypertension, impotence, liver diseases, skin and intestinal diseases, rheumatic diseases, Parkinsonism, chronic bronchitis and pulmonary emphysema
* **Medical Supervision**: permanent medical service
* **Treatments Approval**: Medical Center
* **Email**: termes@ctv.es
* **Web**: www.ctv.es/termes

DESCRIPTION: First class resort and thermal spa in the beautiful Costa Daurada. The complex is a unique harmonious combination of turn-of-the-20th century and modern architecture. Accommodations are in comfortable well appointed rooms and palatial suites. The world class Thermal Center with its own natural thermal source features European revitaliziation and preventive therapies for beauty, pampering and premature aging. An expert team of professionals from the Group Roc Blanc (Andorra) offers up-to-date personalized health programs. A spa vacation at the Hotel Termes Montbrió is recommended for relaxation, beauty and stress reduction. Recreation: 18-hole golf courses nearby, horseback riding, sailing, tennis and sports.

VILA DE CALDES
⟩ 93
✈ Barcelona Airport (BCN) 18 mi. / 28 km.

The Vila de Caldes Spa was completely refurbished for the Barcelona Olympic Games in 1992. The water are sodium-chlorated, lithic at 69.9°c (158°F).

Vila de Caldes Hotel & Spa
❤❤❤❤

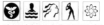

Plaza del Angel, 5 08140 Caldes de Montbui (Barcelona). Tel: (93) 865-4100. Fax: (93) 865-0095. TYPE: Spa Hotel. LOCATION: Historic centre of town just 30 min. from Barcelona city centre. SPA CLIENTELE: Women and men.

* Rooms: 30 w/priv. bath
* Phone, CTV, VCR, A/C, C/H, hair dryer
* Cafeteria, snack bar, private park
* Airport: Barcelona, taxi, bus
* Open: Year round
* Hotel rates: from Pts 15,000
* Spa on premises
* **Spa Facilities**: bubble pools, jacuzzis, vaporarium, showers, swimming pool with rooftop solarium
* **Spa Treatments**: medical, thermal, rapid solarium
* **Indications**: stress, chronic rheumatic, articular, abarticular and neuorological complaints, traumatic effects and neurological complaints, gout, obesity
* **Contraindications**: cardiovascular deficiencies, serious hypertension, cancerous processes, organ-cerebral medular damage.
* **Medical Supervision**: 1 MD, 2 RN
* **Treatments Approved**: Nat'l Assoc. of Thermal Baths

DESCRIPTION: First class Spa boutique hotel with thermal facilities and medical treatments. Recreation: video club, golf course (in town).

ST. LUCIA

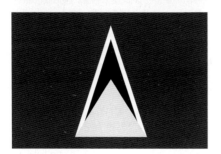

AREA: 238 sq. mi. (616 sq. km.)
POPULATION: 116,000
CAPITAL: Castries
OFFICIAL LANGUAGES: English, French
CURRENCY: East Caribbean Dollar (EC$)
EXCHANGE RATE: 1 US$ = 2.70 EC$
COUNTRY TELEPHONE CODE: 758

The island of St. Lucia, is located midway between Martinique (F.W.I.) to the north, and St. Vincent (B.W.I.) to the south. Shaped like a leaf, the island offers magnificent shorelines, romantic coves, black and white sand beaches, forested mountains, and a bubbling volcano 'La Soufrière'. The island offers natural mineral baths at 'La Soufrière' and European Spas in resort hotels. St. Lucia is connected by flights from New York, Miami and San Juan.

ⓘ St. Lucia Tourist Board

820 2nd Avenue, 9th Fl. New York NY 10017. USA
Tel: (212) 867-2950 or (800) 456-3984.
Fax: (212) 867-2795

✈ Hewandorra Int'l AP (UVF) 42 mi. / 67 km.
Vigie Airport (SLU) 2 mi. / 3 km, north of Castries

Castries, the capital of the island of St. Lucia is a busy port town on the northwest coast of the island. St. Lucia offers fine beaches, tropical climate, and sports: tennis, horseback riding, golf, snorkeling, sailing, and scuba diving. December through April is considered the high season, and June through October is the off season. Temperatures vary between 70°F-90°F (21°c-32°c) with a temperate effect of the cooling trade winds.

The Beach resort and Spa 'Le Sport' is located 9 miles (14 km) north of Castries in a prime beach area with private and secluded beaches. Public transportation is available at the resort for those who wish to go shopping at the duty-free Point Seraphin, or go for horseback riding, scuba, or golf.

Jalousie Hilton Resort & Spa
♥♥♥♥♥

Box 251, Soufriere. Tel: (758) 459-7666. Fax: (758) 459-7667. TYPE: Resort & Spa. LOCATION: Nestled between St. Lucia's famed Piton Mountains on the southwestern coast. SPA CLIENTELE: Women and men.

* Villa Suites: 35
* Villas: 65 1-2BR w/priv. plunge pool
* Phone, CTV, VCR, A/C, veranda w/ocean view computer hook-ups, in-room safe, minibar
* Restaurants, bars, piano lounge, ballroom
* Airport: Vigie Airport Castries, 20 minutes
* Airport Transportation: taxi, bus
* Reservations: deposit required
* Credit Cards: MC/AMEX
* Open: Year round
* Rates: from US$340/day; TAC: 10%; Price include accommodations, all meals, unlimited drinks, water sports, certified spa programs, airport transfers, taxes and service charge
* Spa on premises
* **Spa Facilities:** Spa Center with treatment rooms; Spa restaurant (light cuisine); gym
* **Spa Programs:** Weight Loss, Fitness, Beauty,
* **Spa Treatments:** Thalassotherapy, jet showers, bubbling bath, aqua gym, dynamic swim exercise, seaweed herbal wraps, massage, loofa rubs, mineralization, saunas, facials, hydro massage, aromatherapy, reflexology

DESCRIPTION: Plantation-style all inclusive resort and spa. Enjoy fine low cal Caribbean spa cuisine, and unwind with soothing body treatments by the pool in the tropical sun.

Le Sport
❤❤❤❤

Cariblue Beach, P.O. Box 437, Castries, St. Lucia. Tel: (758) 450-8551. Fax: (758) 450-0368. TYPE: Resort & Spa. LOCATION: On the beach, 8 miles (13 km.) from Castries. Public transportation available to island entertainment and recreation sports. SPA CLIENTELE: Women and men, singles welcome.

* Rooms: 102 w/priv. bath; Suites: 2
* Restaurant & Piano Bar
* Swimming pool, tennis courts (3),
* Airport: Vigie Airport Castries, 20 minutes
* Airport Transportation: taxi, bus
* Reservations: deposit required
* Credit Cards: MC/AMEX
* Open: Year round
* Rates: from US$230, TAC: 10%; rates are per person, per day all inclusive of: accommodations, 3 meals daily, all refreshments and bar drinks, use of all sports equipment, facilities and services of instructors, thalassotherapy, beauty and rejuvenation treatments, full program of daily activities, transfers, hotel and room tax. Single supplement applied.
* Spa on premises: **The Oasis**
* **Spa Facilities**: Spa Center with treatment rooms; Spa restaurant (light cuisine); gym
* **Spa Programs**: Weight Loss, Fitness, Beauty, Stress management
* **Spa Treatments**: Thalassotherapy, aromatherapy, jet showers, bubbling bath, aqua gym, dynamic swim exercise, seaweed herbal wraps, massage, salt loofa rubs, mineralization, saunas, facials, hydro massage, Swedish massage, foot massage, Swiss needle showers, jet nose shower, seaweed wraps, full-body packs, inhalation, mecanotherapy, inemotherapy, reflexology, aerobics, yoga, Clarins beauty products
* Medical Supervision: 1 MD, 1 RN

DESCRIPTION: All inclusive beach resort with European style spa in the tropical climate of the Caribbean. The spa promis-
es to restore your body to feeling its best through a combination of four elements: low calorie diets, beauty treatments, exercise and thalassotherapy. Recreation: water sports, fencing, archery, golf nearby, shopping tour to duty free point Serephin.

Royal St. Lucian
❤❤❤❤

Reduit Beach, PO Box 977, Castries. Tel: (758) 452-9999. Fax: (758) 452-9639. TYPE: Resort & Spa. LOCATION: On the finest stretch of magnificent Reduit Beach. SPA CLIENTELE: Women and men. AGE RESTRICTIONS: No one under 16 will be admitted to the Spa/Fitness area.

* Suites: 98 w/priv. terrace
* Restaurants, cocktail lounge, poolside bar
* Phone, CTV, A/C, in-room safe, minibar, trouser press
* Swimming pool, tennis courts (2)
* Airport: Vigie Airport 6 mi. / 10 km., taxi, bus
* Reservations: deposit required
* Credit Cards: MC/VISA/AMEX/CB/DC
* Open: Year round
* Rates: from US$310; TAC: 10%
* Spa on premises: **The Royal Spa**
* **Spa Hours**: 7:00am-8:00pm daily; therapies 9:00am - 8:00pm daily
* **Spa Facilities**: Spa Center with treatment rooms, Kur baths, eucalyptus steam room, whirlpool, sauna, Swiss shower, in-room massage, outdoor beach treatments, relaxing lounges, cold plunge, Beauty Salon with Kentin Florian beauty products, gym, Cybex Fitness Centre, Restaurant - spa cuisine menu
* **Spa Programs**: Beauty, fitness, weight loss, anti-stress
* **Spa Treatments**: hydrotherapy, body wraps, scrubs, massage, facials, Swedish massage, aromatherpy, fango facial, moor mud,aerobics, personal training, power walks

DESCRIPTION: Superior first class All-Suite resort with full service European Spa and Fitness Center. Enjoy mind-body renewing aromatherapy or massage in the privacy of your room or poolside. Recreation: water sports, scuba, dancing, horseback riding, golf (9 hole) nearby.

ST. MAARTEN

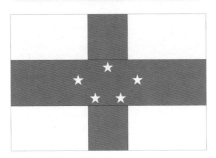

AREA: 21 sq. mi. (70.8 sq. km.)
37 Sq. mi. / 96 sq. km. total area shared with the French
POPULATION: 30,000 (total population)
CAPITAL: Philipsburg
OFFICIAL LANGUAGES: Dutch, French, English
CURRENCY: NA Dfl, FF, US$, Euro
EXCHANGE RATE: 1 US$ = NA Dfl 1.79 = FF 5.60
COUNTRY TELEPHONE CODE: 599

ℹ️ St. Maarten Tourist Bureau

675 Third Ave., Ste 1806, New York NY 10017. USA
Tel: (212) 953-2084. Fax: (212) 953-2145

St. Maarten / St. Martin is a small island in the Caribbean shared by The Netherlands and France. The island lies some 144 mi. / 230 km. southeast of Puerto Rico. This is a lush tropical island with beautiful beaches and year round balmy weather, with temperatures in the 80°sF (29°c).

Some of the beaches on the French side are "clothing optional". US currency is as freely circulating as the Dutch Florin and the French Franc. The Euro will be legal tender for transactions as of January 1999. In St. Martin you will find duty-free shopping, colorful island markets, wonderful beaches, sunny climate, casino excitement, international restaurants, and a variety of sports.

✈️ Princess Juliana Airport, St. Maarten (SXM)
Esperance Airport, St. Martin (SFG)

L'Aqualigne
♥♥♥♥

c/o Box 431 Pelican Key, Pelican Resort, St. Maarten, N.A. Tel: (599) 542503. Fax: (599) 542133. TYPE: Resort & Spa. SPA MANAGER: Marc Van Thielen. LOCATION: At the base of the green mountains in the Pelican Key Estates. SPA CLIENTELE: Women and men. SPECIAL RESTRICTIONS: No Children.

* Suites: 324 at Pelican Resort Club
* Restaurants, bars, open sea marina
* Airport: Juliana Airport, 2 km. / 1 mi.
* Airport Transportation: free pick-up
* Reservations: deposit requested
* Open: Year round
* Hotel Rates: from $115/day
* TAC: 10%
* Spa on premises
* **Spa Facilities**: Complete indoor Spa facilities with treatment rooms, medical center, beauty center, gym, steam room, whirlpools and therapy rooms
* **Spa Programs**: Beauty & Fitness; Cellulite; Weight Loss; Revitalization; Anti-Aging (Dr. Ana Aslan); Rejuvenation; Anti-Wrinkle; Plastic and Reconstructive Surgery; Stimulation of Sexual Potency; Sclerosis of Veins
* **Spa Treatments**: aerobics, drainage, meso, liposuction (anti-cellulite); supervised diet; Gerovital H3, Aslavital (anti-aging); Oligo therapy, vitamin therapy, Dr. Renaud products (beauty); Dr. Simonin treatments (anti wrinkle); acne/scar treatments
* Medical Supervision: 4 MD, professional staff
* Treatments Approved: A.S.P.R.S.

DESCRIPTION: L'Aqualigne Health Spa and Beauty Clinic offers treatments and programs in a deluxe tropical island resort setting. Spa aficionados can choose between American style fitness and pampering programs and a wide range of top-of-the-line European programs. Anti-aging based on the regenerating drug developed by Dr. Ana Aslan; Rejuvenation based on vitamin therapy to fight stress, alcoholism, insomnia, cardiovascular disease, pains, viral diseases and depressions. A Weight Loss program is designed to meet the needs of each individual. The programs last between one and two weeks according to the type of cure required. Recreation: tennis, horseback riding, water sports, casinos nearby

Peter's Health Spa
❤❤❤❤

c/o Maho Beach Hotel & Casino, Box 834 Maho Bay, St. Maarten, N.A. Tel: (599) 552115/6. Fax: (599) 553180. TYPE: Casino Resort & Spa. LOCATION: Beachfront resort on rocky cliff at Maho Beach. SPA CLIENTELE: Women and men.

* Rooms: 602 w/priv. bath. Suites: 40
* Restaurants (9), bars (2), casino, nightclub
* Airport: Juliana Airport, 2 km. / 1 mi.
* Reservations: deposit requested
* Open: Year round
* Hotel Rates: from $115/day
* TAC: 10%
* Spa on premises
* Spa Hours: M-F 7:00am - 8:00pm
  Sat. 8:00am - 6:00pm
* **Spa Facilities**: sauna, therapy baths, beauty salon, Vegetarian cafe, gym, free weights, cardiovascular equipment
* **Spa Programs**: Beauty, wellness and fitness
* **Spa Treatments**: Massages, aromatherapy, reflexology, mud and mineral baths, facials, exfoliation, waxing, aerobics, aqua-gym, yoga, circuit training
* **Spa Packages**: Beauty Day, Mini Beauty Day

DESCRIPTION: First class beachfront resort Casino hotel with full service European Spa. The Health Center offers professional massages, various therapies and body treatments. The Vegetarian cafe serves fresh salads, wholesome meals and guiltless deserts. Recreation: water sports, tennis and entertainment.

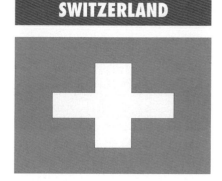

SWITZERLAND

AREA: 15,943 sq. mi. (41,292 sq. km.)
POPULATION: 6,500,000
CAPITAL: Bern
LANGUAGES: German, French, Italian
CURRENCY: Swiss Franc (SF)
EXCHANGE RATE: 1US$ = SF 1.40
COUNTRY TELEPHONE CODE: 41

Switzerland is a favorite destination for wellness holidays. The country is blessed by natural beauty, scenic landscapes and luxurious spa establishments. Swiss spas offer a variety of treatments and programs ranging from classic thermal baths regeneration and fresh cell therapy in modern medical clinics.

🛈 Schweiz Tourismus
Bellariastraße 38, CH-8027 Zurich. Switzerland
Tel: (+41-1) 288-1111. Fax: (+41-1) 288-1205
Email: postoffice@switzerlandtourism.ch

ADELBODEN
🍷 **33**
✈ Belp Airport (BRN) 104 mi. / 65 km.

Park Hotel Bellevue
❤❤❤❤

CH-3715 Adelboden. Tel: (33) 673-4000. Fax: (33) 673-4173. TYPE: Resort Hotel & Spa. LOCATION: Overlooking mountain valley slightly above Adelboden. SPA CLIENTELE: Women and men. DESCRIPTION: Resort hotel with luxurious ambiance featuring a Roman-decor wellness Centre Aqua Vitalis. Spa programs: Aqua Fit and Wellness. Recreation: hiking trails, skiing.

ASCONA
꒐ 91
 Agno Airport, Lugano (LUG) 30 mi. / 48 km.

Hotel Casa Berno
❤❤❤❤

Postfach CH-6612 Ascona. Tel: (91) 791-3232. Fax: (91) 792-1114. TYPE: Resort Hotel & Spa. LOCATION: Perched on a steep hill overlooking the lake. SPA CLIENTELE: Women and men. DESCRIPTION: Modern hotel with golf and health spa programs. 65 rooms, 12 suites. Hotel rates: from Sfr 205.

Hotel Eden Roc
❤❤❤❤❤

Via Albarelle CH-6612 Ascona. Tel: (91) 791-0171. Fax: (91) 792-1571. TYPE: Resort Hotel & Spa. LOCATION: Lakefront on Laggo Maggiore near Piazza Ascona. SPA CLIENTELE: Women and men. DESCRIPTION: Modern hotel with elegant beauty farm, indoor and outdoor pools, private beach, boat landing, sauna, biosauna, steam bath, solarium and fitness room. Spa Package: Clarins Beauty days. 51 rooms, 9 suites, terrace restaurant, piano bar. Hotel rates: from Sfr 280.

Giardino Ascona
❤❤❤❤❤

Via Segnale, CH-6612 Ascona. Tel: (91) 791-0101. Fax: (91) 792-1094. TYPE: Resort Hotel & Spa. LOCATION: In exotic gardens overlooking Lago Maggiore. SPA CLIENTELE: Women and men. DESCRIPTION: Southern country estate hotel with the Vanity Club Health Spa. Seawater baths with pure sea salt, aromatic oils, back massages, facials, solarium, 1000 calorie diet, "Fit for Life" cleansing diet upon

request. 72 rooms, 18 suites, restaurant, bar, tennis. Hotel rates: from Sfr 395.

BAD RAGAZ
꒐ 81
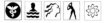 Zurich Int'l Airport (ZRH) 81 mi. / 130 km.

Bad Ragaz, population 3,900, is a famous spa resort at the foot of the Upper Rhin mountains in Eastern Switzerland near the Liechtenstein border. It can be accessed from Zurich, St. Gallen or Winterthur airports.

The acrato-thermal waters contain calcium, magnesium and sodium, hydrocarbonate and fluorine at a temperature of 37°c (98°F), are used in medical treatment of rheumatism, circulatory disturbances, accident ailments and paralysis. The hospital at Valens has a rheumatism and rehabilitation center that caters to both private and general patients.

The medical department of the Thermalbaeder and Grandhotels were established primarily for the guests of the Quellenhof and Hof Ragaz Hotels. The thermal swimming pools, individual thermal baths, massages and underwater massages may be used without medical examination. However, any medical treatment or physiotherapy must be taken only after medical consultation and examination. Special spa treatments offered at the medical department without medical permission include: underwater massage, connective tissue massage, manual lymph drainage, and foot reflex massage.

Grand Hotel Hof Ragaz
❤❤❤❤

CH-7310 Bad Ragaz. Tel: (81) 303-3030. Fax: (81) 303-3033. TYPE: Hotel & Spa. LOCATION: In a quiet but central location with a direct access to the Thermal Baths and medical centre.

* Rooms: 133, Suites:7
* Phone, frigobar, radio, TV, safe
* Restaurant (diet menu), grill room
* Airport: Zurich 130 km. / 81 mi., taxi, limo, train
* Reservations: required

* Credit Cards: AMEX/VISA/DC/EC
* Open: Year round
* Hotel Rates: from SF 280/day; TAC: 8%
* Spa on premises
* **Spa Facilities**: thermal pools (34°c -93°F), thermal baths, fresh water swimming pool (28°c - 82°F), fitness center, sauna, solarium, beauty parlor; medical institute offering special treatments, diet meals on request, Beauty Farm
* **Spa Programs**: Tennis and Ski Weeks (winter) Golf (spring), Bridge Circle (summer), Fitness & Health (winter, spring)
* **Spa Treatments**: medical, health, beauty and slimming cures; diet menus available
* Medical Supervision: 15 MD
* Treatments Approved: Medical Dept.

DESCRIPTION: Old World spa hotel with a human size with direct access to the Thermal Baths and medical center. Recreation: tennis, 18-hole Golf Course.

Grandhotel Quellenhof
♥♥♥♥

CH-7310 Bad Ragaz. Tel: (81) 303-3030. Fax: (81) 303-3033. TYPE: Golf Hotel & Spa. LOCATION: At the foot of the Alps in a private landscaped park with direct access to the Spa and Medical Centre. SPA CLIENTELE: Women and men, family oriented.

* Rooms: 106. Suites: 97 Jr suites
* Phone, frigobar, radio, CTV, in-room safe
* Restaurant, grill room, piano bar
* Airport: Zurich, 130 km. / 81 mi. taxi, limo, train
* Reservations: required
* Credit Cards: AMEX/VISA/DC/EC
* Open: Year round
* Rates: from SF 340/day; TAC: 8%
* Spa on premises
* **Spa Facilities**: thermal pools (34°c -93°F), thermal baths, fresh water pool (28°c - 82°F), fitness room, sauna, solarium, beauty parlor; medical institute offering special treatments, diet meals on request
* **Spa Programs**: Tennis and Ski Weeks (winter)

Golf (spring), Bridge Circle (summer), Fitness & Health (winter, spring)
* **Spa Treatments**: cures can be taken in the connecting medical & cure department of the "Thermalbäder und Grandhotels"; health and slimming cures
* Medical Supervision: 15 MD
* Treatments Approved: Medical Dept.

DESCRIPTION: Landmark Spa hotel offering spacious accommodations in the Grand European tradition. The hotel operates its own thermal spa and offers beauty, fitness and diet programs. For specialized cures, hotel guests have a direct access to the medical department of the "ThermalBaeder und Grandhotels". Special Weekly programs combine spa and sports such as skiing, tennis, golf, fitness, and bridge. Recreation: golf, tennis, swimming, horseback riding, hiking, mountaineering, fishing, downhill and cross-country skiing.

Hotel Tamina
♥♥♥♥

Am Platz 3, CH-7310 Bad Ragaz. Tel: (81) 302-8151. Fax: (81) 302-2308. TYPE: Spa Hotel. MANAGER: Hans Rudolf Schmid. LOCATION: In the centre of town on a large private park with private access to the Thermal Spa. SPA CLIENTELE: Women and men, children accepted.

* Rooms: 38. Suites: 8
* Phone, CTV, C/H, frigobar, radio, in-room safe
* Restaurant (diet menu), grill room, bar
* Airport: Zurich-Kloten 130 km. / 81 mi.
* Train Station: Bad Ragaz (free pick up)
* Reservations: required
* Credit Cards: AMEX/MC/VISA/DC
* Open: Year round
* Hotel Rates: from Sfr 125; TAC: 10%
* Name of Spa: **Tamina Therme**
* Distance to Spa: 500 m / yards
* Year Established: 1990
* **Spa Facilities**: thermal pools (34°c -93°F), thermal baths, fresh water swimming pool (28°c - 82°F), fitness center, sauna, solarium, beauty parlor; medical institute offering special treatments, diet meals on request, beauty farm

* **Spa Programs**: Tennis and Ski Weeks (winter) Golf (spring), Bridge Circle (summer),Fitness & Health (winter, spring)
* **Spa Treatments**: cures can be taken in the connecting medical & cure department
* Medical Supervision: yes
* Treatments Approved: Medical Dept.

DESCRIPTION: Grand hotel with rooms and suites in period or rustic style, those facing south have a large balcony. Recreation: indoor and outdoor tennis and squash, 18-hole golf course nearby. Ski and excursion area around the Pizol.

BAD SCHINZNACH
⟩ 56
✈ Zurich Int'l Airport (ZRH)

Bad Schinznach, population 1,200, is located in northern Switzerland almost half way between Zurich and Basel in the valley of the River Aare. The town spa has a long tradition dating back to the 17th century. The hot springs has the highest sulfur content in Switzerland and are effective in the treatment of rheumatism, post-operational recuperation, diabetes and stress reduction. The thermal healing water works magic on the whole organism and stimulates the body's defense system after illness or exhaustion. The high concentration of minerals have a cosmetic effect and the skin feels softer and healthier looking after taking a bath. Most recommended are three weeks spa cures to keep you in shape with physical and spiritual equilibrium.

To reach Bad Schinznach by car from Zurich, take the Highway to Bern, exit Mägenwil (after Baden) and then through Lupfig to Bad Schinznach. From Bern/Basel, take the highway to Zürich, exit Aarau Ost, follow the signs for Schinznach Bad. By train, all intercity trains from Zürich, Bern and Basel which stop at Brugg. From Brugg take a taxi to Bad Schinznach (about 4 km., 2-1/2 mi. away).

Kurhotel Im Park
♥♥♥♥

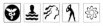

5116 Schinznach Bad. Tel: (56) 463-7777. Fax: (56) 463-7645. TYPE: Hotel & Spa. LOCATION: In a large park

near the River Aare. SPA CLIENTELE: Women and men.

* Rooms: 46 w/private bath. Suite: 1
* Restaurant, grill room, bar
* Airport: Zurich Kloten In'l AP, 18 mi. / 29 km.
* Train Station: Schinznach Dorf, 500m.,1/2m., taxi
* Credit Cards: MC/VISA/AMEX/DC
* Open: Year round
* Hotel Rates: from Sfr 170
* Spa on premises
* **Spa Facilities**: Indoor thermal baths, therapy rooms, individual mineral bath tubs, inhalation rooms, open air thermal pools, sauna, rest rooms, massage rooms
* **Spa Programs**: Rejuvenation, relaxation, stress reduction, general fitness, weight loss, beauty (recommended stay 3 weeks)
* **Spa Treatments**: stimulating baths, inhalations of mineral waters, massages, underwater jet-massage, solarium, physiotherapeutic treatments by in house medical prescription
* **Indications**: rheumatism, post-operational recuperation, stress reduction, skin care
* Medical Supervision: 3 MD, 2 RN
* Treatments Approved: Association of Swiss Health Spas.

DESCRIPTION: Everything at this 19th century spa hotel is provided to meet your needs for comfort, and relaxation. The hotel is directly linked to the thermal cure center which allows one to take the spa treatments in the ambience of a grand hotel. The spa cuisine is excellent and features low calorie menus expertly prepared by dietician. Recreation: tennis courts, 9 hole golf course, and river fishing.

BAD VALS
⟩ 81
✈ Zurich Int'l Airport (ZRH)

Kurhotels Therme Vals
♥♥♥

Bad Vals (Graubunden) CH-7132. Tel: (81) 926-8080. Fax: (81) 926-8000. TYPE: Spa Hotel. LOCATION: Mountain setting. SPA CLIENTELE: Women and men.

DESCRIPTION: Spa hotel with thermal mineral pool, sauna, gym, beauty salon. 148 rooms, 2 suites. Restaurant (diet menus available), grill room, bar, banquet facilities, 3 tennis courts. Hotel rates: from Sfr 110.

BADEN
↳ 56
✈ Zurich Int'l Airport (ZRH) 25 mi. / 40 km.

Baden, population 15,000, is the oldest spa and health resort in Switzerland. The famous international spa and congress town has a unique medieval ambience and is located only 20 km. / 12 mi. northwest of Zürich. The thermal springs contain sodium chloride with a water temperature of 47°c (116°F). The Thermal Baths feature indoor and outdoor pools which are open daily. Treatments include: massages, fango and underwater massages, electrotherapy, gymnastics, connective tissue massage, and hydro-gymnastics under medical direction.

Indications: recuperation after illness, rheumatic diseases, post operative treatments after orthopedic and neurosurgical operations, metabolic disorders, gout, osteoporosis, and neurological illnesses.

Hotel Verenahof
♥♥♥♥

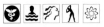

Kurplatz 1, 5400 Baden. Tel: (56) 203-9393. Fax: (56) 203-9394. TYPE: Spa Complex. LOCATION: In the center of the Spa area, directly connected to the Thermal Baths. SPA CLIENTELE: Women and men.

* Rooms: 69; all w/priv. bath. Suites: 3
* Phone, CTV, C/H, minibar, jacuzzi
* Elegant Dining Room, bar, coffee shop
* Airport: Zürich 20 mi. / 32 km.
* Train Station: Baden 1 mi. / 2 km.
* Airport Transportation: taxi, limo, train
* Credit Cards: MC/VISA/AMEX/DC
* Open: Year round
* Hotel Rates: from SF 170; TAC: 10%
* Spa on premises
* Spa Facilities: Thermal Baths directly linked to the

hotel, hot springs (47°) inhouse, medical facilities with gymnastic hall, thermal pool for physiotherapy, facilities for electrotherapy, mud baths, beauty salon
* Spa Programs: Medical, Beauty, Stop Smoking.
* Spa Treatments: massages, physiotherapy, mud baths, fango packs, inhalation, lymph drainage, underwater massage, anti-smoking therapy, special diets, water shiatsu
* Indications: degenerative rheumatic diseases, recuperation after accidents, general beauty, fitness and relaxation, smoking cessation
* Medical Supervision: 2 MD, 4 RN
* Treatments Approved: Health Dept.

DESCRIPTION: Spa hotel in the pedestrians-only thermal bath quarter focusing on wellness. It is the only hotel in town with direct access to medically supervised physiotherapy and training center and to the thermal baths with the most mineral rich springs in Switzerland.

CADEMARIO
↳ 91
✈ Zurich Int'l Airport (ZRH)

Kurhaus Cademario
♥♥♥

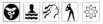

CH-6936 Cademario. Tel: (91) 605-2525. Fax: (91) 604-6128. TYPE: Wellness Hotel. LOCATION: 850 m. / 2,625 ft. above sea level with a view of Lake Lugano. SPA CLIENTELE: Women and men. DESCRIPTION: Charming hotel with Roman thermal baths, sauna, steam room, special showers and effervescent baths, modern fitness centre. Spa treatments: Kneipp treatments, relaxation therapy, massage, Thi-Chi, aerobics, stretching. All treatments are done under the supervision of qualified therapists. Spa Package: Anti-Stress (7 nts) from Sfr 1,435.

CLARENS / MONTREUX
↳ 21
✈ Geneva Int'l Airport (GVA) 56 mi. / 90 km.

Clarens is a small climatic resort near Montreux on Lake

Geneva, known for its magnificent location against the backdrop of the snow covered Alps. The unusual beauty of its location became inspiration to philosophers and poets such as Rousseau and Lord Byron.

The Old Town evokes romantic charms of a bygone era, particularly with the view at distance of the medieval towers of Château Chillon. But Clarens is more than just a beautiful resort, it is an important medical and research center for regeneration and revitalization and plays an important scientific role in the study and treatment of certain disorders associated with the aging process.

Clarens can be reached by car from Lausanne via the Lausanne-Simplon motorway, by train to Montreux, and by air to Geneva Cointrin Airport.

Centre de Revitalisation
Clinique Lémana
❤❤❤❤❤

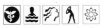

Avenue des Bosquets-de-Julie 21, Clarens-Montreux 1815. Tel: (21) 964-1641. TYPE: Revitalization Clinic. LOCATION: Central location overlooking the Lake. SPA CLIENTELE: Women and men, many celebrities.

* Rooms: w/priv. bath, phone, radio, CTV
* Elegant Dining Room
* Landscaped Garden, tennis court, swimming pool
* Airport: Geneva AP, 90 km. / 56 mi.
* Airport Transportation: taxi, train
* Reservations: deposit required
* Open: Year round
* Rates: from SF 650/day
* Clinic on premises
* **Spa facilities**: Medical clinic, laboratories, treatment center, heated outdoor pool
* **Spa Programs**: Cellvital revitalization, beauty program, 3 day anti-stress break, plastic surgery and post-operative care, removal and treatment of varicose veins, sexual impotency
* **SPA Treatments**: Medical check-up and fat measurement, Cellvital revitalization, active cell facials, hydrothermy with the Dr. Guinot (Paris) method, massages, hydrotherapy, autogenics,

infusion and phyto essence
* **Indications**: loss of vitality, problems from the aging process, stress reduction, beauty care
* Medical Supervision: 3 MD, chemist, biologist
* Treatments Approval: Medical Institution

DESCRIPTION: The Centre de Revitalisation Lémana is an oasis of tranquility on the shores of Lake Geneva. The Clinique offers cellular therapy for revitalization and regeneration according to the techniques developed by Prof. Niehans. The treatments are recommended for problems connected with the aging process, but not limited to it. Some executives undertake the treatments to cope with stressful situations.

Clinic La Prairie
❤❤❤❤❤

Clarens-Montreux 1815. Tel: (21) 989-3311. TYPE: Health Clinic. LOCATION: On Lake Geneva near Montreux. SPA CLIENTELE: Women and men, many celebrities.

* Rooms & Suites: 19 w/private bath
* Restaurant: gourmet dietetic
* Airport: Geneva, 80 km. / 50 mi.
* Airport Transportation: limo, taxi, train
* Reservations: deposit required
* Open: year round
* Rates: on request.
* Clinic on premises
* **Facilities**: Medical Clinic, laboratory
* **Clinic Programs**: Fresh Live Cell (6 night); Slimming Program (7 nights), Special Weight Reduction (10 nights).
* **Clinic Treatments**: Cellular therapy consisting of intramuscular injection of fresh and living fetal cells suspended in a physiological serum; beauty treatments with La Prairie products, biological lifting by anti-wrinkle Chinese acupuncture
* **Indications**: exhaustion, concentration difficulties, weakening memory or sexual drive, troubles of the metabolism and the endocrine system, rheumatism and arteriosclerosislatory resulting from the effect of age.

* Medical Supervision: complete medical surveillance, 4 specialist MD, research scientists, professional nurses
* Treatments Approval: Medical Institute

DESCRIPTION: Clinic La Prairie is an internationally acclaimed scientific and medical center. Top physicians and researchers lead the Medical and Research staff. The Clinic operates a small luxury hotel for a maximum number of 26 patients, who arrive for live cell therapy at the clinic. CLP is the only center in the world that administers intramuscular injection of live cells taken from fetus of sturdy black sheep. This is the procedure pioneered by Dr. Paul Niehans. The treatment is effective wherever the body is deficient or disturbed. All treatments are administered and controlled by top medical staff. Patients who have taken treatments at CLP include many world leaders and celebrities.

CRANS / MONTANA
☽ 27
✈ Geneva Int'l Airport (GVA) 112 mi. / 180 km.

Crans-Montana, population 700, is a small year round resort atop an Alpine plateau overlooking the Rhône Valley. The resort enjoys fine ski conditions and offers excellent skiing facilities including lifts, chairs and aerial cable-ways.The resort offers entertainment, gourmet dining, and sports facilities for tennis and golf.

Hotel Crans Ambassador
❤❤❤❤❤

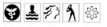

3962 Crans Montana. Tel: (27) 481-4811. Fax: (27) 481-9155. TYPE: Spa Hotel. LOCATION: Hill top with Alpine view. SPA CLIENTELE: Women and men.

* Rooms: 70 w/priv. bath. Suites: 10
* Phone, CTV, radio, fireplaces, minibar, balcony
* Restaurant, bar, disco, wine cellar
* Airport: Geneva, 180 km. / 112 mi. train, taxi
* Reservations: required
* Open: Dec. - April, June - Sept.
* Hotel Rates: from Sfr 195; TAC: 10%
* Spa on premises: **Messegue-Phythotherm**
* Spa Facilities: health center, heated indoor pool,

sauna, jacuzzi,turkish baths, solarium, fitness room, herbal brew room
* **Spa Programs**: Revitalization, anti-aging, slimming, wellness. fitness, beauty, purification, regeneration
* **Spa Treatments**: phythotherapy, nutritherapy, homeopathy, hand and foot baths, phyto-youth serum, pressotherapy, poultices, electro-osmosis, acqua-jogging, pediluve-maniluve, therapeutic baths, mudpacks, LPG massage, manual massage, anti cellulitis, anti-weight, inhalations
* **Spa Packages**: Complete Cure; 4-Day Test Cure; Fitness Week-End; Slimmer's Cure
* Medical Supervision: permanent in house MD

DESCRIPTION: A modern Alpine chalet style hotel complex, with hotel guest rooms and luxury condominium apartments. The Health Centre **Mességué-Phythotherm** accentuates on natural treatments based on plants and herbal brews to disintoxicate, fight illness and premature aging. Their beauty and cosmetic products use O.P.C. + D.N.A. and plant extracts without chemical additions. Recreation: golf, tennis, horseback riding, hiking, skiing.

GSTAAD
☽ 33
✈ Belp Airport (BRN), Bern
Geneva Int'l Airport (GVA), Geneva

Gstaad, population 2,500, is a fashionable summer and winter resort set in the high valley of the Saane, in the most beautiful Western part of the Bernese Oberland. The resort has been for many years favorite with the international jet set and celebrities, yet has been successful to conserve its authentic small village character with lovely Swiss chalets and pristine beauty. Spa aficionados can enjoy the world class spa facilities and Beauty Centre at the glamorous Grand Hotel Park Gstaad for a memorable Spa vacation. Recreation: Alpine golf, tennis, pigeon shooting, ice-rinks, curling, hiking, and ski.

Grand Hotel Park
❤❤❤❤❤

Wispilestrasse, CH- 3780 Gstaad. Tel: (33) 748-9800,

Fax: (33) 748-9808. TYPE: Resort & Spa. LOCATION: On own landscaped park above Gstaad. SPA CLIENTELE: Women and men, popular with celebrities and public figures.

* Rooms: 93 with priv. bath. Suites: 11
* Phone, CTV, C/H, minibar, in-room safe, hair dryer
* Restaurants (3), bar, lounge, meeting facilities
* Airport: Geneva Int'l Airport, 160 km. / 100 mi.
* Train Station: Gstaad, 0.5 km. / 800 yards
* Train Station Transportation: Free pick up (in summer only) on request
* Reservations: Required
* Credit Cards: MC, VISA, AMEX, DC, JCB
* Open: June - September, December - March
* Hotel Rates: from Sfr 180; TAC: 8%
* Spa on premises
* **Spa facilities**: Salt water pool (34° C), whirlpool, outside heated pool (summer), sauna, turkish bath, gymnasium,massages, fitness room, beauty center, salt water pool containing natural Rheinfelden salts at 34˚c (93°F)
* **Spa Packages**: Fit & Beautiful (6 nts) from Sfr 1442 Intensive Beauty (3 nts) from Sfr 736
* **Spa Treatments**: Mud baths, herbal baths, aromatherapy, cellulite treatment, oxygen therapy, massages, acupressure, shiatsu, reflexology, lymph drainage, connective tissue massage, oxygenotherapy, seaweed wraps, body peeling, anti-cellulite, fango and herbal baths,exercise, aerobics, fitness training
* **Indications**: Rejuvenation, regeneration, beauty, anti-stress, well being, relief from many physical problems, from gynecological to respiratory and cardiovascular.

DESCRIPTION: Chalet style grand hotel with a panoramic terrace. The suite-size rooms are tastefully decorated in soft and soothing colors, with sitting area, spacious marble bathroom, and balcony. The Fitness & Aqua Club offers a full program of aerobic, step, stretch and conditioning classes, plus saunas, whirlpools, Turkish baths and various massages. The Beauty Center **Brigitte Glur** is conveniently located inside the hotel for a delightful array of pampering services to relax and rejuvenate your body and soul in the finest tradition of Europe's great Spas. The scenic area provides a variety of summer and winter sports and recreation opportunities for every taste.

HÜTTWILEN
52
Zurich Int'l Airport (ZRH)

Schloss Steinegg
❤❤❤❤❤

CH-8536 Hüttwilen. Tel: (52) 747-1481. Fax: (52) 747-1500. TYPE: Spa Hotel. LOCATION: Sunny southern slope of Lake Constance. SPA CLIENTELE: Women and men. DESCRIPTION: Renovated Baroque Castle with health spa specializing in medically supervised weight loss, beauty and fitness programs. Packages: Fasting Regimen & Beauty/ Fitness from Sfr 1,590 (10 nts); Vitality Diet & Beauty/ Activity from Sfr 159 (1-3 nts).

INTERLAKEN
33
Belp Airport (BRN), Bern

Interlaken, population 13,000, lies between Lakes Thun and Brienz below the north side of the Jungfrau mountains. It is the only one of the three peaks that non-mountain climbers can reach. The train ride provides a spectacular rocky views. This is one of the most popular summer holiday resorts in Switzerland. Recreation: summer skiing, dogsled riding, and mountain climbing.

Victoria-Jungfrau
Grand Hotel & Spa
❤❤❤❤❤

CH-3800 Interlaken. Tel: (33) 828-2828. Fax: (33) 828-2880. TYPE: Spa Hotel. LOCATION: In the exclusive center of Interlaken with sweeping views of the Jungfrau Mt. SPA CLIENTELE: Women and men.

* Rooms: 216 w/private bath. Suites: 64
* Phone, CTV, C/H, minibar

* Restaurants (3), bars (3), nightclub
* Airport: Bern Airport
* Credit Cards: MC, VISA, AMEX, DC, JCB
* Open: Year round
* Hotel Rates: from Sfr 295; TAC: 8%
* Spa on premises
* **Spa Facilities:** Fitness & Beauty Center, pool, sauna, solarium, gyms, indoor golf & tennis center
* **Spa Packages:** Wellness à la carte (2,4 or 6 nts) from Sfr 715; Spa Deluxe (6 nts) from Sfr 2,375
* **Spa Treatments:** body fat analysis, diet plan, 'cuisine minceur' diet, fitness training, medical fitness
* **Indications:** Rejuvenation, regeneration, beauty, anti-stress, well being, weight loss

DESCRIPTION: Deluxe hotel, Interlaken's leading hotel housed in a modernized palace-style building. The elegant spa features a magnificent Hollywood style pool area, fitness training rooms, and a full service beauty department. Recreation: tennis, golf, hiking, adventure excursions in the Jungfrau region.

KASTANIENBAUM
⟩ 41

✈ Zurich Int'l Airport (ZRH)

Seehotel Kastanienbaum Luzern
♥♥♥♥♥

CH-8536 Kastanienbaum. Tel: (41) 340-0340. Fax: (41) 340-1015. TYPE: Spa Hotel. LOCATION: On the shore of Lake Lucerne, 15 min. by car from Lucerne. SPA CLIENTELE: Women and men. DESCRIPTION: Resort hotel with lake and mountain views, 37 rooms. The Kaz Wellness Club offer pampering and weight loss programs. Spa Packages: Wellness Week of Pampering (6 nts) from Sfr 1,490; Trim & Slim Pampering (6 nts) from 2,250.

LAKE GENEVA
⟩ 21

✈ Geneva Int'l Airport (GVA)

Lake Geneva is the largest of the lakes in the Alps shared between Switzerland and France. For centuries the beauty of the northern shores of Lake Geneva has been lauded by famous European poets and writers such as Byron, Voltaire and Rousseau.

The climate in this spectacular Southwestern region of Switzerland is usually within 10°F of Eastern US temperature. During the Summer months, the temperature on Mt. Pelerin normally range from 70°F-80°F (21°c - 27°c) during the day to 60°F - 70°F (16°c - 21 °c) at night. At an altitude of 2,500 ft / 757 m the humidity level is very low.

Le Mirador Resort Hotel & Spa
♥♥♥♥♥

CH-1801 Mont Pelerin, Lake Geneva. Tel: (21) 925-1111, USA (toll free): 1-800-MIRADOR, Fax: (21) 925-1112, TYPE: Deluxe Resort & Spa. SPA DIRECTOR: John R. Herren. LOCATION: Heart of Swiss wine country overlooking Lake Geneva. SPA CLIENTELE: Women and men.

* Rooms: 72 w/priv. bath. Suites: 15 w/jacuzzi
* Phone, CTV, A/C, C/H,minibar
* Restaurants: "Le Trianon" elegant, "Le Patio" informal light low fat spa cuisine
* Airport: Geneva International, 50 minutes
* Train Station: Vevey (10 min.)
* Airport/Train Station Transportation: Taxi / limo
* Reservations: Required
* Credit Cards: MC, VISA, AMEX, DIN
* Open: February 14 - December 31 (1999)
* Rates: Rooms Sfr 220 - Sfr 1,600, Services Sfr 25 - Sfr 130
* TAC: 10% (8% on packages)
* Spa on premises: **Le Mirador Spa**
* Year Established: 1970
* **Spa Facilities:** Indoor/outdoor pools, steam rooms, saunas, whirlpools, swiss showers, fitness room, computerized golf simulator, tennis and volleyball courts, table tennis, billiards, hiking trails, solarium
* **Spa Treatments:** aqua exercises, body massages, herbal wraps, aromatherapy, foot reflexology, natural moor mud hydrotherapy, algotherapy, loofah skin glow, salt-glow, loofah scrub, cellulite / firming

with moor mud or algae, leg treatment, seaweed body mask, facials, eye and neck lifting, back, neck, bust and Décolleté treatment,manicure, pedicure, waxing, make-up consultation and application, revitalizing scalp treatment with seaweed shampoo, anti-stress scalp treatment with moor mud shampoo, scalp massage, cellulite treatments, colortherapy

* **Spa Packages**: "Get away from it all" (3 day) from Sfr 1,680, (6 day) from Sfr 3,025 price per person double occupancy includes full board, up to two treatments each day at choice, airport transfers, unlimited use of fitness and sports facilities
* **Indications**: Stress reduction, weight loss, rejuvenation, pampering
* Email: mirador@ibm.net
* Web: www.mirador.ch

DESCRIPTION: Celebrated as one of Switzerland's finest five-star resorts, Le Mirador is an elegant manor adorned with an exquisite collection of fine art and surrounded by acres of scenic vineyards. The view from 1,200 ft. / 363 m. above the lake is a panoramic vista of Lake Geneva, the Rhone Valley and the Alps. The emphasis at the Health Spa is on healthy living, relaxation and revitalization. The 'sans-regimen' program will teach you how to become healthier and slimmer at your own pace; tone up and trim down with aerobic exercises; or condition your body with a personal fitness trainer. Each day you can choose your meals from low calorie delicious spa dishes or Le Mirador's gourmet cuisine. *Member: The Leading Hotels of the World, Preferred Hotels & Resorts Worldwide, SLH, The Swiss Leading Hotels, SPA, Int'l Association of Conference Centers.*

LAUSANNE
〕 **21**
✈ Geneva Airport (GVA) 42 mi. / 68 km.

Lausanne Palace
♥♥♥♥♥

♨ 🏊 🤸 🕴 ❀

Grand-Chêne 7-9, CH-1002 Lausanne. Tel: (21) 331-3131. Fax: (21) 323-2571. TYPE: Hotel & Spa. LOCA-TION: City center with view of Lake Geneva. SPA CLIEN-

TELE: Women and men. DESCRIPTION: Luxurious Palace hotel in ornate building with wellness centre. The Wellness Center features extensive sports, beauty and anti-stress programs. Spa facilities: indoor pool, jacuzzi, sauna, steam bath, fitness room, meditation room. Spa Packages: Antistress (1 nt) from Sfr 800; Slenderizing (1 nt) from Sfr 900. 150 rooms, 31 suites, restaurant, bars, nightclub, business center. Hotel rates: from Sfr 330.

LENK
〕 **33**
✈ Belp Airport (BRN) Bern

Lenk, population 2,000, is a small spa resort nestling at the foot of Wildstrubel in the Bernese Oberlande about 25 mi. (40 km.) south of Bern. It can be reached from Bern by car or train.

The beautiful mountain setting provides the ideal ambience for relaxation and tranquility. Lenk offers 200 km. (125 mi.) of walks and mountain trails, swimming pools, cable-railway, and a health center with sulfur springs. Winter sports include 130 km. (81 mi.) of downhill ski-runs, ski-lifts, 42 km. (26 mi.) of cross-country ski-runs, free skiing at high altitude and a Swiss ski school. The Health Resort Center of Lenk (open mid-December - late October) offers a complete range of spa treatments.

A preliminary medical examination is required for all therapies, except the use of the mineral indoor pool, solarium, relaxing massages, and sulfur inhalations. Treatments at the center include: mineral indoor pool, sulfur tub-bath, mud bath, remedial gymnastics, spa-gymnastics, massage, Vichy shower, fango and hayseed packs, electro-therapy, sulfur inhalations, ultra modern solarium with intensive face tanning, cosmetics on request.

Kurhotel Lenkerhof
♥♥♥♥

🏥 🏊 🤸 🕴 ❀

CH-3775 Lenk. Tel: (33) 736-3131. Fax: (33) 733-2060. TYPE: Health Resort. LOCATION: Near village center surrounded by gardens. SPA CLIENTELE: Women and men, Family oriented.

* Rooms: 95; 49 w/priv. bath. Suites: 6
* Phone, CTV, C/H, minibar
* Restaurant, bar, lounges, meeting room
* Airports: Berne / Zürich / Geneva
* Train Station: Lenk, 10 min., taxi, hotel bus
* Reservation: Required
* Credit Cards: MC/VISA/AMEX/DC
* Open: 23rd Dec. - 31st Oct.
* Rates on Request: TAC: 8%
* Spa: directly linked to Health Center
* Distance to Health Center: 200 m. (200 yards)
* **Spa Facilities**: Directly linked to The Health Resort Centre of Lenk with spa cure facilities; in the hotel - Anabelle Beauty Studio, mineral indoor pool 34°
* **Spa Programs**: medical, health, fitness, beauty
* **Spa Packages**: Fitness & Feel Good weekends
* **Spa Treatments**: massage, hydrotherapy, exercises, inhalations, lymphatic drainage, physical training, electrotherapy at the Medical Center; facials and cosmetic treatments at the beauty salon
* Medical Supervision: 2 doctor, specially trained and experienced staff
* Treatments Approved: Swiss Health Authority

DESCRIPTION: Elegant hotel with fine Health Center focusing on wellness and modern physiotherapy. Those who wish to indulge in a spa vacation can enjoy the therapeutic effects of Europe's strongest alpine sulfur spring at the thermal swimming pool. Recreation: tennis at the hotel, water sports in nearby lakes and brooks, mountain climbing, and skiing in the winter.

LEUKERBAD
⟩ 27

Leukarbad, population 1,500, is a well known year round high altitude spa resort on a protected south slope in the Alps of Valais. The spa offers elegant resorts and wellness centers and broad programs of summer and winter sports. Three million liters of thermal water flow to the 22 outdoor and indoor baths. The water contain lime and sulphur. The temperature of the baths between 28°c-41°c (82°F-106°F) is helpful in the treatment of rheumatism, gout, and paralysis. Leukerbad can be reached by car from Lenk or Geneva.

In the centre of the resort is **The Alpentherme**, alpine spa for health and relaxation. The Health Centre offers the following treatments: hydrotherapy, electrotherapy, physiotherapy, fango, hayseed, inhalation. Revitalization programs include curative treatments (athrosis, rheumatism), preventive treatments (stress, fatigue, fitness) and slimming cures. All treatments are provided under medical supervision.

Badehotel Bristol
♥♥♥♥

CH-3954 Leukerbad. Tel: (27) 472-7500. Fax: (27) 472-7552. TYPE: Spa Hotel. LOCATION: Town center near the Alpine thermal springs. SPA CLIENTELE: Women and men. DESCRIPTION: Well established spa hotel with Thermal Wellness Park and beauty farm. Spa treatments: thermal baths, beauty treatments, shiatsu, acupressure and body alignment. Spa Packages: Regenerative week (7 nts) from Sfr 2,335; Wellness Weekend (3 nts) from Sfr 595.

Grichting & Badnerhof Hotel
♥♥♥♥

CH-3954 Leukerbad. Tel: (27) 472-7711. Fax: (27) 470-2269. TYPE: Spa Hotel. LOCATION: Village center near Thermal Bath. SPA CLIENTELE: Women and men. DESCRIPTION: Spa hotel with wellness center. Spa facilities: Salt water pool, whirlpool, sauna, solarium, steam room, beauty salon, roman baths, aroma grotto. Spa treatments: sand and light therapy, hay bath, Cleopatra bath, massages. 48 rooms, apartments and junior suites, restaurants and bar. Spa packages: Soft Week (7 nts) from Sfr 901. Trial Weekend (3 nts) from Sfr 511.

Maison Blanche Grand Bain
♥♥♥♥

CH-3954 Leukerbad. Tel: (27) 470-5161. Fax: (27) 470-3474. TYPE: Spa Hotel. LOCATION: Village center near thermal baths. SPA CLIENTELE: Women and men. DESCRIPTION: Traditional spa hotel with the largest thermal bath program in Switzerland. The hotel features a wellness center, three hotel thermal baths, Roman-Irish baths, Clarins beauty center, sun-bathing meadow, tennis courts and restaurant with exquisite cuisine. Spa treatments: hydrotherapy, balneotherapy, acupuncture, full body relaxing massage, daily water gymnastics, beauty treatments. Spa Packages: Anti-stress week (7 nts) from Sfr 1,449. Beauty & Relaxation week (7 nts) from Sfr 1,624.

MONTREUX
↘ 21
✈ Geneva Int'l Airport (GVA)

Montreux, population 20,400, is a cosmopolitan year round climatic resort at the east end of Lake Geneva. As a famous climatic resort, Montreux is a favorite holiday destination for those suffering from age or stress related disturbances.

The city is cherished for its lovely promenades and blossoming parks along the Lake. Adding to this unique, natural setting and mild climate, is the important revitalization clinique: the **Biotonus Center of Medical Regeneration** that specializes in natural and biological treatments of degenerative diseases and aging is located at the Hotel Excelsior Montreux (see description).

Montreux offers recreation, night life, fine dining and tourist attractions such as a pleasure boat cruise on the lake, and a spectacular side trip by train to the nearby Rochers de Naye for a spectacular view of Lake Geneva, and the Alps. Both Lausanne and Geneva with their international flavors are located nearby for city attractions, cultural events, and fine shopping. Montreux can be reached by car or train from Geneva or Lausanne.

Grand Hotel Excelsior
Biotonus Montreux
❤❤❤❤

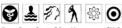

Rue Bon Port 21, Montreux CH-1820. Tel: (21) 963-3231. Fax: (21) 963-7795. TYPE: Hotel & Spa. LOCATION: In a private garden on the shore of Lake Geneva. SPA CLIENTELE: Women and men.

* Rooms: 63 w/private bath. Suites: 4
* Phone, CTV, VCR, A/C, C/H, minibar, balcony

* Restaurant, bar, meeting facilities
* Wheelchair Accessible
* Airport: Geneva AP 50 mi. (80 km.), train, taxi
* Reservations: required
* Credit Cards: MC/VISA/AMEX/DC/CB/EC
* Open: Year round
* Hotel Rates: from Sfr 190; TAC: 8%
* Spa on premises: **Clinique Biotonus**
* **Spa Facilities**: gym, sauna, massage room, heated indoor pool; Biotonus - Center of Medical Regeneration
* **Spa Programs**: Natural & Biological therapies of age related disturbances
* **Spa Treatments**: Organic stimulation based on the concept of Prof. Niehans, stimulation of the connective tissues according to the Filatov method, implantation of fresh placenta, Aslan therapy, gymnastics, hydrotherapy, diet
* Medical Supervision: doctors, nurses, approved dieticians, beauticians, kinesiologist
* Treatments Approved: Medical Institute

DESCRIPTION: The Excelsior Hotel is a fine lakeshore luxury hotel. All guest rooms face south and offer views of the Lake and the Alps. The hotel offers specialized climatic and medical treatments at the famous Biotonus Center for Medical Regeneration. The medical center developed the holistic wellness concept of Biospécifique, which is ideal for treating affections of a physical nature. Treatments are also available for geriatric patients who want to preserve their health and recover their vitality based on methods developed by Prof. Niehans, Dr. Aslan and Denyse Gardinier. Most treatments require a 7 day minimum to be successful. Spa Package: Biotonus Fitness/Health/Beauty (7 nts) from Sfr 2,400. Recreation: tennis, golf, fine dining, sightseeing & shopping.

MORSCHACH
↘ 41
✈ Zurich Int'l Airport (ZRH)

Swiss Holiday Park
❤❤❤❤

CH-6443 Morschach. Tel: (41) 825-5050. Fax: (41) 825-

5060. TYPE: Spa Village. LOCATION: Above Lake Lucerne, 30 min. from Lucerne, 60 min. from Zurich by car. SPA CLIENTELE: Women and men. DESCRIPTION: Holiday park offering the ideal site for fitness and wellness vacation. The complex includes hotel, vacation apartments, and lodgings. Spa facilities: waterworld, sauna world, Roman-Irish thermal baths, indoor and outdoor pools, cosmetic salon, six restaurants. Spa treatments: fitness, sports, balneotherapy, hydrotherapy, massage service, beauty treatments. Spa package: 3 nights from Sfr 599.

RHEINFELDEN
🏂 61
✈️ Basel/Mulhouse Int'l Airport (BSL) 64 mi. /40 km.

Rheinfelden, population 7,000, is a spa resort about 10 miles (17 km) east of Basel, near the Black Forest area in West Germany. Rhinfelden spa is known for the curative properties of its thermal water that include saline deposits that are among the strongest in Europe. The brine water gushes forth from under the ground and is pumped into the spa establishments, the hotels and the spa clinic. The spa's natural brine at a temperature of 33°c (91°F) contains sodium chloride, calcium, magnesium sulfate, magnesium, potassium, and strontium chloride, boric acid and bromide.

Indications: rehabilitation after illnesses, rheumatic diseases, motor disorders following accidents, metabolic disorders, neurological illnesses, illnesses of the respiratory organs, and gynecological disorders (menstrual disorders, sterility).

Park-Hotel am Rhein
❤️❤️❤️❤️

Roberstenstraße 31, 4310 Rheinfelden. Tel: (61) 836-6633. Fax: (61) 836-6634. TYPE: Spa Hotel. LOCATION: Centrally located on a private landscaped park. SPA CLIENTELE: Family oriented

* Rooms: 78 w/private bath. Suites: 7
* Radio, direct dial phone
* Restaurant & Grill Room
* Airport: Basel-Mulhouse 25 km. / 16 mi., taxi, bus

* Train St'n: Rheinfelden 3 km. / 2 mi.
* Credit Cards: MC/VISA/AMEX/DC/EC
* Open: Year round
* Hotel Rates: from Sfr 210; TAC: 8%
* Spa off premises: 30 m. / yards
* **Spa Facilities**: direct access to Rhinfelden Spa in hotel - indoor/outdoor thermal pools, fitness room, sauna, solarium
* **Spa Programs**: Medical, fitness, anti cellulite
* **Spa Treatments**: therapy at the Kurzentrum, diet and fitness at the hotel
* Medical Supervision: 4 MD
* Treatments Approved: Swiss Spa Association

DESCRIPTION: Spa hotel in a garden setting with direct access to the Kurzentrum (Cure Clinic). Own spa program for fitness, diet and general well being. Recreation: tennis, casino gaming and dancing in the New Rheinfelden Casino which is conveniently located nearby.

ST. MORITZ
🏂 81
✈️ Agno Airport, Lugano (LUG) 73 mi. /115 km.

St. Moritz, population 6,000, is located in the Alps of southeast Switzerland, about 150 km. (93 mi.) southeast of Zurich. St. Mortiz is one of Europe's most glamorous ski resorts, where jet setters from all over the world come to spend their vacation. It is also the highest spa town in Europe at 6,000 ft. (1,775 m.) above sea level and its thermal springs have the greatest carbondioxide content in Europe.

Indications: convalescence and rehabilitation after serious accident or a prolonged sickness, rheumatic diseases, mechanical injuries, metabolic disorders, and certain neurological illnesses. The natural thermal water and alpine peat provide the natural cures that made St. Moritz so famous.

Badrutt's Palace Hotel
❤️❤️❤️❤️❤️

7500 St. Moritz. Tel: (81) 837-1000. Fax: (81) 837-2999. TYPE: Resort Complex & Spa. LOCATION: Centrally overlooking the lake. SPA CLIENTELE: Women and men.

* Rooms: 220 w/priv. bath. Suites: 20
* Phone, CTV, A/C, C/H, minibar, private sundecks
* Restaurant, grill room & bar
* Conference and banquets facilities
* Nearest Train St'n: St. Moritz 500 m. / yards
* Train Station Transportation: limo, taxi
* Reservations: 3 nights deposit
* Credit Cards: MC/VISA/AMEX/DC/EC
* Open: December - April & June-Sept.
* Hotel Rates: from Sfr 270
* TAC: 8%
* Spa on premises
* **Spa Facilities**: Health & fitness center, gym, aerobic rooms, jacuzzis/whirlpools, saunas, beauty salon, indoor and outdoor pools,
* **Spa Programs**: Diet/Fitness, Beauty
* **Spa Treatments**: massage, aerobic exercises, beauty treatments
* **Indications**: same as St. Moritz Bad
* Medical Supervision: doctor on premises

DESCRIPTION: The Badrutt's Palace Hotel is a world-renowned health resort with deluxe accommodations, and recreation facilities. The spa program is limited to fitness, weight loss and beauty treatments. International tournaments are organized for bridge, tennis, backgammon and polo on snow. Recreation: swimming, squash, natural ice-rink, skiing, and indoor computer golf. Member: *Leading Hotels of The World*

Kulm Hotel
♥♥♥♥♥

Via Maistra, St. Moritz 7500. Tel: (81) 833-2738. Fax: (81) 833-2738. TYPE: Spa Hotel. LOCATION: A quiet residential area near all sports and spa activities. SPA CLIENTELE: Women and men, family oriented.

* Rooms & Suites: 200 w/priv. bath.
* Phone, CTV, minibar
* Grill room, restaurants, piano bar
* Airport: Zurich, 150 km. (93 mi.) train, taxi
* Credit Cards: MC/VISA/AMEX/EC/ACC
* Open: Dec. 1 - Apr. 12; June 20 - Sept. 10

* Hotel Rates: from Sfr 220
* TAC: 8%
* Spa on premises
* **Spa Facilities**: Heated indoor pool, gym area, sauna, steam room, spa facilities, massage rooms
* **Spa Programs**: Medical, fitness and beauty
* **Spa Treatments**: sauna, massage, Kneipp physiotherapy, peat baths and packs
* **Indications**: same as St. Moritz Bad
* Medical Supervision: in house Medical Clinic
* Treatments Approved: Association of Swiss Health Spas

DESCRIPTION: Luxury hotel that meets a high standard in comfort and service. The hotel offers spa programs from one to two weeks with emphasis on relaxation and beauty. Medical treatments are available under medical supervision. Recreation: tennis, golf, ice skating, bridge games, candle-light dinners, live entertainment and skiing nearby.

Parkhotel Kurhaus
♥♥♥♥

Via Mezdi 27, St. Moritz 7500. Tel: (81) 832-2111. Fax: (81) 833-8861. TYPE: Hotel & Spa. LOCATION: On ski area connected to thermal baths. SPA CLIENTELE: Women and men, family oriented.

* Rooms: 180 w/priv. bath, Suites: 15
* Phone, CTV, C/H
* Dining Room with Terrace
* Airport: Zurich, 150 km. (93mi.), train
* No Credit Cards
* Open: June - Sept, Dec- April
* Hotel Rates: from Sfr 185; TAC: 8%
* Spa on premises
* **Spa Facilities**: Directly connected to mineral baths, cure & diet facilities
* **Spa Programs**: Medical, fitness and beauty
* **Spa Treatments**: sauna, massage, Kneipp physiotherapy, peat baths and packs
* **Indications**: same as St. Moritz Bad
* Medical Supervision: in house Medical Clinic
* Treatments Approved: Assoc. of Swiss Health Spas

DESCRIPTION: First class hotel near ski area. Spa programs focus on medical, fitness, weight loss and beauty. Recreation: tennis and squash. Skiing is available nearby including ski school for first timers.

VALS
) 81

✈ Zürich Int'l Airport (ZRH) 94 mi. / 150 km.

Vals, is an Alpine spa in the Graubünden canton of south-eastern Switzerland. It is an excellent gateway to the sunny Italian canton of Ticino. The area is excellent for year round sports and recreation. In the summer there is mountain climbing and beautiful scenery, and during the winter excellent conditions for skiing.

Vals can be reached from Zurich driving southeast on the N3 to Chur and from there proceeding southwest to Vals.

Hotel Therme
♥♥♥

CH-7132 Vals. Tel: (81) 926-8080. Fax: (81) 926-8000. TYPE: Spa Hotel. LOCATION: In an a mountain setting. SPA CLIENTELE: Women and men.

* Rooms: 150 w/priv. bath. Suites: 2
* Phone, CTV, C/H, balcony
* Restaurant: diet meals available
* Airport: Zürich Airport 150 km. / 94 mi. bus
* Credit Cards: MC/VISA/AMEX/DC/EC
* Open: May 26 - April 20
* Hotel Rates: from Sfr 115; TAC: 8%
* Spa on premises
* **Spa Facilities**: Indoor and outdoor thermal pools; therapy rooms, sauna, fitness studio and spa facilities
* **Spa Programs**: Diet Program, Ski & Spa, Anti-stress (7 nts), Sampler Special (3 nts)
* **Spa Treatments**: medical, diet/fitness, thermal baths, massages, mud packs
* **Indications**: Obesity, rheumatism, recovery after illness/surgery, neuralgia, stress
* **Medical Supervision**: 1 MD, 1 RN
* No of customers per doctor: 200

* Treatments Approved: Swiss Spa Association

DESCRIPTION: A modern spa in the Swiss Alps with direct access to the natural stone thermal bath. The spa offers thermal therapy, and medical diet program. For ski enthusiasts there is a special Spa & Ski package. Recreation: tennis, swimming, hiking.

YVERDON-LES-BAINS
) 24

✈ Geneva Int'l Airport (GVA)

Yverdon-les-Bains, population 22,000, is located at the southern tip of the Lake of Neuchâtel in western Switzerland near the French border. Lausanne and Geneva are only a short drive south.

Yverdon-les-Bains is one of Switzerland's leading spa towns, but its tradition of thermal cure dates back to the Roman time. It houses the central office of the **International Federation of Thermalism and Climatism** which is devoted to the promotion of hydrotherapeutic and health resorts. The spa's unique mineral water gushes forth from a depth of 1,600 ft. (500 m) and emerges at the surface at a temperature of 84°F (29°c). The thermal springs are enriched with sulfur, iodine, bicarbonate, chlorine, sodium and calcium magnesium. The spa's alkaline drinking water are known as 'Arkina' and are used in water drink cure for digestive problems and obesity.

Indications: rheumatic ailments, and problems of the respiratory tract.

Grand Hotel des Bains
♥♥♥♥

22, avenue des Bains, 1400 Yverdon-les-Bains. Tel: (24) 425-7021. Fax: (24) 425-2190. TYPE: Spa Hotel. LOCATION: Surrounded by a magnificent park, adjacent to the Thermal center. SPA CLIENTELE: Women and men.

* Rooms: 125 w/priv. bath. Suites: 4
* Restaurant, dining & banquet room
* Airport: Geneva Int'l Airport, 90 km. / 56 mi.

* Airport Transportation: taxi, limo
* Train Station: Yverdon 3 km. / 2 mi.
* Reservations: 2 nights deposit
* Credit Cards: MC/VISA/AMEX/DC/EC
* Open: Year round
* Hotel Rates: from Sfr 195
* TAC: 8%
* Spa on premises
* **Spa Facilities**: thermal pools (3), fitness center, beauty salon, sauna and solarium; complete thermal and medical center adjacent to the hotel
* **Spa Programs**: Stress Management, Recovery & Relaxation, Theme Week-Ends, Beauty
* **Spa Treatments**: Balneotherapy, kinesiotherapy, massotherapy, mud packs, electrotherapy, Inhalation
* **Spa Packages**: "Opal" Special (2 nts) from Sfr 468; "Emerald" Special (6 nts) from Sfr 1,510
* **Indications**: Rheumatic disorders, traumatic injuries of the locomotory apparatus, re-education following orthopedic surgery, or neurological and cerebrovascular illness, disorders of the peripheral circulation, disorders of the respiratory tract
* Medical Supervision: 2 MD
* Treatments Approved: Swiss Medical Assoc.

DESCRIPTION: First class chateau hotel surrounded by a park near the Thermal Center. The Grand Hotel des Bains offers European spa programs and Week-End themes for those seeking thermal cures, relaxation, body pampering, weight loss and revitalization.

ZURZACH
꒳ 56

✈ Zurich Int'l Airport (ZRH) 16 mi. / 25 km.

Zurzach, population 3,200, is a medieval spa town in northern Switzerland right in the Black Forest region. One of the youngest spa towns in Switzerland, Zurzach has developed rapidly and acquired international recognition since the mid

50's. Today, the spa boasts a modern rheumatic clinic, an ambulatorium and thermal establishments. The thermal center is directly connected with the Kurhotel, the Turmhotel and the Trumpavillion. The hot springs have a temperature of 40°c (104°F) and contain sodium sulfate and hydrocarbonate with lithium and fluorine.

Indications: for treatment at Bad Zurzach: recuperation from accident or sickness, rheumatic diseases, motor disorders, metabolic disorders, and neurological illnesses.

Parkhotel Golden Tulip
♥♥♥♥

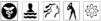

Badstraße 44, Bad Zurzach 8437. Tel: (56) 249-0151. Fax: (56) 249-3808. TYPE: Spa Hotel. LOCATION: Centrally located at the corner of Badstraße and Kornblumenweg, near the thermal pool and the rheumatic clinic. SPA CLIENTELE: Women and men, family oriented.

* Rooms: 170 w/pri. bath, suites
* Cafeteria, grill room, piano bar, restaurant
* Airport: Zurich / Kloten, 30 km. / 19 mi. taxi, bus
* Open: Year round
* Hotel Rates: Sfr 135
* Spa on premises
* **Spa Facilities**: Saline pool and therapeutical department, fitness center, beauty salon; direct access to the Rheumatologic Clinic
* **Spa Programs**: Medical, health, fitness, beauty
* **Spa Treatments**: medical treatments, beauty treatments, exercises, balneotherapy
* **Indications**: see Bad Zurzach
* Medical Supervision: Resident Physician
* Treatments Approved: Association of Swiss Health Spas

DESCRIPTION: Spa hotel with relaxing atmosphere. It is conveniently situated for those who wish to take the cure at the nearby thermal facilities.

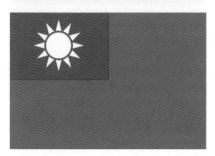

TAIWAN

AREA: 13,971 sq. mi. (36,185 sq. km.)
POPULATION: 20,204,880
CAPITAL: Taipei
OFFICIAL LANGUAGES: Chinese, Formosan
CURRENCY: Taiwan dollar (T$)
EXCHANGE RATE: 1 US$ = T$ 32.30
COUNTRY TELEPHONE CODE: 886

ℹ️ Taiwan Tourism Bureau
9 Fl. 280 Chunghsiao . Rd., Section 4, Taipei, Taiwan
tel: (+886-2) 721-8541. Fax: (+886-2) 773-5487

KAOHSIUNG
�’ 7
✈ Kaohsiung Int'l AP (KHH) 7 mi. / 11 km.

Grand Hi-Lai Hotel
♥♥♥♥♥

266 Cheng-Kung 1st Rd., Kaohsiung 800. Tel: (7) 216-1766. Fax: (7) 216-1966. TYPE: Hotel & Spa. LOCATION: In business and financial district. SPA CLIENTELE: Women and men. DESCRIPTION: Luxury business hotel with full service health spa, gym, sauna, massage, whirlpool, solarium, steam room, exercise equipment, aerobics, jacuzzi, outdoor pool, squash and health consultant. 450 rooms, floor for women travellers, floor for non smokers, restaurants (25), steakhouse, pizza pub, business services, executive club.

Hotel rates: from T$4,800.

TAIPEI
�’ 2
✈ Chiang Kai Shek Int'l AP (TPE) 25 mi. / 40 km.
Sung Shan AP (TSA) 5 mi. / 8 km.

Grand Formosa Regent Taipei
♥♥♥♥♥

41 Chung Shan North Road, Section 2, Taipei. Tel: (2) 2523-8000. Fax: (2) 2523-2828. TYPE: Hotel & Spa. LOCATION: Downtown Taipei business district. DESCRIPTION: Deluxe high-rise downtown hotel with health spa. Full service health spa, body/beauty treatments, aerobics, exercise equipment, steam room, whirlpool, sauna, massage, hair salon. 490 rooms, 60 suites, 2 nonsmoker floors, women travellers floor, wheelchair access. 10 restaurants, bars, lounge, meeting facilities. Hotel rates: from T$6,900.

TAITUNG
�’ 89
✈ Taitung Airport 13 mi. / 20 km.

Hotel Royal Chihpen Spa
♥♥♥♥

41 Chung 23 Lane 113, Long Chuien Rd., Wen Chuien Village, Peinan Hsiang, Taitung Hsien. Tel: (89) 510-666. Fax: (89) 510-678. Reservations (Taipei office) Tel: (2) 2523-9681. Fax: (2) 2523-3396. TYPE: Spa Resort. LOCATION: In Hot Springs area on the eastern coast. DESCRIPTION: Elegant Spa resort full of aboriginal round rattan designs, presenting a combination of modern and traditional styles. The health complex include hot spring baths, hot & cold whirlpools, sauna, solarium, beauty salon, jogging track and a full health club. 183 rooms each with a spa bath tub, 10 suites, 18 Japanese rooms, wheelchair access. Restaurants (2), piano bar, meeting facilities, swimming pool, tennis court. Hotel rates: from T$5,400.

THAILAND

AREA: 198,455 sq. mi. (513,998 sq. km.)
POPULATION: 46,455,000
CAPITAL: Bangkok
OFFICIAL LANGUAGES: Thai, Lao, Chinese
CURRENCY: Baht
EXCHANGE RATE: 1US$ = B 36
COUNTRY TELEPHONE CODE: 66

ⓘ Tourism Authority of Thailand
5 World Trade Center, Suite 3443,New York NY 10048
Tel: (212) 432-0433/5. Fax: (212) 912-0920

BANGKOK
✈ Bangkok Int'l Airport (BKK) 18 mi. / 29 km. NE

Bangkok, Krung Thep in Thai, is the orient in its mystical sense. The city sits on endless web of klongs (water canals) that serve communication, transportation and commerce. Explore the city's exquisite blend of richly ornate pagodas, modern hotels and exotic veils of colors and smells. Bangkok is a heaven for shoppers and bargain hunters. Many exotic wears, jewelry, arts and crafts can be imported to the US duty free.

Climate: There are three well defined seasons: the Hot Season (March - April); the Rainy Season (May - October) and the Cool Season (November - February). Average temperatures are about 83°F (28°c) ranging from 96°F (34°c) in April to 62°F (14°c) in December.

Oriental Bangkok
♥♥♥♥♥

48 Oriental Ave., Bangkok 10500. Tel: (2) 236-0400. Fax: (2) 236-1937/9. TYPE: Hotel & Spa. LOCATION: City center near major tourist attractions. SPA CLIENTELE: Women and men.

* Rooms: 396 w/priv. bath. Suites: 34
* Restaurants, bars and lounges
* Airport: Bangkok Int'l, 15 mi. / 24 km.
* Train Station: Hua Lampong, 3 km. / 2 mi.
* Credit Cards: MC/VISA/AMEX
* Open: Year round
* Hotel Rates: from B 6,800; Spa packages from $1,400 (3 nts) to $3,700 (7 nts); TAC: 10%
* Spa on premises
* Spa Facilities: Health & beauty spa, health club, pools (2), hydrotherapy and massage rooms, sauna, whirlpools, jogging track
* Spa Programs: Beauty, fitness and wellness
* Spa Treatments: body wraps, aromatherapy, Thai herbal treatments, reflexology, facials, Thai massage, European hydro treatments, Thai Spa cuisine, aerobics

DESCRIPTION: The Oriental Bangkok is one of the world's most beautiful hotels. The rooms and suites are luxuriously decorated. Some of the deluxe suites are equipped with a private sauna and elegant whirlpool. The health & beauty spa offers a variety of Thai and European treatments from exclusive herbal and exotic fruit treatments to relaxing massages and hydrotherapy.

Sheraton Grande Sukhumvit Grande Spa & Fitness Club
♥♥♥♥

250 Sukhumvit Rd. Bangkok. Hotel Tel: (2) 653-0333. Fax: (2)653-0400. SPA Tel: (2) 653-0333. Fax: (2) 653-0400. TYPE: Hotel & Spa. LOCATION: Heart of the business area. DESCRIPTION: Elegant hotel in the heart of the business area with Health Club and Spa. SPA: spa therapies using all-natural organic "E" spa products, health club. 439 rooms, 26 suites, nonsmoker rooms, wheelchair

access. Restaurants (4), lounge, meeting facilities, business center, outdoor pool. Hotel rates: from B 5,200.

The Westin Banyan Tree & Banyan Tree Spa
❤❤❤❤❤

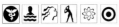

21/100 South Sathorn Road, Sathorn, Bangkok 10120. Hotel Tel: (2) 679-1200. Fax: (2) 679-1199. Spa Tel: (2) 679-1052. Fax: (2) 679-1053. TYPE: Hotel & Spa. LOCATION: In the Wah Tower in the central business district. DESCRIPTION: All-suite business hotel fitness and spa center, spa treatments, yoga, crystal therapy, sauna, steam room, pool, jacuzzi. 216 suites, nonsmoker rooms, wheelchair access. Restaurants (2), lounges (2), meeting rooms, business center. Hotel rates: from B 6,200.

CHIANG MAI
✈ 53
Chiang Int'l Airport (CNX) 3.5 mi. / 6 km.

The Regent Chiang Mai
❤❤❤❤❤

502 Mae Rim, Samoeng Road, Chiang Mai 50180. Tel: (53) 298-181. Fax: (53) 298-190. TYPE: Hotel & Spa. LOCATION 25 minutes to downtown & airport. DESCRIPTION: All-suite luxury hotel with health spa. Aromatherapy, facials, massage, exercise room, sauna, jacuzzi. 72 units, nonsmoker rooms. Restaurants (2), bar, entertainment, meeting room, business services, outdoor pool. Hotel rates: from US$280.

HUA-HIN
✈ 32
Hua Hin Airport 6 mi. / 10 km.

Chiva-Som International Health Resort
❤❤❤❤❤

73/4 Petchkasem Rd., Hua Hin 77110. Tel: (32) 536-

536. Fax: (32) 511-615. TYPE: Health Resort. LOCATION: Set on 7 acres of beach side land near the King's summer palace at Hua Hin, 210 km. / 131 mi. south of Bangkok. SPA CLIENTELE: Women and men.

* Rooms: 33 ocean view. Suites: 7
* 17 Thai-style Pavilion rooms
* Restaurant: Emerald Room - fine dining seaside restaurants, Open style lounges (2)
* Airport: Hua Hin, taxi
* Credit Cards: MC/VISA/AMEX/DC
* Open: Year round
* Hotel Rates: from US$420; TAC: 10%
* Spa on premises
* **Spa Facilities**: Yoga & Tai Chi pavilions, outdoor massage pavilions (3), bathing pavilion, steam room, cold plunge pool, large hydro jacuzzi, gym, exercise and dance studios (2), treatment rooms (12), medical consultation rooms (5), hydrotherapy suite, beauty salon
* **Spa Programs**: Beauty, fitness and wellness, Rejuvenation, oxygen training, thalassotherapy
* **Spa Treatments**: massage therapies, traditional thai, swedish, shiatsu, aromatherapy, back and shoulder, reflexology, oriental foot massage, G5 vibro, hydro therapies and body treatments, underwater massage, deluxe hydrotherapy with essential oils, body blitz hydro jet, body contour and firming therapy, body polish and hydro therapy, thai body glow, loofah scrub, slim and slender therapy, flotation therapy, Kneipp baths, bust firming therapy, facials, aerobics, aqua aerobics, yoga, tai chi, meditation, beach power walk, mountain biking, iridology, allergy testing, physiotherapy, spa cuisine, health & beauty workshops
* Staff to guests ratio: 4 to 1
* Medical Supervision: medical department on premises

DESCRIPTION: Specialized health resort on the Gulf of Siam the brainchild of Thailand's former Deputy Prime Minister Mr. Boonchu Rojanastien. Chiva-Som translates as "Haven of Life" and it is Asia's first health resort. The spa offers comprehensive and holistic approach spa treatments that are complemented by medical wellness programs. The medical programs are biological and non-toxic and combine western and traditional Chinese medicine. Alternative medicine programs are also available. Chiva-Som provides an immense choice of treatments and consultations for health, fitness, body & soul. Member: *SLH*

PHUKET

76

 Phuket Int'l Airport 19 mi. / 30 km.

Banyan Tree Phuket & Banyan Tree Spa
❤❤❤❤

33 Moo 4, Srisoonthorn Rd. Cherngtalay, Amphur Talang, Phuket 83110. Tel: (76) 324-374. Fax: (76) 324-375. TYPE: Villa Resort & Spa. LOCATION: On Bang Tao Bay on Phuket's northwest coast. DESCRIPTION: Deluxe resort with full service spa, massage, rejuvenation treatments, aerobics, exercise equipment, meditation, lap pool. 98 villas. Restaurants (5), cafe, bars (3), lounge, meeting facilities, pool, tennis courts (3), 18-hole golf course. Hotel rates: from B 6,500.

RANONG

77

Ranong Airport 15 mi. / 24 km.

Ranong, population 10,300, is an up and coming resort town featuring the only potable geo-thermal hot mineral-water spring in Thailand. The town is located some 312 mi. (500 km.) southwest of Bangkok, on the beach of the Andaman Sea. The climate is temperate year round thanks to cooling breezes from the Indian Ocean and China Seas surrounding the narrow strip of land on which Ranong sits.

The major attraction in Ranong is the Public Park with its three natural Hot Springs. Other tourist attraction and recreation include a Marine sightseeing by boat, and Deep Sea fishing for the great Marlin and the fighting Sailfish. For nightlife, guests can enjoy the high-tech dance Disco at Jansom Thara and join the friendly local Thai patrons. Ranong can be reached by air from Bangkok, Surat Thani, and Phuket. There is air-conditioned bus service to Ranong from Bangkok which takes 8 hours.

Jansom Thara Hot Spa Health Resort
❤❤❤❤

2/10 Moo Petchasam Road, Bangrin, Ranong 85000. Tel: (77) 823-350/2. Fax: (77) 821-821. TYPE: Hot Springs Resort. LOCATION: At the foot of 1,000 ft. (300 m.) hills, besides a mountain fed stream and separated by a ridge from the city. SPA CLIENTELE: Women and men.

* Rooms: 220 standard & superior with private hot bath, mineral spa en suite
* Suites: 16 luxury style w/jacuzzi and cooking facilities
* Restaurant: delicious seafood meals
* Airport: Ranong's AP, 12 km. / 8 mi. taxi, bus
* Reservations: deposit required
* Credit Cards: MC/VISA/AMEX
* Open: Year round
* Rates: from US$50 (room only); TAC: 10%
* Spa on premises, hot springs off premises (1 km)
* **Spa Facilities:** 2 large semi-public natural, hot mineral water jacuzzis (42°c/108°F) the largest in Southeast Asia, accommodates 40 people each (Separate men and women bathing); fully equipped health club, gym, jogging track, huge mineral water swimming pool
* Spa Programs: Western style structured and disciplined jogging programs, diet, exercise & health programs, Special group programs; Flexible Asian style programs for those who are not accustomed to spa disciplines
* **Spa Treatments:** Bathing in mineral water, supervised exercise, calisthenics and aerobics, nutritious and delicious diet meals, massages
* Medical Supervision: 2 MD, 2 RN; experienced European health supervisor, fully trained instructors

DESCRIPTION: Jansom Thara is a charming health resort and the only hot-springs spa in Thailand. It is marketed to international travelers interested in wellness vacation. The hotel is elegant and combines Western and Thai architecture. The spa programs are American and European style. They feature state-of-the-art techniques and equipment to help you keep in shape and loose weight while being pampered in an exotic and relaxing ambience. Recreation: tennis courts, horseback riding, mini golf, and deep-sea fishing.

TRINIDAD & TOBAGO

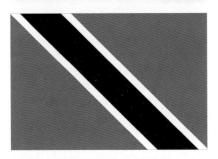

AREA: 1,980 sq. mi. (5,128 sq. km.)
POPULATION: 1,212,000
CAPITAL: Port of Spain
OFFICIAL LANGUAGES: English, Hindi
CURRENCY: Trinidad & Tobago dollar (T$)
EXCHANGE RATE: 1 US$ = T$ 6.25
COUNTRY TELEPHONE CODE: 868

ℹ️ Tourism & Industry Dept.

10-14 Philipps St., Port of Spain, Trinidad
Tel: (868) 623-1932. Fax: (868) 623-3848

Trinidad and Tobago are twin-island nation in the Caribbean near the northern coast of Venezuela. Tobago is the smallest of the two with a population of 100,000 and mostly Caribbean flair. The capital of Tobago is Scarborough, a tiny creole village on Rockly Bay.

Climate: The weather is sunny and tropical year round tampered by the cool trade winds. The average temperature is 74°F (23°c) at night and 84°F (29°c) during the day. The rainy season lasts from May to November.

BLACK ROCK

✈️ Crown Point Int'l Airport 5 mi. / 8 km.

Le Grand Courlan Resort & Spa
♥♥♥♥

PO Box 25, Black Rock, Tobago. Tel: 639-9667, Fax: 639-9292. TYPE: Beachfront Hotel & Spa. LOCATION: On Stonehaven Bay. DESCRIPTION: Beach resort hotel with fulll service spa & health club, sauna, massage, steam room, jacuzzi. 68 rooms, 10 suites, nonsmoker rooms, wheelchair access. Restaurants (2), bar, meeting facilities, business center, tennis courts (2), pool, beach, watersports. Hotel rates: from US$200.

SCARBOROUGH

✈️ Crown Point Int'l Airport 2 mi. / 3 km.

Coco Reef Resort & Spa
♥♥♥♥

P.O.Box 434, Scarborough. Tel: 639-8571. Fax: 639-8573. TYPE: Beachfront Hotel & Spa. LOCATION: Overlooking the Caribbean. DESCRIPTION: Beachfront resort with full service spa, gym, sauna, steam room, massage. 135 rooms & suites, nonsmoker rooms. Restaurant (2), bars (2), entertainment, meeting facilities, pool, tennis courts, beach water sports. Hotel rates: from US$198.

TUNISIA

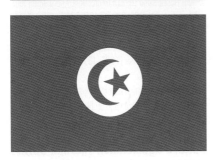

AREA: 63,378 sq. mi. (164,149 sq. km.)
POPULATION: 7,465,000
CAPITAL: Tunis
OFFICIAL LANGUAGES: Arabic, French
CURRENCY: Tunisian dinar (TD)
EXCHANGE RATE: 1 US$ = TD 1.10
COUNTRY TELEPHONE CODE: 216

ℹ️ Office National du Tourisme
Avenue Mohamed V, 1001 Tunis, Tunisia
Tel: (+216-1) 341-077. Fax: (+216-1) 350-977

SOUSSE
✈ Monastir Int'l Airport (MIR) 10 mi. / 15 km.

Abou Nawas Diar El Andalouss Hotel
♥♥♥♥

BP 40, Sousse 4089, Sousse. Tel: (3) 246-200. Fax: (3) 246-348. TYPE: Resort Complex. LOCATION: 7 km. / 4 mi. to Sousse, 25 km. / 16 mi. to Monastir/Skanes Airport. DESCRIPTION: Bayside resort complex with beauty & health center, body treatments, exercise, sauna. 291 rooms, 10 suites, nonsmoker rooms. Restaurants (3), coffee shop, piano bar, disco, meeting facilities, indoor & outdoor pools, tennis courts (12), bowling. Hotel rates: from TD 50.

TUNIS
✈ Carthage Airport (TUN) 5 mi. / 8 km.

Le Palace Tunis
♥♥♥♥

BP 68 La Marsa, les Cotes de Carthage 2078. Tel: (1) 748-445. Fax: (1) 748-442. TYPE: Hotel & Spa. LOCATION: In Cap Gammarth overlooking the Mediterranean Sea, 15 km. / 9 mi. to Tunis airport & 17 km. / 10 mi. to Tunis city center. DESCRIPTION: Modern hotel with balneotherapy center, body treatments, indoor & outdoor pools, gym, sauna, turkish bath, tennis courts (2), squash courts (3). 246 rooms, 45 suites, nonsmoker rooms, wheelchair access. Restaurants (2), coffee shop, bars (2), disco, meeting facilities,business center, beach club. Hotel prices: from TD 100.

TURKEY

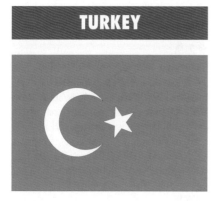

AREA: 300,946 sq. mi. (779,450 sq. km.)
POPULATION: 46,000,000
CAPITAL: Ankara
OFFICIAL LANGUAGES: Turkish
CURRENCY: Turkish Lira (T£)
EXCHANGE RATE: 1US$ = T£ 301,000*
* unstable currency, high inflation rate
COUNTRY TELEPHONE CODE: 90

Turkey has more than 1,000 geothermal sources, 190 thermal springs. The total facilities for thermal tourism which have obtained investment and operation permissions from the Tourism Ministry is 34. The better known spas are located along the Aegean Coast. The health giving properties of Turkey's natural hot springs and mineral baths have been renowned since antiquity. Health vacation in Turkey can be combined with visits of fascinating historic sites, skiing in winter resorts, or relaxing at the country's beautiful Aegean or Mediterranean beach resorts.

ⓘ Turkish Tourist Office
821 United Nations Plaza, New York NY 10017 USA
Tel: (212) 687-2194. Fax: (212) 599-7568

BALÇOVA - IZMIR
🕓 **232**
✈ Adnan Menderes Airport (ADB), Izmir

The Balçova Hot Springs are located on the site of the Baths of Agamemnon in the Aegean Coast east of Cesme. The hot

springs are known since ancient times for the therapeutic qualities of the water. The thermal water are composed of sodium chloride and calcium bicarbonate with a water temperature between 62°c-80°c (143°F-176°F). The climate is mild and pleasant year round. The average temperatures in the winter is 9°c (48°F) in January; the average temperatures in the summer is 28°c (82°F) in July.

Indications: rheumatic diseases, digestive maladies, post-injuries and post-operational problems, calcification and metabolic disorders.

Balçova Agamemnon Thermal Baths
❤❤❤

Balçova - Izmir. Tel: (232) 259-0102. Fax: (232) 259-0829. TYPE: Hotel & Spa. LOCATION: Near the thermal pools at the feet of the rolling verdant hills. SPA CLIENTELE: Women and men.

* Rooms: 215 w/priv. bath. Suites: 13
* Restaurants, bars and lounges
* Airport: Izmir
* Open: Year round
* Hotel Rates: from $100
* Spa on premises
* **Spa Facilities**: hot mineral pools and springs, Turkish bath
* **Spa Treatments**: balneotherapy, massages, underwater massage, electro-physical therapy,
* **Indications**: see general indications

DESCRIPTION: The Balçova hot baths complex, with a total capacity of 1,000 persons per day, provides hot mineral pools and baths, therapy pools and massages.

Thermal Prenses
❤❤❤❤❤

Ilica Mah, 112 Zeytin Sok, Nahdere - Izmir. Tel: (232) 238-5151. Fax: (232) 239-0939. TYPE: Hotel & Spa. LOCATION: Near the thermal pools at the feet of the rolling verdant hills. SPA CLIENTELE: Women and men.

* Rooms: 278 w/priv. bath
* Restaurants, bars and lounges
* Airport: Izmir
* Open: Year round
* Hotel Rates: from $180
* Spa on premises
* **Spa Facilities**: hot mineral pools and springs, Turkish bath
* **Spa Treatments**: balneotherapy, massages, underwater massage, electro-physical therapy,
* **Indications**: see general indications

DESCRIPTION: Elegant 5-star hotel part of the Balçova hot baths complex, provides new park, hot mineral pools and baths, therapy pools and massages.

BURSA
☽ 224
✈ Ataturk Airport (IST), Istanbul

Bursa, the first capital of the Ottoman dynasty is Turkey's 6th largest city. Located in Northwestern Anatolia, it is one hour drive from Istanbul. Bursa offers alpine setting, and winter skiing on the slopes of the 8,300 ft. / 2,515 m. Mt. Uludag. **The Ottoman Baths**, known as Eski Kaplica, function as part of the **Hotel Kervansaray**. The 5-star Celik Palas Hotel has luxuriously appointed facilities with natural hot springs and baths. The water composition of the Cekirge hot springs are: calcium, magnesium, sulfate and bicarbonate at water temperature from 39°c - 58°c (102°F - 136°F). The climate is mild year round with winter average temperatures of 5°c (41°F) in January, and summer average temperatures are 24°c (75°F) in July.

Indications: rheumatic diseases, hepatic and gall bladder diseases, metabolic disorders, gynecological diseases, and post-operational problems.

Celik Palas Hotel Thermal
❤❤❤❤❤

Cekirge Caddesi 79, Bursa. Tel: (224) 233-3800. Fax: (224) 236-1910. TYPE: Hotel & Spa. LOCATION: City cen-

ter near major tourist attractions. SPA CLIENTELE: Women and men.

* Rooms: 234 w/priv. bath. Suites: 13
* Restaurants, bars and lounges
* Airport: Istanbul, 1 hour
* Open: Year round
* Hotel Rates: from $120 (room only)
* Spa on premises
* **Spa Facilities**: hot mineral pools and springs, Turkish bath
* **Spa Treatments**: balneotherapy, massages, underwater massage, electro-physical therapy
* Indications: see general indications

DESCRIPTION: 5-star art-deco spa hotel featuring thermal springs and baths for recreation and medical therapy. The hotel feature luxuriously appointed facilities with natural hot springs and baths.

Kervansarai Hotel
❤❤❤❤❤

Cekirge Caddesi, Bursa. Tel: (224) 233-9300. Fax: (224) 233-9324. TYPE: Deluxe Hotel & Spa. LOCATION: City center near major tourist attractions. SPA CLIENTELE: Women and men.

* Rooms: 200 w/priv. bath. Suites: 13
* Restaurants, bars and lounges
* Airport: Istanbul, 1 hour
* Open: Year round
* Hotel Rates: from $120 (room only)
* Spa on premises
* **Spa Facilities**: hot mineral pools and springs, Turkish bath
* **Spa Treatments**: balneotherapy, massages, underwater massage, electro-physical therapy
* **Indications**: see general indications

DESCRIPTION: 5-star hotel featuring thermal springs and baths for recreation and medical therapy. The domed baths run by the hotel are an excellent example of early Ottoman architecture.

CESME

) 232

✈ Adnan Menderes Airport (ADB), Izmir

Cesme, is located on a peninsula at the Aegean Coast overlooking the Greek island of Chios, 70 km. / 44 mi. west of Izmir. Cesme means fountain in Turkish. The resort is famous for its therapeutic hot springs and natural sea spa. **Turban Cesme hot springs** contain high levels of sodium chloride and calcium bicarbonate at 55°c (131°F).

Cesme enjoys a mild climate year round. The average temperatures in the winter is 9°c (48°F) in January; the average summer temperatures is 25°c (77°F) in July. Cesme is conveniently located to the Turkish Aegean Coast. Both Izmir and ancient Ephesus are easily accessible.

Indications: Thermal and thalassotherapy are used for treating rheumatic, dermatological and gynecological diseases. They are also recommended for neurological exhaustion and to help strengthen the muscles.

Altinyunus Holiday Resort
❤❤❤❤❤

Boyalik Mevkii, Altinyunus Tatil Koyu, Cesme. Tel: (232) 723-1250. Fax: (232) 723-2252. TYPE: Resort & Spa. LOCATION: Set on a long sandy beach on the Aegean Coast. SPA CLIENTELE: Women and men.

* Rooms: 515 w/priv. bath
* Restaurants, bars and lounges
* Airport: Izmir, 1 hour
* Season: Year round
* Hotel Rates: from $110 (room only)
* Spa on premises
* **Spa Facilities**: Sea Spa, hot mineral pools and springs, Turkish bath, gym, geriatric units
* **Spa Treatments**: balneotherapy, massages, underwater massage, electro-physical therapy, thalassotherapy, physical rehabilitation. geriatric treatments
* **Indications**: see general indications

DESCRIPTION: Holiday resort on a cove along the sea front. Its natural Sea Spa can handle 500 people per day.

Turban Cesme Hotel
❤❤❤❤

Ilica Mevkii, Cesme-Izmir. Tel: (232) 723-1240. Fax: (232) 723-1388. TYPE: Resort & Spa. LOCATION: Beachfront on the Aegean Coast. SPA CLIENTELE: Women & men.

* Rooms: 210 w/priv. bath
* Restaurants, bars and lounges
* Airport: Izmir, 1 hour
* Open: Year round
* Hotel Rates: from $90 (room only)
* Spa on premises
* **Spa Facilities**: hot mineral pools and springs, Turkish bath, Thermal Bath, gym
* **Spa Treatments**: balneotherapy, massages, underwater massage, electro-physical therapy, thalassotherapy, physical rehabilitation, geriatric treatments
* **Indications**: see general indications

DESCRIPTION: Modern 4-star hotel with thermal pools and treatment facilities.

PAMUKKALE

) 258

✈ Adnan Menderes Airport (ADB), Izmir

Pamukkale "Cotton Castle" is one of the most popular tourist destination in Turkey. For thousands of years an underground hot spring has been pouring out hot mineral water that created a magnificent snow white plateau, almost 400 ft. / 121 m. high with a curtain of white stalagmites and shallow pools. To the ancients this was a holy place. The grand hellenic city of Hierapolis attracted pilgrims to bath in the curative waters. The mineral-rich hot springs contain calcium-magnesium sulfate and bicarbonate and have a radioactive content.

The climate is pleasant during winter, fall and spring.

Summers can be extremely hot. The average temperatures in the winter is 6°c (43°F); the average temperatures in the summer is 31°c (88°F).

Indications: the waters, used for drinking and bathing, are recommended for the treatment of rheumatic, dermatological and gynecological diseases, neurological and physical exhaustion, digestive maladies and nutrition disorders.

Club Colossea
❤❤❤❤

Karahayit - Pamukkale, Denizli. Tel: (258) 271-4373. Fax: (258) 271-4050. TYPE: Resort & Spa. LOCATION: Near the hot springs. SPA CLIENTELE: Women and men.

* Rooms: 230 w/priv. bath
* Restaurant, bar and lounges
* Airport: Izmir, 250 km. / 160 mi.
* Open: Year round
* Hotel Rates: from $90 (room only)
* Spa on premises
* **Spa Facilities**: Hot springs, Turkish bath, gym
* **Spa Treatments**: balneotherapy, massages, underwater massage, electro-physical therapy, thalassotherapy, geriatric treatments
* **Indications**: see general indications

DESCRIPTION: Health Spa Resort.

Hierapolis Thermal
❤❤❤❤❤

Karahayit - Pamukkale Denizli. Tel: (258) 271-4105. Fax: (258) 262-4816. TYPE: Resort & Spa. LOCATION: Near the hot springs. SPA CLIENTELE: Women and men.

* Rooms: 180 w/priv. bath
* Restaurant, bar and lounges
* Airport: Izmir, 250 km. / 160 mi.
* Open: Year round
* Hotel Rates: from $130 (room only)
* Spa on premises
* **Spa Facilities**: Hot springs, Turkish bath, gym
* **Spa Treatments**: balneotherapy, massages, underwater massage, electro-physical therapy, thalassotherapy, geriatric treatments
* **Indications**: see general indications

DESCRIPTION: Health Spa Resort.

SILIVRI
✈ Ataturk Int'l AP (IST), Istanbul 15 mi. / 24 km.

Klassis Golf & Country Club & Thalgo Health Farm
❤❤❤❤

Seymen Koyu, Altintepe Mevkii, Silivri 34930. Hotel - Tel: (212) 727-4050. Fax: (212) 727-4049. SPA - Tel: (212) 748-4600. Fax: (212) 748-4643. TYPE: Seaside Resort & Health Farm. LOCATION: On the beach of the Marmara Sea, 65 km. / 40 mi. to Istanbul. DESCRIPTION: Deluxe seaside resort hotel with health and beauty spa, Lavnium & Clarins Institutes with doctors, nurses, dieticians, aestheticians & sport instructors. Treatments emphasize beauty, positive health, fitness and relaxation. 263 rooms, 9 suites, 19 villas. Restaurants (3), coffee shop, bars (7), nightclub, meeting facilities, business center, private beach, swimming pools, tennis, squash. Hotel rates: from US$150.

TURKS & CAICOS

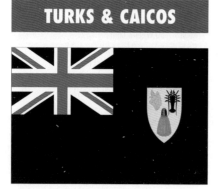

AREA: 193 sq. mi. (500 sq. km.)
POPULATION: 8,000
CAPITAL: Cockburn Town
OFFICIAL LANGUAGES: English
CURRENCY: US dollar (legal tender)
EXCHANGE RATE: 1 US$
COUNTRY TELEPHONE CODE: 649

❶ Turks & Caicos Islands Tourist
Board, P.O. Box 128, Pond St. Grand Turk BWI
Tel: (800) 241-0824. Fax: (649) 946-2321/1

Turks & Caicos islands is an archipelago of eight large islands and a large number of small cays spreading for 50 mi. / 80 km. about 575 mi. / 920 km. southeast of Miami (Florida/USA). The islands are sunny and peaceful, with beautiful sandy beaches

Climate: The weather is sunny and tropical year round tampered by the cool trade winds. The average temperature is 77°F (25°c) at night and 85°F (29°c) during the day. The rainy season lasts from May to November.

PROVIDENCIALES ISLAND
✈ Povidenciales Int'l Airport (PLS)

Beaches Resort & Spa
♥♥♥♥

Lower Bight Rd., Providenciales Island. Tel: 946-8000, Fax: 946-8001. SPA - Tel: 946-8000. Fax: 946-8001. SPA MANAGER: Christine Hays. TYPE: All-inclusive Resort & Spa. LOCATION: On a 12 mi. / 19 km. stretch of beach fo beach, nestled amidst palm grove. SPA CLIENTELE: Women and men. SPECIAL RESTRICTIONS: Persons under the age of 16 are not permitted to use the spa.

* Rooms: 177 w/priv. bath
* Suites: with 4-poster beds
* Phone, minibar, CTV, hair dryer, in-room safe
* Restaurants (5), pastry shop, grill room
* Airport: 15 minutes
* Reservations: required
* Credit Cards: AMEX/VISA/DC/EC
* Open: Year round
* Hotel Rates: from US$800 (2 nts plan); TAC: 10%
* Spa on premises: **Ultra Spas Sandals**
* **Spa Hours**: 8am-8pm daily
* **Spa Facilities**: fitness center with cardiovascular machines and CYBEX weight equipment, hot and cold plunge pools, saunas, showers, treatment rooms, beauty salon, fully stocked vanity area
* **Spa Programs**: beauty, pampering, fitness
* **Spa Treatments**: swedish massage, aromatherapy, reflexology, body scrubs, body wraps, moor mud, facials, hydrotherapy, hungarian kur bath, thalasso bath, aromatherapy mineral bath, power walks, aquacise, beach jog, aerobics, circuit training, stretch

DESCRIPTION: Elegant all-inclusive beach resort with a full service spa featuring the very best in spa treatments and facilities. Enjoy exercise regimen at the fitness center or indulge in revitalizing hydrotherapy or thalasso bath, exfoliating body scrub or a relaxing swedish massage. Spa treatments can be reserved for additional charge, subject to availability.

U.S.A.

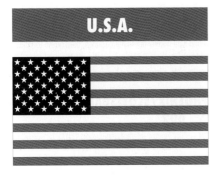

CURRENCY: Dollar (US$)
EXCHANGE RATE: 1 US$ = 100¢
COUNTRY CODE: 1

America spas are famous for their emphasis on healthy life style. Unlike European spas which have historically developed around thermal springs with restorative powers, American Spas draw their strength from a large spectrum of resources and ideas, They cater to the growing needs of Americas living the high paced lifestyle of the end of the 20th century and suffering from environmental pollution, job stress, and dietary over indulgence. American spas and resorts create the right environment for those who wish to loose weight, get in shape, revitalize, or simply enjoy the exotic body pampering. American spas are diverse and most teach long term lifestyle changes.

AREA: 3,623,420 sq. mi. (9,384,658 sq. km.)
POPULATION: 228,000,000
CAPITAL: Washington, D.C.
OFFICIAL LANGUAGE: English

ALASKA

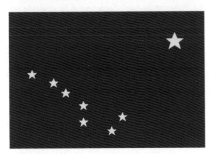

AREA: 591,004 sq. mi. (1,531,700 sq. km.)
POPULATION: 552,000
CAPITAL: Juneau
TIME ZONE: Alaska Time

ARCTIC CIRCLE
907

Circle Hot Springs Airport, 1/4 mi. / 400 m.

Circle Hot Springs Resort
♥♥♥

Circle Hot Springs Rd., P.O. Box 254, Central, AK 99730, Tel: (907) 520-5113. Fax: (907) 520-5442. TYPE: Rustic lodge with Hot Springs Spa. LOCATION: 50 mi. / 80 km. south of Arctic Circle off Steese Highway. DESCRIPTION: Hot springs spa with outdoor hot mineral pool and jacuzzi. 45 rooms, 18 suites, 9 cabins w/kitchenette, restaurant, bar, business center. Hotel rates: from $60.

CHENA HOT SPRINGS
907

✈ Fairbanks Int'l Airport (FAI)
65 mi. / 104 km.

Chena Hot Springs Resort
♥♥♥

56 1/2 Mile Chena Hot Springs Rd., Chena Hot Springs AK 99701. Mailing address: 331 7th Ave., Bakersfield; P.O. Box 73440, Fairbanks, AK 99707. Tel: (907) 452-7867, Fax: (907) 456-3122. TYPE: Rustic Lodge & Hot Springs Spa. LOCATION: On 440 wooded acres, 1/4 mi. / 400 m. to airport, 60 mi. / 96 km. to Fairbanks, 50 mi. / 80 km. south of the Arctic Circle. DESCRIPTION: Hot Spings Spa with outdoor mineral pool, hot tub, massage. 27 rooms, 18 suites & cabins with kitchenette, restaurant, coffee shop, cocktail lounge. Hotel rates: from $60.

ARIZONA

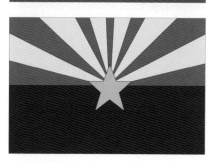

AREA: 114,000 sq. mi. (295,260 sq. km.)
POPULATION: 3,680,000
CAPITAL: Phoenix
TIME ZONE: Mountain Time

CAREFREE
ᒉ 602
✈ Sky Harbor International AP (PHX) 45 mi. / 70 km.

Golden Door Spa at The Boulders
♥♥♥♥♥

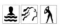

34631 N. Tom Darlington Drive, PO BOX 2090, Carefree, AZ 85377. Tel: (602) 488-9009. Fax: (602) 488-4118. TYPE: Resort & Spa. LOCATION: In the Sonoran Desert foothills, 45 min. from Phoenix. DESCRIPTION: Deluxe Southwestern style resort hotel with Golden Door Spa, body treatments, gym, massage, whirlpool, aerobics. 202 units including 42 villas. Restaurants (4), lounge, business center, 18-hole golf courses (2), tennis courts (8). Hotel rates: from $195.

MESA
ᒉ 602
✈ Sky Harbor Int'l Airport

Buckhorn Mineral Wells Spa
♥♥♥

5900 E. Main St., Mesa, AZ 85205. Tel: 602-832-1111. TYPE: Hot Springs Motel. DESCRIPTION: Old world desert motel with natural hot mineral springs, bath house facilities, whirlpool baths (2), massage offices (9), massages. 12 apartments. restaurant & shopping center next door.

PHOENIX/SCOTTSDALE
ᒉ 602
✈ Sky Harbor International Airport (PHX)
Scottsdale Municipal Airport (SCF)

Phoenix with Scottsdale, Tempe, Mesa, and Paradise Valley form a large metropolis area 60 mi. (96 km.) in diameter known as the "Valley of the Sun". Scottsdale is an affluent suburb and a major art center. Part of the town **The Rawhide** was built as a replica of an 1880 old Western town with a genuine frontier ambience and daily rodeo. Scottsdale and Phoenix offer world class health resorts, cosmopolitan nightlife, classy restaurants, unique saloons, and fashionable shopping centers. The sun always shines in the "Valley of the Sun". Summers can be extremely hot with temperatures reaching 95°F (35°c) and over. Fall, winter and spring are the best for vacation with comfortable temperatures in the 70°sF (21°c).

The Arizona Biltmore Resort & Spa
♥♥♥♥♥

24th & Missouri, Phoenix, AZ 85016. Tel: (602) 955-6600. Fax: (602) 381-7600. SPA Tel: (602) 381-7632. Fax: (602) 381-7683. TYPE: Resort & Spa. SPA DIRECTOR: Lorraine Park. LOCATION: Next to Aquaw peak mountain, 10 mi. / 16 km. to airport. SPA CLIENTELE: Women and men. SPECIAL RESTRICTION: Guests 16 years or younger must be accompanied by an adult.

* Rooms & Villas: 650
* Phones (2), Cellcom door lock security, balcony
* Dining Room, lounge
* Airport: Sky Harbor Int'l, taxi, limo
* Open: Year round
* Credit Cards: MC/VISA/AMEX/DC/DIS
* Hotel Rates: from $160
* Spa on premises: **The Biltmore Spa**

* **Spa Hours**: 5:30am - 10pm (fitness hours); 8am - 8pm treatments and salon hours
* **Spa Facilities**: 20,000 sq.ft. / 1820 sq.m. spa complex, retreat areas, spa whirlpool treatment pool, men's and women's locker and grooming facilities, steam room, sauna, whirlpools
* **Spa Programs**: beauty, fitness, well-being
* **Spa Packages**: Various daily spa packages starting at $125 for women and men
* **Spa Treatments**: massage, swedish massage, aromatherapy, reflexology, lymphatic massage, shiatsu in-room massage, cellulite treatments, gel packs, self-heating therapy pack, Ayurvedic elemental balancing, Ayurvedic bath, hydro massage, body glow, aloe body wraps, exfoliation, balneotherapy, slimming hydrotherapy, herbal body treatments, mud, facials, and sculp treatments, foot treatments, walking, hiking, jogging, aerobics, water, aerobics, yoga, qi chong

DESCRIPTION: Arizona Biltmore is a distinguished desert resort on landscaped grounds. Accommodations consist of hotel rooms and spacious 2BR and 2 bathroom villas. The Arizona Biltmore Spa features an array of facial and body treatments emphasizing natural healing and pampering and a wide variety of massage techniques. Ayurveda products and treatments are offered as well as products indigenous to the land. Recreation: golf, tennis.

Hyatt Regency Scottsdale
❤❤❤❤❤

7500 East Doubletree Ranch Rd., Scottsdale AZ 85258. Tel: (602) 991-3388. Fax: (602) 483-5550. TYPE: Resort & Spa. LOCATION: Southwestern resort hotel on 560-acre Gainey Ranch, set against the magnificence of the Sonoran Desert. SPA CLIENTELE: Women and men.

* Rooms: 493, suites: 25, Casitas: 7
* Phone, CTV, A/C, C/H, in-room safe, hair dryer minibar, balcony, fireplace (in casita)
* Restaurants (3), lobby bar, poolside bars
* Airport: Sky Harbor Int'l, 15 mi. / 24 km., taxi, limo
* Open: Year round
* Credit Cards: MC/VISA/AMEX/DC/DIS

* Rates: $155-$2,500 (room only)
  Spa Treatments: $100-$300 (per treatment)
* TAC: 10%
* Spa on premises: **The Sonwai Spa**
* **Spa Facilities**: fitness center, steam room, sauna, massage rooms, beauty salon
* **Spa Programs**: Beauty, wellness & fitness
* **Spa Treatments**: massage, body wraps, fitness counselling

DESCRIPTION: A glittering desert oasis with a complete health and fitness center offering everything from relaxing massage to an invigorating work out. Recreation: 27 hole championship golf course and tennis courts.

Marriott's Camelback Inn
❤❤❤❤

5402 E. Lincoln Dr., Scottsdale, AZ 85253. Tel: (602) 948-1700. Toll Free (800) 24-Camel. Fax: (602) 951-8469. TYPE: Moderate Deluxe Resort, Golf Club & Spa. MANAGING DIRECTOR: Jim Marks. LOCATION: Heart of Scottsdale in the Sonoran Desert. SPA CLIENTELE: Women & men adults oriented, must be 16 years or older.

* Rooms: 453, suites: 27
* Dining Room, lounge
* Nearest Airport: Sky Harbor Int'l
* Airport Transportation: taxi, limo
* Open: Year round
* Credit Cards: MC/VISA/AMEX/DC/DIS
* Rates: $125-$2,000 (room only)
  Spa Treatments: $100-$300 (per treatment)
* TAC: 10%
* Spa on premises: **The Spa at Camelback Inn**
* Year Established: 1989
* Spa Hours: open daily 6:15am-7:30pm
* **Spa Facilities**: European health spa, exercise & fitness facilities, aerobics rooms, multi-lane heated outdoor lap pool, cold plunge pools, whirlpool baths, private massage rooms, private facial rooms, relaxation rooms, Turkish steam rooms, Finnish saunas, outdoor solarium for sunbathing, beauty salon, wellness center
* **Spa Programs**: Pampering, wellness & fitness,

beauty, stress management

* **Spa Packages**: Gentleman's Day Packages $105-$200; Day Packages $140-$230
* **Spa Treatments**: Swedish body message, therapeutic massage, aromatherapy, maternity massage, foot massage, shiatsu, Hot Stone massage, European facials, body care, adobe clay treatments, Vitamin C facial, herbal wrap, Southwestern Botanical facial, brush & glow, loofah, full body mud musk, herbal body treatment, Para-joba body moisturizer, Aloe Vera body treatments, Tranquility treatment, personal training, aerobics, exercise, daily walks
* **Web:** www.camelbackinn.com

DESCRIPTION: The Spa at Camelback Inn is the most extensive freestanding resort spa in the Southwest. Set on 120 private acres at the elegant Marriott's Camelback Inn Resort, the Spa offers a full range of services and activities from soothing massages to energizing fitness classes and rejuvenating body treatments. Enjoy creative Spa cuisine at Sprouts Restaurant, featuring delicious Arizona-inspired, healthy low calorie dishes.

The Mist Spa
❤❤❤❤❤

c/o Radisson Resort & Spa Scottsdale, 7171 North Scottsdale Rd., Scottsdale AZ 85253. Tel: (602) 991-3800. Toll Free 877-MIST-SPA. Fax: (602) 948-9843. TYPE: Deluxe Resort & Spa. SPA DIRECTOR: Karen Steidl. LOCATION: In the heart of Scottsdale's cultural district. SPA CLIENTELE: Women & men. AGE RESTRICTION: no persons under 18.

* Rooms: 318 w/priv. bath. Suites: 32
* Phone, CTV, A/C, minibar, hairdryer, private patios
* Restaurants: **Andre's** - gourmet cuisine, **Oasis** - French-style patisserie; **Orchids** - healthy cuisine with Oriental flair; **Taps** - Micro Pub
* Airport: Sky Harbor Int'l, 12 mi. / 19 km.
* Airport/Train Transportation: taxi / shuttle service
* Reservations: suggested
* Credit Cards: All major credit cards
* Open: Year round

* Spa on premises: **The Mist Spa**
* Year Established: 1998
* **Spa Facilities**: Fitness center, hair salon, aerobics studio, lighted tennis courts; treatment rooms (15), meditation atrium, whirlpool (2), steam sauna (2), sunbathing terrace, lap pool, Orchids spa restaurant (healthy cuisine)
* **Spa Programs**: relaxation, detoxifying, rejuvenation and renewal programs
* **Spa Treatments**: hydrotherapy, massage, skin & body care, body wraps,
* **Spa Packages**: 1/2 and full day programs ranging from $123 - $447
* **Indications**: beauty, pampering, fitness, stress reduction, general well-being
* Web: www.radisson.com/scottsdaleaz

DESCRIPTION: Radisson Resort & Spa Scottsdale offers gracious hospitality in a south-western ambiance. Over 30,000 sq. ft. (2,727 sq.m.) of function space is available for meeting and corporate events. Accommodations are in luxurious guest rooms and suites. The Mist Spa is a full service destination spa. The impressive 20,000 sq. ft. (1,818 sq. m.) health and beauty center is set amidst an oriental zen garden complete with mens and ladies locker areas each have herbal steam, sauna and whirlpool. Relaxation lounges allow peaceful meditation. Fitness and Aerobics studios complete with state-of-the-art equipment and private terraces for relaxation and sunbathing. It is a perfect place to enjoy therapeutic body massage and revitalizing treatments. Our helpful, multilingual staff is always happy to assist you.

The Phoenician
❤❤❤❤❤

6000 East Camelback Rd., Scottsdale, AZ 85251. Tel: (602) 941-8200. Fax: (602) 947-4311. TYPE: Resort & Spa. LOCATION: In the heart of Camelback Mountain. SPA CLIENTELE: Women and men.

* Rooms: 605 w/priv. bath. Suites: 31, Casitas: 131
* Phone, CTV, A/C, hair dryer, minibar
* Rooms for non-smokers, wheelchair access

* Restaurants (6), lounges (5), business center
* Airport: Sky Harbor Int'l 20 minutes, taxi, limo
* Open: Year round
* Credit Cards: MC/VISA/AMEX/DC/DIS
* Hotel Rates: from $200; TAC: 10%
* Spa on premises
* **Spa Facilities**: Health & Beauty Spa, outdoor heated and cooled pools, sauna, beauty salon, athletic room, whirlpool and steam baths, jogging and biking trails
* **Spa Treatments**: health, beauty and fitness

DESCRIPTION: An ultra modern year-round resort on 130 acres featuring a centre for well being. Recreation: championship 18-hole golf course, 11 lighted tennis courts, six miles of hiking, jogging and biking on property.

Scottsdale Hilton Resort & Villas
♥♥♥♥

6333 N. Scottsdale Road, Scottsdale, AZ 85250. Tel: (602) 948-7750. Fax: (602) 443-9702 or 948-2232. TYPE: Resort Hotel & Spa. LOCATION: 5 minutes from downtown Scottsdale. SPA CLIENTELE: Women and men.

* Rooms: 187 w/priv. bath. Villas: 45
* Wheelchair Accessibility
* Restaurant, lounge, live entertainment
* Airport: Sky Harbor Int'l 20 minutes, taxi, limo
* Open: Year round
* Credit Cards: MC/VISA/AMEX/DC/CB
* Hotel Rates: from $110; TAC: 10%
* Spa on premises
* **Spa Facilities**: Health Spa, beauty salon, pools
* **Spa Treatments**: health and beauty

DESCRIPTION: Southwestern resort featuring spacious air-conditioned rooms, suites and two bedroom villas. Full service health Spa. Recreation: tennis, entertainment and shopping.

Scottsdale Princess Spa
♥♥♥♥♥

7575 East Princess Dr., Scottsdale, AZ 85255, Tel: (602) 585-4848. Fax: 602-585-0086. TYPE: Resort & Spa. LOCATION: 45 min. to Phoenix Airport. DESCRIPTION: Luxurious resort with spa & fitness Center, sauna, gym, and spa treatments. 650 rooms suites and casitas, restaurant (4), bars/lounges (3), heated pools (3), tennis courts (7), 36 holes of golf. Hotel rates: from $160.

The Spa at Gainey Village
♥♥♥♥

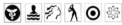

7477 E. Doubletree Ranch Road, Scottdale, AZ 85258. Tel: (602) 609-6980. Fax: (602) 609-6976. TYPE: Day spa and sports-medical complex. SPA DIRECTOR: Judy Snow. LOCATION: SW corner of Doubletree and 74th Way. SPA CLIENTELE: Women and men. RESTRICTIONS: Age 12 to 16 accepted for treatment, but must be accompanied by parent or guardian.

* Rooms & suites: neighboring hotels
* Airport: Phoenix Sky Harbor 30 minutes, shuttle service
* Open: Year round
* Reservations: Required
* Credit Cards: MC/VISA/AMEX/DC/DISC
* **Spa Facilities**: 25 rooms including movement and pilates studio, hydrotherapy, VIP couple treatment room
* **Spa Programs**: Alternative healing, rehabilitation, nutrition, fitness, pilates - based training, meditation, tai chi, yoga
* **Spa Treatment**: Massage, facials, mud, ayurvedic, hydrotherapy, vichy, VIP couple massage, shiatsu, salon hair, nails, makeup, waxing
* **Spa Packages**: Men's package $85 - 175; Day package from $195
* **Contraindications**: Guest limited to those not needing attendant assistance
* **Medical Supervision**: Rehab complex with holistic and standard medical service.
* Web: www.dmbclubs.com

DESCRIPTION: A day spa and sports-medical complex featuring alternative healing, rehabilitation, fitness and pampering treatments. Opening June 1999.

SEDONA

) **520**

✈ Sedona Airport

Enchantment Resort & Spa
♥♥♥♥♥

525 Boynton Canyon Road, Sedona, AZ 86336, Tel: (520) 204-6260 or (800) 826-4180, Fax: (520) 204-2936. TYPE: Adobe-style resort & Spa. LOCATION: In Boynton Canyon, 9 mi. / 14 km. to Sedona Airport. DESCRIPTION: Full Service Spa & Fitness Center with massages, body wraps, facials, Tai Chi and yoga. 162 rooms and casitas, restaurants (2), meeting pavilion, outdoor heated pools (4), tennis courts (9). Hotel rates: from $195.

Los Abrigados
♥♥♥♥

160 Portal Lane, Sedona, AZ 86336. Tel: (520) 282-1777. Fax: (520) 282-2614. TYPE: Resort & Spa. LOCATION: Nestled between the red rocks and canyons. SPA CLIENTELE: Women and men. DESCRIPTION: A Spanish-style All-suite resort complex with health spa. Hotel rates: from $210.

TUCSON

) **520**

✈ Tucson Int'l Airport (TUS) 7 mi. / 11 km. South

Tucson, population 330,000, has a year round sunny dry desert climate. The unique climate has contributed to the city's development as a popular winter health resort. In spite of the massive modernization and development the city maintains a rich mix of Spanish and Mexican heritage which is reflected in old monuments of the period. The local native Indians add color with their traditional art and culture.

Canyon Ranch
♥♥♥♥

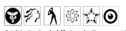

8600 E. Rockcliff Road, Tucson, AZ 85715. Tel: (520)

749-9000. Fax: (520) 749-7555. TYPE: Health and Fitness Resort. LOCATION: At the base of the Santa Catalina Mountains near Tucson. SPA CLIENTELE: Women and men.

* Rooms: 76 w/private bath. Suites
* Airport: Tucson Int'l AP, 20 mi. (32 km.)
* Airport Transportation: taxi, rent-a-car
* Credit Cards: AMEX/VISA/MC
* Open: Year round
* Hotel Rates: from $260
  $1,120-$1,860/ (4 nights), $1,990-$3,190/
  (7 nights) , $2,740-$4,450/ (10 nights)
  Rates include: accommodations, 3 meals, use
  of Spa facilities, nutrition and fitness classes
* TAC: 10%
* Spa on premises
* **Spa Facilities**: outdoor and indoor facilities - 4 indoor Racquetball courts, 5 gyms, 4 Jacuzzis, saunas, steam & inhalation rooms, 6 tennis courts, 3 swimming pools, therapy & exercise pools, fully equipped weight room
* **Spa Programs**: 10, 7, or 4 nights packages; week long programs in healthy living: Life enhancement, healthy heart, ElderCamp, executive women's week, living with arthritis, new directions in diabetics
* **Medical Supervision**: nurses, exercise physiologist, registered dieticians, psychologists, certified fitness instructors, skin care specialists, massage therapists

DESCRIPTION: A 60-acre desert oasis where people of all ages come to relax and make healthy lifestyle changes. The Spa program includes weight control, fitness and a variety of personal services - such as herbal wraps, soothing massages and relaxing facials. Guests may consult with professional staff how to improve their lifestyles through good eating habits, enjoyable exercise and relaxation. The Canyon Ranch has twice as many employees as guests to insure the quality of service and individual attention.

Golden Door Spa
♥♥♥♥

c/o The Lodge at Ventana Canyon, 6200 North Clubhouse Lane, Tucson, AZ 85750. Tel: (520) 577-1400. Fax:

(520) 577-4065. TYPE: All-suite hotel & Spa. LOCATION: Catalina foothills, 21 mi. / 34 km. to Tucson Airport. DESCRIPTION: Resort hotel with a Golden Door Spa, body treatments, beauty salon. 1/2BR suites (45). restaurant, poolside bar, business center, pool, two 18-hole golf courses, tennis. Hotel rates: from $135.

Loews Ventana Canyon Resort
♥♥♥♥♥

7000 N. Resort Drive, Tucson, AZ 85750. Tel: (520) 299-2020. Fax: (520) 299-6832. TYPE: Resort hotel & Spa. LOCATION: Foothills of the Catalina Mountains, 20 mi. / 32 km. to airport. DESCRIPTION: Self-contained resort hotel with a full service health spa, treatment rooms (8), beauty salon, workout room, aerobic studio, saunas, walking and jogging trails. 398 rooms, 27 suites, nonsmoker rooms, wheelchair access, restaurant, cafe, lobby lounge, bar & grill, business services, pools (2), tennis courts (8), 36 holes of golf. Hotel rates: from $145.

* Rooms: 398 w/priv. bath. Suites: 27
* Phone (3), CTV, A/C, C/H, minibar, hair dryers
* Wheelchair Accessible
* Dining rooms, grill, lounges, coffee shop
* Airport: Tucson Int'l Airport, 8 mi. / 13 km.
* Reservations: Credit Card guarantee
* Credit Cards: MC/VISA/AMEX/DC/CB
* Open: Year round
* Hotel Rates: from $149; TAC: 10%
* Spa on premises
* Year Established: 1997
* **Spa Facilities**: 7,000 sq. ft. / 636 sq. m. full service spa, treatment rooms (8), work-out room, free-weight area, locker rooms with steam and dry saunas, lap pool, jacuzzi, walking/jogging trail, hiking and mountain biking areas
* **Spa Program**: beauty, wellness, fitness
* **Spa Treatments**: wet treatments, body wraps, body polishes, mud and seaweed dips, facials (men and women), massage, shiatsu, aromatherapy, reflexology personal fitness training
* **Other Packages**: Tennis clinics for children and adults

DESCRIPTION: Deluxe Self-contained resort hotel with full service Spa & Tennis center, PGA golf courses and a myriad of recreational activities for adults and children. The renovated Spa & Tennis Center offers up-to-date equipment, facilities and services in an ideal setting. The spa employees are fully trained, certified and licensed in his/her area of expertise.

Miraval Life in Balance
♥♥♥♥

5000 East Via Estancia Miraval, Catalina, AZ 85739, Tel: (520) 825-4000. Toll Free: (800) 232-3969. Fax: (520)792-5870. TYPE: Spa Resort. DESCRIPTION: Unique all-inclusive spa resort housed in Santa-Fe style Adobe building. Meditation, yoga, nutrition & fitness classes, trail rides, hot stone massage. 106 rooms, pools (3), tennis courts (3). Hotel rates: from $360.

Omni Tucson National Golf Resort & Spa
♥♥♥♥♥

2727 West Club Drive, Tucson, AZ 85741. Tel: (520) 297-2271. Fax: (520) 742-2452. TYPE: Resort & Spa. LOCATION: 10 mi (16 km) from Tucson's business district on 650 desert acres overlooking the Tucson Valley. SPA CLIENTELE: Women and men.

* Villa Suites: 167
* Wheelchair Accessible
* Dining room, grill & coffee shop
* Nearest Airport: Tucson Int'l Airport
* Distance to the Airport: 25 minutes
* Reservations: Credit Card guarantee
* Credit Cards: MC/VISA/AMEX/DC/CB
* Open: Year round
* Hotel Rates: from $120; TAC: 10%
* Spa on premises
* **Spa Facilities**: large pool, health & beauty Spa with showers, sauna and steam cabinets, hydrotherapy pools, Finnish sauna, inhalation rooms, Russian bath (for men), gym, tanning beds, skin care salon
* **Spa Program**: Personalized programs in exercise,

diet, beauty and overall fitness for men and women; Special SPA Getaway Plan for 4 nights
* **Spa Treatments**: exercises, workout, aerobic classes,water aerobics, massages, pulsation baths, European Scandinavian hydro-tour, Finnish sauna, Russian bath (men only), herbal wraps, mud packs, loofah, salt glow, Swiss shower, Scotch water massage, panthermal (women only), inhalations, skin and beauty care, facials, low calorie meals
* **Other Packages**: Championship Golf Getaway (2-6 nts)

DESCRIPTION: A superb resort and Spa at the foothills of the Santa Catalina Mountains in a peaceful desert environment. Accommodations consist of tastefully decorated guest rooms and suites. The luxurious Spa combines European tradition with American technology. A large variety of beauty and pampering treatments, some exotic, are available for men and women. Recreational facilities include the championship USGA 27-hole golf course, and tennis center.

Stepping Stone Spa Resorts
❤❤❤

4740 E. Sunrise Dr, #241, Tucson, AZ 85718, Tel: (888) 216-1110. Fax: (520) 577-2755. TYPE: Resort & spa. SPA CLIENTELE: Women and men. DESCRIPTION: Beauty & body treatments, fitness classes.

The Westin La Paloma
❤❤❤❤❤

3800 E. Sunrise Dr., Tucson AZ 85718. Tel: (520) 742-6000. Fax: (520) 577-5878. SPA - Tel: (520) 742-7866. Fax: (520) 722-2292. SPA MANAGERS: Robert &

Leah Kovitz. PROGRAMS DIRECTOR: Beth McIlrath. TYPE: Resort & Spa. LOCATION: At the foot of the Santa Catalina Mountains. SPA CLIENTELE: Women and men. Teenagers accepted.

* Rooms: 487 w/priv. bath. Suites: 31
* Phone, CTV, A/C, C/H, safe, minibar, coffee maker
* Rooms for non smokers
* Dining Rooms (5), lounges (5), meeting facilities
* Freedom pool with swim up bar, adults only pool
* Airport: Tucson Int'l Airport, 25 mi. / 40 km.
* Open: Year round
* Credit Cards: MC/VISA/AMEX/DC/DIS
* Hotel Rates: from $120
* TAC: 10%
* Spa on premises: **The Personal Services Center**
* Year Established: 1985
* **Spa Facilities**: 3 therapy pools, beauty salon, Spa and exercise facilities
* **Spa Treatments**: massage, skin care, nail care, body treatments, aromatherapy, waxing, make up

DESCRIPTION: Deluxe Spanish mission-style convention resort with a full service health and beauty spa. Recreation: golf, tennis.

Westward Look Resort
❤❤❤❤❤

245 E. Ina Road, Tucson, AZ 85704. Tel: (520) 297-1151, Fax: (520) 297-9023. TYPE: Resort & Wellness Center. LOCATION: Catalina Mountain foothills 10 mi. / 16 km. to downtown. DESCRIPTION: Deluxe year round resort with wellness center, fitness club, herbal treatments, jogging trail. 244 rooms, restaurant, cafe, lounge, outdoor pools (3) and tennis courts (8). Hotel rates: from $120.

ARKANSAS

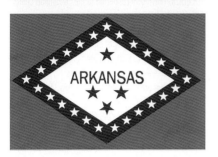

AREA: 53,187 sq. mi. (137,754 sq. km.)
POPULATION: 2,362,000
CAPITAL: Little Rock
TIME ZONE: Central Time

EUREKA SPRINGS
 501

✈ Little Rock Regional Airport (LIT)

Palace Hotel & Bath House
❤❤❤

[icons]

135 Spring St., Eureka Springs, AR 72632, Tel: (501) 253-7474, Fax: (501) 253-7494. TYPE: Inn and bath house. LOCATION: Downtown within walking distance of shops and galleries. DESCRIPTION: Victorian-era all suite Inn & Spa with licensed therapist, whirlpool mineral baths and antique oak steam cabinets. Suites (8) with coffee bar, CTV, jacuzzi & direct dial phone, complimentary breakfast and evening refreshments. Hotel rates: from $100.

HOT SPRINGS
501

✈ Memorial Field Airport (HOT) 3 mi. / 5 km. SW

The city of Hot Springs, population 35,000, is a popular year round hot springs resort located in the Hot Springs National Park in the scenic Ouachita Mountains. The main attraction here is the thermal hot springs which gush out at an average temperature of 143°F (62°c). The water is then cooled down to a bearable 90°F (32°c) for therapeutic purposes without being exposed to air or mixed with regular water during the cooling process. Like most Spa towns with medicinal waters, the town has its own cure center - **The Libbey Memorial Physical Medicine Center**. The Medical Center operates its own equipment, facilities and thermal pools; it specializes in hydrotherapy treatments under medical supervision for arthritis sufferers, or those suffering from injury-paralysis. Some of the treatments include: options of showers, sitz tubs, steam cabinets, packs and prescription baths. There is a Health Spa at the center which offers relaxing, and stress reduction treatments for recreational and enjoyment purposes only. Hot Springs can be reached by car from Little Rock via I-30 south, then SR 270 west.

Water Composition: The water chemical composition of the 45 hot springs is naturally sterile as follows: silica, calcium, magnesium, sodium, potassium, bicarbonate, sulfate, chloride and fluoride. Radioactivity through radon gas emanation is 0.81 millimicrocurie per liter.

Indication: Rheumatic and gouty conditions, neuralgiam neuritis, arthritis, anemia, cardio-vascular disease with high blood pressure, prostate and kidney disorders.

Arlington Resort Hotel & Spa
❤❤❤❤

[icons]

239 Central Avenue, P.O. Box 5652, Hot Springs, AR 71901. Tel: (501) 623-7771. Fax: (501) 623-6191. TYPE: Resort Complex & Spa. MANAGER: Horst Fischer, GM. LOCATION: In downtown Hot Springs. SPA CLIENTELE: Women and men, family Oriented.

* Rooms: 484 w/private bath. Suites: 42
* Phone, CTV, A/C, C/H
* Rooms for non smokers, wheelchair access
* Restaurants, bar & entertainment
* Airport: Memorial Field AP, 5 mi. / 9 km., bus
* Credit Cards: MC/VISA/AMEX
* Open: Year round
* Hotel Rates: from $58; TAC: 10%
* Spa on premises
* **Spa Facilities**: Bath House with thermal mineral

baths, thermal pools (2), massage rooms, whirlpool, private hot tubs, vapor cabinets, exercise room, beauty salon

* **Spa Programs**: Thermal Baths, Beauty Care, Masculine Fitness, Pampering; medical therapy is available at the Libbey's Memorial Center
* **Spa Treatments**: Thermal mineral water baths, whirlpool, massages, sauna
* **Indications**: relief of tension, relaxation

DESCRIPTION: A landmark hotel in a mountain setting overlooking downtown Hot Springs. Spacious accommodations include all modern amenities. The Spa offers natural hot springs for therapeutic and recreational use. Beauty treatments are available to complement the hot springs experience. Recreation: tennis, golf, and nightly entertainment.

Downtowner Hotel & Spa
♥♥♥

135 Central Ave., Hot Springs, AR 71901. Tel: (501) 624-5521. Fax: (501) 624-4635. TYPE: Spa Hotel. LOCATION: In downtown business district. SPA CLIENTELE: Women and men.

* Rooms: 150 w/priv. bath. Suites: 15
* Dining Room & Coffee Shop
* Airport: Memorial Field 15 min., limo service/charge
* Open: Year round
* Credit Cards: MC/AMEX/DC/CB
* Hotel Rates: from $54; TAC: 10%
* Spa on Premises
* **Spa Facilities**: Bathhouse with thermal facilities, heated pool, beauty salon
* **Spa Treatments**: balneotherapy

DESCRIPTION: A moderate first class 10 story resort hotel with in house complete Bathhouse with thermal water. Recreation: golf privileges.

Hot Springs Park Hilton Hotel
♥♥♥

305 Malvern Ave., Hot Springs, AR 71901. Tel: (501) 623-6600. Fax: (501) 623-6600. TYPE: Hotel & Spa. LOCATION: Downtown connected to the Convention Center. SPA CLIENTELE: Women and men.

* Rooms: 200 w/priv. bath. Suites: 16
* Phone, CTV, A/C, C/H, minibar
* Restaurants, lounge, meeting facilities
* Airport: Hot Springs Memorial AP, 5 min., taxi
* Open: Year round
* Credit Cards: MC/VISA/DIS/DC/CB
* Rates: from $70
* Spa on Premises
* **Spa Facilities**: Thermal mineral baths, hot tubs, massage rooms, indoor/outdoor heated pools
* **Spa Treatments**: balneotherapy, massages

DESCRIPTION: Business oriented hotel with thermal baths.

Majestic Hotel & Spa
♥♥♥

101 Park Avenue, Hot Springs, AR 71901. Tel: (501) 623-5511. Fax: (501) 624-4737. TYPE: Spa Resort. LOCATION: Downtown at Central Avenue. SPA CLIENTELE: Women and men.

* Rooms: 228 rooms w/priv. bath. Suites: 23 superior
* Phone, CTV, A/C, C/H, wet bar, refrigerator, balcony
* Wheelchair Accessibility
* Dining room, cocktail lounge, meeting facilities
* Airport: Hot Springs Memorial AP, 4 mi. / 6 km.
* Airport Transportation: shuttle service
* Open: Year round
* Credit Cards: MC/VISA/AMEX/DIS
* Hotel Rates: from $50
* TAC: 10%
* Spa on Premises
* **Spa Facilities**: Thermal Baths, whirlpool, massage room, heated outdoor pool, beauty salon
* **Spa Treatments**: balneotherapy, massages

DESCRIPTION: First class spa resort with thermal baths. Recreation: water sports on Lake Hamilton.

CALIFORNIA

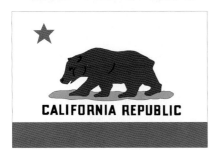

CALIFORNIA REPUBLIC

AREA: 158,706 sq. mi. (411,049 sq. km.)
POPULATION: 30,000,000
CAPITAL: Sacramento
TIME ZONE: Pacific Time

BIG SUR
 831
✈ Monterey Airport, 35 mi. / 56 km.

Post Ranch Inn and Spa
❤❤❤❤

Hwy 1,PO Box 219 , Big Sur, CA 93920. Tel: (831)667-2200. Fax: (831) 667-2824. TYPE: Inn & Spa. LOCATION: Set in 98 acres overlooking dramatic Big Sur coastline. SPA CLIENTELE: Women and men. DESCRIPTION: Exclusive Inn with complete health spa facilities, hiking, yoga, massage, basking & swimming pools. 30 rooms, restaurant, bar. Hotel rates: from $285.

Ventana Inn
❤❤❤❤

Highway 1, Big Sur, CA 93920. Tel: (831) 667-2331. Fax: (831) 667-2419. TYPE: Romantic Inn & Spa. LOCATION: Above the Pacific, 35 mi / 56 km from Monterey Airport. SPA CLIENTELE: Women and men. DESCRIPTION: Deluxe Inn with complete spa services, fitness room, 2 heated pools, 2 Japanese hot baths, hiking, horseback rid-

ing. 62 rooms in 12 buildings, each with terrace, air conditioning, phone & wet bar, most with fireplace, some with hot tubs. Restaurant, complimentary breakfast, afternoon wine & cheese. Hotel rates: from $215.

CALABASAS
 818
✈ Los Angeles Airport (LAX)

The Ashram Health Retreat
❤❤

Box 8009, Calabasas, CA 91372. Tel: (818 222-6900. TYPE: "No-frills" health retreat. SPA CLIENTELE: Women and men. DESCRIPTION: Small health retreat, 6 rooms, maximum 12 guest, dining room (vegetarian meals). Activities from 6am to 7pm: yoga, hiking, weights, waterworks, massage. Rates: on request.

CALISTOGA
 707
✈ Sonoma County Airport

Calistoga, population 4,000, is a small health resort in northern California which has developed around the town's hot mineral springs mud baths. Commercial bottling of Calistoga's own mineral water has become a successful enterprise.

Nestled in the beautiful wine country just north of the Napa Valley, it maintains a quaint charm for those who wish to indulge in a spa experience at a very reasonable prices. Many hotels in Calistoga offer various spa programs and treatments. Calistoga is located 75 mi. / 120 km. north of San Francisco.

Dr. Wilkinson's Hot Springs
❤❤❤

1507 Lincoln Avenue, Calistoga, CA 94515. Tel: (707) 942-4102. Fax: (707) 942-6110. TYPE: Spa Motel. MANAGER: M. Wilkinson, GM. LOCATION: In Calistoga at the northern end of the Napa Valley. SPA CLIENTELE: Women and men.

* Rooms: 42 w/private bath
* Phone, CTV, C/H, A/C, refrigerator
* Airport: opposite local airport
* Credit Cards: VISA/MC
* Open: Year round
* Hotel Rates: from $74
* TAC: 10%
* Distance to the Spa: 300 mtrs.
* **Spa Facilities**: indoor facilities - bathhouse, 3 pools, hot mineral whirlpool (104°F / 40°c); outdoor facilities - warm mineral pool (92°F / 33°c), beauty salon
* **Spa Treatments**: mud baths, mineral baths, natural mineral steam, blanket wraps, massage, facials, body massage, Cerofango
* **Indications**: arthritis and stress
* **Contraindications**: pregnant women, heart patients, some diabetics

DESCRIPTION: Small motel with spa services. The naturally heated mineral waters and steam combined with volcanic ash (mud bath) provide natural relief from arthritis and tension. Complimentary Calistoga Mineral water is offered upon check-in. Spa treatments are not included in the room rate and the cost of each individual treatment may vary between $27 - $195.

Golden Haven Hot Springs Spa
❤❤

1713 Lake Street, Calistoga CA 94515. Tel: (707) 942-6793. Fax: (707) 942-1563. TYPE: Motel & Spa. LOCATION: In Calistoga, corner of Lake and Grant Myrtledale. SPA CLIENTELE: Women and men.

* Rooms: 28 w/priv. bath. Suites: 10
* Phone, CTV, A/C,refrigerator
* Airport: Santa Rosa, 20 mi. / 32 km.
* Reservations: 48 hrs. cancellation (room)
* Credit Cards: MC/VISA/AMEX
* Hotel Rates: from $55 (room only)

* TAC: 10% mid week only
* Spa on Premises
* **Spa Facilities**: Health & beauty spa, mineral pools, private therapy and massage rooms
* **Spa Programs**: Pampering, weight loss, cellulite reduction
* **Spa Treatments**: mud bath, sea mud wrap, herbal wrap, massages, skin glow rub, body wrap, herbal facial, acupressure
* **Spa Packages**: The Ultimate; Pamper Packages
* **Indications**: stress, fatigue, obesity
* No Medical Supervision

DESCRIPTION: Motel accommodations ranging from deluxe to economic. Spa treatments include mineral and mud baths, and European body wraps with a weight loss guarantee.

Mount View Hotel
❤❤❤

1457 Lincoln Ave., Calistoga, CA 94515. Tel: (707) 942-6877. Fax: (707) 942-6904. TYPE: Hotel & Spa. LOCATION: Downtown Calistoga. SPA CLIENTELE: Women and men. DESCRIPTION: Stylish hotel with European spa, private deck & hot tub. 33 rooms with CTV, phone. Restaurant, saloon. Hotel rates: from $115.

Silver Rose Inn
❤❤❤

351 Rosedale Road, Calistoga, CA 94515. Tel: (707) 942-9581. Fax: (707) 942-0841. TYPE: County Inn and Spa. LOCATION: Set in vineyards minutes from downtown Calistoga. SPA CLIENTELE: Women and men. DESCRIPTION: Country lodge Inn with full service spa, exercise equipment. 20 rooms, lounge, sitting room. Hotel rates: from $150.

Village Inn & Spa
❤❤❤

1880 Lincoln Ave., Calistoga 95405. Tel: (707) 942-4636, Toll Free 1-800-543-1923 (Northern CA). Fax: (707) 942-5262. TYPE: Inn & Spa. LOCATION: At the extreme north end of Calistoga, on Lincoln Ave at the Silverado Trail. SPA CLIENTELE: Women and men.

* Rooms: 42 w/priv. bath. Suites: 3
* Phone, CTV, A/C, C/H
* Restaurant
* Airport: Calistoga 1/4 mi. / 400 m., walking distance
* Reservations: credit card guarantee
* Credit Cards: MC/VISA/AMEX
* Open: Year round
* Hotel Rates: from $65 - $105
* Spa on premises
* **Spa Facilities**: Mineral water swimming and wading pool, mineral water whirlpool, sauna and steam rooms
* **Spa Programs**: Revitalization
* **Spa Treatments**: mud baths, mineral baths, massages, skin glow rub, natural facial
* **Spa Packages**: $65-$150; also available Spa & Lodging Packages. Rates on request
* **Contraindications**: none
* Medical Supervision: no. Any person with health conditions requiring medical care should check with their physicians prior to taking any treatment

DESCRIPTION: The Village Inn & Spa offers accommodations with pleasant decor. Some rooms have Roman tubs. Non smoking rooms are available. The health spa features mineral water and mud treatments for relaxation, stress reduction, beauty and revitalization. Their Ultimate Spa Package (cost $120) offers a revitalizing four hours of mud treatment, full body massage, skin glow rub and facial.

CARLSBAD
︶ 760
✈ Palomar Airport (CLD) 4 mi. / 6 km.

Carlsbad, population 36,000, north of San Diego along the Gulf of Santa Catalina, derives its name from the famous Karlsbad Spa in the Czech Republic because of the similar mineral water composition. It is a blossoming beach side health resort town which turns exceptionally pleasant during the spring season. Carlsbad, is easily accessible from San Diego or Los Angeles.

La Costa
❤❤❤❤❤

Costa del Mar Rd., Carlsbad, CA 92008. Tel: (760) 438-9111, CA (800) 542-6200, USA (800) 854-6564. Fax: (760) 438-9007. TYPE: Resort & Spa. LOCATION: 2 mi. (3km.) from the ocean, 30 mi. (48 km) north of San Diego. SPA CLIENTELE: Women and men.

* Rooms: 479 w/private bath
* Suites, chateau suites, executive homes
* Phone, CTV, A/C, C/H, minibar, hair dryer, balcony
* Restaurants (5), lounges (2), meeting rooms (15)
* Airport: San Diego 30 mi. / 48 km., limo
* Credit Cards: MC/VISA/AMEX/DC
* Open: Year round
* Hotel Rates: from $250
* TAC: 10%
* Spa on premises
* **Spa Facilities**: Luxurious Spa; mineral whirlpool baths, rock steam rooms, saunas, Swiss showers, Roman baths, solariums, exercise pools, beauty salon
* **Spa Programs**: Fitness, lifestyle management, stress reduction, weight loss, beauty care
* **Spa Treatments**: body conditioning, steam baths, aerobics, power walking, weight training, low calorie meals, nutrition education, herbal wraps, body scrubs, loofah massage, collagen facial
* Medical Supervision: Resident physician (MD), dietician

DESCRIPTION: Deluxe Resort with a European Spa for men and women. The village like resort sprawls over a landscaped 1000 acres of parks, gardens and golf course. The accommodations vary in size and style but all offer high standard and comfort. There are separate spa facilities for men only and women only. Low calorie meals are available for weight watchers. Each item on the menu lists its caloric value and guests are in complete control of their own diet. La Costa specializes in Lifestyle management for executives, nutrition education and stress reduction. Recreation: tennis, golf and horseback riding.

Four Seasons Resort Aviara
❤❤❤❤

7100 Four Seasons Point, Carlsbad, CA 92009. Tel: (760) 603-6800. Fax: (760) 603-6801. TYPE: Resort & Spa. LOCATION: Overlooking the Pacific Ocean and Batiquitos Lagoon. SPA CLIENTELE: Women and men. DESCRIPTION: Golf & Tennis resort with full service spa, saunas, steam rooms, whirlpools, cool-down lounge, exercise room, aerobics. 331 rooms & suites, rooms for nonsmokers. Restaurants (4), bars (3), business center, outdoor pool, 18 hole golf course.Hotel rates: from $275.

Olympic Resort Hotel & Spa
❤❤❤

6111 El Camino Real, Carlsbad, CA 92009. Tel: (760) 438-8330. Spa Tel: (760) 931-1411. Fax: (760) 431-0838 TYPE: Resort & Spa. SPA MANAGER: Wolfgang Seitzer. LOCATION: 4 mi. (6 km.) from the Pacific Ocean, about 2 hours south of Los Angeles. SPA CLIENTELE: Women and men.

* Rooms: 80 w/private bath. Suites: 8
* Nearest Airport: San Diego 35 mi. / 56 km.
* Airport Transportation: limo, Hotel Van
* Reservations: 25% or Credit Card #
* Credit Cards: MC/VISA/AMEX
* Open: Year round
* Hotel Rates: from $85
* TAC: 10%
* Spa on premises: **Baden-Baden Spa**
* **Spa Facilities**: Beauty salon, massage & facial rooms, exercise rooms, steam room, sauna, swimming pool, therapy pool
* **Spa Programs**: Diet, fitness, beauty, stress mgmt
* **Spa Treatments**: massages, under water massage, hydrotherapy, skin care, Fango mud, European herbal wraps, relaxation, exercise pool, body-shaping, yoga, low impact aerobics

DESCRIPTION: An intimate Spa at the Olympic Resort Hotel. Accommodations feature rooms in French country style. Baden-Baden specializes in European health and skin care.

Individual programs offer many options. Diet meals are prepared in a Swiss continental fashion. Recreation: 5 tennis courts, 27-hole golf course at the nearby Whispering Palms Country Club.

CARMEL VALLEY
⟩ 408
✈ Monterey Peninsula Airport (MRY) 6 mi. / 9 km.

Carmel Valley, population 4,000, is a small community snuggled in a picturesque valley near Carmel and Monterey south of Santa Cruz and San Francisco. Carmel was established at the turn of the century by a group of artists and writers as a cultural retreat community. The small village maintains a unique flavor with its international and individual architectural style. The town's business center has many interesting shops and boutiques that specialize in the trade of local arts and crafts. Carmel Valley can be reached by car using Hwy 1 and exiting onto Carmel Valley Road south of Carmel-by-the-Sea.

Carmel Country Spa
❤❤

10 Country Club Way, Carmel Valley, CA 93924. Tel: (408) 659-3486. Toll Free (800) 568-6879. Fax: (408) 659-5022. TYPE: Weight Reducing Resort MANAGER: Carl Trigilio. LOCATION: In a valley, 10 miles (16 km.) southeast of Carmel. SPA CLIENTELE: Women and men.

* Rooms: 26 w/private bath
* Dining Room: diet menus
* Airport: Monterey AP 20 mi. / 32 km., bus, taxi
* Reservations: 1 night deposit req'd
* Credit Cards: MC/VISA/AMEX
* Hotel Rates: from $95
* TAC: 10%
* Spa on premises
* **Spa Facilities**: Olympic size pool, hot spa, gym, activity room, beauty salon
* **Spa Programs**: Weight Loss, Group Weight Therapy, Health & Fitness, Beauty Care
* **Spa Treatments**: aerobics, aqua-thinics, toning, yoga, facials, body wrap, cellulite control wraps, massage,

salt rub, collagen treatment w/ionizer, low cal meals, herbal consultation, hair & nail treatments

DESCRIPTION: A country Spa with rustic accommodations specializing in weight reduction. Daily scheduled routines include exercises, low calorie meals, spartan diets (600 calories per day), and à la carte beauty treatments at the beauty salon. Recreation: tennis, golf, jogging trails and horseback riding.

CITY OF INDUSTRY
🤙 626
✈ Los Angeles Int'l Airport (LAX) 40 mi. / 64 km.

Industry Hills Sheraton Resort & Spa
♥♥♥♥

1 Industry Hills Parkway, City of Industry, CA 91744. Tel: (626) 810-4455. Fax: (626) 964-9535. TYPE: Resort hotel & Spa. LOCATION: Overlooking the San Gabriel Mountains, 25 min. to downtown Los Angeles. SPA CLIENTELE: Women and men. DESCRIPTION: Modern resort hotel with separate men's and women's spas, sauna. 273 rooms and 21 suites, nonsmokers room. Restaurants (4), lounges (2), entertainment, pools (2), 18-hole golf courses (2), tennis courts (17), equestrian center. Hotel rates: from $140.

CORONA
🤙 909
✈ Ontario Int'l Airport (ONT) 30 mi. / 48 km.
   Los Angeles Int'l (LAX) 1 hr. 15 min.

Corona, population 38,000, became a popular spa resort for south Californians thanks to the **Glen Ivy Hot Springs** - a natural hot mineral spa 8 miles (13 km.) south on I-15. Glen Ivy was opened as a spa resort in 1885 and reached the peak of its popularity in the 30's and 40's. Hollywood stars came to the spa for relaxation and rejuvenation. Today, Glen Ivy is popular with people from all walks of life who visit the spa for a day of relaxation and fun.

The main attraction is the red clay mud rich with sulfur and

other minerals for a do-it-yourself mud packs. Besides the famous mud baths the hot springs resort offers a selection of spa facilities and treatments.

Since Glen Ivy operates as a day spa only from 10 a.m. to 6 p.m. overnight accommodations can be arranged at the Kings Inn of Corona near the spa.

Glen Ivy is accessible from Los Angeles via the I-15 (Santa Ana Fwy.), or from San Diego, taking the I-15 north towards Corona. Driving distance is about 1 hour from either city.

Glen Ivy Hot Springs
♥♥♥♥

25000 Glen Ivy Road, Corona, CA 91719. Tel: (909) 277-3529. Toll Free: (800) 454-8772. Fax: (909) 277-1202. TYPE: Day Spa. MANAGER: John C. Gray, CEO. PROGRAM DIRECTORS: Ron Bahner, Pamela Gray. LOCATION: Corona, 1 hr. southeast of Los Angeles, exit 15 fwy southbound at Temescal Canyon Rd. SPA CLIENTELE: Men & Women. Age 16 and over.

* Accommodations: Best Western Kings Inn
   Tel: (909) 734-4241
* Train Station: Anaheim (CA)
* Credit Cards: VISA/MC/AMEX
* Open: Year round
* Rates: Mon-Thu $19.50 / Sun. Holidays: $25.00
   rates include: pools, spas, sauna and mud bath;
   Massage from $35-$100; Salon: $10-$80
* Year Established: 1977
* **SPA Facilities**: 15 warm mineral spas, Olympic-size swimming pool, sauna, red clay mud bath, massage & salon service available by reservation for additional fee
* **SPA Treatments**: Swedish & Shiatsu massage, eucalyptus body wraps, loofah body scrubs, cellulite wraps, aromatherapy massages, men's manicures, deep cleansing & regenerating European facials based on the spa's own line of skin and body care products
* **Length of Stay Recommended**: 4 - 6 hrs.
* Maximum Number of Guests: 1,000
* **Web**: http://www.glenivy.com

DESCRIPTION: A hundred year-old mineral springs Spa retreat, internationally acclaimed for its unique red clay mud bath'. The accent is on relaxation, revitalization and beauty care. Mud treatments are used to draw out toxins, and help relieve arthritis and rheumatic pains.

CORONADO
⅂ 619

✈ Linderbergh Field Int'l AP (SAN) 2 mi. / 3 km.
Montgomery Field AP (MYF) 7 mi. / 11 km.
Gillespie Field Airport (SEE) 12 mi. / 19 km.

Coronado, population 19,000, lies across the bay from San Diego and is connected to the mainland by the beautiful Coronado Bridge. Nearby San Diego is a popular year round vacation destination known for its fine climate, beautiful beaches, cosmopolitan culture and nightlife, excellent shopping centers, and fine restaurants. Mexican flavor is dominant due to the proximity to the Mexican border.

Le Meridien San Diego
❤❤❤❤❤

2000 Second St., Coronado, CA 92032. Tel:(619) 435-3000. Toll Free (800) 543-4300. Fax: (619) 435-3032. TYPE: Resort & Spa. LOCATION: On Coronado Island across the Bay Bridge from San Diego. SPA CLIENTELE: Women and men.

* Rooms: 300 w/private bath. Suites: 35
* Phone, CTV, A/C, C/H, minibar, hair drier
* Restaurants, cocktail lounge, business center,
* Airport: San Diego Int'l (10 mi. / 16 km.)
* Train Station: Amtrak (10 mi. / 16 km.)
* Airport/Train Station Transportation: taxi, limo
* Credit Cards: MC/VISA/AMEX/DC/EC
* Open: Year round
* Hotel Rates: from $195
* TAC: 10%
* Spa on premises
* Name of spa: **Clarins Institut de Beauté**
* **Spa Facilities**: Beauty Center, heated swimming pools, saunas, exercise rooms
* **Spa Programs**: beauty and fitness, skin care

* **Spa Treatments**: hydrotherapy, herbal wrap, massages, hatha yoga, facials, body treatments, aquacize, low calorie spa meals
* **Spa Packages**: Rejuvenator (1 day); Clarins Day of Beauty; Executive Package (1 day); Spa Package (2-3 days)

DESCRIPTION: French ambience on a sixteen waterfront landscaped acres. Deluxe accommodations vary from large villas to lavish hotel rooms. The resort features the famous **Clarins Institut de Beauté** - world famous for its skin care products and treatments. Aerobics and aquacize classes are available for those interested in shaping up. Recreation: jet skiing, sailing, deep sea fishing, sun bathing, tennis, and 18-hole championship golf course across the street.

DEL MAR
⅂ 619

✈ Lindbergh Field Int'l Airport (SAN) 16 mi. / 26 km.

L'Auberge Del Mar Resort & Spa
❤❤❤

1540 Camino Del Mar, Del Mar CA 92014. Tel: (619) 259-1515. Toll Free (800) 553-1336. Fax: (619) 793-6492. TYPE: Hotel & Spa. LOCATION: Overlooking the Pacific Ocean 25 mi / 40 km north of San Diego. DESCRIPTION: Gracious European Cottage style resort hotel with complete European spa & health club, gym, sauna, massage, whirlpool, steam room, aerobics & jacuzzi. 112 rooms, 8 suites, nonsmoker rooms. Dining room, bar, outdoor pools (2). Hotel rates: from $159.

DESERT HOT SPRINGS
⅂ 760

✈ Municipal Airport (PSP) Palm Springs

Desert Hot Springs, population 6,000, is a rapidly growing spa resort town in the desert just a few miles north of Palm Springs. The town is blessed with hot natural mineral springs with temperatures varying between 110°F - 207°F (43°c - 97°c) which are then cooled to a bearable 102°F -

110°F (39°c - 43°c) for therapy or recreation. The hottest springs are known to have higher mineral content which increase their therapeutic value.

Water Composition: The water contain calcium, sulfate, phosphate, magnesium-sulfate, sodium bi-carbonate, lithium chloride, and potassium chloride have a soothing, relaxing beneficial effect. Their natural softening properties leave the skin feeling soft and smooth.

Winter is the best time for a spa vacation in Desert Hot Springs; the summers are extremely hot with temperatures in the high 100°F (37°c). Desert Hot Springs is accessible by car from nearby Palm Springs or Los Angeles.

Desert Hot Springs Spa
❤❤❤

10805 Palm Drive, Desert Hot Springs 92240. Tel: (760) 329-6495, CA Toll Free (800) 843-6053. Fax: (760) 329-6915. TYPE: Motel & Spa. LOCATION: 5 mi. / 8 km. north of I-10 / Palm Drive interchange. SPA CLIENTELE: Women and men, family oriented.

* Rooms: 48 w/priv. bath. Suites: 2
* Phone, CTV, A/C, C/H
* Nearest Airport: Palm Springs 12 mi. / 19 km.
* Airport Transportation: free pick up
* Reservations: 1 night deposit
* Credit Cards: MC/VISA/AMEX/DC/CB
* Open: Year round
* Hotel Rates: from $69; TAC: 10%
* Spa on premises
* **Spa Facilities**: Heated pool, 8 hot therapy pools, sauna, massage rooms, beauty shop
* **Spa Treatments**: massages (Shiatsu or Swedish) European facials bathing in mineral waters, aerobics, low-cal meals; fitness and diet seminars
* **Indications**: relaxation of muscular tension, body circulation improvement,
* No Medical Supervision
* Treatments approved: professional licensed attendants

DESCRIPTION: A two-story hotel with rooms facing the thermal pool complex. The mineral pools come in different sizes and vary in their water temperature. This is basically a family type recreational spa 'to take the water' for relaxation and recreation. The spring waters are rich in minerals and natural gases but they contain no sulfur and therefore are odorless and pleasant. A one-day Daytime Spa Relaxer Package is available. The package includes: massage, natural hot mineral springs soaks, sauna, fruit juice, and a delicious low-cal Spa lunch. Recreation: area golf, tennis and horseback riding privileges.

Lido Palms Spa Resort
❤❤

12801 Tamar Drive, Desert Hot Springs, CA 92240. Tel: (760) 329-6033. Fax: (760) 329-6033. TYPE: Spa Hotel. DESCRIPTION: Intimate spa hotel with natural hot mineral swimming pool, two therapy pools. 11 rooms.

Mineral Springs Hotel & Spa
❤❤❤❤

11000 Palm Drive, Desert Hot Springs, CA 92240. Tel: (760) 329-6485. Fax: (760) 329-6484. TYPE: Spa Hotel. DESCRIPTION: European style hotel and mineral spa with mineral baths, bodywraps, mud baths, facials, massages, herbal rubs, steam room, sauna. 97 rooms & suites. Restaurants (2), lounge, sports bar, acabna bar, cafe, gift shop, jewelry shop.

Miracle Springs Hotel & Spa
❤❤❤❤

10625 Palm Drive, Desert Hot Springs, CA 92240. Tel: (760) 251-6000. Toll Free (800) 400-4414. Fax: (760) 251-0460. TYPE: Resort Hotel & Spa. LOCATION: Set among the majestic San Jacinto Mountains, 12 mi / 19 km from Palm Springs. SPA CLIENTELE: Women and men. DESCRIPTION: Desert resort hotel with health spa featuring natural hot mineral waters, massages, body treatments, aromatherapy, reflexology and herbal wraps. Hotel rates: from $89.

Two Bunch Palms Resort & Spa
♥♥♥

67425 Two Bunch Palms Trail, Desert Hot Springs, CA 92240. Tel: (760) 329-8791. (800) 472-4334. Fax: (760) 329-1874. TYPE: Beauty Spa. LOCATION: 13 mi. / 21 km. from Palm Springs Airport. SPA CLIENTELE: Women and men. DESCRIPTION: First class beauty spa with hot mineral pool, hair & skin treatments, massage, sauna. 44 rooms, studios, villas 1 & 2 bedroom condos. Restaurant, lounge, pool, 2 tennis courts. Hotel rates: from $145.

We Care Health Retreat
♥♥

18000 Long Canyon Road, Desert Hot Springs, CA 92240. Tel: (760) 251-2261. Toll Free (800) 888-2523. Fax: (760) 251-5399TYPE: New Age Health Retreat. SPA DIRECTOR: Susana Lombardi. LOCATION: Coachella Valley surrounded by mountains. SPA CLIENTELE: Mixed

* Rooms 6; 2 w/priv. bath
* Airport: Palm Springs, 20 min., free pick up
* Reservations: deposit required
* Credit Cards: MC/VISA/AMEX
* Open: Year round
* Hotel Rates: from $75; TAC: 15%
* Spa off premises: distance 2 mi. (3 km.)
* **Spa Facilities**: indoor and outdoor facilities
* **Spa Programs**: Deluxe Revitalization, Colon Hygiene, Healthful Vacationing
* **Spa Treatments**: colon hygiene, reflexology, massages, herbal wraps, clay packs, facials, yoga, meditation, vegetarian diets, iriodology, fasting with raw vegetable juices, lymphatic exercises, hot mineral water
* Spa Packages: from $1,199 Deluxe Revitalization Program (6 days/5 nights) including accommodations, meals, 10 treatments, and daily classes; other packages vary from $700

DESCRIPTION: An holistic/New Age health center where healthy people come to learn how to better take care of their body, mind, and spirit through improved diet and self awareness. The main program consists of fasting with liquid meals or light cleansing food, colon hygiene, hot mineral baths, cooking lessons, and group therapy teaching trust and love sharing.

ESCONDIDO
〉 760
✈ Linderbergh Field Int'l AP (SAN)
Montgomery Field AP (MYF)
Gillespie Field Airport (SEE)

Escondido, population 64,500, is a ranger district of the Cleveland National forest some 29 miles (47 km.) north of San Diego. The area is typical southern California, mostly rocky and rugged mountainous wilderness. Some 420,000 acres of dense forests are nearby with natural trails for hiking, jogging and horseback riding, the popular beach health resort of Carlsbad is only few miles to the west. Escondido can be reached by car from San Diego or Los Angeles. Driving time from San Diego Airport in about 1 hour.

Castle Creek Inn Resort & Spa
♥♥♥♥♥

29850 Circle R Way, Escondido, CA 92026. Tel: (760) 751-8800. Fax: (760) 751-8787. TYPE: Resort & Spa. LOCATION: In the mountains, 40 min. from San Diego Airport. SPA CLIENTELE: Women and men. DESCRIPTION: European style resort with health spa, gym, sauna, massage, exercise equipment, jacuzzi. 30 rooms & 1-3 bedroom cottage with CTV, phone, coffee maker. Restaurant, tavern, business center, tennis courts (2), 18-hole golf courses. Hotel rates: from $135.

Golden Door
♥♥♥♥♥

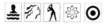

P.O. Box 1567, Escondido, CA 92025. Tel: (760) 744-5777. Fax: (760) 471-2393. TYPE: Health & Beauty Spa. LOCATION: North of San Diego in Escondido, a Ranger District office of the Cleveland National Forest. SPA CLIENTELE: Women and men. Open to women only 39 weeks yearly, other weeks for couples or men only.

* Rooms: 39 Japanese style
* Large dining room, Organic gardens
* Airport: San Diego 35 mi. / 56 km., free pick up
* Reservations: deposit required
* Credit Cards: MC/VISA/AMEX
* Season: Year round
* Rates: from $3,950/week
* Spa on premises
* **Spa Facilities**: 2 pools, Japanese hot tub, saunas, Camstar-equipped gym, beauty salon
* **Spa Programs**: Diet, fitness, beauty, stress reduction
* **Spa Packages**: Mother/Daughter's Week; Women's Weeks, Men's Weeks, Couples Week, Inner Door Weeks
* **Spa Treatments**: exercises, aerobics, under water aerobics, weight lifting, hiking, movement assessment, water exercises, beauty treatments, massages, heated herbal wraps, body scrubs, low cal spa cuisine (1,000 - 1,200 calories), yoga

DESCRIPTION: The most famous and most luxurious health resort in the USA. The Japanese-inspired complex is set in 200 country acres with serene Japanese Zen gardens, waterfalls, koi ponds and a one story stucco building modeled in the tradition of the Honjin inns that were favorites of the Japanese nobility. Each room is equipped with a complete set of spa clothing and a comfortable kimono. The bathroom is stocked with Golden Door creams and a variety of beauty soaps. Daily structured programs consist of a rigorous regimen of stretching & water exercises, low calorie meals, physical activity, and it is complemented by a soothing and revitalizing beauty and relaxation treatments. The program emphasizes a holistic approach to fitness and well being rather than weight loss alone. The guest-staff ratio is 3:1 one of the best in the Spa business. The spa has a worldwide reputation for results. There are special weeks for women only, and special weeks for men only. Recreation: tap dancing, water games, tennis.

GARBERVILLE
⊃ 707

✈ Eureka/Arcadia AP 80 mi. / 128 km. North

Heartwood Institute
❤❤

220 Harmony Lane, Garberville, CA 95440. Tel: (707) 923-2021. Fax: (707) 923-4906. TYPE: Wellness Retreat LOCATION: Rural mountain setting. DESCRIPTION: Massage therapies, oriental healing arts & hypotherapies. Dining room (Vegetarian meals).

GRASS VALLEY
⊃ 530

✈ Metropolitan AP (SMF) 62 mi. / 100 km.

Sivananda Ashram Yoga Farm

14651 Ballantree Ln, Grass Valley, CA 9594.Tel: (530) 272-9322. Fax: (530) 477-6054. TYPE: Yoga Farm. LOCATION: In the Sierra foothills. DESCRIPTION: Budget yoga retreat on 80 acres with vegetarian meals, yoga, meditation positive thinking and relaxation techniques.

INDIAN WELLS
⊃ 760

✈ Municipal AP (PSP) Palm Springs

Hyatt Grand Champions Resort
❤❤❤❤

44-600 Indian Wells Lane, Indian Wells, CA 92210. Tel: (760) 341-1000. Fax: (760) 568-2236. TYPE: Resort & Spa. LOCATION Base of the San Jacinto Mountains 15 minutes to downtown Palm Springs. DESCRIPTION: Deluxe golf and tennis resort with fully equipped health spa and fitness club, sauna, steam room, whirlpool spas, massage. 338 suites, 20 garden villas, 26 penthouse suites, Regency Club Floor. Hotel rates: from $145.

Renaissance Esmeralda Resort Spa
❤❤❤❤❤

44-400 Indian Wells Lane, Indian Wells, CA 92210. Tel: (760) 773-4444. Fax: (760) 773-9250. TYPE: Mega

Resort & Spa. LOCATION: 13 mi. / 21 km. to Palm Springs Airport. SPA CLIENTELE: Women and men. DESCRIPTION: Deluxe mega resort with a full service spa, swedish & deep tissue massage, facials, manicure, pedicures, aerobics exercise equipment, steam room, sauna. 560 rooms 7 suites, nonsmoker rooms, wheelchair access. Restaurants (2), lounge, entertainment, business center, pools (3), tennis courts (7), 36-holes of golf. Hotel rates: from $175.

LA JOLLA
619

✈ Lindbergh Field Int'l AP (SAN)

Chopra Center For Well Being
❤❤

7630 Fay Avenue, La Jolla, CA 92037. Tel: (619) 551-7788. Toll Free (888) 424-6772. Fax: (619) 551-9570. LOCATION: Near town center. SPA CLIENTELE: Women and men. DESCRIPTION: Small hotel (24 rooms) with multiply day wellness programs for enhanced physical, emotional, and spiritual well being.

LA QUINTA
760

✈ Municipal Airport (PSP) Palm Springs

Spa La Quinta
❤❤❤❤

c/o La Quinta Resort & Club, 49-499 Eisenhower Drive, La Quinta CA 92253. Tel: (760) 564-5757. Toll Free (800) 598-3828. Fax: (760) 564-7625. TYPE: Spa Resort Complex. LOCATION: an 800 acre garden oasis in foothills of Santa Rosa mountains, just 19 mi. / 30 km. southeast of Palm Springs, 120 mi. / 192 km. east of Los Angeles. SPA DIRECTOR: Linda Richey. SPA CLIENTELE: Men & women. No age or gender restriction.

* Accommodations: **La Quinta Resort & Club**
  Hotel Tel: (760) 564-4111
* Rooms: 640 guest casitas w/priv. bath. Suites: 27
* Phone, CTV, minibar, hairdryer

* Restaurants: Montañas (innovative Mediterranean); Morgans (American/Mexican); light cuisine at the Golf & Tennis Clubhouses
* Airports: Palm Springs or Los Angeles
* Airport/Train Transportation: taxi, limo
* Reservations: required
* Credit Cards: VISA/AMEX/MC/DIN
* Open: Year round
* Hotel Rates: $140 - $360. Tax: 9%
* TAC: 10%
* Spa on premises: **Spa La Quinta**
* Year Established: 1998
* **Spa Facilities**: 23,000 sq. ft. (2,090 sq. m.) health spa sanctuary, 48 treatments areas, open air Spa La Quinta Celestial showers, seven outdoor aromatherapy garden tubs, swimming pools, beauty salon, 4,000 sq. ft. (364 sq. m.) fitness center, mind & movement studio, hiking trails
* **Spa Programs**: Skin Care, Beauty, Fitness, revitalization, water therapy
* **Spa Packages**: from day spa to 3 nights; Desert Celebration (2 nights); Golf & Spa (3 nights); Couple's Hide-a-Way (3 nights). Packages include: accommodations, treatments and breakfast daily Rates: from $610 - $1,765 (p.p. double occupancy)
* **Spa Treatments**: facials, aromatherapy, Cahuilla Sage wrap, lavender wrap, grape seed crush glow, desert rose polish, sports pack body rub, solar body bronzer, luxurious paraffin wraps, massages, hydrotherapy, carnio sacral therapy, Shiatsu, celestial shower treatment, fango bath, serenity bath, desert rose bath, yoga, aerobics, weight training, Creative treatment combinations from $80 - $290.
* **Indications**: stress reduction, body pampering, general well being, revitalization
* Web: www.laquintaresort.com

DESCRIPTION: La Quinta Resort is an elegant complex in classic Spanish architectural style and welcoming ambiance. The world class Spa La Quinta offers unique services and treatments exclusively for resort guests and club members. The Spa is committed to the concept of overall "wellness" through the beauty and serenity of nature. Ancient healing arts are combined with the latest in beauty and pampering treatments. The Spa focuses on the benefits of being outside by featuring its signature open-air Celestial Showers. Recreation: golf (72 holes of championship golf) and tennis (24 courts). Nearby attractions: hot air ballooning, desert tours, polo, horseback riding, shopping and casinos.

LOS ANGELES
213
✈ Los Angeles Int'l AP (LAX) 10 mi. / 16 km.

Miyako Inn & Spa
❤❤❤

328 East First St., Los Angeles, CA 90012. Tel: (213) 617-2000. Fax: (213) 617-2700. TYPE: Hotel & Spa. LOCATION: In the heart of Little Tokyo, adjacent to civic center. SPA CLIENTELE: Women and men. DESCRIPTION: Pleasant hotel with Japanese style health spa, jacuzzi, sauna and massage. 172 rooms, 2 suites, rooms for nonsmokers, wheelchair access. Japanese Restaurant, bar, business center. Hotel rates: from $115.

The New Otani Hotel & Garden
❤❤❤

120 S. Los Angeles St., Los Angeles CA 90012. Tel: (213) 629-1200. Fax: (213) 629-1200. TYPE: Executive Hotel & Spa. LOCATION: Downtown near Civic Center. SPA CLIENTELE: Women and men.

* Rooms: 434 w/priv. bath. Suites: 20
* Phone, CTV, VCR, A/C, C/H, refrigerator fax/computer hook ups
* Restaurants (3), bar, lounge, business center
* Airport: LAX
* Train Station: Union Station (Amtrak)
* Reservations: required
* Open: Year round
* Hotel Rates: from $190
* TAC: 10%
* Spa on premises: **Sanwa Health Spa**
* **Spa Facilities**: massage room, jacuzzi, sauna, lockers, beauty salon
* **Spa Programs**: Royal, regular, facials

* **Spa Treatments**: sauna, shiatsu, acupressure, anma massage, facials

DESCRIPTION: Sanwa Health Spa is located on the 4th floor of the New Otani Hotel & Gardens in downtown Los Angeles. It is a relaxing escape with Japanese and oriental massages and treatments.

MURRIETA
909
✈ Ontario Int'l AP

Murrieta is a southern California resort with pleasant and sunny climate the year round. It is located north of Temecula (CA), off I-15 almost halfway between San Diego and Los Angeles. Built on a site of a Temacula Indian village, it is most famous for its mineral hot springs with some therapeutic properties. Murrieta can be reached by car from Los Angeles in 90 minutes, or from San Diego in about 75 minutes.

Murrieta Hot Springs Resort & Health Spa
❤❤❤

39405, Murrieta Hot Springs Road, Murrieta, CA 92362. Tel: (909) 677-7451, Toll Free (CA) (800) 458-4393. Fax: (909) 677-2124. TYPE: Resort & Spa. LOCATION: In Murrieta, on 45 acres of landscaped grounds. SPA CLIENTELE: Women and men. SPECIAL RESTRICTIONS: Limited smoking rooms and smoking areas, beer & wine only no liquor.

* Rooms: 242 w/private bath. Suites: 4
* Dining Rooms: vegetarian and non-vegetarian cuisine
* Night Club/ Theatre
* Nearest Airport: Ontario Airport 60 minutes
* Airport Transportation: taxi, airporter
* Reservations: recommended
* Credit Cards: MC/VISA/AMEX/DC/CB
* Open: year round
* Hotel Rates: from $90/day.
* TAC: 10%
* **Spa Facilities**: mineral pools and private indoor

mineral baths, private mud baths, saunas, beauty and skin care salons, aerobic rooms; fitness center

* **Spa Programs:** Health programs, self-awareness, one week health & fitness, Fit'n trim nutritional program , relaxation, communication
* **Spa Treatments:** aerobic exercises, relaxation, traditional and polarity massages, mineral and mud baths, body wraps, lymphatic massage European facials
* **Spa Packages:** Hot Springs Special; Spa Royale

DESCRIPTION: Hot Springs Resort & Health spa in an historic turn of the century renovated building. The resort offers hot springs balneotherapy, European spa treatments and various health programs. Recreation: live entertainment and comedy shows, tennis, shuffleboard, basketball, water volleyball, folk dancing and golf nearby.

NEVADA CITY
ꓛ **530**
✈ Nevada Air Park 4 mi. / 6 km.

The Expanding Light at Ananda
♥♥

🕴 ◉

14618 Tyler Foote Rd, Nevada City, CA 95959. Tel: (530) 478-7518. Toll Free (800) 346-5350. Fax: (530) 478-7519. DESCRIPTION: Small hotel (26 rooms) offering stress management through yoga & meditation workshops. Dining room (vegetarian cuisine).

OAKLAND
ꓛ **510**
✈ Oakland Int'l Airport (OAK) 10 mi. / 16 km.
San Francisco Int'l AP (SFO) 24 mi. / 38 km.

The Claremont Resort & Spa
♥♥♥♥♥

41 Tunner Rd., Berkeley, CA 94623. Tel: (510) 843-3000. Fax: (510) 843-6208. TYPE: Resort & Spa. LOCATION: Amid the Oakland/Berkeley Hills surrounded by land-

scaped gardens with views of San Francisco.

* **Rooms:** 279 w/priv. bath. Suites: 26
* **Restaurant** & cocktail lounges, meeting rooms
* **Wheelchair** accessibility
* **Airport:** Oakland 20 mi. / 32 km.
* **Train Station:** Oakland 10 minutes
* **Airport/Train Transportation:** free pick up, limo
* **Reservations:** Credit Card # guarantee
* **Credit Cards:** MC/VISA/AMEX/DC/CB/DIS
* **Open:** Year round
* **Hotel Rates:** from $169
* **TAC:** 10%
* **Spa** on Premises
* **Spa Facilities:** exercise room, weight room, whirlpools, saunas, steam rooms, Olympic size pools, spa restaurant (low cal cuisine)
* **Spa Programs:** Diet/fitness, pampering, lifestyle enhancement
* **Spa Treatments:** aerobics, stretching exercises, massages, aromatherapy, hydrotherapy, reflexology, salt glo, loofah, herbal wrap, yoga, meditation, low calorie spa cuisine

DESCRIPTION: Moderate deluxe landmark resort and convention hotel with long tradition of service and quality. Accommodations range from standard hillside rooms to luxury suites. The full service European spa offers facilities for fitness, pampering, revitalization and stress reduction. Recreation: tennis courts (6 lighted) and Olympic size swimming pools (2).

OJAI
ꓛ **805**
✈ Santa Barbara Airport (SBA) 40 mi. / 64 km.

Ojai, population 6,800, is a quite winter resort and retreat for artists in a beautiful valley surrounded by mountains. The nearby Lake Casitas provides excellent recreational opportunities for those who enjoy water sports such as boating and fishing. Tennis lovers can enjoy the oldest tennis tournament in the US that takes place in Ojai each year in April 24-27. The fine ocean beaches of Santa Barbara are only a few miles away. Ojai, can be reached by car from Los Angeles or Santa Barbara.

The Oaks at Ojai
❤❤❤

122 E. Ojai Avenue, Ojai, CA 93023. Tel: (805) 646-5573. Fax: (805) 640-1504. TYPE: Health Resort Complex. MANAGER: Sheila Cluff (owner). LOCATION: 20 minute drive from the city of Ventura on Hwy. 150. SPA CLIENTELE: Women and men (no children).

* Rooms: 46 w/private bath. Cottages: 19
* Airport: LAX/Santa Barbara
* Distance to the Airport: 70/30 mi. 112/48 km.
* Airport Transportation: taxi, limo, bus, Oaks Van service (Mon. - Fri.)
* Reservations: deposit required
* Credit Cards: AMEX/VISA/MC
* Open: Year round
* Hotel Rates: from $195; TAC: 10%
* Spa on premises
* **Spa Facilities**: whirlpool, sauna, gym, weight room, swimming pool, beauty salon,
* **Spa Programs**: Fitness, weight loss
* Medical Supervision: 1 nurse on duty

DESCRIPTION: Country Inn built in 1918, nestled among oak trees. Lobby with large stone fireplace, relaxed, casual atmosphere. The Spa owned and managed by Sheila Cluff, a physical fitness specialist offers health, fitness and weight loss programs. Recreation: boating & fishing at Lake Casitas, golf, tennis and horseback riding nearby.

Ojai Valley Inn and Spa
❤❤❤❤

Country Club Road, Ojai, CA 92032. Tel: (805) 646-5511. Toll Free (800) 422-6524. Fax: (805) 646-7969. TYPE: Resort Hotel & Spa. LOCATION: 35 minutes from Santa Barbara. SPA CLIENTELE: Women and men. DESCRIPTION: Attractive mission-style resort with full service health spa, aerobics, exercise room, sauna, steam room. 192 rooms, 15 suites, rooms for nonsmokers. Restaurants (2), lounges (2), live entertainment, pools (2), tennis courts (8), 18 hole golf course. Hotel rates: from $195.

PALM DESERT
❱ 760

✈ Municipal Airport (PSP) Palm Springs

Palm Desert, population 12,000, is located at the foot hills of the Santa Rosa Mountains, about 20 miles (32 km.) southwest of Palm Springs. Palm Desert hosts various famous golf tournaments including the Bob Hope Desert Golf Tournament (mid. January), and the Dinah Shore-Colgate Winners Circle Invitational Golf Tournament (early April).

The major tourist attraction in town is the Living Desert Reserve, located at 47-900 S. Portola Avenue. The Reserve is actually a huge public garden with a fascinating display of desert flora and fauna, including some rare botanical species. Palm Desert can be reached from Palm Springs, Los Angeles or San Diego by car.

Marriott's Desert Springs
❤❤❤❤

74855 Country Club Drive, Palm Desert, CA 92260. Tel: (760) 341-2211, Toll-free (800) 255-0848. Fax: (760) 341-1872. TYPE: Resort & Spa. LOCATION: In the center of southern California's famous desert retreat. SPA CLIENTELE: Women and men.

* Rooms: 884 w/priv. bath. Suites: 51 deluxe
* Phone, CTV, A/C, C/H, minibar, patio/balcony
* Restaurants (5), lounges (4), meeting facilities
* Airport: Palm Springs 20 mi. / 32 km.
* Airport Transportation: taxi, limo, shuttle
* Reservations: 1 night credit card guarantee
* Credit Cards: AMEX/VISA/MC/DC/CB
* Open: Year round
* Hotel Rates: from $160
* TAC: 10%
* **Spa Facilities**: European Spa with separate facilities for men and women; lap and exercise pool, hot and cold plunge pools, individual whirlpool baths, Turkish steam room, Finnish sauna, 22-station fitness gym, aerobics room with resilient floor and high-tech sound system, locker rooms, walking/jogging paths; full service beauty salon for men and women by

José Eber of Rodeo Drive

* **Spa Programs**: Fitness, beauty, weight control and health programs; medically supervised Spa programs in conjunction with the Eisenhower Medical Center
* **Spa Treatments**: exercise, aerobics, calisthenics, yoga, water exercise, fitness classes, swedish and shiatsu massages, skin care, biological peels, herbal wrap, aromatherapy, loofah body buff, whirlpool, underwater massage, calorie controlled spa cuisine
* **Spa Packages**: Deluxe Spa Program (4-7 day); Men's Spa Day; Lady's Beautiful Day.
* **Medical Supervision**: 1 RN on duty, MD on call

DESCRIPTION: A European spa and resort on 400 acres of landscaped gardens overlooking a blue lagoon and surrounded by mountains. Deluxe rooms and suites with excellent service and amenities. The programs emphasize fitness, exercises, beauty care and pampering for men and women. Recreation: terraced swimming pools, huge sunbathing and lounging beach, golf, tennis, croquet court, and fashion boutiques.

Palm Valley Country Club
❤❤❤❤

76-200 Country Club Drive., Palm Desert, CA 92260. Tel: (760) 345-2737. Fax: (760) 360-9633. TYPE: Resort Complex & Spa. LOCATION: 15 mi. (24 km.) southeast of Palm Springs, 5 mi. (8 km) from Palm Desert Town Center. SPA CLIENTELE: Women and men.

* Vacation homes: 1-3 bedrooms
* Dining & grill rooms
* Airport: Palm Springs, 20 minutes, taxi
* Credit Cards: MC/VISA
* Open: Year round
* Hotel Rates: from $180
* Spa on premises
* **Spa Facilities**: expanded weight room with Nautilus Universal equipment, Racquetball courts, swimming pool, jogging trail, saunas, steam rooms, jacuzzis, Juice Bar
* **Spa Packages**: Racquetball & Spa, Golf/Racquetball

& Spa, Tennis/Racquetball & Spa

* **Spa Treatments**: aerobics, fitness classes, aqua classes, fitness seminars, yoga and stretching, nature hikes, walking club, fun runs, prenatal fitness, massages - swedish, acupressure, shiatsu and sport, salt glow rub, herbal wrap, bindi treatment, foot reflexology, facial treatment, back treatment
* **Indications**: general fitness, prenatal fitness, sports conditioning, stress reduction

DESCRIPTION: Vacation complex featuring 1-3 bedroom condominiums and 1-2 story condominiums with patios. The resort offers club house, 2 restaurants, meeting banquet facilities, 36-holes of golf and 19 tennis courts (10 lighted). The Spa and racquetball club features racquetball courts, weight and aerobic rooms, separate men's and women's locker rooms with saunas, steam rooms and whirlpools. Spa treatments are available a la carte or as a special Spa package.

PALM SPRING
ﾱ **760**
✈ Municipal AP (PSP) Palm Springs 2 mi. / 3 km.

Palm Springs, population 33,000, is a fashionable resort at the foot of the San Jacinto mountains in the Upper Colorado Desert. During the 30's many of the first Hollywood celebrities chose Palm Springs as their favorite winter retreat. The town's mineral springs were discovered by local Indians, then by the Spanish in 1774. The site was named "Agua Caliente" (hot water). The Palm Springs area is a favorite winter vacation haven for Californians and international visitors who come to escape the stress of every day urban life and relax in the magnificent scenery surrounded by exotic palm trees and pure clean desert air. Palm Springs can be reached from Los Angeles in about 2 hours driving time.

Merv Griffin's Resort Hotel & Givenchy Spa
❤❤❤❤❤

4200 E. Palm Canyon Drive, Palm Springs CA 92264. Tel: (760) 770-5000. Toll Free (800) 276-5000. Fax: (760) 324-7280. TYPE: Resort Hotel & Spa. LOCATION: 2 mi. /

3 km. from downtown Palm Springs. SPA CLIENTELE: Women and men.

* Rooms & Suites
* Phone, CTV, VCR, A/C, C/H, refrigerator
* Rooms for non smokers, wheelchair access
* Restaurants (2), lounge, business center
* Airport: Palm Springs, 3 mi. / 5 km. limo, bus,
* Reservations: deposit required
* Credit Cards: AMEX/VISA/MC
* Open: Year round
* Hotel Rates: from $195
* TAC: 10%
* Spa on premises: **Givenchy Spa**
* **Spa Facilities**: spa building, whirlpool, sauna, gym, weight room, swimming pools, beauty salon
* **Spa Programs**: beauty, fitness, weight loss
* **Spa Treatments**: body scrubs, marine mud wrap, seaweed wrap, hydrojet, swedish massage, deep tissue massage, foot reflexology, slimming, lymphatic drainage, aromatherapy, shiatsu, hydrotherapy, multijet bath with seaweed, under water massage with Givenchy oils, hydromassage
* **Spa Packages**: A day of splendor (pampering, health and well being, fitness)

DESCRIPTION: Elegant hotel of contemporary French renaissance style with Givenchy Spa building and fitness facilities. Enjoy a large selection of unique beauty and pampering treatments using Givenchy oils and creams for the ultimate in spa experience.

Palm Springs Hilton Resort
❤❤❤❤

400 E. Tahquitz Canyon Way, Palm Springs CA 92262. Tel: (760) 320-6868. Fax: (760) 320-2126. TYPE: Resort Hotel & Spa. LOCATION: One half block from convention center. SPA CLIENTELE: Women and men. DESCRIPTION: Desert resort hotel with full service spa, body treatments, health club, sauna, jacuzzis (2), pool. 189 rooms, 71 suites, rooms for nonsmokers, wheelchair access. Restaurant, poolside cafe & bar, cocktail bar, pool, 6 tennis courts. Hotel rates: from $175.

Spa Hotel & Casino
❤❤❤

100 North Indian Avenue, Palm Springs, CA 92262. Tel: (760) 325-1461. Toll Free (800) 854-1279. Fax: (760) 325-3344. TYPE: Resort & Spa Complex. MANAGER: Gabor Komyathy, GM. LOCATION: Downtown Palm Springs, near the center of Palm Springs. SPA CLIENTELE: Men, Women.

* Rooms: 230 w/private bath
* Suites: 20; Apartments: 1
* Phone, CTV, A/C, minibar, many w/balcony
* Dining room, cafe, casino, meeting facilities
* Airport: Palm Springs 2 mi. / 3 km.
* Airport Transportation: courtesy car service
* Reservations: 1 night deposit req'd
* Credit Cards: AMEX/VISA/MC/DC/CB
* Open: Year round
* TAC: 10% (hotel rooms only)
* Spa on premises
* **Spa Facilities**: freshwater pool, hot mineral water outdoor pools (2), health club with spa facilities, russian steam room, private natural hot mineral spring baths (34), Beauty services & products by Ilona of Hungary, Paramount gym with trained instructor
* **Spa Programs**: Spa Sampler (2 nights/3 days), Discover the Springs (5 nights/6 days)
* **Spa Treatments**: mineral baths, massage, herbal wrap, exercise program, eucalyptus inhalation, weight training, tennis/swimming, complimentary mineral water, hydrotherapy, health lifestyle lectures, low calorie spa cuisine
* **Spa Packages**: Spa Sampler (2 nights); Discover The Springs (5 nights); Spa/Golf

DESCRIPTION: A resort hotel in the centre of Palm Springs with European spa facilities and ambience. The spa offers exotic body pampering, stress reduction, relaxation and beauty care for men and women. Recreation: casino, tennis and golf available.

The Palms at Palm Springs
❤❤❤

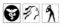

572 N. Indian Avenue, Palm Springs, CA 92262. Tel: (760) 325-1111. Fax: (760) 327-0867. TYPE: Spa Resort. LOCATION: Near downtown Palm Springs, 5 minutes stroll to the Desert Fashion Plaza. SPA CLIENTELE: Women and men. No children under 16.

* Rooms & Bungalows: 43, 31 w/private bath
* Phone, CTV, A/C, hair dryer, balcony
* Airport: Palm Springs 4 mi. / 6 km.
* Airport Transportation: taxi, limo
* Reservations: required
* Credit Cards: AMEX/VISA/MC
* Open: Year round
* Hotel Rates: from $195; TAC: 10%
* **Spa Facilities**: pool, saunas, spa & fitness center,
* **Spa Programs**: Weight loss - approx. 750 calories, fitness program, beauty care
* Medical Supervision: 1 nurse on duty

DESCRIPTION: The Palms offers a wide range of accommodations, from poolside rooms, to bungalows with private patio. The Spa programs emphasize weight loss and fitness. Recreation: tennis, golf, hot air ballooning, celebrity tours, bicycle & horseback riding.

RANCHO MIRAGE
 760

✈ Municipal Airport (PSP) Palm Spgs 8 mi. / 13 km.

The Spa at the Ritz Carlton
♥♥♥♥♥

68-900 Frank Sinatra Drive, Rancho Mirage, CA 92270. Tel: (760) 321-8282. Toll Free (888) 748-9772. Fax: (760) 321-6928. TYPE: Resort Hotel & Spa. LOCATION: Foothills of the Santa Rosa mountains. SPA CLIENTELE: Women and men. DESCRIPTION: Luxurious resort hotel with a full service health & fitness spa. 219 rooms, 21 suites, room for nonsmokers. Dining room, cafe, poolside restaurant & bar, business center, swimming pool, 10 tennis courts. Hotel rates: from $120.

REDWOOD CITY
🢂 650

✈ San Francisco Int'l Airport (SFO) 7 mi. / 112 km.

Sandra Caron European Spa
♥♥♥♥♥

c/o Hotel Sofitel SF Bay, 223 Twin Dolphin Drive, Redwood City, CA 94065. Tel: (650) 598-9000. Fax: (650) 598-0459. TYPE: European style Spa. MANAGER: Sandra Caron. YEAR ESTABLISHED: 1986. LOCATION: Hotel Sofitel near the San Mateo Convention Center. CLIENTELE: Women & men.

* Accommodations: Hotel Sofitel San Francisco Bay
* Rooms: 319 w/priv. bath; Suites: 28
* Phone, A/C, C/H, CTV, minibar
* Restaurants (2), lounge, bar, business center
* Airport: San Francisco Int'l. 7mi. / 12 km.
* Train Station: San Carlos/Caltrans
* Airport/Train Transportation: free pick up
* Open: Year round
* Reservation: deposit required
* Hotel Rates: from $175
* TAC: 10%
* Spa on premises
* **Spa Facilities**: Sauna, multijet tub, cascade showers, heated swimming pool overlooking lagoon, jogging trail, workout studio
* **Spa Treatments**: Mud, seaweed, mineral and milk baths (hydrojets); mud, seaweed and paraffin wraps; parafango packs, body polish, cascade showers, underwater massage, massages (various styles), facials, waxing, sea weed, mud and royal jelly scalp treatments and hair design, Spa pedicure with hydrojet, spa manicure, cellulite treatments, body composition, nutrition
* **Spa Programs**: Relax and unwind, cellulite, body care, facial care
* **Spa Packages**: 2-4 days

DESCRIPTION: Elegant Spa at the Hotel Sofitel with a touch of France on San Francisco bay. The spa offers a wide range of European treatments. Sandra Caron specializes in relaxing, pampering and cellulite treatments. Low calorie Spa cuisine is available.

SAN DIEGO
⟩ 619

✈ Lindbergh Field Int'l Airport (SAN) 2 mi. / 3 km.
Montgomery Field Airport (MYF) 7 mi. / 11 km.
Gillespie Field Airport (SEE) 12 mi. / 19 km.

San Diego Hilton Resort & Spa
❤❤❤❤❤

1775 East Mission Bay Drive, San Diego, CA 92109. Tel: (619) 276-4010. Fax: (619) 275-7991. TYPE: Resort & Spa. LOCATION: On Mission Bay, 10 min. to the airport. DESCRIPTION: Mediterranean-style resort with a full service European spa providing a variety of services, exercise equipment and treatments. 360 rooms, 17 suites, rooms for non smokers, wheelchair access. Restaurants (3) and cafes, bars (2), outdoor pool, tennis courts, gift shop. Hotel rates: from $165.

SAN FRANCISCO
⟩ 415

✈ San Francisco Int'l Airport (SFO) 16 mi. / 25 km.
Oakland Int'l Airport (OAK) 18 mi. / 29 km.

San Francisco, metro area population 3,255,000, is one of the most beautiful cities in the world. Its architecture is a mixture of Victorian, Edwardian, Oriental and Mediterranean. Here you can explore the charm of San Francisco's "Painted Ladies" - Victorian houses with endlessly varied faces, shapes and colors in the tradition of the 19th century. The city's financial center is known as the "Wall Street of the West", and the port is one of the busiest in the USA. Whether you come for business or pleasure there is always plenty to see and do in and around San Francisco.

Hotel Nikko San Francisco
❤❤❤❤

222 Mason St., San Francisco, CA 94102. Tel: (415) 394-1111. Fax: (415) 394-1106. TYPE: Tower Hotel & Spa. LOCATION: In the business district, 13 mi. / 21 km. to San Francisco Airport. SPA CLIENTELE: Women and men. DESCRIPTION: Modern tower hotel with a unique blending of high-

tech and Japanese designs with health club & spa, glass enclosed swimming pool. Restaurant, sushi bar, lobby bar, business. 523 rooms, 22 suites. Hotel rates: from $225.

SANTA BARBARA
⟩ 805

✈ Municipal airport (SBA) 10 mi. / 16 km.

Radisson Hotel Santa Barbara
❤❤❤❤

1111 E. Cabrillo Blvd., Santa Barbara, CA 93103. Tel: (805) 963-0744. Fax: (805) 962-0985. TYPE: Resort Hotel & Spa. LOCATION: Across from the Pacific Ocean at East Beach. SPA CLIENTELE: Women and men. DESCRIPTION: Elegant Spanish style resort with a full service health & beauty spa, separate facilities for men & women, saunas, whirlpool, massage, and gym. 171 rooms, 2 suites, rooms for nonsmokers. Restaurant, poolside deli, heated swimming pool. Hotel rates: from $179.

SANTA MONICA
⟩ 310

✈ Los Angeles Int'l AP (LAX) 13 mi. / 21 km.

Santa Monica, population 90,000, is a rapidly growing beach resort west of Los Angeles facing the Santa Monica Bay. Of interest to visitors is the Santa Monica Pier and the magnificent turn-of-the century carousel which was restored in 1984. The promenade along the beach offers opportunities for recreation and shopping.

Pritikin Longevity Center & Spa
❤❤❤❤

c/o Loews Santa Monica Beach Hotel, 1700 Ocean Avenue, Santa Monica, CA 90401. Hotel - Tel: (310) 458-6700. Fax: (310) 458-6761. Longevity Center - Tel: (310) 899-4040. Fax: (310) 899-4045. Pritikin Program reservations (800) 421-9911. TYPE: Longevity Center. SPA DIRECTOR: Nicola Evans. LOCATION: Near the Ocean beach in Santa monica. SPA CLIENTELE: Women and men.

* Rooms: 350 w/priv. bath. Suites: 38
* Phone, CTV, A/C, C/H, minibar, patio or balcony
* Airport: Los Angeles, 20 minutes
* Airport Transportation: free pick up
* Reservations: deposit required
* Credit Cards: MC/VISA/AMEX
* Open: Year round
* Hotel Rates: from $245; TAC: 10%
* Spa on premises
* **Center Facilities**: 6000 sq. ft. / 545 sq. m. spa, treatment rooms (8), cardiovascular room, strength-training room with Life Fitness resistance training circuit, fitness studio, beauty salon, locker rooms with steam and dry saunas, glass-domed indoor/outdoor pool, jacuzzi, several walking / jogging trails
* **Center Programs**: Diet & weight management, cardiovascular exercise evaluation program, comprehensive medical management program
* **Center Treatments**: Pritikin diet, exercise and fitness therapy, body treatments, moor muds, body wraps, body polish, aromatherpay salt glo, facials, massage therapy, swedish massage, shiatsu massage, reflexology, yoga, Pilates classes
* **Indications**: Overweight with health problems such as heart disease and diabetes; degenerative diseases, astheroclerosis, angina, claudication, stroke, diabetes, obesity, arthritis, gout, high blood cholesterol and triglyceride levels, general fitness, well being and pampering at the spa
* Special Restrictions: applications and medical acceptance required
* Treatments Approval: Doctors Board Certified in specialties of Cardiology, Endocrinology, and internal medicine.

DESCRIPTION: The Pritikin Longevity Center is a medically oriented institute which specializes in weight loss programs based on the Pritikin Diet. The Pritikin diet consists of 80% complex carbohydrates (fresh fruit, vegetables, whole grain), 7% - 8% fat, and 12% - 13% protein from vegetable and lean animal sources. The diet is also helpful for individuals who wish to lower their cholesterol and triglyceride levels. There are special demonstrations how to prepare Pritikin meals in order to continue with the diet after leaving

the center. The New Pritikin Longevity Center & Spa offer healthy lifestyle change with pampering and pleasure of a European spa.

SONOMA
⟩ 707
✈ San Francisco Int'l Airport (SFO) 60 mi. / 96 km.
Oakland Int'l Airport (OAK) 60mi. / 96 km.

Sonoma is located 40 mi. / 64 km. north of San Francisco in the heart of the famous California's Wine country. Many of the Sonoma wineries are open to the public and have facilities. Visits are encouraged with complimentary wine tasting. The countryside is post-card beautiful with quaint, picturesque villages, delightful bed-and-breakfasts, country bistros and restaurants. Many travelers enjoy a panoramic scenic float above the vineyards in colorful hot-air balloons.

Sonoma Mission Inn & Spa
❤❤❤❤❤

18140 Sonoma Hwy, P.O. Box 1447, Sonoma, CA 95476. Tel: (707) 938-9000. Fax: (707) 938-4250. TYPE: Hotel & Spa. LOCATION: 2 1/2 miles (4 km.) north of Sonoma. CLIENTELE: Women and men. SPECIAL RESTRICTION: Non smoking policy.

* Rooms: 198 w/private bath
* Suites: 33, 32 with fireplace
* Phone, CTV, A/C, minibar, hair dryer
* Dining room, cafe, lobby bar, pool bar
* Airport: San Francisco, 1-1/2 hours
* Airport Transportation: rent-a-car
* Reservations: required
* Credit Cards: MC/VISA/AMEX/DC/CB
* Open: Year round
* Hotel Rates: from $165
* TAC: 10%
* **Spa Facilities**: Co-ed bathhouse, aerobic studio, sauna, steam rooms, whirlpools, exercise pool, two gyms, locker rooms, thermal mineral pools
* **Spa Programs**: from 1 to 5 day programs; Executive Stress Buster, Fitness Program, SPA Sampler

* **Spa Treatments**: aerobics, morning hikes, swedish and underwater massages, aromatherapy, herbal wraps, marine salt scrub, facials, hair and scalp treatments, 1000 - 1200 calorie diet meals, reflexology
* **Professional Supervision**: exercise physiologist, trained masseuses, fitness, nutrition & diet experts

DESCRIPTION: Elegant Spanish Mission-style Inn with a desert pink and pastel decor. The spa programs are for both men and women and emphasize fitness, weight loss and beauty. Over 40 spa treatments are offered. Guests are invited to sample local wines which is natural for a spa amidst the richest wine producing region in the USA. Recreation: tennis courts (2), nearby golf, hot-air-ballooning and horseback riding. Member: *Preferred Hotels Worldwide.*

SOUTH LAKE TAHOE
⟩ 530
✈ Lake Tahoe Airport (TVL) 7 mi. / 11 km.

The Keys at Lake Tahoe
❤❤❤❤

589 Tahoe Keys Blvd., #E5, South Lake Tahoe, CA 96150. Tel: (530) 541-3355. Toll Free (800) SHAPE-UP. Fax: (530) 931-7569. TYPE: Marina Spa Resort. LOCATION: On the marina at the base of Heavenly Valley Ski resort. SPA CLIENTELE: Women and men. DESCRIPTION: Resort with skin & beauty center, massage, gym, weight-loss, longevity, skin rejuvenation & plastic surgery clinic. 35 rooms. Indoor/outdoor pools, tennis, beach.

ST. HELENA
⟩ 707
✈ San Francisco Int'l AP (SFO) 90 mi. / 140 km.

Inn at Southbridge's
Health Spa Napa Valley
❤❤❤

1030 Main Street, St. Helena, CA 94574. Tel: (707) 967-8800. Fax: (707) 967-8801. TYPE: County Inn & Spa. LOCATION: Downtown St. Helena, 75 mi. / 120 km. from SF Airport. SPA CLIENTELE: Women and men. DESCRIPTION: Charming country inn with a full service health club & spa, body treatments, facials, Ayurvedic treatments, fitness facilities, whirlpool, steam rooms, massage, pool. 20 rooms, 1 suite, rooms for nonsmokers. Restaurant, meeting room. Hotel rooms: from $120.

Spa at Meadwood Resort
❤❤❤❤❤

900 Meadwood lane, St. Helena, CA 94574. Tel: (707) 963-3646. Fax: (707) 963-3532. TYPE: Resort & Spa. LOCATION: In the Napa Valley, 90 minutes to San Francisco. SPA CLIENTELE: Women and men. DESCRIPTION: New-England style resort with full health spa, exercise equipment, sauna, whirlpool, jacuzzi, aerobic, massage. 99 rooms with CTV, phone (fax & computer hookup), minibar, coffee maker. Restaurant, grill, pool cafe, bar, 2 outdoor pools, 7 tennis courts, 9-hole golf course. Hotel rates: from $310. Member: *Small luxury hotels.*

White Sulfur Springs Resort and Spa
❤❤❤

3100 White Sulphur Springs Road, St. Helena, CA 94574. Tel: (707)963-8588. Fax: (707) 963-2890. TYPE: Unstructured Health Retreat. LOCATION: Near Napa Valley wineries. DESCRIPTION: Retreat with natural sulfur pool, mud wraps, facials, massage, jacuzzi, sauna. 37 rooms.

UKIAH
⟩ 707
✈ Ukiah Airport, 3 mi. / 5 km.

Vichy Hot Springs Resort Inn
❤❤❤

2605 Vichy Springs Rd. Ukiah CA 95482. Tel: (707) 462-9515. Fax: (707) 462-9516. TYPE: Inn & Spa. LOCATION: 3 mi. / 5 km. east of Ukiah in the Mendocino foothills. SPA CLIENTELE: Women and men. DESCRIPTION: Historic landmark bed & breakfast inn with naturally carbonated mineral baths, olympic-size swimming pool. 20 rooms and 1 & 2 bedroom cottages. Breakfast room, lounge, business center. Hotel rates: from $115.

VISTA

⟩ **760**

✈ Lindbergh Field Int'l AP (SAN)

Vista, population 36,000, is located between Escondido and Oceanside north of San Diego. Oceanside, at the mouth of San Luis Rey Valley, has a fine beach, harbor facilities, main port for deep sea fishing, and a marina where whale watching cruises are available from December to March.

Cal - A - Vie
♥♥♥♥

2249 Somerset Rd., Vista, CA 92084. Tel: (760) 945-2055. Fax: (760) 630-0074. TYPE: European style Spa Resort. LOCATION: North of San Diego near Vista. SPA CLIENTELE: Women and men. Special weeks for men only, couples only and co-ed groups.

* Cottages: 24 w/private bath
* Phone, CTV, A/C, C/H, balcony
* Airport: San Diego Int'l, 35 mi. (56 km.)
* Transportation: free pick up
* Reservations: $1,000 deposit required
* Credit Cards: MC/VISA/AMEX
* Open: Year round
* Rates: from $3,500/week for a structured 7 day program from Sunday to Sunday
* TAC: 10%
* Spa on premises
* **Spa Facilities**: gym, swimming pool, beauty salon, therapy & massage rooms
* **Spa Programs**: Fitness, Exercise plan, beauty, diet

* **Spa Treatments**: European body & skin care, seaweed wraps, herbal wrap, hydrotherapy, aromatherapy, thalassotherapy, massages, facials, body glo, yoga and Tai Chi, stretching, dancersise, low calorie meals

DESCRIPTION: Elegant Spa combining European tradition with American fitness and nutrition programs. Accommodations are in private cottages with a French Provincial motif recreating a Mediterranean ambience. The spa specializes in European body detoxification treatments: thalassotherapy, aromatherapy and hydrotherapy. Diet Fitness and Beauty programs are offered and tailored to the individual's need. The daily menu is a satisfying gourmet 800-1000 calorie meals prepared by a well known Belgian Chef. Recreation: golf at a nearby private club.

WOODSIDE

⟩ **650**

✈ San Francisco Int'l Airport (SFO)

The Lodge at Skylonda
♥♥♥♥

16350 Skyline Blvd., Woodside CA 94062. Tel: (650) 851-6625. Toll Free Reservations: (800) 851-2222. Fax: (650) 851-5504. TYPE: First Class Health Resort. LOCATION: Nestled in the redwoods of Woodside California. SPA CLIENTELE: Men and Women. DESCRIPTION: The Lodge at Skylonda offers a relaxing getaway or an active adventure far from the complexities of daily living. Facilities and services include: indoor swimming pool, outdoor hot tub and deck, sauna and steam rooms, fully equipped exercise room, guided hikes to many of the Bay Area's most picturesque trails, spa treatments, massages, and healthy gourmet cuisine. Complimentary classes are offered daily in Tai Chi, Yoga, stretching, aqua aerobics and cooking (Tue/Sat only).

COLORADO

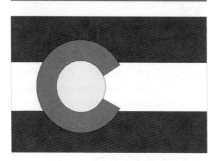

AREA: 104,091 sq. mi. (269,596 sq. km.)
POPULATION: 3,308,000
CAPITAL: Denver
TIME ZONE: Mountain Time

BEAVER CREEK
) **970**
✈ Eagle Country Airport, 20 mi. / 30 km.

Hyatt Regency Beaver Creek & Allegria Spa
❤❤❤❤❤

136 East Thomas Place, Beaver Creek CO 81620. Hotel - Tel: (970) 949-1234. Fax: (970) 949-4164. SPA Tel: (970) 748-7500. SPA CLIENTELE: Women and men. DESCRIPTION: Deluxe European style mountain resort with a 20,000 sq. ft. / 1,820 sq. m. health and beauty spa with Vichy shower, hydrotherapy, cold plunge, massages, circuit training, aerobics, yoga, salon, make up studio. Hotel rates: from $140.

The Charter At Beaver Creek & Spa Struck
❤❤❤❤

120 Offerson Rd., Beaver Creek, CO 81620. Hotel - Tel: (970) 949-6660. Fax: (970) 949-6709. SPA Tel: (970) 476-2225. SPA CLIENTELE: Women and men. DESCRIP-

TION: Appealing condominium lodge at the base of Beaver Creek Ski mountain with health spa, beauty salon, spa treatments include facials, wraps body polishes, hydrotherapy, full salon, massages. Hotel rates: from $135.

BRECKENRIDGE
) **970**
✈ Denver Int'l Airport (DEN)

The Lodge at Breckenridge
❤❤❤❤

112 Overlook Drive, P.O. Box 391, Breckenridge, CO 80424. Tel: (970) 453-9300, Fax: (970) 453-0625. TYPE: Mountain Lodge & Spa. LOCATION: On a forested cliff overlooking Breckenridge. DESCRIPTION: Intimate mountain lodge with a full service athletic club & spa with indoor pool, sauna & jacuzzis. 36 room, 9 suites, rooms for nonsmokers, restaurant, bar, meeting facilities. Hotel rates: from $160.

COLORADO SPRINGS
) **719**
✈ Municipal Airport (COS) 7 mi. / 11 km. SE

Colorado Springs, population 247,700, is one of the most popular vacation spots in Colorado. Nestled at the foot of Pikes Peak it offers dry mountain air, sunshine, beautiful scenery and skiing facilities. The weather from May through September is mild but can be cool in the evenings, temperatures vary from high 80°sF to low 50°sF (28°c-12°c). December - March are the coldest months with plenty of snowfall. Sports and Recreation: skiing, ice skating, golf, swimming, fishing, horseback riding & Greyhound racing.

The Spa At The Broadmoor
❤❤❤❤❤

1 Lake Avenue, Colorado Springs, CO 80901. Tel: (719) 634-7711. Toll Free: (800) 634-7711. Fax: (719) 577-5700. TYPE: Resort & Spa. LOCATION: On the front range of the Rocky Mountains. SPA CLIENTELE: Women and men, teenagers accepted.

* Rooms 700, Suites 80 all with private bath
* Phone, CTV, A/C, C/H, minibar, jacuzzi
* Restaurant, bar, nightclub
* Airport: Colorado Springs, 10 mi. / 16 km.
* Nearest Train Station: Colorado Springs
* Airport / Train Transportation: Taxi / limo
* Reservations: Required, one night's prepayment
* Credit Cards: MC, VISA, AMEX, DC, DISC, CB
* Open: Year round
* Hotel Rates: from $195; TAC: 10%
* Spa on premises
* **Spa Facilities**: Steam room, sauna, weight resistance and cardiovascular rooms, locker facilities, aerobics studio, indoor pool, lap pool & jacuzzi, massage therapy, aromatherapy, skin care, therapeutic baths, body treatments
* **Spa Programs**: Health, beauty, and fitness
* **Spa Packages**: Spa Splurge; Spa Spectacular.
* **Spa Treatments**: Mud bath, milk/whey bath, aromatherapy bath, Broadmoor Falls shower and spray, salt glo, loofah, herbal wrap, mud wrap, body polish, paraffin body moisturizer wrap, massages; reflexology, swedish, sports, shiatsu, aromatherapy, facials; mini, Colorado cleansing, specialty, depilatory waxing, brow tweezing, make-up application, body composition analysis, exercise prescription, personal training, step, stretch, yoga, tai chi ch'uan, aquacise, body sculpting, specialty dance-themed classes; salon services

DESCRIPTION: Resort & spa in the Colorado Mountains. Revitalizing mountain water is used in showers, baths and whirlpools. A wide range of treatments are used for the renewal of the body, mind & spirit. Pampering treatments and a health-conscious cuisine are available. The spa offers skin and body care treatments that feature natural Rocky Mountain elements. There is an abundance of exercise alternatives, classes, and fitness programs for the fitness enthusiasts. Recreation: World-class tennis, golf, hiking trails, and horseback riding.

DENVER
303
Denver Int'l Airport (DEN) 23 mi. / 37 km.

Oxford Aveda Spa and Salon
♥♥♥♥

c/o Oxford Hotel, 1616 Seventeenth St.. Denver, CO 80202. Tel: (303) 628-5435. Fax: (303) 628-5448. TYPE: Hotel & Spa. LOCATION: Downtown Denver, 4 blocks from Larimer Square. SPA CLIENTELE: Women and men. DESCRIPTION: Historic grand-style hotel with a full service spa & health club, body treatments, fitness, weight loss. 81 rooms & suites, restaurant, lounges (2). Hotel rates: from $149.

GLENWOOD SPRINGS
970
Sardy Field Airport (ASE) 45 mi. / 72 km.

Glenwood Hot Springs Lodge
♥♥♥

415 E. 6th St., PO Box 308, Glenwood Springs, CO 81601. Tel: (970) 945-6571. Fax: (970) 945-6683.TYPE: Hotel & Spa. LOCATION: Opposite Amtrak station 1 block from downtown. DESCRIPTION: Downtown hotel with natural hot springs pool with year round lifeguards, jacuzzi. 107 rooms, 28 suites, nonsmoker rooms. Restaurant, coffee shop. Hotel rates: from $90.

GUNNISON
970
Gunnison Airport 6 mi. / 10 km.

Waunita Hot Springs Ranch
♥♥♥

8007 Country Road 887, Gunnison, CO 81230. Tel: (970) 641-1266. TYPE: Dude Ranch & Spa. SPA CLIENTELE: Women and men. DESCRIPTION: Family-owned dude ranch high in the Colorado Rockies with hot springs fed swimming pool, 26 units, non smoking policy, dining room, TV and library area, log barn with recreation room, horseback riding, cookouts, hayrides, raft trips, fishing. Hotel rates: from $1,090 (per week).

IDAHO SPRINGS
ͻ 303

✈ Denver Int'l Airport (DEN) 35 mi. / 56 km.

Indian Springs Resort
❤❤❤

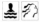

PO Box 1990, Idaho Springs, CO 80452. Tel: (303) 567-2191, Fax: (303) 567-9304. DESCRIPTION: Hot mineral springs, geothermal cave, mineral pool, mud baths, body wraps, swedish massage, stone massage, facials. 68 rooms, restaurant, lounge.

OURAY
ͻ 970

✈ Montrose County Airport 35 mi. / 56 km.

Box Canyon Lodge & Hot Springs
❤❤

45 Third Ave., PO Box 439, Ouray, CO 81427, Tel: (970) 325-4981. Fax: (970) 325-0223. TYPE: Spa Motel. LOCATION: Mouth of canyon, 45 min. to Montrose Airport. DESCRIPTION: Economy motel with outdoor hot mineral spring spa. 34 rooms, 4 suites, nonsmoker rooms, complimentary coffee, near restaurant, discount Telluride downhill skiing tickets available, cross-country & snowmobiling available. Hotel rates: from $60.

Wiesbaden Hot Springs Spa & Lodgings
❤❤

PO Box 349, 625 5th Street, Ouray, CO 81427, Tel: (970) 325-4347, Fax: (970) 325-4845. TYPE: Small lodge & Spa. LOCATION: 2 blocks from town center. DESCRIPTION: Intimate lodge with vapor cave, geothermal mineral pool, mineral swimming pool, massage, body wraps, facials, reflexology. 13 rooms, 3 suites, 2 condos, no smoking policy, complimentary coffee and tea. Hotel rates: from $95.

TELLURIDE
ͻ 970

✈ Regional Airport 5 mi. / 9 km.

The Peaks at Telluride & Golden Door Spa
❤❤❤❤❤

136 Country Club Dr., P.O. Box 2702, Telluride CO 81435. Tel: (970) 728-6800. Toll Free: (800) 789-2220. Fax: (970) 728-6567. TYPE: Deluxe Elegant Hotel Spa Resort. LOCATION: In the exclusive Telluride Mountain Village. SPA CLIENTELE: Women and men. DESCRIPTION: Elegant spa hotel with the Golden Door Spa treatment programs, massage, pools (3), jacuzzis, saunas, gym, squash, racquetball. 149 rooms w/priv. bath, 28 suites, restaurant, cafe, sports bar, 18-hole golf course, tennis courts (5). Hotel rates: from $190.

VAIL
ͻ 970

✈ Vail/Eagle County Airport (EGE) 30 mi ./ 48 km.

Vail, population 2,500, is a year round mountain resort in the White River National Forest. The resort offers European-style village, sophisticated shopping, restaurants and entertainment. Skiing is available in the winter at the nearby Vail Ski Resort. The rest of the year outdoor activities are: golf, tennis, hot-air balloon rides, river rafting, scenic gondola rides, hunting and fishing. The Vail Valley is located two hours drive west of Denver Colorado on the Interstate 70. Starting with the 90/91 ski season, Vail's Eagle County Airport will have daily non-stop service to and from Chicago and Dallas. America West flies non-stop daily to and from Phoenix and weekly to and from Los Angeles.

The Lodge & Spa At Cordillera
❤❤❤❤

2205 Cordillera Way, Edwards, P.O. Box 1110, Vail, CO 81632. Tel: (970) 926-2200. Toll Free (800) 548-2721. Fax: (970) 926-2714. TYPE: Hotel & Spa. LOCA-

TION: In Edwards, 20 mi (32 km) west of Vail. SPA CLIEN-TELE: Women and men.

* Rooms: 28 w/priv. bath
* Restaurant: Picaso "New French" cuisine
* Airport: Avon Stolport 10 mi. / 16 km.
* Airport transportation: taxi, limo
* Credit Cards: AMEX/MC/VISA
* Open: Year round
* Hotel Rates: from $160; TAC: 10%
* Spa on premises
* **Spa Facilities:** Beauty salon, hydrotherapy tubs, exercise and weight room, steam room, indoor and outdoor pools and Jacuzzis
* **Spa Programs:** Fitness, beauty, weight loss
* **Spa Treatments:** massages, hydrotherapy, aromatherapy, facials, exercise,aerobics, water aerobics, low calorie spa cuisine
* **Spa Packages:** Fitness Four Winter (4 nights); Classically Colorado (7 night)

DESCRIPTION: Elegant mountain retreat modeled after a French manor house, amidst 2,000 acres of private Rocky Mountain wilderness. Accommodations are in oversized rooms furnished with European antiques, many with fireplaces. The spa specializes in fitness, and stress management for executives. Recreation: mountain trails for hiking, tennis, 15 mi. / 24 km. of cross country ski trails, golf and rafting nearby. *Member: Small Luxury Hotels & Resorts.*

Marriott Vail Mountain Resort & Spa Struck
❤❤❤❤❤

715 West Lionshead, Vail CO 91657. Hotel - Tel: (970) 476-4444. Fax: (970) 476-1647. Spa Tel: (970) 476-2225. DESCRIPTION: Country club like resort hotel with full service athletic club and spa. Spa treatments include facials, wraps body polishes, hydrotherapy, full salon, massages. Hotel rates: from $99.

Sonnenalp Resort of Vail
❤❤❤❤

20 Vail Road, Vail, CO 81657, Tel: (970) 476-5656, Toll Free: (800) 654-8312. Fax: (970) 476-1639. TYPE: Alpine-style Hotel & Spa. LOCATION: On Gore Creek, near major ski lifts. DESCRIPTION: Full service European spa with beauty treatments, gym, sauna, pool. 94 room, 94 suites, nonsmoker rooms, restaurants (4), lounge, business center, 18-hole golf course, tennis courts (4). Hotel rates: from $145.

Vail Athletic Club Hotel & Spa
❤❤❤❤

352 East Meadow Drive, Vail, CO 81657. Tel: (970) 476-6451. Fax: (970) 476-6451. TYPE: Hotel & Athletic Club. LOCATION: In Vail Village, 25 mi / 40 km from Vail Beaver Creek Airport. DESCRIPTION: Health club & spa with massages, baths, wraps, sauna, jacuzzi, gym, indoor pool. 31 rooms, 5 suites, 2 condos, limited wheelchair access, restaurant, meeting room. Hotel rates: from $120.

Vail Cascade Hotel Club & Spa
❤❤❤❤❤

1300 Westhaven Dr., Vail, CO 81657, Tel: (970) 476-7111. Fax: (970) 479-7020. TYPE: Superior mountain resort. DESCRIPTION: Spa treatments including massages, manicures, facials, pedicures, weight rooms, exercise equipment, aerobics, basketball courts, racquetball, squash, indoor track. 289 rooms & suites. Hotel rates: from $120.

WARD
⟩ 303
✈ Denver Int'l Airport (DEN)

Four Seasons Spa at Gold Lake Mountain Resort
❤❤❤

3371 Gold Lake Road, Ward, CO 80538. Tel: (303) 459-3544, Fax: (303) 459-9080. TYPE: Mountain resort & hot springs spa. LOCATION: on the Continental Divide. DESCRIPTION: Mineral hot-springs, pool, massage. 17 rooms, restored cabin lodging.

CONNECTICUT

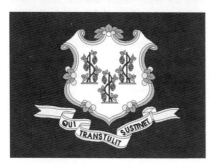

AREA: 104,091 sq. mi. (269,596 sq. km.)
POPULATION: 3,308,000
CAPITAL: Denver
TIME ZONE: Eastern Time

NORWICH
🌙 860
✈ Groton/New London Airport

Norwich, population 38,000, is a small historic New England town located at the confluence of three rivers. Nearby Fort Shantok State Park on the west bank of the Thames River offers recreational facilities and interesting relics of an Indian fort and burial ground. From Norwich you are within easy reach of Mystic Port, Essex and Old Lyme, popular summer resorts and art centers. Norwich can be reached by car from New York City via I-95 to New London (CT), and then Rte. 12 to Norwich.

Norwich Inn & Spa
❤❤❤❤

607 W. Thomes St. (Route 32), Norwich CT 06360. Tel: (860) 886-2401. Toll Free: (800) 892-5692. Fax: (860) 886-9483. TYPE: Inn & Spa. LOCATION: Set on landscaped grounds overlooking the Norwich Golf Course. SPA CLIENTELE: Women and men. SPECIAL RESTRICTIONS: No children under 18 in Spa. No pets.

* Rooms: 65, Villas: 60, Suites: 20

* Phone, CTV, A/C
* Grill Restaurant & Prince of Wales Bar
* Train Station: New London (CT) 20 mi. (32 km.)
* Train Station Transportation: free pick up
* Reservations: required
* Credit Cards: MC/VISA/AMEX
* Open: Year round
* Hotel Rates: from $125
* TAC: 10%
* Spa on premises
* **Spa facilities**: Indoor exercise pool, whirlpool, sauna, steam rooms, treatment rooms, beauty & skin care rooms
* **Spa Programs**: beauty, health, diet & fitness
* **Spa Treatments**: facials, massage, aromatherapy, hydrotherapy, body scrub, thalassotherapy, hand & foot treatments, workout, waterworks, stretching exercises, fitness evaluation, body composition, whirlpool, sauna and steam rooms;

DESCRIPTION: Elegant New England Inn & Spa offering deluxe accommodations with restored antique furniture, Chippendale mirrors and hand woven rugs. The Spa offers body and skin care treatments, fitness programs, nutritional counselling and thalassotherapy. Fine dining is available with classic American cooking. Recreation: golf, tennis, and jogging. Visits to nearby historical and art centers are recommended.

WESTBROOK
🌙 860

Water's Edge Inn & Resort
❤❤❤❤

1525 Boston Post Road, Westbrook, CT 06498. Tel: (860) 399-5901. Fax: (860) 399-6172. TYPE: Waterfront Resort & Spa. LOCATION: Overlooking the beach, 4 mi. / 6 km. from Old Saybrook. DESCRIPTION: Contemporary resort hotel with full service health spa, gym, aerobics. 121 rooms, 15 suites, 67 beachfront villas, nonsmoker rooms, wheelchair access, restaurant, grill, bar, meeting facilities, indoor & outdoor pools, jacuzzis, 2 tennis courts. Hotel rates: from $125.

FLORIDA

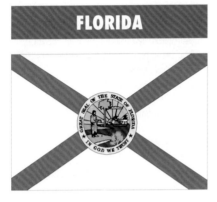

AREA: 58,664 sq. mi. (151,940 sq. km.)
POPULATION: 13,000,000
CAPITAL: Tallahassee
TIME ZONE: Eastern Time

BONITA SPRINGS
ⅎ 914
✈ Southwest Florida Regional AP (RSW)

Shangri-La Resort & Spa
♥♥

27580 Old 41 Road, Bonita Springs, FL 34135, Tel: (941) 992-3811. Toll Free: (800) 279-3811. Fax: (941) 947-9079. TYPE: unpretentious vacation & health resort. LOCATION: 17 mi. / 27 km. from Fort Myers or Naples. DESCRIPTION: Health resort with with health rejuvenation, weight control, beauty & fitness programs, massage, facials, solarium, yoga, meditation. 50 rooms & suites, nonsmoker rooms, vegetarian meals, chicken & fish available, outdoor heated pool, tennis courts (2). Hotel rates: from $115.

CLEARWATER
ⅎ 813
✈ St. Petersburg/Clearwater Int'l AP (PIE)
Tampa Int'l Airport (TPA)

Clearwater, population 86,000, is a beach resort city north of St. Petersburg and west of Tampa. Nearby Clearwater Beach offers a 4-mile-long (6 km.) white sand beaches con-

nected to the mainland by Memorial Causeway. Recreation: fishing pier, marina, water sports, sailing, sport fishing, skin diving and shelling. Nearby attractions include: Disney World, Epcot Center, Boardwalk & Baseball, Sea World and Cypress Gardens (90 minutes away); Busch Gardens (45 minutes away); Tarpon Springs, a century old Greek sponge diving and fishing village, is just 30 minutes away. Clearwater can be reached from Tampa Int'l Airport in about 30 minutes drive west.

Belleview Biltmore Resort & Spa
♥♥♥♥♥

25 Belleview Blvd., Clearwater, FL 34616. Tel: (813) 442-6171. Toll Free (800) 237-8947. Fax: (813) 443-6361. TYPE: Resort Complex. LOCATION: On a high bluff overlooking the Gulf of Mexico. SPA CLIENTELE: Women and men.

* Rooms: 292 w/priv. bath. Suites: 50
* Phone, CTV, A/C, hair dryer, minibar
* Restaurant, cafe & veranda bar
* Convention facilities: 12 meeting rooms
* Airport: Tampa Int'l 30 minutes
* Airport Transportation: free hotel shuttle
* Reservations: required
* Credit Cards: MC/VISA/AMEX/DC/CB
* Season: Year round
* Hotel Rates: from $150; TAC: 10%
* Spa on premises
* **Spa Facilities**: spa & fitness club, steam room, Sauna baths, needle swiss showers, hot Whirlpool, indoor heated lap pool, gym, aerobics rooms
* **Spa Treatments**: massage, facial care, cosmetology, hand and foot treatments
* **Spa Programs**: beauty, pampering, fitness

DESCRIPTION: Elegant turn-of-the-century Victorian style resort overlooking the Gulf of Mexico. Hotel rooms or suites are decorated with period furniture and designer fabrics. The European style spa provides beauty and pampering treatments. Low calorie spa menus are available for slimming. Recreation: beach, deep sea fishing, sailing, golf, tennis, shuffleboard, volleyball, croquet, and bicycling.

CORAL GABLES

⟩ 305

✈ Miami Int'l Airport (MIA) 4 mi. / 6 km.

Coral Gables, population 44,000, is one of the 26 separate municipalities that make up Metropolitan Miami. The town was originally laid out in the 1920's as an "American Riviera" with homes and mansions in Mediterranean-Florida style. Coral Gables is an affluent community, a cosmopolitan leisure destination and a major business headquarter for large multinational corporations that deal with Latin America.

The Biltmore Hotel
♥♥♥♥

1200 Anastasia Ave., Coral Gables, FL 33134. Tel: (305) 445-1926. Toll Free: (800) 877-36437. Fax: (305) 913-3159. TYPE: Resort Complex & Spa. LOCATION: Set in 55 acres in the mediterranean residential suburb of Coral Gables. Downtown Miami and the beaches are all within 30 minutes drive. SPA CLIENTELE: Women and men.

* Rooms: 240 w/private bath. Suites: 35
* Restaurant: four star dining
  gourmet spa menus available
* Nearest Airport: Miami Int'l (4 mi. / 6 km.)
* Nearest Train Station: Amtrak (1/2 hr. drive)
* Reservations: required
* Credit Cards: MC/VISA/AMEX
* Open: Year round
* Hotel Rates: from $290; TAC: 10%
* Spa on premises
* Name of Spa: The Biltmore Club & Spa
* Spa Facilities: European spa, aerobics and work out rooms, 34,200 sq. ft pool for laps and pool games
* Spa Programs: fitness, pampering, stress reduction, weight control, nutrition
* Spa Packages: 1-5 day packages
* Spa Treatments: massages, shiatsu, aromatherapy, body wraps, hydrotherapy, Vichy shower, hydro-massage, fangocean mud, exercise, computerized fitness test
* Medical Supervision: MD on call
* Treatments Approved: Florida State Licensed

DESCRIPTION: Mediterranean style resort on 55 landscaped acres in the affluent suburb of Coral Gables. The Spa offers European style fitness, pampering and relaxation programs and Elizabeth Arden beauty treatments. The Biltmore's restaurant creates low calorie gourmet meals. A balanced three-course meal contains less than 500 calories. Recreation: swimming pool, golf, and tennis.

FORT LAUDERDALE

⟩ 954

✈ Ft. Lauderdale/Hollywood Int'l AP (FLL) 4 mi. / 6 km.
  Ft. Lauderdale Executive AP (FXE) 6 mi. / 10 km.

Ft. Lauderdale is a year round beach resort on the famous Gold Coast north of Miami. Man made sea water canals give this town a "Venice" like flavor. Fashionable boutique can be found on Las Olas Blvd. Many excellent restaurants that specialize in seafood or French cuisine are available for elegant and exquisite dining. Ft. Lauderdale is easily accessible by air from any US major city.

Hyatt Regency Pier 66 & Spa
♥♥♥♥♥

2301 SE 17th Street Causeway, Fort Lauderdale, FL 33316, Tel: (954) 525-6666. Fax: (954) 728-3541. TYPE: Resort hotel & Spa. LOCATION: On the Intra-Coastal Waterway, 3 blocks from the beach, 3 miles to the airport. DESCRIPTION: Resort hotel with health club and full service spa with gym, sauna, massage, whirlpool, steam room aerobics, beauty salon. 388 rooms and suites, cafe, grill, 3 bars, entertainment, 3 outdoor heated pools, 2 tennis courts, marina. Hotel rates: from $199.

Wyndham Resort & Spa
♥♥♥♥♥

250 Racquet Club Road, Ft. Lauderdale, FL 33326. Tel: (954) 389-3300. Toll Free: (800) 327- 8090. Fax: (954) 384-1416. Spa - Tel: (954) 349-5515. TYPE: Resort & Spa. LOCATION: Lake location near Ft. Lauderdale. SPA CLIENTELE: Women and men.

* Rooms: 492 w/private bath. Suites: 96, 1 - 2 BR

* Phone, CTV, A/C, minibar, balcony
* Restaurants (4) and spa restaurant
* Airport: Ft. Lauderdale, 20 minutes
* Airport Transportation: taxi, limo
* Reservations: required
* Credit Cards: MC/VISA/AMEX/DC
* Open: Year round
* Hotel Rates: from $145
* TAC: 10%
* Spa on premises
* **Spa Facilities**: Health spa facilities, swimming pools (3), solariums, gyms, whirlpools, saunas, turkish steam rooms, swiss showers, finnish saunas, complete Lancôme Beauty Center; Horizons - spa dining room
* **Spa Programs**: fitness, beauty, pampering
* **Spa Treatments**: swedish massage, aromatherapy, shiatsu, thermal mineral massage, reflexology, loofah body treatment, herbal wrap, body wrap. moor mud, Xerstin skin care treatments, glycolic services, fitness classes, personal training, aerobics, conditioning and water exercises
* **Spa Packages**: full day and 1/2 day packages; InSparartion (3 nts); Ultimate Spa (7 nts)
* Medical Supervision: 1 MD, 2 RN; careful medical screening, individual evaluation

DESCRIPTION: Elegant resort and spa with a complete fitness resort, separate facilities for men and women. The spa, one of America's top ten, emphasizes body pampering, weight loss and well-being. A wide array of pampering and Kur treatments are available. Recreation: tennis, racquetball, squash, golf and horseback riding.

FORT MYERS
ל 942
✈ Southwest Florida Regional AP (RSW) 10 mi. / 16 km.

Fort Myers, population 40,000, is a rapidly growing winter resort and commercial center of southwest Florida. The city is sprawling between the beautiful beaches of the Gulf of Mexico, and the wide Caloosahatchee River. Nearby Sanibel Island, is a beautiful resort and recreation island which is popular with international celebrities. Ft. Myers/Sanibel island can be reached through the Ft. Myers International Airport.

Sonesta Sanibel Harbour Resort
❤❤❤❤

17260 Harbour Pointe Dr., Ft. Myers FL 33908. Tel: (941) 466-4000. Fax: (941) 466-2150. TYPE: Resort Complex & Spa. LOCATION: On San Carlos Bay. SPA CLIENTELE: Women and men, family oriented..

* Rooms: 240 w/priv. bath. Suites: 42
* Condominiums: 80 w/cooking facilities
* Restaurants, Bar & Grill
* Function and Meeting Rooms
* Airport: Ft. Myers International, 16 mi. (25 km.)
* Airport Transportation: taxi, limo, bus
* Reservations: required
* Credit Cards: MC/VISA/AMEX/DC/CB/DIS/EC
* Open: Year round
* Hotel Rates: from $140; TAC: 10% (on room only)
* Spa on premises
* **Spa Facilities**: spa and fitness center, keiser strength training equipment, indoor pool, whirlpools, steambaths, sauna, plunge tubs, tanning beds, showers and massage rooms, beauty salon
* **Spa Programs**: Beauty and fitness
* **Spa Treatments**: skin care, body care, full body massage, herbal wrap, loofa bath/salt glo, swiss shower, cellulite treatment, body contour wrap, exercise classes, calisthenics, water exercise
* Medical Supervision: Doctor on call

DESCRIPTION: A resort complex at the gateway to the Sanibel and Captiva Islands. The Spa and Fitness Center offers individual beauty and fitness treatments at the 40,000 sq. ft. state-of-the-art facility. Recreation: Tennis Center w/13 lighted tennis courts, golf courses nearby, Yacht & Country Club 5 minutes away, boating, fishing, swimming, sailing, canoeing.

HALLANDALE
ל 954
✈ Ft. Lauderdale / Hollywood Int'l AP (FLL)

Hallandale, population 37,000, is located half way between Miami and Ft. Lauderdale. Like nearby Hollywood, it is a popular seaside resort with a pleasant residential area and palm-lined fine sand ocean beaches. The town's vicinity to Miami and Ft. Lauderdale makes it an ideal vacation spot with most of Florida's best attractions within driving distance. Hallandale can be reached from either Miami or Ft. Lauderdale by car or taxi.

Regency Spa
❤❤❤

2000 South Ocean Dr., Hallandale, FL 33009. Tel: (954) 454-2220. Toll Free: (800) 454-0003. FAX: (954) 454-4637. TYPE: Resort & Spa. MANAGER: Mr. Dejnega. SPA DIRECTOR: Joan Switalski. LOCATION: Beach front, 15 min. south of Ft. Lauderdale. SPA CLIENTELE: Women and men.

* Rooms: 50 w/private bath
* Phone, CTV, A/C
* Airport: Ft. Lauderdale AP, 15 minutes
* Airport Transportation: taxi
* Reservations: deposit required
* Credit Cards: AMEX/MC/VISA
* Open: Year round
* Rates: from $795/week and up; TAC: 10%
* Spa on premises
* **Spa Facilities**: outdoor heated pool, sauna, whirlpool, lecture room, exercise room, Nautilus equipment room, two massage rooms, beauty salon
* **Spa Programs**: weight loss, nutritional counselling, stress reduction, lifestyler modification, exercise
* **Spa Treatments**: massages, body wraps, exercise, water exercise, stretchercise, low impact aerobics, reflexology, low cal meals, vegetarian diets, relaxation workshops, juice/water fasting (medically supervised)
* Medical Supervision: MD & Professional staff

DESCRIPTION: Health Resort offering natural weight loss programs based on vegetarian diet consisting of fresh fruit, nuts, vegetables, seeds and grains, designed for a substantial weight reduction (10 - 20 lbs per week) without diet pills or calorie counting. Other programs include: Detoxification through water or juice fasting, overcome habits such as smoking, alcohol, caffeine, food addiction. Weekly rates include: accommodations, three nutritious

vegetarian meals, relaxation workshop, health lectures, food preparation classes, full exercise program, medically supervised water or juice fast.

KEY WEST
〕 **305**
✈ Key West Int'l Airport (EYW)

Key West, population 24,300, is the southernmost city in the continental USA. Its particular location, deep in the sea and secluded, made Key West an ideal retreat for many writers, artists and poets such as Ernest Hemingway, Tennessee Williams and Robert Frost. Today, it is a year round resort with a thriving tourist industry. Key West can be reached from Miami by following Overseas Highway (US1) to the end, or flying to Key West's small airport.

Caribbean Spa
The Pier House Resort
❤❤❤

Pier House, 1 Duval St., Key West, FL 33040. Tel: (305) 296-4600. Fax: (305) 296-4600. Toll Free (800) 327-8340. TYPE: Resort & Spa. LOCATION: at the Pier House. SPA CLIENTELE: Women and men.

* Rooms: 142 w/priv. bath
* Phone, CTV, VCR, A/C, hair dryer
* Restaurant & Bars
* Airport: Key West 3 mi. / 5 km.
* Open: Year round
* Hotel Rates: from $195
* Spa on premises
* **Spa Facilities**: 5,000 sq. ft. spa, steam room, beauty salon, exercise circuit
* **Spa Treatments**: loofah rub, massage, exercise, aerobics, weight training, facials, body wraps

DESCRIPTION: Casual elegant resort in tropical setting with a European spa for pampering and exercise.

LAKE BUENA VISTA
〕 **407**
✈ Orlando Int' Airport

Buena Vista Palace Resort & Spa
❤❤❤❤❤

1900 Buena Vista Drive, Lake Buena Vista, FL 32830. Tel: (407) 827-2727, Fax: (407) 827-6034. TYPE: Deluxe Walt Disney World Resort Hotel & Spa. LOCATION: Across the street from the downtown Disney Village Marketplace. DESCRIPTION: Deluxe resort in distinctive architectural design situated in the heart of Walt Disney World Resort. The resort features a magnificent 10,000 sq. ft. / 910 sq. m. European style spa, beauty salon, fitness center, sauna, whirlpool, hydrotherapy treatments. 1,014 rooms & suites, wheelchair access, 9 restaurants and lounges, meeting rooms, business center, 3 pools, children's pool, tennis courts, private marina.

Grand Floridian Spa Health Club
❤❤❤❤❤

4111 North Floridian Way, Lake Buena Vista, FL 32830. Tel: (407) W-DISNEY, Fax: (407) 824-2346. TYPE: Resort Hotel & Spa. LOCATION: Walt Disney World Resort on the South Sea Lagoon. DESCRIPTION: Health club and spa, sauna, jacuzzi. 897 rooms & suites, nonsmoker rooms, wheelchair access, 4 restaurants and lounges, convention center, pool, beach, tennis courts, private marina.

Hilton at Walt Disney World Village
❤❤❤❤❤

1751 Hotel Plaza Blvd., Lake Buena Vista, FL 32830, Tel: (407) 827-4000, Fax: (407) 827-3890. TYPE: Resort hotel & Spa. LOCATION: Downtown near Disney Village Marketplace. DESCRIPTION: Impressive resort hotel with health club & spa. 814 rooms and suites, restaurants (7), lounges (2), bars, deli, meeting rooms, business center, pools (2). Hotel rates: from $200.

Spa at the Disney Institute
❤❤❤❤

1920 Magnolia Way, Lake Buena Vista, FL 32830. Tel:

(407) 827-1100. Toll Free: (800) 282-9282 ext MG66. Fax: (407) 354-2709. TYPE: Lakeside resort with small town america motif. Disney institute with spa, fitness, culinary, golf & tennis programs. LOCATION: Disney World. DESCRIPTION: All natural spa treatments and fitness programs, spa cuisine lunches & dinners. 457 rooms, bungalows and townhouses. Hotel rates: from $790 (3 nts).

MIAMI / MIAMI BEACH
↘ 305

✈ Miami Int'l Airport (MIA) 7 mi. / 11 km.

Miami, population 346,000 - Metro 1,600,000, is the largest city in Florida. Located on the popular Gold Coast. The city is a major attraction for vacationers who come to Miami to enjoy the mile long, palm-lined sandy beaches, sunny weather and resort hotels. Miami is also a cosmopolitan city, a cultural and commercial center and the headquarter for hundreds of Multinational corporations. Latin influence is prominent and the Spanish language is widely used. Miami offers many recreational and tourist attractions such as: boating, yachting, fishing, night clubs, elegant restaurants, Seaquarium, Monkey jungle, Parrot Jungle, horse racing, plane or helicopter tours. It is convenient for visiting other major South Florida attractions. Miami can be accessed by domestic and international flights through Miami International Airport.

Agua at the Delano Hotel
❤❤❤

1685 Collins Avenue, Miami Beach, FL 33139, Tel: (305) 672-2000. Fax: (305) 674-6499. TYPE: Hotel & Spa. LOCATION: South Miami Beach Art Deco District. DESCRIPTION: Beachfront resort hotel with a rooftop women's bathhouse, solarium, gym, physical trainers. 208 rooms, suites, lofts, penthouse and poolside bungalows, restaurant, bar, business center pool.

Doral Golf Resort & Spa
❤❤❤❤❤

4400 NW 87th Avenue, Miami, FL 33178. Tel: (305) 592-2000, Toll Free (800) 331-7768. Fax: (305) 591-

6630. TYPE: Resort & Spa. LOCATION: In the heart of Miami adjacent to the Doral Country Club. SPA CLIENTELE: Women and men.

* Rooms: 694 w/priv. bath. Suites: 48 spa suites
* Phones (2), CTV, A/C, hair dryer, terrace
* Airport: Miami Int'l Airport 8 mi. /13 km.
* Airport Transportation: limo, Free pick up
* Reservations: deposit required
* Credit Cards: MC/VISA/AMEX/DC
* Open: Year round
* Hotel Rates: from $125; TAC: 10%
* Spa on premises
* **Spa Facilities**: Workout studios, outdoor exercise course, pools (3), massage rooms, beauty salon
* **Spa Programs**: Health, fitness, beauty, sports
* **Spa Packages**: 4-7 night Spa Packages, 7 night cellulitis program, tennis/spa studio
* **Spa Treatments**: yoga, steam, saunas, massages, hydromassages, body polish, herbal wraps, Fango treatments, mineral and plankton baths, facials, lifestyle consultations, detoxification, skin, hair, scalp, nail grooming, image-wardrobing (for men), European cellulite treatments, skin care, low cal spa cuisine, body composition, blood cholesterol analysis
* Indication: Fitness, relaxation, pampering
* Medical Supervision: Associated with a doctor's hospital, RN

DESCRIPTION: Elegant resort and spa. The lavish villa style accommodations include two marble bathrooms, living rooms, jacuzzi, and gold plated fixtures. A wide range of European spa treatments and American lifestyle programs are available.

Eden Roc Resort & Spa
♥♥♥♥

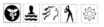

4525 Collins Avenue, Miami Beach, FL 33140. Tel: (305) 531-0000. Fax: (305) 674-5555. TYPE: Resort hotel, Marina and Spa. LOCATION: 5 minutes to the convention center and 12 mi. / 19 km. to Miami Int'l Airport. DESCRIPTION: Oceanfront resort hotel with an impressive 50,000 sq. ft. / 4,550 sq. m. spa complex offering a wide

selection of beauty, massage, body treatments, exercise equipment. 300 rooms, 50 suites, nonsmoker rooms, restaurant, coffee shop, lounge, piano bar, outdoor pools. Hotel rates: from $115.

Fontainbleau Hilton Resort & Spa
♥♥♥♥♥

4441 Collins Avenue, Miami Beach, FL 33140, Tel: (305) 538-2000. Toll Free: (800) 445-8667. Fax: (305) 673-5351.TYPE: Landmark Hotel & Spa. LOCATION: On the Atlantic Ocean, 8 blocks from the Convention Center. SPA CLIENTELE: Women and men.

* Rooms: 1224 w/priv. bath. Suites: 61
* Phone, CTV, A/C, minibar, balcony
* Restaurants (7), lounges & nightclub
* Airport: Miami Int'l 12 mi. / 19 km.
* Airport Transportation: taxi, limo
* Reservations: 1 night deposit
* Credit Cards: MC/VISA/AMEX/DC/CB
* Open: Year round
* Hotel Rates: from $160; TAC: 10%
* Spa on premises
* **Spa Facilities**: Free Weight Center, Cardiovascular Center, free form pool, exercise pool, whirlpools, gym, aerobic class rooms, sauna, beauty salon
* **Spa Programs**: beauty, pampering & fitness
* **Spa Treatments**: aerobics, body sculpture, conditioning, yoga, aqua-aerobics, massage, sauna, mineral baths, herbal wrap, skin care, aromatherapy, salt glow loofa, individual whirlpool, byogenic treatments, ultra-live cell treatments, fresh herbal or fruit masks, beauty treatments for men, skin care
* Medical Supervision: Mount Sinai's Medical Center's Sports Medicine Institute

DESCRIPTION: The Spa at the Fontainebleau Hilton is a 40,000 sq. ft. (3,650 sq. m.) health and fitness complex. Accommodations consist of elegant rooms and suites. The Spa offers a computerized fitness evaluation and a wide range of beauty, skin care and pampering treatments for men and women. Low calorie spa meals are available at the Spa Eatery. Recreation: tennis, golf, and water sports.

The Spa Internazionale
at Fisher Island Club
❤❤❤❤

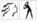

1 Fisher Island Dr., Fisher Island, Miami, FL 33109. Tel: (305) 535-6021. Toll Free (800) 537-3708, Fax: (305) 535-6037. TYPE: Mediterranean-style resort & Spa. LOCA-TION: 3 miles offshore from Miami, access by helicopter, private boat or auto ferry. DESCRIPTION: Elegant resort with a complete beauty & fitness spa with body and skin care treatments. 60 rooms, suites, villas & cottages, nonsmoker rooms, wheelchair access, restaurants (6), bars, lounges, meeting rooms, indoor/outdoor pools, tennis courts (18), 9-holes of golf, marinas (2).

Hotel Inter-Continental Miami
❤❤❤❤❤

100 Chopin Plaza, Miami, FL 33133. Tel: (305) 577-1000, Fax: (305) 577-0380. TYPE: Hotel & Spa. LOCA-TION: On Biscayne Bay within the financial and commercial district. DESCRIPTION: New 1997 health club & spa, jogging path. 644 rooms & suites, nonsmoker rooms, 3 restaurants. 2 lounges, poolside bar, business center, meeting rooms, outdoor pool. Hotel rates: from $169.

Lido Spa Hotel
❤❤❤

40 Island Ave, Miami Beach, FL 33138. Tel: (305) 538-4621. Toll Free (800) 327-8363. Fax: (305) 534-3680. TYPE: Spa Resort. OWNER: Mr. Chuck Edelstein. MANAGER: Mr. Don Robinson. LOCATION: The heart of Miami Beach on the Venetian Causeway, near Convention Center. SPA CLIEN-TELE: Women and men. SPECIAL RESTRICTIONS: No pets.

* Rooms: 140 w/private bath. Suites: 25. Apts: 36
* Phone, CTV, A/C
* Dining Room: Kosher cuisine
* Airport: Miami Int'l Airport, 8 mi./ 13 km.
* Train Station: Amtrak 6 mi. / 10 km.
* Airport / Train Transportation: taxi, limo
* Reservations: deposit required

* Credit Cards: MC/VISA/AMEX/DC/DIS
* Open: Year round
* Rates: from $68
* TAC: 10%
* Spa on premises
* **Spa Facilities:** 2 heated pools with hydro whirlpools (one salt), outdoor solaria, gym, saunas (2), steam rooms & cabinets, diagnostic laboratory
* **Spa Programs:** Health & Diet Program
* **Spa Treatments:** exercises, massages, mineral & steam baths, sauna, whirlpool, low calorie and special diet meals (salt free, sugar free)
* Medical Supervision: 1 MD, 1 RN

DESCRIPTION: Ocean-side resort featuring lanai-type rooms and suites. The spa one of the oldest in the south, offers economic programs emphasizing health and weight loss under medical supervision for mature clientele. All meals are salt free and low fat. Rates include initial medical examination, relaxing whirlpool baths, steam baths and daily massages. Recreation: entertainment at the 'Spa Theatre', dancing, movies, bingo & bridge games.

Turnberry Isle Health Spa
❤❤❤❤

19999 W. Country Club Drive, Aventura, North Miami, FL 33180-2401. Tel: (305) 932-6200, Toll Free: (800) 327-7028. Fax: (305) 933-6560. TYPE: Resort & Spa. LOCA-TION: The heart of South Florida's Gold Coast, minutes from Miami and Ft. Lauderdale. SPA CLIENTELE: Women and men. SPECIAL RESTRICTIONS: no children allowed at the spa.

* Rooms: 340 rooms & suites
* Phone, CTV, minibar, in-room safe, balcony
* Restaurants, disco, lounges, piano bar
* Airports: Miami, Ft. Lauderdale
* Distance to the Airport: minutes away
* Airport Transportation: limo service
* Reservations: 1 night deposit
* Credit Cards: AMEX/MC/VISA/DC
* Open: Year round
* Hotel Rates: from $165
* Spa on premises

* **Spa Facilities**: Finish Sauna, turkish steam rooms, swimming pool, whirlpools, nautilus room, workout studio, beauty salon
* **Spa Programs**: beauty, pampering, fitness
* **Spa Treatments**: Swedish massage, skin care, loofa salt glow, Swiss shower, individual vita bath, herbal wrap, derma peels, exercise, personal fitness class, nutrition consultation
* **Spa Packages**: Pamper Day; Spa Weekender (3 day/2 nights); Spa Nutrition & Fitness Plan
* Medical Supervision: staff physician, nutritionist, and physical therapist

DESCRIPTION: Well designed Resort on the Intercoastal Waterway north of Miami Beach. Luxurious rooms and suites with private jacuzzis, solarium and redwood hot tub. Casual elegant rooms at the Country Club Hotel. The spa emphasizes relaxation, body pampering, and beauty care, but fitness and diet programs are available. Recreation: golf, tennis, racquet, and pleasure boat yachting.

PALM BEACH / WEST PALM BEACH
⟩ 561

 Palm Beach Int'l Airport (PBI)

West Palm Beach, population 64,000, is an affluent winter resort north of Fort Lauderdale on the beautiful Gold Coast. Baseball fans can watch famous baseball teams training in the spring at the West Palm Beach Municipal Stadium. Nearby is the exclusive resort of Palm Beach 'the jewel of the American Riviera'. Palm Beach caters almost exclusively to its privileged residents and their guests. The tiny town is famous for its expensive properties, elegant shops, and golf courses. West Palm Beach enjoys clean and healthy air and is therefore a perfect location for a Health Spa.

Four Seasons Palm Beach
❤❤❤❤❤

2800 South Ocean Blvd., Palm Beach, FL 33480, Tel: (561) 582-2800. Fax: (561) 547-1557. TYPE: Oceanfront Resort & Spa. LOCATION: On the ocean, 12 mi from Palm Beach Airport. DESCRIPTION: Health club & spa. 198 rooms, 12 suites, nonsmoker rooms, wheelchair access, 2 restaurants, poolside bar & grill, meeting facilities, business center, outdoor pool 3 tennis courts, beach.

Hippocrates Health Institute
❤❤❤

443 Palmdale Court, West Palm Beach, FL 33411. Tel: (561) 471-8876. Fax: (561) 471-9464. TYPE: Vegetarian Health Resort. SPA DIRECTOR: Mr. Brian Clement. LOCATION: In West Palm Beach, 10 miles (16 km.) from the ocean. SPA CLIENTELE: Men, Women, Families. SPECIAL RESTRICTIONS: Non-ambulatory people and unaccompanied children.

* Rooms: 12 w/private bath, Suites: 2; Cottages: 4
* Airport: West Palm Beach 5 mi. /8 km.
* Airport Transportation: taxi, limo
* Reservations: 50% deposit required
* Credit Cards: MC/VISA/AMEX
* Open: Year round
* Rates: from $788 - $3,420 1 week program. Rates include room, meals, daily maid service, massage, facials, medical exam, blood monitoring, chiropractic exam, psychological exam, lectures, classes and excursions
* Spa on Premises
* **Spa Facilities**: swimming pool, sauna, whirlpool, exercise rooms
* **Spa Programs**: Health Encounter Program - a personalized health and nutrition program
* **Spa Treatments**: blood monitoring, exercise classes, aerobics, stretches, health improvement classes, special diets, wheatgrass juice therapy, all-raw diet, water exercise
* **Indications**: degenerative diseases, digestive problems, high blood cholesterol and triglyceride levels, tension, fatigue
* **Contraindications**: non-ambulatory, AIDS
* Medical Supervision: 1 MD on call
* Number of Customers per Doctor: 20

DESCRIPTION: Alternative health center with program that promotes emotional stability, balanced diets, and non-stressful exercises. The program can be effective in the treatment of high cholesterol levels. Some individuals show a significant drop after a 21 day therapy. The center has formulated its own Diet Program - The Hippocrates Diet which is based on enzyme-rich living food that help clean and detoxify the digestive tract. Fresh wheatgrass juice supplements the diet and helps the body get rid of dangerous toxins. The Health programs are monitored by consultants and health professionals.

PGA National Resort & Spa
❤❤❤❤

400 Avenue of The Champions, Palm Beach Gardens, FL 33418. Tel: (561) 627-2000. Toll Free (800) 633-9150. Fax: (561) 627-6056. TYPE: Mediterranean-style Resort & Spa. LOCATION: Part of PGA National Community, 15 minutes to the airport. DESCRIPTION: Full service spa and fitness center. 339 rooms, 61 suites & 80 cottages, nonsmoker rooms, wheelchair access, 7 restaurants, lounges, business center, five 18-hole golf courses, 19 tennis courts, outdoor pools. Hotel rates: from $119.

Ritz-Carlton Palm Beach
❤❤❤❤❤

100 S Ocean Blvd., Palm Beach, FL 33462. Tel: (561) 533-6000. Fax: (561) 588-4555. TYPE: Deluxe Mediterranean-style resort hotel. LOCATION: On the beach, 11 miles to the airport. DESCRIPTION: Spa treatments, fitness center, steam room, sauna. 214 rooms, 56 rooms, 3 restaurants, lobby lounge & bar, meeting facilities, business center, outdoor pool, jacuzzi, 7 tennis courts. Hotel rates: from $250.

POMPANO BEACH
⌐ 954

✈ Fort Lauderdale Int'l Airport (FLL)

Pompano Beach is a fashionable resort town along Florida's Gold Coast a few miles north of Fort Lauderdale. The beaches are lovely. Many water sports are available year round. Pompano Beach is easily accessible from Ft. Lauderdale, Miami, or West Palm Beach.

Spa Atlantis
❤❤❤

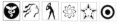

1460 S. Ocean Blvd., Pompano Beach, FL. Tel: (954) 941-6688. Toll free (800) 583-3500. Fax: (954) 943-1219. TYPE: Oceanfront heath resort and spa. LOCATION: On 200 feet of private Florida beach. SPA CLIENTELE: Women and men.

* Rooms: 70 (hotel room and efficienccy style)
* Phone, CTV, A/C
* Restaurant: 3 meals daily featuring gourmet vegetarian cuisine
* Airport: Ft. Lauderdale Int'l
* Distance to the Airport: minutes away
* Airport Transportation: Free pick up
* Reservations: required
* Credit Cards: AMEX/MC/VISA
* Open: Year round
* Spa Rates: Daily from $188.42 Double & $219.85 Single; Weekly from $899 Double & $1,099 Single
* Service/Tax Charge: 18%
* Spa on premises
* **Spa Facilities**: Fully equipped gym, free-weigths, exercise room, cardio room, sauna, pool, whirlpool, massage rooms, beauty salon
* **Spa Programs**: beauty, pampering, fitness, weight loss, smoking cessation, nurition
* **Spa Treatments**: facials, massages, herbal wraps, manicures, pedicures, shiatsu, reflexology, seaweed cellulite treatment, aromatherapy, neuro-muscular massages, step aerobics, water aerobis,
* **Spa Packages**: Fit For life, Fitness Plus, Supervised Weight Loss Intensive, Smoking Cessation
* **Medical Supervision**: Qualified health care specialist services include Acupuncture, Deep Tissue Massage, Osteopathic Manipulation, Chinese Herbology, Bioelectric Medicine, Nutraceuticals, Behavioral Consultations, Medical Assessment, Nutritional Assessment, Fitness Assesment

DESCRIPTION: Spa Atlantis is a total health and fitnes resort where you can relax and renew your mind, body and spirit or safely lose weight, get in shape and stay in shape.

The Spa at Palm-Aire
♥♥♥♥♥

2501 Palm-Aire Drive North, Pompano Beach, FL 33069. Tel: (954) 972-3300. Toll Free USA (800) 327-4960. Fax: (954) 972-3300. TYPE: Resort & Spa. LOCATION: On a beautiful 1,500 acres of landscaped grounds near the ocean. SPA CLIENTELE: Women and men. SPECIAL RESTRICTIONS: Children under 16 not allowed in spa.

* Rooms & Suites: 192 w/private bath
* Phone, CTV, A/C, minibar, balcony
* Restaurants (2), bar, meeting facilities
* Airports: Ft. Lauderdale - Miami, 15 - 30 min.
* Airport Transportation: taxi, limo
* Credit Cards: MC/VISA/AMEX/DC
* Open: Year round
* Hotel Rates: from $95
* TAC: 10%
* Spa on premises
* **Spa Facilities**: separate men's & women's spa pavilions, co-ed exercise area, scandinavian saunas, junior Olympic size pool, turkish steam baths, plunge pools, solarium & sundecks
* **Spa Treatments**: thalassotherapy, calorie controlled cuisine, daily massage, facial, herbal wrap, loofah massage, manicure, pedicure, hair treatment, paraffin treatment, calisthenics, stretch & water exercises, aerobics
* **Spa Programs**: 4 to 8 days beauty, fitness & recreation programs for men and women.
* Medical Supervision: doctor, fitness counselors

DESCRIPTION: Elegant Resort & Spa popular with international celebrities. The emphasis is on fitness, nutrition and stress management. The spa offers a combination of European pampering treatments and American fitness programs. The trained staff will assist you achieving your personal goals.

PONTE VERDA BEACH
🕭 **904**
✈ Jacksonville Int'l Airport (JAX) 35 mi. / 56 km.

Ponte Vedra Inn and Club
♥♥♥♥

200 Ponte Vedra Blvd, Ponte Vedra Beach, FL 32082. Tel: (904) 285-1111. Toll Free: (800) 234-7842, Fax: (904) 285-2111. TYPE: Resort & Spa. LOCATION: Beachfront, 25 min. from downtown Jacksonville. DESCRIPTION: Elegant resort with full service health club and spa; complete pampering services, jacuzzi, sauna. 280 rooms, 20 suites, nonsmoker rooms, wheelchair access. 4 restaurants, bars (6), entertainment, meeting facilities, business center, pools (4), 36-holes of golf, tennis courts (15). Hotel rates: from $130.

ST. PETERSBURG
🕭 **813**
✈ St. Petersburg/Clearwater Int'l AP (PIE)

The Don CeSar Beach Resort & Spa
♥♥♥♥♥

3400 Gulf Blvd. St. Petersburg Beach, FL 33706, Tel: (813) 360-1881. Toll Free: (800) 282-1116 or 800-637-7200. Fax: (813) 367-3609. TYPE: Beach Resort & Spa. LOCATION: On the Gulf beach, 29 mi. / 46 km. to Tampa Airport. DESCRIPTION: Deluxe Mediterranean style beach resort with spa & health club. 226 rooms, 49 suites, nonsmoker rooms, wheelchair access. Restaurants (3), lobby bar, lounges (3), entertainment, outdoor pools (2), beach club, water sports. Hotel rates: from $195.

SARASOTA
🕭 **941**
✈ Sarasota-Bradenton Int'l AP (SRQ) 6 mi. / 10 km.

Sarasota, population 50,000, is a thriving resort town on Florida's West Coast with tourism and holiday making as a major mainstay. The city is known for its pleasant climate year round. The average temperatures are 76°F (24°c) in the spring, 81°F (27°c) in the summer, and 60°F (10°c) in the winter. The city offers fine beaches, water sports, boating, fishing, golf, tennis, and various recreation parks for children and adults. Longboat Key, an island resort in the

Sarasota Bay, can be reached by car from the Sarasota/Brandon Airport in about 30 minutes.

The Colony
Beach & Tennis Resort
❤❤❤❤❤

1620 Gulf of Mexico Drive, Longboat Key, FL 34228. Tel: (941) 383-6464. Toll Free (800) 237-9443. Fax: (941) 383-7549. TYPE: Resort & Spa. LOCATION: On Longboat Key island in the Sarasota Bay. SPA CLIENTELE: Women and men, family oriented. SPECIAL RESTRICTIONS: Must be 18 or older to use the Spa.

* Suites: 235 w/priv. bath; Cottages: 3
* Phone, CTV, A/C, kitchens, "mini spas", sun balcony
* Restaurants, bistro, lounge, entertainment
* Credit Cards: MC/VISA/AMEX/DIS
* Open: Year round
* Hotel Rates: from $190
* TAC: 10%
* Spa on premises
* **Spa Facilities**: Aerobic center and fitness center, men's and women's health clubs, watersports center, beach side heated pool
* **Spa Programs**: no structured programs, daily classes in shape-up and performance training
* **Spa Treatments**: massage therapy, neuromuscular therapy, shiatsu, body wrap, facial massage, mud packs, sauna, aerobics
* **Indications**: general fitness, revitalization
* **Contraindications**: high blood pressure, heart disease must check with physician before using sauna, steam or whirlpool
* Medical Supervision: none
* Treatments Approved: all staff are licensed massage therapists in State of Florida

DESCRIPTION: The Colony Beach & Tennis Resort is a family type resort complex with emphasis on leisure, sports and recreation. The accommodations are spacious, fully equipped one or two bedroom suites with all the amenities including "mini spas" and marble master bath. The Spa offers a variety of massages, beauty and pampering treat-

ments that are offered on à la carte basis. Shape-up classes are available daily at the Aerobic center, and a variety of workout equipment with certified instructors at the Fitness Center. Recreation: watersports, tennis, golf nearby. A supervised program is available for children age 4-12.

TAMPA
⌐ 813

✈ Tampa Int'l Airport (TPA) 20 mi. / 32 km.
  St. Petersburg/Clearwater Int'l AP (PIE)

Tampa, population 272,000, is Florida's third largest city. Located on a beautiful Bay across from St. Petersburg, it has rapidly grown to become the main business and vacation hub of Florida's West Coast. Among the main nearby tourist attractions are: **Busch Gardens** - "The Dark Continent" (45 min. drive), **Clearwater Beach** (20 min. drive), **Disney world** (1-1/2 hours drive). The excellent area climate was declared very healthy by the American Medical Association. Tampa is easily accessible by air from any major USA and some international cities through the Tampa International Airport.

Safety Harbor Resort & Spa
❤❤❤❤

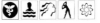

105 N. Bayshore Drive, Safety Harbor, FL 34695. Tel: (813) 726-1161. Toll Free (800) 237-1055. Fax: (813) 726-4268. TYPE: Resort Hotel & Spa. LOCATION: 10 mi. / 16 km. from Tampa Airport, near the Ruth Eckerd Hall (Performing Arts Center). SPA CLIENTELE: Women and men. SPECIAL RESTRICTIONS: No pets. No children under 16 allowed in the spa area.

* Rooms: 182 w/priv. bath. Suites: 120
* Airport: Tampa International, 15 minutes
* Airport Transportation: taxi, limo
* Reservations: 1 night deposit req'd
* Credit Cards: MC/VISA/AMEX
* Open: Year round
* Hotel Rates: from $110/day
* TAC: 10%
* Spa on premises

* **Spa Facilities**: Heated mineral water jacuzzis, saunas, steam room, group jacuzzis, aerobic and exercise rooms, equipment rooms, indoor exercise pool, outdoor lap pool, beauty salon
* **Spa Programs**: Fitness, beauty, weight loss
* **Spa Treatments**: body massage, loofah salt-glow, herbal wrap, whirlpool baths, Lancôme facials, hair care, coloring, nail care, depilatory waxing, diets
* **Spa Packages**: Total Fitness Plan; Fitness Weekend Smoking Cessation
* **Contraindications**: for exercise - back problems, heart disease, high blood pressure, All guests receive medical screening prior to their participation
* **Medical Supervision**: 2 full time doctors, 2 part time doctors, 2 nurses

DESCRIPTION: Spanish style 60,000 sq. ft. resort and spa complex. Guest rooms are comfortable, mostly in modern design with the famous Old Florida atmosphere. The spa emphasizes fitness, weight loss, and beauty care. It features a supervised and medically sound weight loss program, and beauty treatments by the Lancôme Skin Care Institute. The main ideology is to educate guests to make long lasting behavior changes regarding nutrition, physical fitness and skin care. The spa has its own natural mineral springs. Mineral waters are served daily to promote digestion and lubricate the joints. They are also used in the spa's water-based beauty services. Recreation: tennis and golf.

The Spa at Saddlebrook Resort Tampa
❤❤❤❤

5700 Saddlebrook Way, Wesley Chapel, FL 33543-4499. Tel: (813) 973-1111. Toll Free: (800) 729-8383. Fax: (813) 973-4505. TYPE: Conference Resort & Spa. LOCATION: 15 mi. / 24 km. north of Tampa. DESCRIPTION: Resort complex with spa & health salon, sports village & fitness center. 790 rooms & suites, wheelchair access. Restaurants (4), sports bar, pool bar, lounge entertainment, 36-holes of golf, tennis courts (45), pools (3). Hotel Rates: from $110.

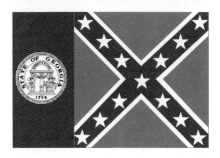

GEORGIA

AREA: 58,910 sq. mi. (152,577 sq. km.)
POPULATION: 6,508,000
CAPITAL: Atlanta
TIME ZONE: Eastern Time

ATLANTA
➲ **404**
✈ Hartsfield Atlanta Int'l Airport (ATL)
9 mi. / 14 km. South

Ritz-Carlton Buckhead
❤❤❤❤❤

3434 Peachtree Road NE, Atlanta, GA 30326, Tel: (404) 237-2700. Fax: (404) 239-0078. TYPE: Superior Deluxe Hotel. LOCATION: Opposite Lenox Square Mall, 17 mi. / 27 km. to airport. DESCRIPTION: Deluxe hotel with health spa & sauna, heated indoor pool. 452 rooms, 72 club rooms, 29 suites, nonsmoker rooms, wheelchair access, restaurant, cafe, lobby lounge, meeting facilities, business center. Hotel rates: from $195.

Swissotel Atlanta
❤❤❤❤

3391 Peachtree Rd. NE, Atlanta, GA 30326. Tel: (404) 365-0065. Fax: (404) 365-8787. TYPE: Hotel & Spa. LOCATION: In the Buckhead area, adjacent to the Lenox Square Mall, 10 minutes to downtown Atlanta, 17 minutes to the airport. DESCRIPTION: Stylish hotel with a complete beauty spa and fitness center; indoor pool, sauna, steam bath & gym. 348 rooms, 15 suites, nonsmoker rooms, wheelchair access, restaurants, lounge, business center.

BRASELTON
⟩ 770
✈ Hartsfield Atlanta Int'l AP (ATL) 55 mi. / 88 km.

Chateau Elan Winery and Resort
❤❤❤❤

♨ 🏃 🏊 ❀

100 Rue Charlemagne, Braselton, GA 30517. Tel: (770) 271-6064 or 932-0900. Fax: (770) 271-6069. TYPE: Chateau-style Resort Hotel & Spa. LOCATION: In a winery of the foothills of northern Georgia, 55 mi. to the airport. SPA CLIENTELE: Women and men.

* Rooms: 300 w/private bath
* Suites: 14 spa suites, 9 villas
* Restaurants (6), Irish pub, meeting and business center
* Airport: Atlanta Int'l, 1 hour
* Reservations: deposit required
* Credit Cards: MC/VISA/AMEX
* Open: Year round
* Hotel Rates: from $145
* TAC: 10%
* Spa on premises: **The Spa st Château Élan**
* **Spa Facilities**: European spa, treatment rooms, unique guest rooms, service rooms (30), spa restaurant - Fleur-de-Lis

* **Spa Programs**: beauty, pampering, fitness
* **Spa Treatments**: swedish massage, aromatherapy, foot reflexology, aroma glow, salt glow, herbal wraps, thalassotherapy, hydrotherapy, skin care, facials
* **Spa Packages**: day packages available. Prices start at $212.

DESCRIPTION: World class resort in Georgia's premier winery. The European spa features a wide range of beauty treatments, stress elimination and rejuvenation programs. Men and women alike benefit from the Spa services. Recreation: golf, tennis.

SEA ISLAND
⟩ 912
✈ Brunswick's Glynco Jet Port, 15 mi. / 24 km.

The Sea Island Spa At The Cloister
❤❤❤❤❤

🏃 🏊

100 First Street, Sea Island, GA 31561. Tel: (912) 638-3611. Toll Free: (800) 732-4752. Fax: (912) 638-5814. TYPE: Resort & Spa. LOCATION: On five miles of private beach, 8 miles off the coast of Brunswick, 15 mi. to the airport. DESCRIPTION: Sea Island beach club with full service spa & fitness center with pools, lounges & food service. 262 rooms in main hotel, guest houses, river houses & beach homes, dining rooms (4), lounges, bars meeting rooms, pools (2), tennis courts (18), 54 holes of golf, fishing, boating, horseback riding, private beach. Hotel rates: from $240.

HAWAII

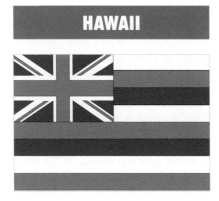

AREA: 6,471 sq. mi. (16,760 sq. km.)
POPULATION: 1,115,274
CAPITAL: Honolulu
TIME ZONE: Hawaii-Aleutian Time

HAWAII (Island)

KAMUELA/KOHALA
⟩ 808

 Keahole-Kona Airport (KOA) 8 mi. / 13 km.
NW of Kailua-Kona

Four Seasons Resort Hualalai
Spa & Sports Club
❤❤❤❤❤

🧍🏃

100 Ka'upulehu Dr., PO Box #1269, Kailua-Kona, Hawaii, HI 96745. Tel: (808) 325-800, Fax: (808) 325-8100. TYPE: Deluxe Resort & Spa. LOCATION: On the beach, 10 minutes to Keahole-Kona Airport. DESCRIPTION: Tropical resort on the exclusive North Kona Coast with 15,000 sq.ft / 1,294 sq. m. sports club & spa with innovative fitness and spa facilities, 17 treatment rooms, lap pool, aerobic studio, and exercise studio. 243 bungalow-style rooms, 31 suites, nonsmoker rooms, wheelchair access. Restaurants (3), bars (2), meeting facilities, business center, outdoor pools (3), tennis courts (8), 18-hole golf course. Hotel rates: from $450.

Kohala Spa
Hilton Waikoloa Village
❤❤❤❤❤

🧍🏃🌸◎

425 Waikoloa Beach Drive, Waikoloa, Hawaii, HI 96738. Tel: (808) 886-2828. Toll Free (800) HILTONS. Fax: (808) 885-2953. TYPE: Deluxe Resort & Spa. SPA MANAGING DIRECTORS: Suzy Bordeaux Johlfs. LOCATION: Nestled on 62 oceanfront acres on the sunny Kohala coast. CLIENTELE: Women and men. SPECIAL RESTRICTIONS: Must be 16 years or older to use the Spa.

* Rooms: 1,240 w/priv. bath; 57 suites
* Phone, CTV, A/C, minibar
* nonsmoker rooms, wheelchair access
* Restaurants (6), lounges, bar, nightclub, meeting rooms, pools (2), 36-holes of golf, 8 tennis courts
* Airport: Kona Int'l 18 mi. / 29 km.
* Airport transportation: rental cars, taxi
* Open: Year round
* Credit Cards: MC/VISA/AMEX/JTB/DISC/DC/CB
* Hotel rates: from $250; TAC: 10%
* Spa on premises: **Kohala Spa**
* Year Established: 1988
* Spa Hours: from 6:00am - 8:00pm daily
* **Spa Facilities**: European style spa, weight and cardiovascular workout rooms, Keiser weight equipment, free weights, Olympic weights,stairmasters and life cycles. Men's and women's locker lounge with Turkish steam, Finish sauna, outdoor whirlpool, relaxation lounges, spa wardrobe and amenities
* **Spa Treatments**: Full and half-session massages including Swedish, Lomi-Lomi Hawaiian, Shiatsu and Aromatherapy. Body care treatments include baneotherapy, aromatherapy, limu, herbal and Kur baths, herbal wraps and body polish. Facials include European, aromatherapy, Hawaiian and others
* **Spa Programs**: beauty, fitness, revitalization, holistic
* **Spa Packages**: Pleasures in Paradise; 7 nights $5,557 for two; 4 nights $3,024 for two à la carte treatments available on request
* Medical Supervision: available if needed

DESCRIPTION: Elegant oceanfront resort with a 4-acre

swimming and snorkeling lagoon and beach where you can see tropical fish or swim with the dolphins. The resort consists of luxurious hotel rooms and suites divided among the three low-rise Ocean, Lagoon and Palace towers. The Kohala Spa is a luxury 25,000 ft / 2,272 sq,m. European style spa designed to promote health and well being. The Spa offers a wide range of beauty and body treatments ranging from lomi-lomi massages to body wraps and aromatherapy. The Spa added to its services the LaStone therapy, a powerful age old massage technique that combines the healing power of heat and the energies of stones. The emphasis at the Kohala Spa is on self-renewing, toning, stress-reduction and beauty treatments.

Kona Village Resort
❤❤❤❤

PO Box #1299, Kailua-Kona, Hawaii, HI 96745. Tel: (808) 325-5555. Fax: (808) 325-5124. TYPE: Resort & Spa. LOCATION: On a secluded sandy beach at Kaupulehu. SPA CLIENTELE: Women and men. DESCRIPTION: Resort village situated on 82 acres encompassing a sandy beach and lagoons with a fitness spa, massage area, sauna, outdoor pools, tennis. 125 rooms. Hotel rates: from $425.

The Orchid at Mauna Lani
❤❤❤❤❤

One North Kaniku Drive, Kohala, Hawaii, HI 96743. Tel: (808) 885-2000, Fax: (808) 885-5778. TYPE: Beachfront Hotel & Spa. LOCATION: Pauoa Bay coast. SPA CLIENTELE: Women and men.

* Rooms: 539 w/priv. bath
* Suites: 20 oceanview
* Phone, CTV, A/C, hair dryer, minibar, refrigerator
* Restaurants (3), bars (6), lounges, meeting facilities, business center, wheelchair access
* Airport: Keahole Kona Int'l AP, 20 mi. / 32 km.
* Open: Year round
* Credit Cards: MC/VISA/AMEX/DIS/JCB
* Hotel Rates: from $350; TAC: 10%
* Name of Spa: **The Orchid Centre for Well Being**
* Spa Facilities: spa without walls, sauna, fitness center,

jogging track, pools, whirlpools
* Spa Treatments: tai chi, seaside meditation, water-dance, mind/body conditioning, seaside yoga, aerobics, pilates method, swim classes, personal training, power walk, massage, body and beauty treatments
* Spa Programs: beauty, pampering, fitness

DESCRIPTION: Beachfront luxury resort featuring a health spa and fitness centre with traditional Hawaiian healing techniques, massage, movement, meditation classes and a variety of beauty and body spa treatments. The "Spa Without Walls" is a wellness spa program that capitalizes on Hawaii's therapeutic natural environment and ancient healing arts. Recreation: 36 holes of golf, tennis courts (10).

KAUAI (Island)

KOLOA
↙ **808**
✈ Lihue Municipal Airport (LIH), 2 mi. / 3 km.

Hawaiian Wellness Holiday
❤❤❤❤

PO Box 279, Koloa, Kauai HI 96756. Tel: (808) 332-9244. Tel: (800) 338-6977. Fax: (808) 332-5941. TYPE: Wellness Resort. SPA DIRECTOR: Grady Deal Ph.D. LOCATION: Sunny Poipu Beach. SPA CLIENTELE: Women and men. Teenagers and children accepted.

* Rooms: 60 w/priv. bath
* Phone, CTV, A/C, cooking facilities
* Airport: Lihue AP, 10 min. by car
* Open: Year round
* Credit Cards: MC/VISA
* Rates: from $895 (3 days); TAC: 10%
* Name of Spa: **Hawaiian Wellness Holiday**
* Year Established: 1986
* Spa Facilities: we do not have our own spa facilities we take our guests to the Spa at the Hyatt Hotel in Poipu Beach
* Spa Treatments: yoga, breathing techniques, aerobics, aquacize, walks, and hikes

* **Spa Programs**: holistic wellness, weight loss, workshops on astrology, numerology, spiritual and physical healing, yoga diet
* **Spa Packages**: 3 days to 2 weeks
* Maximum number of guests: 10
* Number of clients per Doctor: 10
* Medical Supervision: 1MD + 1 D.C.
* Documentation from Doctor: required

DESCRIPTION: Hawaiian Wellness Holidays offer holistic and methapysical programs. The programs teach lifestyle changes, personal transformation and holistic body, mind and spirit techniques. Guests stay in condominiums in sunny Poipu Beach while using the spa facilities at the Hyatt Hotel Poipu Beach.

Hyatt Regency Kauai Resort & Spa
❤❤❤❤❤

1571 Poipu Road, Koloa, Kauai, HI 96756. Tel: (808) 742-1234. Fax: (808) 742-1557. Toll Free (800) 55-HYATT. TYPE: Oceanfront Resort & Spa. SPA MANAGING DIRECTOR: Holly Porter. LOCATION: 30 minutes to Lihue Airport. SPA CLIENTELE: Women and men. SPECIAL RESTRICTION: Children under 16 are not permitted to use the Spa facilities.

* Rooms: 602 w/priv. bath. Suites: 37
* Phone, CTV, A/C, minibar
* Restaurants (5), lounges (5), bar, nightclub, jacuzzi
* Airport: Lihue AP 16 mi. / 26 km.
* Open: Year round
* Credit Cards: MC/VISA/AMEX/DC
* Hotel rates: $310-$520 (rooms) $785-3,550 (suites); TAC: 10%
* Spa on premises: **Anara Spa**
* Year Established: 1990
* Spa Hours: 6:00am - 8:00pm; salon 8:00am - 6:00pm
* **Spa Facilities**: 25,000 sq. ft. / 2,272 sq. m. spa, separate men's and women's showers, treatment rooms (20), aerobics & fitness facilities, weight room, lap pool
* **Spa Treatments**: botanical baths, swedish massage, lomi lomi hawaiian massage, aromatherapy, shiatsu, reflexology, facials, body treatments, herbal wraps,

fitness classes, aerobics, yoga, tai chi, personal training
* **Spa Programs**: fitness; day packages
* **Spa Packages**: Day spa packages and unlimited fitness classes from $135-$350.
* **Web**: www.hyatt.com

DESCRIPTION: Classic Hawaiian oceanfront resort with a full service **Anara Spa**. The spa is committed to a new age restorative approach focusing on Hawaiian healing. The spa offers opportunity to deal with stress, maintain good health, to pamper and cleanse the soul in an open-air tropical setting.

LIHUE
🌙 **808**
✈ Lihue Municipal Airport (LIH), 2 mi. / 3 km.

Kauai Marriott Resort & Beach Club
❤❤❤❤❤

Kalpakaki Beach, Lihue, Kauai, HI 96766. Tel: (808) 245-5050. Fax: (808) 245-5049. TYPE: Resort Hotel & Spa. LOCATION: Overlooking Kalapaki Bay. DESCRIPTION: Full service spa, pool, hot tubs, jogging track. 588 rooms & suites, nonsmoker rooms, wheelchair access. Restaurants (3), snack bar, lounge, entertainment, meeting rooms,

MAUI (Island)

HANA
🌙 **808**
✈ Hana Municipal Airport (HNM) 4 mi. / 6 km. NW

Hana-Maui Wellness Center
❤❤❤❤❤

PO Box 9, Hana, Maui, HI 96713. Tel: (808) 248-8211. Fax: (808) 248-7202. TYPE: Deluxe Resort & Spa. LOCATION: Hana Ranch, 3 mi / 5 km to Hana Airport. DESCRIPTION: Exclusive resort with Maui Wellness center. Spa services include yoga, aquacise, and massage treatments. 55 rooms, 35 suites, nonsmoker rooms, wheelchair access, restaurants (2), lounge, business center, outdoor pool, tennis courts (2). Hotel rates: from $395.

KAPALUA
] 808
✈ Kapalua-West Maui Airport (OGG)
3.5 mi. / 5.6 km. south of Kapalua

Ritz Carlton-Kapalua
♥♥♥♥♥

1 Ritz Carlton Drive, Kapalua, Maui, HI 96761. Tel: (808) 669-6200. Fax: (808) 665-0026. TYPE: Resort & Spa. LOCATION: 3 mi. / 5 km. from airport. SPA CLIENTELE: Women and men. DESCRIPTION: Deluxe resort with full service spa; body wraps, facials, manicures, fitness center, steam sauna, massage, 548 rooms. Hotel rates: from $285.

WAILEA BEACH
] 808
✈ Kahului Airport (OGG), 20 mi. / 32 km.

Wailea-Beach, population 83,000, is a superb beach resort on the south-western shore of Maui. Maui is rapidly becoming one of the best resort destinations in the world. Wailea offers tourist hotel complexes and resorts on its magnificent sunny beaches. It is located 50 mi. / 80 km. from the **Halakela National Park** and 65 mi. / 104 km. from Wailua Falls.

Grand Wailea Resort & Spa
♥♥♥♥♥

3850 Wailea Alanui Drive, Wailea, Maui, HI 96753. Tel: (808) 875-1234. Toll Free: (800) 888-6100. Fax: (808) 874-2411. TYPE: Deluxe Oceanfront Resort & Spa. SPA DIRECTOR: David Erlich. LOCATION: On 40 acres of Maui's south shore. SPA CLIENTELE: Women and men. SPECIAL RESTRICTIONS: Must be 16 years or older to get treatments at the spa.

* Rooms: 761 w/priv. bath. Suites: 51
* Phone, CTV, A/C, minibar, safe, ocean view

* Restaurants, Spa cuisine cafe, nightclub, lounges
* Wheelchair Access
* Airport: Kahului AP 8 mi. / 13 km.
* Airport Transportation: public transportation
* Open: Year round
* Credit Cards: MC/VISA/AMEX/JCB/DC
* Hotel Rates: from $380
* Spa on premises: **Spa Grande**
* Year Established: 1991
* **Spa Facilities**: 40,000 sq. ft. / 3,636 sq. m. Spa Grande, sauna, steam, gym, aerobics, weight training, exercise and facilities
* **Spa Treatments**: hydrotherapy (Termé Wailea); moor mud, body detoxification, meditation, weight control, stress reduction, skin care, S.A.D. seasonal affective disorder, full spectrum light, aromatherapy, music & sound therapy, traditional and Japanese massages, facial and herbal wraps, milk, mineral and fruit baths, loofah scrub, aerobics, weight training
* **Spa Packages**: Hawaiian Holiday (full day); First Time Spa Goer (3 hrs.); Anti-cellulite (3 hrs.)
* Medical Supervision: medical and dietary staff

DESCRIPTION: Elegant beach resort featuring the luxurious Spa Grande. A full array of Hawaiian, European, American and Oriental spa treatments and therapies are offered at the spa. Recreation: beach bathing, water sports, whale-catching, scuba diving, Catamaran cruises, billiard, card rooms, children's recreation center.

OAHU (Island)

KAPOLEI
] 808
✈ Honolulu Int'l Airport (HNL), 20 mi. / 32 km.

Ihilani Resort & Spa
♥♥♥♥♥

92-1001 Olani Street, Kapolei, Oahu, HI 96707. Tel: (808) 679-0079. Fax: (808) 679-0080. TYPE: Deluxe atrium hotel. SPA DIRECTOR: Ann Emich. LOCATION: On the western shore of Oahu in a pristine area renowned for its

unspoiled beaches. SPA CLIENTELE: Women and men. SPE-
CIAL RESTRICTION: Teenagers accepted, but must be 16
years or older to use the spa.

* Rooms: 387 w/priv. bath. Suites: 36
* Deluxe Spa Rooms: 6 w/priv. garden terrace
* Phone, CTV, A/C, minibar, safe, ocean view
* Restaurants, spa cuisine cafe, nightclub, lounges
* Wheelchair Access
* Airport: Honolulu Int'l AP 25 min.
* Open: Year round
* Credit Cards: MC/VISA/AMEX/JCB/DC
* Hotel Rates: from $295
* Spa on premises: **Inhilani Spa**
* Spa Hours: 7:00am - 11:00am / 2:00pm - 7:00pm
* **Spa Facilities**: 35,000 sq. ft. / 3,180 sq. m. Spa
  Roman pools, fitness center, treatment rooms,
  baths and showers, saunas, steam baths, beauty
  salon 3 mi. / 5 km. fitness trail
* **Spa Treatments**: thalassotherapy, herbal wraps,
  hydrotherapy, swiss showers, grand jets, vichy
  showers, swedish, sports, shiatsu, reflexology, lomi
  lomi hawaiian massage, exercise classes, aerobics
* **Spa Programs**: beauty, pampering, stress reduction,
  weight loss, nutritional program
* **Spa Packages**: Hawaiian Harmony; 3-7 night stay
  with spa treatments
* Medical Supervision: 1RN

DESCRIPTION: Deluxe resort hotel with full service destination Spa. The Ihilani Spa, considered one of the top spas in
the USA, offers authentic thalassotherapy, full range body
treatments,underwater massage, herbal wraps, swiss
showers, grand jets, needle showers, roman pools and a
low cal spa cafe. The fitness center offers exercise class,
exercise equipment,weight loss and nutritional programs.
Amenities include: lap pool, steam bath, whirlpool and fitness trail.

IDAHO

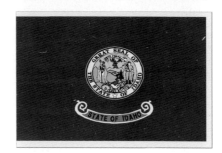

AREA: 83,564 sq. mi. (216,431 sq. km.)
POPULATION: 1,011,986
CAPITAL: Boise
TIME ZONE: Mountain Time

COEUR D'ALENE
208

✈ Spokane Int'l Airport, WA (GEG)
40 mi. / 64 km. West

Spa at Coeur D'Alene Resort on the Lake
♥♥♥♥♥

115 S. 2nd St., PO Box #7200, Coeur D'Alene, ID
83814, Tel: (208) 765-4000, Fax: (208) 667-2707.
TYPE: Superior first class marina hotel & golf resort. LOCA-
TION: On Lake Couer d'Alene. DESCRIPTION: Full service
spa, fitness center with sauna, 2 whirlpools,pool, steam
room, and racquetball. 221 rooms, 22 suite, nonsmoker
rooms, wheelchair access, 2 restaurants, 3 lounges, bars,
entertainment, convention center, indoor pool, marina.

ILLINOIS

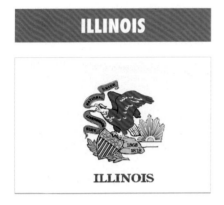

ILLINOIS

AREA: 56,345 sq. mi. (145,934 sq. km.)
POPULATION: 11,466,682
CAPITAL: Springfield
TIME ZONE: Central Time

CHICAGO
ϡ 312

✈ O'Hare Int'l Airport (ORD), 18 mi. / 29 km. NW
Midway Airport (MDW), 11 mi. 18 km. SW

Four Seasons Hotel Chicago
♥♥♥♥♥

120 East Delaware Place, Chicago, IL 60611. Tel: (312) 280-8800. Fax: (312) 280-1748. TYPE: Deluxe Hotel & Spa. LOCATION: In the 900 North Michigan Avenue Complex Above Bloomingdale's. DESCRIPTION: Deluxe hotel with complete health spa, nautilus equipment, indoor pool, sauna, jogging path. 205 rooms, 138 suites, non-smoking rooms, Restaurant, cafe, lounge, bar, meeting facilities. Hotel rates: from $395.

GILMAN
ϡ 815

✈ O'Hare Int'l Airport (ORD), 80 mi. / 128 km.

Gilman, population 2,000, is a small rural community located half way between Chicago and Champaign (IL) along I-57. Nearby Kankakee (28 mi./45km. south), is an interesting small town which continues to preserve its original

French heritage which is manifested in the old buildings and local culture. Chicago, the magnificent industrial, financial, and cultural center of the Midwest, is located some 80 miles (128 km.) north on the shores of Lake Michigan. Gilman can be reached from Chicago via I-57 driving south.

The Heartland
♥♥♥

Gilman, IL. Mailing Address: 20 E. Jackson, Chicago, IL 60938. Tel: (815) 683-2182. Toll Free 1-800-545-4853. Fax: (815) 683-2144. TYPE: Health & Fitness Retreat. MANAGER: Audrey Weinberg, Dir. LOCATION: On a landscaped 31-acres around a small lake. SPA CLIENTELE: Women and men .(minimum age: 18).

* Rooms: 14 w/private bath
* Dining Room: low calorie vegetarian
* Airport: O'Hare Airport/Chicago 90 mi. (144 km.)
* Airport Transportation: free transfers from down town Chicago, bus
* Reservations: 50% deposit required
* Credit Cards: MC/VISA/AMEX
* Open: Year round
* Rates: from $540; TAC: 10%
* **Spa facilities**: Health Spa; exercise rooms, Pneumatic resistance weight equipment, cardiovascular workout equipment, steam rooms, saunas, whirlpools, massage rooms, indoor pool
* **Spa Programs**: Fitness, weight loss, nutrition, stress management, body shaping
* **Spa Treatments**: low-impact aerobics, water works, sauna, massages, facials

DESCRIPTION: Health retreat nestled in the rural country side and surrounded by 31 acres of woodland. The mansion is furnished with 2 large lounges/wood burning fireplaces. The accommodations consist of nicely appointed twin-bedded guest rooms. The Spa is housed in a renovated multi-level barn. The emphasis is on long term behavior modification which leads to better nutrition, permanent weight loss and lasting improvement of the quality of life. Recreation: tennis (summer), Cross-Country skiing in nearby trails (winter).

INDIANA

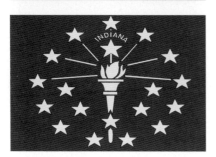

AREA: 36,185 sq. mi. (93,719 sq. km.)
POPULATION: 5,564,228
CAPITAL: Indianapolis
TIME ZONE: Central Time

CHESTERTON
219

✈ Midway Airport, IL (MDW), 52 mi. / 83 km. West

Indian Oaks Resort & Spa
♥♥♥

558 Indian Boundary Road, Chesterton, IN 46304. Tel:
(219) 926-2200. Toll Free (800) 552-4232. Fax: (219)
929-4285. LOCATION: On Lake Chubb, one hour driving
time from South Bend or Chicago. SPA CLIENTELE: Women
and men. Teenagers and children accepted.

* Rooms: 100 w/priv. bath. Suites: 12
* Phone, CTV, A/C, balcony, fireplace, jacuzzi
* Restaurant, Irish Pub, banquet center
* Airport: O'Hare & Midway, Chicago
* Train Station: Dune Park, South Shore train
* Transportation: free pick up from train station
* Reservations: required
* Open: Year round
* Hotel rates: from $75
* TAC: 10%
* Spa on premises
* Year Established: 1983

* **Spa Facilities**: fitness center, indoor pool, sauna,
  steam room, walking trails, treatment rooms (8)
* **Spa Treatments**: loofah scrub, sea salt glo, body wrap,
  seaweed body mask, Sedona mud, anti-stress back
  treatments, hydrotherapy bath treatments, tranquility
  treatments, hydrotherapy cellulite treatments,
  La Stone therapy, massages, vichy shower,
  scrub & rub, reflexology, hydro drainage,
  Aveda make up, work out, Qi Gong, Aqua exercise
* **Spa Programs**: health, beauty and wellness
* **Spa Packages**: 1 - 5 nights from $99 - $350

DESCRIPTION: Lakefront resort with graciously oversized
lakeside or woodside rooms some with a fireplace or a
jacuzzi. The Indian Oak spa feature a wide range of revitalizing and holistic beauty and health treatments for both
women and men. Only high quality, all natural products
are used by professionally licensed and certified spa tech-
nicians. Special workshops are offered during the year on
wellness, nutrition and meditation topics.

FRENCH LICK
812

✈ French Lick Airport 3 mi. / 5 km.
  Indianapolis Int'l AP (IND) 108 mi. / 172 km. N.

French Lick, population 2,300, is famous health and vacation resort. The spa's artesian spring contains a high concentration of minerals with revitalizing benefits. French Lick
was the site of the early 18th century French trading post.

French Lick Springs Resort
♥♥♥♥

Hwy 56, French Lick, IN 47432. Tel: (812) 936-9300,
Toll Free (800) 457-4042. Fax: (812) 936-2100. TYPE:
Resort & Spa. LOCATION: On 1,200 landscaped acres in
French Lick, 2 hours from Indianapolis. SPA CLIENTELE:
Women and men.

* Rooms: 485 w/priv. bath. Suites: 20
* Phone, CTV, A/C, rooms for non smokers
* Dining rooms, lounge with dancing
* Airport: French Lick AP 3 mi. / 5 km., or

Indianapolis Int'l AP 108 mi. / 172 km.
* Transportation: courtesy car from French Lick AP
* Open: Year round
* Credit Cards: MC/VISA/AMEX/DC/DIS/CB
* Hotel Rates: from $99
* TAC: 10%
* **Spa Facilities**: mineral baths, pools, saunas, whirlpools, locker rooms, massage and facial rooms, exercise rooms, beauty salon
* **Spa Programs**: Weight loss, fitness, beauty
* **Spa Packages**: 2-7 night packages
* **Spa Treatments**: balneotherapy, massages, facials, cellulite body wraps, low calorie diets

DESCRIPTION: Turn of the century grand hotel, and convention center, the largest of its kind in the Midwest. The co-ed health spa offers revitalizing mineral water baths, European pampering treatments, weight loss programs and plenty of exercises to stay in shape. Recreation: tennis, scenic trail rides, game room, children activities, lake water sports and winter skiing nearby.

MAUCKPORT
) 812
✈ Louisville, KY (SDF) 48 mi. / 77 km. East

Orbis Farm
❤❤

8700 Ripperdan Valley Rd SW, Mauckport, IN 47142. Tel: (812) 732-4657. TYPE: 75 acre health retreat. LOCATION: Just north of the Ohio River. DESCRIPTION: Kundalini meditation, yoga, t'ai chi, spiritual and therapeutic journeys, two dormitories.

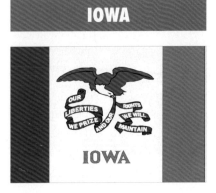

AREA: 56,275 sq. mi. (145,752 sq. km.)
POPULATION: 2,787,424
CAPITAL: Des Moines
TIME ZONE: Central Time

DES MOINES
) 515
✈ Des Moines Int'l Airport (DSM), 5 mi. / 8 km.

Savery Hotel & Spa
❤❤❤

401 Locust Street, Des Moines, IA 50309, Tel: (515) 244 2151, Fax: (515) 244-1408. TYPE: Hotel & Spa. LOCATION: Downtown next to convention center. DESCRIPTION: Complete health spa with whirlpool, sauna, jogging track. 205 rooms 14 suites, penthouse suite, 3 restaurants, meeting facilities, indoor pool.

FAIRFIELD
) 515
✈ Cedar Rapids Municipal Airport (CID), 80 mi. / 128 km.

The Raj Maharishi Ayur - Veda Health Center
❤❤❤

1734 Jasmine Ave., Fairfield, IA 52556. Tel: (515) 472-9580. Toll Free: (800) 248-9050. Fax: (515) 472-2496. TYPE: Hotel & health center. LOCATION 100 acres of rolling meadows & woodland, 90 minutes to Cedar Rapids Airport. DESCRIPTION: Health Center with a selection of rejuvenation, cellulite reduction, & beauty regimens, yoga & transcendental meditation programs. 24 rooms, no smoking policy, wheelchair access, restaurant with separate vegetarian menu for health center guest.

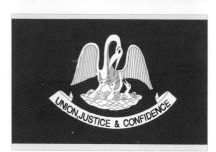

LOUISIANA

AREA: 47,752 sq. mi. (123,678 sq. km.)
POPULATION: 4,238,216
CAPITAL: New Orleans
TIME ZONE: Central Time

NEW ORLEANS
〕 504

✈ New Orleans Int'l Airport (MSY), 12 mi. / 19 km.

New Orleans, population 558,000, is a colorful and romantic city on the Mississippi River. Old New Orleans traditions have always celebrated the 'Good Life' with soulful Jazz, fun filled Mardi Gras, and the delicious Cajun Cuisine. The city still conserves a unique blend of cultures, resulting from a long and dramatic history. French and Spanish influence can be observed in the architectural style of many buildings in the picturesque Old Town, better known as "Le Vieux Carré".

New Orleans protects its heritage with the careful restoration of historic quarters, and the construction of tourist oriented recreation facilities and shopping malls. New Orleans Airport is directly served by regular flights from all major US cities.

Avenue Plaza Hotel & Spa
♥♥♥♥

2111 St. Charles Avenue, New Orleans, LA 70130. Tel: (504) 566-1212. Toll free (800) 535-9575.Fax: (504) 525-6899. TYPE: Hotel & Spa. LOCATION: Garden District, 5 min. from the French Quarter by streetcar. SPA CLIEN-

TELE: Women and men. Family oriented.

* Suites: 250 w/private bath
* Phone, CTV, A/C, wet bar & refrigerator
* Sidewalk café & cocktail lounge
* Airport: New Orleans Int'l, 16 mi. / 26 km.
* Airport Transportation: taxi, limo
* Reservations: suggested
* Credit Cards: MC/VISA/AMEX/DC/CB
* Open: Year round
* Hotel Rates: from $99
* TAC: 10%
* Spa on premises
* **Spa Facilities**: European Spa, scandinavian saunas, turkish steam baths, swiss showers, individual whirlpools, tanning solarium, unisex beauty Salon, co-ed workout gym with universal and paramount machines, heated swimming pool, rooftop sundeck with hot tub
* **Spa Programs**: Stress Reliever; Day of Beaut; Perfect Day of Pampering, SPA Sampler (2 nts), Energizer (3 nts), Shape Up (6 nts)
* **Spa Treatments**: Swedish and shiatsu massages, acumassage, facial, herbal wrap, fitness class, low-impact aerobics tanning, loofa salt glo, nutritional profile, fitness evaluation, wellness profile, hair & skin care, low calorie meals

DESCRIPTION: Charming all-suite hotel with a lobby furnished with European antiques. Rooms are spacious and well appointed. The EuroVita spa combines high standard hotel service with a fully equipped health and fitness Spa. The Spa specializes in fitness, weight loss, body pampering and stress reduction. A full range of skin and hair care services are available at the unisex beauty salon.

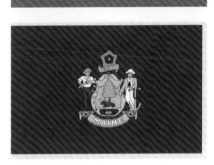

MAINE

AREA: 47,752 sq. mi. (123,678 sq. km.)
POPULATION: 4,238,216
CAPITAL: New Orleans
TIME ZONE: Central Time

POLAND SPRINGS
) 207
✈ Portland Int'l Jetport (PWM)

Poland Spring Health Institute
32 Summit Springs Road, Poland, ME 04274. Tel: (207) 998-2894, (207)998-2795. Fax: (207) 998-2164.

RAYMOND
) 207
✈ Portland Int'l Jetport (PWM)

Raymond, population 2,250, is located about 25 mi. (15 km.) north of Portland (ME) in the beautiful Sabago Lake Region of Southern Maine. Nearby Portland, the largest city in the state, is a popular summer resort with historic houses, and rich with cultural events year round.

Northern Pines Health Resort
❤❤

559 Route 85, PO Box 279, Raymond, ME 04071. Tel: (207) 655-7624. Fax: (207) 655-3321. TYPE: Holistic Health Retreat. MANAGER: Marlee T. Coughlan. LOCATION:

In the Sabago Lake region north of Portland (ME). SPA CLIENTELE: Women and men (no children).

* Rooms: 15; 3 w/priv. bath. Cottages: 2
* Airport: Portland (ME)
* Reservations: deposit required
* Credit Cards: MC/VISA/AMEX
* Rates: $375-$650/week
* TAC: 10%
* Spa on premises
* **Spa Facilities**: lakeside hot tub, sauna, hiking and jogging trails, aerobic room, gym
* **Spa Programs**: Stress management, exercise, weight loss, fasting ,Spa/Ski (winter)
* **Spa Treatments**: massage, hair treatments, facials, reflexology

DESCRIPTION: Northern Pines offers a healthful vacation in the scenic lake and mountain country of southern Maine. Accommodations are rustic style and all but the cottages share bath. Four daily exercise programs are offered and include: walking, jogging, aerobic dance, workouts and yoga. The low calorie spa cuisine consists of fresh fruits and vegetables. Special classes are offered in holistic and natural health to develop better nutritional habits. Winter program includes ski activities.

MASSACHUSETTS

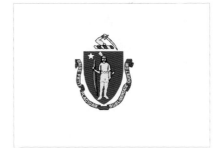

AREA: 8,284 sq. mi. (21,456 sq. km.)
POPULATION: 6,030,000
CAPITAL: Boston
TIME ZONE: Eastern Time

BOSTON / CAMBRIDGE
↱ **617**
✈ Logan Int'l Airport (BOS) 3 mi. / 5 km.

Boston, population 560,000 (City), 2,760,000 (Metro) is the Capital of Massachusetts. Located on the Boston Harbor, at the confluence of the Charles and Mystic Rivers, the city has a prominent historical heritage dating back to the days of early settlements and their fight for independence. Boston is a magic combination of Old restored residential and commercial districts with ultra modern high rise buildings and modern shopping and tourist recreation areas. Boston can be reached through the Logan International Airport or by car via I-90 the major east-west highway that leads to Boston, or I-95 for north - south access.

Boston Harbor Hotel
♥♥♥♥♥

70 Rowes Wharf, Boston, MA 02110. Tel: (617) 439-7000. Fax: (617) 330-9450. TYPE: Hotel & Spa. LOCATION: At Rowes Wharf in the heart of downtown Boston. SPA CLIENTELE: Women and men.

* Rooms: 230 w/private bath. Suites: 28

* Phone, CTV, A/C, life safety systems, mini-bar,
* Restaurants, Lounges w/harbor views
* Airport: Logan Int'l 7 min., taxi, water shuttle
* Reservations: One night deposit
* Credit Cards: MC/VISA/AMEX/DC
* Open: Year round
* Hotel Rates: from $220
* Spa on premises
* **Spa Facilities**: 60 ft. lap pool, fully equipped gym with weight and computerized aerobic equipment, large whirlpool, sauna, steam, spa & beauty treatment rooms, aerobic rooms
* **Spa Programs**: Diet/fitness, beauty, fitness weekend, spa weekend
* **Spa Treatments**: exercises, aerobics, weight training, aqua waterworks, massage, herbal wrap, hydrotherapy, facials, various spa treatments, diet natural and fresh foods

DESCRIPTION: Luxury hotel on the Boston Harbor with harbor views. Accommodations are spacious in New England design. The Spa features health club for exercise, aerobics, weight training and body building. Spa treatments for body pampering and relaxation are available.

Four Seasons Hotel Boston
❤❤❤❤❤

200 Boylston St., Boston, MA 02116. Tel: (617) 338-4400. Fax: (617) 423-0154. TYPE: Hotel & Spa. LOCATION: Overlooking the Public Gardens and Beacon Hill. DESCRIPTION: Superior deluxe downtown hotel with spa services, indoor pool, gym, sauna, whirlpool. 275 rooms, 15 suites, nonsmoker floors, wheelchair access, restaurant, 2 private dining rooms, lounge, meeting facilities. Hotel rates: from $310.

The Charles Hotel
❤❤❤❤

1 Bennett St., Charles Square, Cambridge, MA 02138. Tel: (617) 864-1200. Fax: (617) 864-5715. TYPE: Hotel & Spa. LOCATION: In Harvard Square. SPA CLIENTELE: Women and men.

* Rooms: 296 w/priv. bath
* Phone, CTV, hair dryer, mini-bar, room safe
* Restaurants (2), bars (2), live jazz
* Airport: Logan Int'l 20 min., taxi
* Open: Year round
* Credit Cards: AMEX/MC/VISA
* Hotel Rates: from $260
* Spa on premises: **Le Pli** (day spa)
* **Spa Facilities**: exercise studio, weight room, showers and lockers, spa cafe, beauty salon, glass enclosed pool area, suntan booth, whirlpool, sun terrace
* **Spa Programs**: Weight loss, fitness, beauty
* **Spa Treatments**: exercises, body conditioning, yoga, aerobics, hydro-exercise, massages, fango mud, hydrotherapy, European beauty treatments

DESCRIPTION: Fashionable hotel with Urban Spa. The Spa occupies three different levels and offers a variety of European pampering treatments and American fitness and weight loss programs.

LANCASTER
➲ **508**

✈ Municipal Airport (ORH)

Lancaster, is a small town near Worcester the second largest city in Massachusetts. Worcester is an industrial center, but it also has good museums, craft centers, colleges, and it is the home of the famous Worcester Music Festival, the oldest festival of its kind in the country. Lancaster can be reached by car from Boston via Worcester or Fitchburg.

Maharishi Ayur-Veda
❤❤❤

P.O. Box 344, 679 George Hill Rd., Lancaster, MA 01523. Tel: (508) 365-4549. Fax: (508) 368-0674. TYPE: Holistic Health Center. LOCATION: Amidst 200 acres of secluded woodland. SPA CLIENTELE: Women and men.

* Rooms: 12; 10 w/priv. bath. Suites: 3
* Elegant Dining Room
* Health Center on premises
* Airport: Logan Int'l 55 mi. / 88 km.

* Train St'n: Worcester 25 mi. / 40 km.
* Airport/Train St'n Transportation: taxi, limo
* Reservations: deposit req'd
* Open: Year round (closed Christmas week)
* Rates: from $2,900
* **Spa Facilities**: Maharishi Ayur-Veda Health Center
* **Spa Programs**: meditation, natural health care, stress mgmt, natural weight loss,
* **Spa Treatments**: rejuvenation therapy, aromatherapy, herb and oil massages, herbal steam baths, relaxing therapy, marma therapy, breath awareness therapy
* Indications: stress, obesity, high blood pressure, insomnia, PMS, lower back pain
* Medical Supervision: 3 MD, 3 RN
* Number of customers per doctor: 3
* Treatments: not approved by medical/professional association

DESCRIPTION: Elegant holistic health center with a traditional system of health approach from India known as Maharishi Ayur-Veda. The center offers luxury rooms and suites in a tranquil environment. The therapies and programs are based on age old natural health care that promotes balance to the mind, body and spirit.

LENOX
↳ 413
✈ Albany Airport (NY)

Lenox, population 1,800, is a year round resort in the southern Berkshires. The town became famous when the Boston Symphony Orchestra made its summer home in Tanglewood one mile west. Lenox is located about 180 mi. / 290 km. west of Boston via I-90.

Canyon Ranch
♥♥♥♥

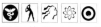

16 Kemble Street, Lenox, MA 01240. Tel: (413) 637-4100. Toll Free (800) 326-7100. Fax: (413) 637-0057. TYPE: Health & Fitness Resort. LOCATION: 120 acre Bellefontaine estate in Lenox. SPA CLIENTELE: Women and men.

* Rooms: 120 w/priv. bath. Suites: 24

* Phone, CTV, VCR
* Dining room, meeting room
* Airport: Albany (NY) 60 mi. / 96 km.
* Reservation: 3 night minimum stay
* Open: Year round
* Credit Cards: MC/VISA/AMEX
* Hotel Rates: from $310; TAC: 10%
* Spa on premises
* **Spa Facilities**: exercise areas, weight-training rooms, men's and women's facilities complete with steam, sauna, inhalation rooms, whirlpool baths, lockers and showers, therapy rooms, trails for walking, biking, swimming pool
* **Spa Programs**: exercise, nutrition, stress reduction, lifestyle improvement, special programs for arthritics, stop smoking, substantial weight loss, living with medical limitations
* **Spa Treatments**: exercise, aerobics, full body massages, herbal and aroma wraps, skin care, fitness classes, presentations by fitness, nutrition, stress management and medical experts
* **Indications**: weight loss, life enhancement, preventive medicine
* Medical Supervision: 1 MD, 4 RN

DESCRIPTION: Health resort and spa offering the same comprehensive program as the original Canyon Ranch Spa in Tucson AZ. The 100,000 sq. ft Spa complex has beauty treatments and therapy area, sports facilities, 75-foot enclosed swimming pool and exercise areas. The spa focuses on fitness, nutrition, stress reduction and Lifestyle changes. Recreation: tennis, racquetball, squash, basketball, skiing is available nearby. Evening activities include bingo and game rooms.

Kripalu Center for Yoga and Health
♥♥♥

PO Box 793, Lenox, MA 01240, Tel: (413) 448-3400 ext.224. Toll Free: (800) 967-3577. Fax: (413) 448-3384. TYPE: Health Resort. LOCATION: In the Berkshires on a private lake. DESCRIPTION: Health retreat offering yoga, massage, sauna, whirlpool, vegetarian meals. 174 rooms.

MINNESOTA

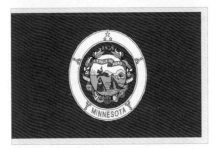

AREA: 84,402 sq. mi. (218,601 sq. km.)
POPULATION: 4,387,000
CAPITAL: Minneapolis
TIME ZONE: Central Time

LITCHFIELD
320
✈ Minneapolis/St. Paul AP (MSP) 60 mi. / 96 km.

Litchfield, population 6,200, is a rural town 60 miles (96 km.) west of Minneapolis/St. Paul.

Birdwing Spa
♥♥♥

R.R. 2, Box 104, Litchfield MN 55355. Tel: (320) 693-6064. Fax: (320) 693-7026. TYPE: Spa Hotel. LOCATION: 60 mi. / 96 km. west of Minneapolis/St. Paul. SPA CLIENTELE: Women and men. SPECIAL RESTRICTIONS: No children or pets.

* Rooms: 13, 1 w/priv. bath. Suites: 3
* Spa Facilities: sauna, jacuzzi, beauty room, gym
* Spa Programs: Diet, fitness, beauty
* Spa Packages: Ultimate Spa (7 days), Revitalizing (5 day); Pampered Weekend, SPA Day
* Spa Treatments: nutrition and fitness, exercise, aerobics, beauty treatment, spa cuisine

DESCRIPTION: Country style European inspired spa for relaxation, beauty treatments, exercise and recreation. A 900-1,100 calories diet program is available for a sensible weight loss.

MINNETONKA
612
✈ Minneapolis/St. Paul AP (MSP) 16 mi. / 26 km.

Spa at The Marsh
♥♥♥

15000 Minnetonka Blvd., Minnetonka, MN 55345. Tel: (612) 935-2202. Fax: (612) 935-9685. TYPE: Destination Spa. MANAGING DIRECTOR: Jessica Lyman. PROGRAM DIRECTOR: Hilman Wagner. LOCATION: Urban setting. SPA CLIENTELE: Women and men, teenagers accepted.

* Rooms: 6 w/priv. bath
* Phone, CTV, A/C, C/H
* Dining Room, conference center
* Airport: 30 minutes
* Reservations: deposit required
* Credit Cards: MC/VISA/AMEX
* Open: Year round
* Rates: from $100
* Spa on premises
* Year Established: 1985
* Spa Facilities: sauna, jacuzzi, full service salon, pools, studios, training center, indoor/outdoor track, wooded trails
* Spa Programs: Wellness, rehab, relaxation
* Spa Treatments: acupuncture, thai massage, shiatsu, swedish massage, sports massage, trigger point therapy, nutrition and fitness, exercise, aerobics, skin treatments, hydrotherapy, spa cuisine
* Spa Packages: Beauty care; Spa Sampler, Spa Experience, 24 hrs Getaway
* Email: visionary@sprintmail.com

DESCRIPTION: A day and destination spa in an urban setting providing an integrated, enriched program. Referrals by medical practitioners are common for body work, acupuncture and skin treatments to facilitate the healing process.

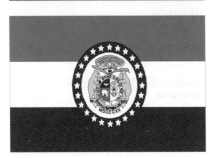

MISSOURI

AREA: 69,697 sq. mi. (180,515 sq. km.)
POPULATION: 5,137,800
CAPITAL: St. Louis
TIME ZONE: Central Time

EXCELSIOR SPRINGS
🤙 816
✈ Kansas City Int'l AP (MCI)

The Elms Resort & Spa
♥♥♥

Regent & Elms Blvd., Excelsior Springs, MO 64204. Tel: (816) 630-2141 or (816) 630-4738. Fax: (816) 637-0752, (816) 637-1222. DESCRIPTION: Resort with health spa.

OSAGE BEACH
🤙 573
✈ Lee Fine Airport
   15 mi. / 24 km.

The Lodge of Four Seasons
♥♥♥♥

Lake Road, PO Box 215, Lake of the Ozarks, MO 65049. Tel: (573) 365-3001. Fax: (573) 365-8525. TYPE: Golf & Spa Resort. LOCATION Tip of Horseshoe peninsula on the Lake of then Ozarks. DESCRIPTION: Health spa including massage therapy. 149 rooms, 12 suites, 150 one to 3-bedroom condos, nonsmoker rooms, wheelchair access, selection of restaurants, lobby bar, lounge entertainment, meeting facilities, pools (5), 27-hole of golf, tennis courts (17).

Marriott's Spa at Tan Tar A Resort
♥♥♥♥

State Road KK, PO Box, Osage Beach, MO 65065. Tel: (573) 348-3535, Toll Free: (800) 826-8272. Fax: (573) 348-3535. TYPE: Resort & Spa. LOCATION: On the shore of the Lake of the Ozarks, 15 miles to Lee Fine Airport. DESCRIPTION: Self-contained mega resort with a complete health spa. 190 rooms, 175 suites, 565 condos. non smoker rooms, wheelchair access, restaurants, bars, lounges, entertainment convention facilities, 5 pools, 27-holes of golf, 6 tennis courts, 4 racquetball courts. Hotel rates: from $75.

WASHBURN
🤙 417
✈ Pomona Airport

Wholistic Life Center
♥♥

Route 1, Box 1783, Washburn, MO 65773. Tel: (417) 435-2212, Fax: (417) 435-2211. DESCRIPTION: Holistic retreat offering a cleansing and rebuilding nutritional program, massage. Nine 10-bed cabins.

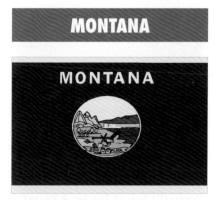

MONTANA

AREA: 147,046 sq. mi. (380,849 sq. km.)
POPULATION: 803,655
CAPITAL: Billings
TIME ZONE: Mountain Time

ANACONDA
⟩ 406
✈ Butte's Bert Mooney Airport (BTM) 25 mi. / 40 km.

Fairmont Hots Springs Resort
♥♥♥♥

1500 Fairmont Rd., Anaconda, MT 59711. Tel: (406) 797-3241, Fax: (406) 797-3337. TYPE: Resort & Spa. LOCATION: 18 miles form Butte. DESCRIPTION: Convention resort with mineral springs spa, indoor/outdoor mineral water pools, steam room, jacuzzi, and gym. 128 rooms, 24 suites, nonsmoker rooms, wheelchair access, dining room, coffee shop, lounge, meeting facilities, 18-hole golf course, 2 tennis.Hotel rates: from $79.

BOULDER
⟩ 406
✈ Butte's Bert Mooney Airport (BTM) 25 mi. / 40 km.

Boulder Hot Springs Hotel
♥♥♥♥

PO Box 930, Boulder, MT 59632, Tel: (406) 225-4339, Fax: (406) 225-4345. TYPE: Restored 1888 Hot Springs Hotel. DESCRIPTION: Natural hot springs for soaking and swimming. 33 rooms. Hotel rates: from $69.

PRAY
⟩ 406
✈ Livingston Airport

Chico Hots Springs Lodge
♥♥

PO Drawer D, Pray, MT 59065, Tel: 406-333-4933, Fax: 406-333-4694. TYPE: Resort & Spa. LOCATION: In Paradise Valley, 26 mi / 42 km to Livingston, and 38 mi. / 60 km. to Yellowstone Nat'l Park. DESCRIPTION: Rustic resort in Paradise Valley with hot mineral spring pools. 81 motel rooms, 2 cottages, 4 cabins, 3 log homes, restaurant, poolside grill, saloon with entertainment. Recreation: cross-country skiing, hay rides, dog sled treks, fishing. Hotel rates: from $45.

NEVADA

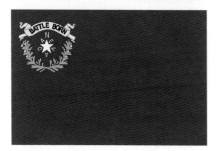

AREA: 110,561 sq. mi. (286,353 sq. km.)
POPULATION: 1,206,152
CAPITAL: Carson City
TIME ZONE: Pacific Time

CRYSTAL BAY
☽ **775**
✈ Reno Cannon Int'l AP (RNO), 30 mi. / 48 km. NE

Cal-Neva Resort Hotel, Spa & Casino
♥♥♥♥

2 Stateline Rd., PO Box 368, Crystal Bay, NV 89402. Tel: (775) 832-4000. Fax: (775) 831-9007. TYPE: Casino Resort Hotel & Spa. LOCATION: On Lake Tahoe's north shore, 40 mi. / 64 km. to Reno's Cannon Int'l Airport. DESCRIPTION: Landmark resort hotel and casino with a European style health spa. 200 rooms, 18 suites, 20 chalets, nonsmoker rooms, wheelchair access. restaurant, coffee shop, bar, casino, meeting facilities, pool, tennis, gift shop. Hotel rates: from $69.

GENOA
☽ **775**
✈ Lake Tahoe Airport (TVL)

Walley's 1862 Hot Springs Resort
♥♥

P.O. Box 26, Genoa, NV 89411. Tel: (775) 782-8155.

Toll Free (800) 628-7831. Fax: (775) 782-2103. TYPE: Renovated natural hot springs resort. LOCATION: At the base of the Sierra Mountains. DESCRIPTION: Mineral springs spa with massage yoga, aquacise, weight room, pool, whirlpools, tennis. 5 rooms.

LAS VEGAS
☽ **702**
✈ McCarran Int'l Airport (LAS), 7 mi. South

Las Vegas, population 183,000, is a desert Fantasyland for grown ups in the Nevada desert near the Hoover Dam and Lake Mead. It is world famous for its gambling casino palaces and plush mega resorts that offer non stop entertainment 24 hours a day. The Strip is where the big action is in Las Vegas. Many couples flock to town to get married in one of the little chapels along the strip that offer instant wedding services. Las Vegas has an International Airport and is served by air from any major US city, or by car from Los Angeles via Interstate -15.

Bellagio - The Resort Spa Bellagio
♥♥♥♥♥

3600 Las Vegas Blvd. S., Las Vegas, NV 89109. Hotel Tel: (702) 693-8771. Toll Free: (888) 744-7687. Fax: (702) 693-8777. Spa - Tel: (702) 693-7472. TYPE: Deluxe Resort Hotel & Casino. LOCATION: Mid Las Vegas Strip, 4 mi. / 6 km. to the airport. DESCRIPTION: Italian village themed mega resort with a full service spa & health club, open 6am to 8pm. 3,005 rooms & suites, nonsmoker rooms, wheelchair access, gourmet restaurants, bars, entertainment, casino, meeting facilities, business center, heated pools, lake, art exhibit, shopping.

Caesars Palace
♥♥♥♥♥

3570 Las Vegas Blvd. S., Las Vegas, NV 89109. Tel: (702) 731-7110. Fax: (702) 731-6636. TYPE: Deluxe Casino Resort & Spa. LOCATION: On the Las Vegas Stripe, 4 mi. / 6 km. to the airport. DESCRIPTION: Landmark casino resort with a roof garden Roman themed health spa, mud baths, mineral soaks, seaweed wraps, massage, sauna, jacuzzi. 2,360 rooms, 140 suites, nonsmoker rooms, wheelchair access, 9 restaurants & bars, 24 hr. coffee shop, lounge, entertainment, casino, meeting facilities, 2 heated pools, 6 tennis courts, Forum Shops. Hotel rates: from $110.

Cenegenics Anti-Aging enter
❤️❤️❤️❤️❤️

851 South Rampart Blvd., Las Vegas, NV 89128. Tel: (702) 240-4200. Toll Free (888) YOUNGER. Fax: (702) 240-7320. TYPE: Anti-Aging Center. LOCATION: Las Vegas. SPA CLIENTELE: Women and men. DESCRIPTION: Proactive medical facility dedicated to individual optimal health and anti-aging management. Treatment: Ceregenics therapies, human growth hormone (hGH); sex hormones and other hormonal supplements. Optimal nutritional programs are developed after extensive nutritional history and laboratory testing. The Cenegenics Anti-Aging Center can coordinate your exercise plan with a local fitness facility and a National Academy of Sports Medicine certified personal trainer. **Indications**: decreased energy level, reduced muscle strength, decreased sexual drive and performance, reduction in mental and visual acuity, lean muscle, changing body fat, hair loss, hair loss, reduced moisture content of the skin, osteoporosis.

Desert Inn Hotel & Casino
❤️❤️❤️❤️❤️

3145 Las Vegas Blvd. South, Las Vegas, NV 89109. Tel: (702) 733-4444 or USA (800) 634-6906. Fax: (702) 733-4676. TYPE: Deluxe Casino Resort & Spa. LOCATION: In the heart of the Las Vegas Strip, across the street from Fashion Show shopping Center, 5 min. from I - 15. SPA CLIENTELE: Women and men.

* Rooms: 715 w/priv. bath. Suites: 50
* Phone, CTV, A/C, wet bar, patio
* Casino, restaurants & grill rooms
* Crystal room: All Star Entertainment
* Airport: McCarran Int'l, 4 mi. (6 km.)
* Airport Transportation: taxi, limo

* Reservations: 1 night deposit req'd
* Credit Cards: MC/VISA/AMEX/DC/CB
* Open: Year round
* Hotel Rates: from $175; TAC: 10%
* Spa on premises: **The Desert Inn Spa**
* **Spa Facilities**: Hot, warm and cold spa pools, private whirlpools, turkish steam room, finnish sauna, beauty salon, spa gym & weight training center, cardiovascular fitness center, fitness track
* **Spa Programs**: fitness, nutrition, diet & beauty
* **Spa Treatments**: Hydrotherapy, salt glow body scrub, loofah body scrub, freshwater underwater massage; thermotherapy, fango therapy, hot herbal linen wrap; massages; skin care - treatment with non-allergenic 100% natural products; exercises - aerobics, stretch and water classes; calorie counted meals

DESCRIPTION: Upscaled, glamorous, Casino Hotel in the center of the Las Vegas Strip. The accommodations are superb, and there is plenty going on: entertainment, gambling, shopping and sports. The Desert Inn Spa was created to offer sophisticated, state-of-the-art facilities and that measure up to those found in Europe's finest health resorts. The Spa caters to men and women and offer a wide range of treatments and facilities to relax, shape up, revitalize, and rejuvenate the body and the spirit alike. The personnel at the Spa is well trained and personal attention is guaranteed. Special fitness or beauty programs can be recommended upon request. Recreation: tennis and golf.

Golden Nugget Hotel/Casino
❤️❤️❤️❤️❤️

129 E. Fremont Street, Las Vegas, NV 89125. Tel: (702) 385-7111. Toll Free (800) 634-3454. Fax: (702) 386-8362. TYPE: Hotel Complex & Spa. LOCATION: In the heart of Las Vegas Casino Center, 2 blocks from Union Plaza. SPA CLIENTELE: Women and men.

* Rooms: 1,907 w/private bath. Suites: 102
* Phone, CTV, A/C
* Casino, restaurants & coffee shops
* The Cabaret - spectacular nightclub
* Airport: McCarran AP, 8 mi. (13 km.)

* Airport Transportation: taxi, limo, bus
* Reservations: 1 night deposit req'd
* Credit Cards: AMEX/VISA/MC/DC/CB
* Open: Year round
* Hotel Rates: from $69
* TAC: 10% (room rate only)
* Spa on premises
* **Spa Facilities**: massage rooms, spa's float tank, steam bath, sauna, swedish showers, whirlpool bath, gymnasium, beauty salon, outdoor olympic size swimming pool & jacuzzi
* **Spa Programs**: fitness programs, beauty care for men and women, hair care, facials, massages
* Medical Supervision: MD on call

DESCRIPTION: Elegant Hotel & Casino with custom designed rooms and suites featuring the 'Golden Nugget Spa' - a luxurious fitness and beauty center for men and women. The Beauty Salon offers personal skin and hair care with the latest electronic equipment. The emphasis here is on body pampering in an atmosphere of total grandeur. Recreation: All star entertainment, casino, and gourmet dining in the 5 excellent hotel restaurants and the Coffee Shop.

Luxor Las Vegas
❤❤❤❤❤

3900 Las Vegas Blvd. S., Las Vegas, NV 89119-1000. Tel: (702) 262-4000, Fax: (702) 262-4405. TYPE: Mega Casino Resort & Spa. LOCATION: On the south Las Vegas Strip, 10 minutes to the airport. DESCRIPTION: Deluxe Egyptian-themed mega resort with 12,000 sq.ft / 1,090 sq.m Oasis Spa, beauty treatments, aromatherapy, massage, exercise equipment, whirlpool, sauna. 4,427 rooms & suites, 236 suite w/jacuzzi, nonsmoker rooms, wheelchair access. Restaurants (9), bars, lounges, casino, entertainment, Imax 3D theatre, meeting space, outdoor pool. Hotel rates: from $149.

MGM Grand Hotel/Casino
❤❤❤❤❤

3799 Las Vegas Blvd. S., Las Vegas, NV 89109. Tel:

(702) 891-1111. Fax: (702) 891-1112. TYPE: Mega Casino Resort & Spa. LOCATION: South Las Vegas Strip, 3 mi. / 5 km. to the airport. DESCRIPTION: Deluxe highrise mega resort hotel & casino with a Shangri-la pool and spa complex, heath club, gym, sauna, massage, steam room, jacuzzi. 4,254 rooms, 751 suites, nonsmoker rooms, wheelchair access. Restaurants (9), food court, lounges, entertainment, casino, meeting facilities, pools, MGM Grand Adventures Theme Park. Hotel price: from $89.

The Mirage
❤❤❤❤❤

3400 Las Vegas Blvd., So. Las Vegas, NV 89125. Tel: (702) 791-7111. Toll Free (800) 627-6667. Fax: (702) 791-7446. SPA - Tel: (702) 791-7472. TYPE: Casino Resort Hotel & Spa. LOCATION: Las Vegas Strip adjacent to the Caesars Palace. SPA CLIENTELE: Women and men. SPECIAL RESTRICTION: Children under 18 not permitted.

* Rooms: 3,044 w/priv. bath. Suites: 279
* 6 Lanai bungalows w/priv. garden & pool
* Phone, CTV, VCR, A/C, jacuzzi, bidet
* Restaurants, ballrooms & convention facilities
* Airport: McCarran AP 2 mi. / 3 km., taxi, limo
* Open: Year round
* Credit Cards: MC/VISA/AMEX/DC/CB
* Hotel Rates: from $89
* TAC: 10%
* Spa on premises
* **Spa Facilities**: separate men's and women's facilities, exercise room, aerobic studio, sauna, steam bath, beauty salon, co-ed weight training center
* **Spa Programs**: fitness, beauty, pampering
* **Spa Treatments**: aerobics, exercise, weight training, sauna, massages, tanning, beauty treatments

DESCRIPTION: The Mirage 31-story tower contains over 3,000 luxury rooms. The landscaping is a tropical fantasyland with lush gardens, lagoons, waterfalls and a simulated erupting volcano. The Spa at the Mirage features men's and women's facilities with a wide array of treatments and therapies for pampering and stress reduction.

Monte Carlo Resort & Casino
❤❤❤❤

3770 Las Vegas Blvd. S., Las Vegas, NV 89109. Tel: (702) 730-7000. Fax: (702) 730-7250. TYPE: Casino Resort & Spa. LOCATION: Southern Las Vegas Strip, 3.5 mi. / 6 km. to the airport. DESCRIPTION: Neo-classical resort and casino with health, whirlpool and sauna. 2,743 rooms, 259 suites, nonsmoker rooms, wheelchair access, variety of restaurants, pub & brewery, lounge, entertainment, casino, meeting rooms, pools, tennis courts (3). Hotel rates: from $69.

Treasure Island at The Mirage
❤❤❤❤❤

PO Box 7711, Las Vegas, NV 89177-0711. Tel: (702) 894-7111. Fax: (702) 894-7466. TYPE: Casino Hotel & Spa. LOCATION: Mid Las Vegas Strip, 4.5 mi. / 7 km. to airport. DESCRIPTION: Deluxe tower hotel & casino with full service health spa. Separate men's and women's spas and salon, saunas, steambaths, whirlpools, fitness, massage. 2,688 rooms, 212 suites, nonsmoker rooms, wheelchair access, 6 restaurants, bars, lounges, entertainment, casino, tropical pool, meeting facilities, wedding chapels (2). Hotel rates: from $69.

MESQUITE
🌙 702
✈ McCarran Int'l Airport (LAS), 43 mi. / 69 km. SW

CasaBlanca Resort Golf Spa
❤❤❤❤

950 West Mesquite Blvd., Mesquite, NV 89027. Tel: (702) 346-6760. Toll Free: (800) 459-PLAY. Fax: (702) 346-6777. TYPE: Casino Resort & Spa. LOCATION: Downtown Mesquite, 36 mi. / 58 km. from Lake Mead & Las Vegas. DESCRIPTION: Downtown casino resort with a co-ed full service health club & spa, soaking pools, inhalation steam room, exercise, body care, mudbaths, massage. 486 rooms, 18 suites, 4 detached 3-bedroom bungalows, nonsmoker rooms, wheelchair access, restaurant, coffee shop, lounge, entertainment, casino, ballroom, pool, tennis courts (3). Hotel rates: from $59.

RENO
🌙 775
✈ Reno Cannon Int'l Airport (RNO), 4 mi. / 6 km. SE

Silver Legacy
❤❤❤❤

407 N. Virginia St., PO Box 3920, Reno, NV 89501. Tel: (702) 329-4777. Fax: (702) 325-7474. TYPE: Casino Resort & Spa. LOCATION: In downtown Reno between 4th and 5th Streets. DESCRIPTION: Superior first class resort & casino with a full service health spa & salon. 1,563 rooms, 149 spa suites, 8 executive suites, nonsmoker rooms, wheelchair access. Restaurants (5), bars (3), entertainment, casino, meeting facilities, pool. Hotel rates: from $69.

NEW JERSEY

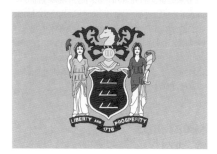

AREA: 7,787 sq. mi. (20,168 sq. km.)
POPULATION: 7,748,630
CAPITAL: Trenton
TIME ZONE: Eastern Time

ATLANTIC CITY
609

✈ Bader Municipal Airport (AIY), 1 mi. / 0.6 km. W
Atlantic City Int'l Airport, Pomona (ACY)
12 mi. / 19 km. NW

Atlantic City, population 40,000 was a sleepy fishing town and a seaside resort. Today it is the East Coast most popular Casino destination town with a lively casinos strip, boardwalk, sandy beaches, shopping and entertainment. Atlantic City is easily accessible by flights, cars or bus service from New York City or Philadelphia.

The Spa at Bally's Park Place
♥♥♥♥♥

Boardwalk & Park Place, Atlantic City, NJ 08401. Tel: (609) 340-2000. Toll Free (800) BALLYS7. Fax: (609) 340-4713. TYPE: Casino Hotel & Spa. LOCATION: Centrally located between Park Place and Michigan Avenue on 8.5 acres of oceanfront property along the Boardwalk. SPA CLIENTELE: Women and men.

* Rooms: 1,265 w/priv. bath. Suites: 110
* Phone, CTV, A/C, minibar

* Restaurants (9), lounges (2)
* Casino & cabaret with live entertainment
* Nearest Airport: Atlantic City
* Airport: 3 mi. / 5 km., limo, taxi
* Reservations: required
* Credit Cards: MC/VISA/AMEX/DC/CB
* Open: Year round
* Hotel Rates: from $135; TAC: 10%
* Spa on premises
* **Spa Facilities**: exercise room, sport courts, Olympic style swimming pool, whirlpool park with jacuzzis, sauna and inhalation room, massage rooms, massage and spa treatment area for handicapped members and guests, separate men and women's locker room area with spa facilities, MVP Suites, beauty salon
* **Spa Programs**: Individual Membership Corporate Membership program
* **Spa Treatments**: exercises, conditioning and stretching, Swiss needle showers, Swedish massages, herbal wraps, loofah treatments
* Medical Supervision: no, but a medical station is located at the hotel

DESCRIPTION: The elegant Bally Park Place Casino Hotel offers contemporary hotel rooms and lavish suites. The rooftop Spa, with great ocean views combines 40,000 sq. ft. / 3,636 sq. m. of health and fitness facilities on two levels. The emphasis is on fitness and pampering. The spa operates on membership basis, but hotel guests can use the facilities for an admission fee. Recreation: Casino, fine restaurants including the health oriented Spa Café, and live cabaret entertainment.

The Spa at Trump Plaza
♥♥♥♥♥

Mississippi Ave. & Boardwalk, Atlantic City, NJ 08401. Tel: (609) 441-6000. Toll Free (800) 677-7378. Fax: (609) 441-6917. TYPE: Casino Hotel & Spa. LOCATION: On the Boardwalk. SPA CLIENTELE: Women and men.

* Rooms: 1,395 w/ocean view. Suites:73
* Phone, CTV, A/C

* Casino, theatre, lounges, restaurants
* Airport: Atlantic City 3 mi. / 5 km., limo, taxi
* Open: Year round
* Credit Cards: MC/VISA/AMEX/DC
* Hotel Rates: from $90; TAC: 10%
* Spa on premises
* **Spa Facilities**: Health Spa with saunas, glass enclosed swimming pool, gym, beauty shop
* **Spa Treatments**: massage, herbal wrap, salt-glo loofah, facial and cosmetic treatments

DESCRIPTION: Trump Plaza is Atlantic City's tallest atrium hotel & casino complex at the center of the Boardwalk. All guest rooms have fine amenities and great ocean view. The Health Spa features a variety of fitness and pampering treatments.

LONG BRANCH
⟩ 732

✈ Newark Int'l Airport (EWR), 40 mi. / 64 km.

The Spa at Ocean Place Hilton Resort
❤❤❤❤

One Ocean Boulevard, Long Branch, NJ 07740, Tel: (732)

571-4000. Toll Free: 800-HILTONS. Fax: (732) 571-3314. TYPE: Resort & Spa Hotel. LOCATION: Overlooking the ocean. DESCRIPTION: Highrise resort hotel with a full service spa, European skin and body treatments, facials, detoxifying body masks, reflexology, thalassotherapy, 4 whirlpools, indoor & outdoor pools. 244 rooms, 5 suites, nonsmoker rooms, wheelchair access. Restaurants (2), sports lounge, piano bar, entertainment, meeting facilities, business center. Hotel rates: from $99.

SHORT HILLS
⟩ 973

✈ Newark Int'l Airport (EWR), 12 mi. / 19 km.

The Hilton at Short Hills
❤❤❤❤❤

41 John F. Kennedy Pkwy, Short Hills, NJ 07078. Tel: (973) 379-0100. Fax: (973) 379-6870. TYPE: Hotel & Spa. LOCATION: Opposite Short Hills Mall. DESCRIPTION: Deluxe hotel with a full service spa; massage, sauna, gym, indoor & outdoor pools, hair salon. 263 rooms, 37 suites, nonsmoker rooms, wheelchair access. Restaurants (3), lounge, entertainment, meeting facilities. Hotel rates: from $225.

NEW MEXICO

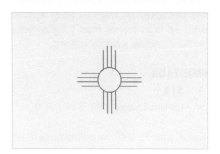

AREA: 7,787 sq. mi. (20,168 sq. km.)
POPULATION: 7,748,630
CAPITAL: Trenton
TIME ZONE: Eastern Time

GALISTEO
) 505
✈ Santa Fe's Municipal Airport (SAF)
33 mi. / 53 Km. East

Vista Clara Ranch Resort & Spa
❤❤❤❤

HC 75 Box 111 County Road 41, Galisteo, NM 87540.
Tel: (505) 466-4772. 888 NMEXSPA. Fax: (505) 466-
1942. TYPE:Resort & Spa. LOCATION: 20 minutes to
Santa Fe. DESCRIPTION: Full service 4-star resort and destination spa with 3, 5, and 7 night packages.

OJO CALLENTE
) 505
✈ Gallup's Municipal Airport (SAF), 50 mi. / 80 km.

Callenete Mineral Springs Spa
❤❤❤

PO Box 68, Ojo Callente, NM 87549. Tel: (505) 583-
2233. Toll Free: (800) 222-9162. Fax: (505) 583-
2464. TYPE: Mineral Springs Spa. DESCRIPTION: Mineral
spring pools, spa treatments, massage. 36 rooms.

SANTA FE
) 505
✈ Santa Fe's Municipal AP (SAF), 10 mi. / 16 km.

Ten Thousand Waves
❤❤❤

3451 Hyde Park Road, PO Box 10200, Santa Fe, NM
87504. Tel: (505) 982-9304. Fax: (505) 989-5077.
TYPE: Japanese Day Spa. YEAR ESTABLISHED: 1981. MAN-
AGING DIRECTOR: Duke Klauck. LOCATION: 3.5 mi. / 6
km. from downtown Santa Fe on Hyde Park Road, in the
Santa Fe Mountains. SPA CLIENTELE: Women and men.
Teenagers and children accepted. DESCRIPTION: Intimate
hotel with Japanese style treatments, facials, massage,
aquatic massage, hot tubs, sauna, east-indian treatments,
aromatherapy, salt glows, watsu. 8 rooms, 5 suites at the
Houses of the Moon.

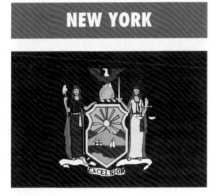

NEW YORK

AREA: 41,108 sq. mi. (127,190 sq. km.)
POPULATION: 18,045,000
CAPITAL: Albany
TIME ZONE: Eastern Time

BOLTON LANDING
518
✈ Albany County Airport (ALB) 60 mi. / 96 km.

The Sagamore
♥♥♥♥

110 Sagamore Rd., Bolton Landing, NY 12814. Tel: (518) 644-9400. Fax: (518) 644-2626. TYPE: Conference Center & Spa. LOCATION: In the Adirondack on Lake George. DESCRIPTION: Deluxe resort complex with complete spa and & fitness center, indoor pool. 220 rooms & 130 suites in main hotel & seven lodges, nonsmoker rooms, wheelchair access. Restaurants (5), lobby lounge, meeting rooms, tennis courts (7), 18-hole golf course. Hotel rates: from $99.

HUNTER
518
✈ Albany County Airport (ALB) 54 mi. / 86 km.
Stewart Int'l Airport, Newburgh, 80 mi. / 128 km.

Vatra Mountain Valley Lodge & Spa
♥♥♥

Route 214, Hunter, NY 12442. Tel: (518) 263-4919. (800) 232-2772. Fax: (518) 263-4994. TYPE: European Weight Loss Spa. LOCATION: In the Catskill Mountains. DESCRIPTION: Weight loss through vegetarian dieting and fitness programs, indoor & outdoor heated pools, tennis, massage and beauty treatments.

MONTAUK
516
✈ East Hampton Airport (HTO) 15 mi. / 24 Km.

Montauk, population 3,000, is a small fishing town at the easternmost tip of Long Island. The area including Amagansett and East Hampton is a favorite summer resort for affluent New Yorkers.

Guerney's Inn Resort & Spa
♥♥♥♥

Old Montauk Highway, Montauk, New York NY 11954. Tel: (516) 668-2345. Fax: (516) 668-3576. TYPE: Resort & Spa. LOCATION: On the Atlantic Ocean with private wide sandy beach. CLIENTELE: Women and men. RESTRICTIONS: Pets not allowed.

* Rooms: 128 w/priv. bath; Suites: 19; Cottages: 5
* Restaurant & spa dining room
* Train station: Montauk, 6 mi. / 10 km.
* Train Station Transportation: free pick up
* Credit Cards: MC/VISA/AMEX/DC/DIS
* Open: Year round
* Hotel Rates: from $245
* Spa on premises
* **Spa Facilities**: heated salt-water indoor pool, finnish rock saunas, russian steam-rooms, swiss showers, gym, full service beauty salon, physical therapy center
* **Spa Programs**: Rejuvenation, marine renewal, health & beauty, executive longevity, stress reduction
* **Spa Treatments**: Thalassotherapy, hydro relaxation, Italian fango packs, seaweed cell-fluid wrap, brush & tone therapy,herbal wrap, french vichy treatments, salt glow, norwegian sponge rub, massotherapy, swedish massage, lymph drainage (cosmetic), Aroma therapy, shiatsu therapy, roman baths, swiss showers,

group exercise, weight training, swimming, aerobics, calisthenics, slimnastics, cardiovascular exercises, marinotherapeutic services, reflexology, low calorie gourmet cuisine for weight loss, marinoVital nutritional supplements, stress reduction

* **Spa Package**: Rejuvenation Plan: Executive Longevity Program: Marine Renewal; Health & Beauty; Day of Beauty (ladies); Day of Vitality (men)
* **Indication**: revitalization, stress reduction, weight loss, beauty
* **Contraindications**: pregnancy, illness
* **Medical Supervision**: none; 3 RN one on duty

DESCRIPTION: Health & Beauty Spa and conference center. The resort consists of luxury accommodations with ocean view, some have private terraces. The European spa offers a wide selection of beauty, health and fitness treatments including thalassotherapy or marinotherapeutic treatments in sea water. A nutritionally balanced international cuisine is offered providing an average of 800 to 1200 calories for weight loss or weight maintenance . The spa cuisine is high in fibre, low in fat and cholesterol, sugar, salt and refined carbohydrates and strictly adheres to the Federal Government's dietary guide lines.

LAKE PLACID
✈ 518
✈ Saranac Lake Airport (SLK) 16 mi. / 26 km.

The Spa at The Mirror Lake Inn
❤❤❤❤

5 Mirror Lake Drive, Lake Placid, NY 12946, Tel: (518) 523-2544, Fax: (518) 523-2871. TYPE: Country Inn & Spa. LOCATION: North shore of Lake Mary, 2 blocks to Village center. DESCRIPTION: Historic Inn with health and beauty spa; seaweed collagen and salt treatments, facials, body nail and hair treatments, gym, sauna, jacuzzi. 128 rooms, nonsmoker rooms, wheelchair access, dining room, cafe, cocktail lounges (2), meeting rooms, outdoor pool, tennis court, private beach. Hotel rates: from $99.

NEVERSINK
✈ 914

✈ Stewart In'l Airport, Newburgh, 60 mi. / 96 km.

Neversink is a small village on the edge of the Catskill Forest Preserve. Here you can discover the serenity of country living, quaint villages and fine antique shops. The Catskill area offers year round recreational activities: hunting, trout fishing, hiking, and sightseeing. Neversink can be reached by car from New York City taking the I-87 north, then follow route 17 west to Exit 100 (Liberty). Neversink is about 9 mi. (14 km.) northeast of Liberty near the Rondout Reservoir. By bus, use the Short Line Terminal for Liberty. Driving time from New York City is about 2-1/2 hours.

New Age Health Spa
❤❤

Route 55, Neversink, NY 12765. Tel: (914) 985-7601, Toll Free (800) 682-4348. Fax: (914) 985-2467. TYPE: New Age Health Spa. MANAGER: Stephanie Paradise & Werner Mendel, Dir. LOCATION: The hills of the Catskill Mountains. SPA CLIENTELE: Women and men. SPECIAL RESTRICTIONS: No Smoking, no alcohol, no children, no pets.

* Rooms: 39 w/private bath
* No TV or phone in room
* Dining Room
* Airport: New York/Newark, 100 mi. (160 km.)
* Airport Transportation: limo, bus
* Reservations: 2 night deposit req'd
* Credit Cards: MC/VISA/AMEX
* Open: Year round
* Rates: from $199
* TAC: 10%
* Spa on premises
* **Spa Facilities**: indoor/outdoor pools, solarium, exercise/therapy rooms, beauty salon
* **Spa Programs**: Exercise, weight loss, beauty
* **Spa Treatments**: exercise, yoga, stretching, calisthenics, aerobics, weight training, massage: swedish, shiatsu, aquatics, Dead Sea mud treatments, reflexology, aromatherapy, facials, paraffin body treatments, herbal wraps, body

scrubs, fresh juice fasting, diets (350 -1,200 calories per day), low-cal vegetarian meals for non-fasters, chicken and fish available, colonic therapy
* Medical Supervision: Nurse on duty

DESCRIPTION: Casual new age retreat in the Catskill Mountains. Accommodations are rustic, but well appointed. The spa emphasizes holistic approach to health, fitness and beauty. The daily routine includes a check up at the nurse's office, meditation, exercise classes, power walking, hiking, fasting or low-cal meals, yoga meditation, and various daily lectures or workshops on topics of health, stress reduction, and nutrition.

NEW YORK CITY
) 212
✈ John F. Kennedy Int'l AP (JFK) 15 mi. / 9 km.
La Guardia Int'l AP (LGA) 8 mi. / 13 km.
Newark Int'l AP, NJ (EWR) 16 mi. / 26 km.
to Manhattan

The Barbizon Hotel
♥♥♥♥

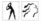

140 East 63rd St. New York, NY 10021. Tel: (212) 838-5700. Fax: (212) 888-4271. TYPE: Hotel & Spa. LOCATION: Fashionable Upper east side neighborhood near midtown. DESCRIPTION: First class new-classical landmark hotel with a full service spa & fitness center. 287 rooms, 20 suites, nonsmoker rooms, wheelchair access, dining room, lounge. Hotel rates: from $190.

Essex House - Hotel Niko
♥♥♥♥♥

160 Central Park South, New York, NY 10019, Tel: (212) 247-0300. Fax: (212) 315-1839. TYPE: Hotel & Spa. LOCATION: Midtown overlooking Central Park. DESCRIPTION: Deluxe midtown hotel with spa services, gym & sauna. 595 rooms, non smoker rooms, wheelchair access. Restaurants (2), bars, meeting facilities, business center. Hotel rates: from $295.

The Peninsula New York & Spa
♥♥♥♥♥

700 Fifth Avenue, 21st Floor, New York, NY 10019. Tel: (212) 903-3985. Toll Free (800) 262-9467. Fax: (212) 903-3859. TYPE: Hotel & Spa. LOCATION: Midtown, business, shopping, entertainment district. DESCRIPTION: Classic sophisticated deluxe hotel with spa & health club; beauty pampering & personalized fitness programs. 201 rooms, 42 suites w/jacuzzi & wetbar, nonsmoker rooms, wheelchair access, 2 restaurants, lounge, 3 bars, meeting facilities. Hotel rates: from $365.

SARATOGA SPRINGS
) 518
✈ Albany County Airport (ALB) 25 mi. / 40 km. S

Gideon Putnam Hotel
♥♥♥♥

Saratoga Spa State Park, PO Box 476, Saratoga Springs, NY 12866. Tel: (518) 584-3000, Fax: (518) 584-1354. TYPE: Resort Hotel. LOCATION: In Saratoga Spa State Park. DESCRIPTION: Resort hotel with spa services, massages and mineral baths provided at the nearby Lincoln Mineral Bath center (tel: 518-583-2880). 120 rooms, 12 suites, nonsmoker rooms, wheelchair access, dining room, cocktail parties, dancing, meeting facilities, business center, 27-holes of golf, 8 tennis courts. 3 pools. Hotel rates: from $99.

SHANDAKEN
) 518
✈ Albany County Airport (ALB) 54 mi. / 86 km. NE
Stewart Int'l Airport, Newburgh, 80 mi. / 128 km. S

Cooperhead Inn & Spa
♥♥♥♥

Route 28, Shandaken, NY 12480. Tel: (518) 688-2460. Fax: (518) 688-7484. LOCATION: Near Woodstock, NY. DESCRIPTION: European spa with herbal wraps massages, hydrotherapy, indoor pool, sauna, jacuzzis.

NORTH CAROLINA

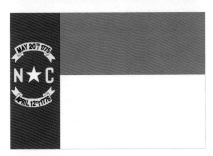

AREA: 52,669 sq. mi. (136,413 sq. km.)
POPULATION: 6,658,000
CAPITAL: Raleigh
TIME ZONE: Eastern Time

BLOWING ROCK
) 828

✈ Douglas Int'l Airport (CLT) Charlotte

Blowing Rock is a quaint mountain village with some of the finest naturescapes in America. Recreation: unique shops, restaurants, golf, skiing and horseback riding.

Westglow Spa
♥♥♥♥

2845 US Hwy 221 South, Blowing Rock, NC 28605. Tel: (828) 295-4463. Toll Free (800) 562-0807. Fax: (828) 295-5115. TYPE: Intimate Spa Retreat. SPA MANAGER: Mr. Mark Higby. LOCATION: Just outside Blowing Rock. SPA CLIENTELE: Women and men.

* Rooms: 7 w/priv. bath. Cottages: 2
* A/C, C/H, jacuzzi, restaurant
* Airport: Charlotte (NC)
* Train Station: Charlotte (NC)
* Airport/Train Transportation: taxi
* Reservations: required
* Credit Cards: VISA/MC
* Open: Year round

* Spa on premises
* Year Established: 1991
* **Spa Package Rates**: Day Packages $120-$250 Resort Package All-Inclusive Programs: High Season: April-October, Thanksgiving, Christmas, and New Year. Off Peak rates: November - March One Night Package: $330-$469; Two-Night Package $638-$918; Three-Night Package $836-$1,294; Four-Night Package $1,111-$1,714; Five-Night Package $1,364-$2,108; Six-Night Package $1,584-$2,464; Seven-Night Package $1,760-$2,772 price is per person single/double occupancy. Rates include spa services, sales tax and gratuities. Two-nights minimum on week-ends
* TAC: 10%
* **SPA Facilities**: Life Enhancement Center with the latest in advanced fitness and therapeutic spa equipment, indoor pool, whirlpools, wet/dry saunas, body treatment rooms, hair and nail salon, fitness center, aerobics studio, cardiovascular conditioning center
* **SPA Programs**: Day Spa; All Inclusive Spa Programs from one to seven night packages
* **Spa Treatments**: aromatherapy, body massage, herbal body wraps, Parisian body polish, detoxification treatment and lymphatic drainage massage, foot reflexology, upper back acne treatment, European facials, facial scar and brown spot treatment, manicure, pedicure, hair care, fitness and nutrition assessment, low fat cooking class, carnal sacral work, exercise, aerobics, supervised hikes in in the Blue Ridge Mountains.
* **Indications**: good health, diet, well being
* **Maximum Number of Guests**: 20
* **Email**: westglow@appstate.campus.mci.net
* **Web**: www.westglow.com

DESCRIPTION: Westglow Spa is an intimate spa retreat in an elegant mansion. Guests can enjoy beautifully restored guest rooms and cottages each unique in its design and vintage period furnishings. The Spas's Life Enhancement Center helps the guests with all the factors of good health, diet, physical activity, and emotional well being. Recreation: tennis, croquet, and nearby horseback riding. Westglow Spa pledges to become your favorite getaway for leisure, recreation and rejuvenation.

DURHAM

↷ 919

✈ Raleigh/Durham Airport (RDU) 13 mi. / 21 km.

Durham, population 100,000, owes much of its prosperity to the growth of the tobacco industry since the late 19th century. Today new economic sectors are rapidly replacing the tobacco industry. Durham places a priority in developing new educational, medical and research oriented services. The Durham County was elected to be the site of the Research Triangle Park. The Duke Medical Center and other fine medical institutes contribute to Durham's new reputation as the "City of Medicine". Duke University, founded in 1838, is an important university sprawling on 8,000 acres of green lawns and manicured gardens with a beautiful Gothic-style chapel.

Nearby Raleigh, is the state's historic capital and an important government and educational center. Both cities share the same airport - the Raleigh-Durham Airport which is located 15 miles (24 km.) northwest of Raleigh on US 70.

Duke University Diet & Fitness Center
❤❤❤❤

804 West Trinity Ave., Durham, N.C. 27701. Tel: (919) 684-6331. Fax: (919) 684-6176. TYPE: Diet & Fitness Medical Center. LOCATION: In mid-town Durham. SPA CLIENTELE: Women and men.

* Accommodations: not included
* Airport: Raleigh/Durham Airport, 20 minutes
* Airport Transportation: bus, taxi
* Reservations: required
* Credit Cards:MC/VISA/AMEX
* Open: Year round
* Rates: from $2,400 (2 week program)
* Complete Medical Center, dining facilities, large gym, indoor pool, beauty salon
* **Center Programs**: Diet & weight management, Lifestyle management, nutrition education, fitness, pulmonary rehab, diabetes mgmt.
* **Center Treatments**: special diets from 750

calories to 2,000 calories per day based on well-balanced low salt, low fat, and no sugar, exercises, therapeutic massages, acupressure, and physical therapy

* **Indications**: obesity, high blood pressure, high level of cholesterol, intestinal disorders, osteoporosis,
* Medical Supervision: 11 health professionals
* Treatments Approval: Medical Center

DESCRIPTION: Duke University Diet & Fitness Center offers medically supervised weight loss program for those who suffer from obesity and health related problems. Substantial weight loss can be achieved with a well balanced low calorie meals which are prescribed by a registered dietitian according to the needs of each individual. Daily exercise activities help burn fat. Nutritional education is provided to help participants achieve a better understanding of their diet needs in order to maintain a lasting weight-loss after they leave the center.

Structure House
❤❤❤❤

3017 Pickett Road, Durham, NC 27705. Tel: (919) 493-4205. Toll Free (800) 553-0052. Fax: (919) 490-0191. TYPE: Treatment, diet & fitness center. MANAGER: Gerard J. Musante, Ph. D. LOCATION: In Durham (NC), a mid sized urban center northwest of Raleigh (NC). SPA CLIENTELE: Women and men.

* Apartments: 74 fully furnished
* Phone, Voice Mail, CTV, A/C, Washer-Dryer
* Airport: Raleigh/Durham, 20 mi. / 32 km.
* Airport Transportation: private limo
* Reservations: $500 deposit required
* Credit Cards: VISA/MC
* Season: Year round
* Open: from $1000/wk all inclusive
* TAC: Negotiable
* **Center facilities**: Outdoor Facilities - recreation areas and trails; Indoor Facilities - gym, weight training room, exercise pool, massage facilities
* **Center Programs**: Weight loss, behavior modification, dietary re-education, exercise, health education

* Medical Supervision: 1 doctor, 2 nurses, psychotherapists, exercise physiologists, dietician, nutritionist, massage therapists. 35 treatment & support personnel
* Email: info@structurehouse.com
* Web: structurehouse.com

DESCRIPTION: The Structure House is an interconnected campus of apartments, health & fitness facilities and the gracious main Structure House. The weight loss program emphasizes and treats the psychological and physical causes of excess weight. The spa menu is based on a nutritional low sodium, low cholesterol meals, providing a total of 1,000 to 1,400 calories. Aqua aerobics are used for health improvement and decrease body fat. The recommended stay is 4 weeks.

LAKE TOXAWAY
☽ 828

✈ Ashville Airport, 50 mi. / 80 km.

The Spa at the Greystone Inn
❤❤❤❤

Greystone Lane, Lake Toxaway, NC 28747. Tel: (828) 966-4700. Toll Free: (800) 824-5766. Fax: (828) 862-5689. TYPE: Intimate Inn & Spa. LOCATION: On landscaped grounds off US HWY 64. DESCRIPTION: Carefully restored Inn with a complete spa. Treatments include massages, reflexology, aromatherapy, hair and skin care. 33 units, afternoon tea, restaurant, library lounge, meeting room, outdoor heated pool, 18-hole golf course, clay tennis courts (5), water sports. Hotel rates: $245.

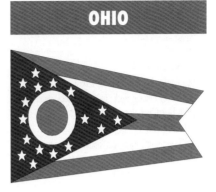

OHIO

AREA: 41,330 sq. mi. (107,045 sq. km.)
POPULATION: 10,887,325
CAPITAL: Cleveland
TIME ZONE: Eastern Time

AURORA
☽ 330

✈ Hopkin's Int'l Airport (CLE), 10 mi. / 16 km.

Aurora, population 8,700, is an urban community in northeastern Ohio just outside of Cleveland. The town preserves its heritage by imposing strict architectural standards on all new residential and commercial construction. Nearby Cleveland, population 574,000, is Ohio's largest city. Aurora can be reached by car from Cleveland via SR 43 southeast, then SR 82 east.

Mario's Int'l Spa & Hotel
❤❤❤

35 E. Garfield Road, Aurora, OH 44202. Tel: (330) 562-9171. Toll Free: (888) 464-7721. Fax: (330) 562-5380. TYPE: Spa Hotel. MANAGERS: Mario and Jo Ann Liuzzo (owners). LOCATION: Countryside location in Aurora (corner of SR 82 and SR 306). SPA CLIENTELE: Women and men. SPECIAL RESTRICTIONS: No children under 18.

* Rooms: 14 w/priv. bath
* Airport: Cleveland Hopkins 35 mi. / 56 km.
* Reservations: deposit required

* Credit Cards: MC/VISA/AMEX
* Open: Year round
* Rates: from $145
* TAC: 10%
* Spa on premises
* **Spa Facilities**: Finnish sauna, Turkish bath, hot tub, indoor running track, swimming pool, natural foods health bar, Beauty Salon
* **Spa Programs**: Beauty, Fitness & Weight Loss
* **Spa Treatments**: exercises, aerobics, aqua-fitness, massages, aromatherapy, thalassotherapy, dulse scrub, salt glo, body wrap

DESCRIPTION: Western reserve style victorian manor. Graciously decorated rooms with imported antiques. The co-ed spa program emphasizes fitness, stress reduction, relaxation and body pampering. Low-cal spa nouvelle cuisine (600-1000 calories per day) is available. *(Formerly: The Aurora House Spa).*

GRAND RAPIDS
) 419

 Toledo Express Airport (TOL), 17 mi. / 27 km.

Grand Rapids, population 1,000, is a small town on the Maumee River in northwestern Ohio. Extensive restoration is giving the village a turn of the century ambiance. Grand Rapids can be reached by car from Toledo (OH) driving southwest along the scenic Maumee River.

The Kerr House
♥♥♥

17777 Beaver St., Grand Rapids, OH 43522. Tel: (419) 832-1733. Fax: (419) 832-4303. TYPE: Spa Retreat.

MANAGER: Laurie Hostetler, Dir. LOCATION: In the tiny village of Grand Rapids, 38 mi / 61 km southwest of Toledo. SPA CLIENTELE: Mainly women; co-ed weeks, men only weeks and family weeks available.

* Rooms: 25; 5 w/private bath
* Cafe for Lunch & Formal Dining Room
* Airport: Toledo/Detroit Metro
* Distance to the Airport: 20 mi. (32 km.)
* Airport Transportation: Free Pick Up, limo
* Reservations: 50% deposit Required
* Credit Cards: MC/VISA/AMEX
* Open: Year round
* Rates: from $469
* TAC: 10%
* Spa on premises
* **Spa Facilities**: Whirlpool, sauna, massage area, beauty salon, exercise room
* **Spa Programs**: Holistic Program, Rejuvenation, Stress Management, Weight Loss & Beauty
* **Spa Treatments**: Hatha yoga exercises, stretching exercises, massage, facials, herbal wraps, mineral baths, low calorie meals (750 - 1,000 calories per day, no salt, fresh fruit & vegetables), kinesiology

DESCRIPTION: Victorian style restored mansion with elegant rooms, parlors and guest bedrooms decorated with antiques. The spa with its holistic approach, is owned and directed by Laurie Hostetler, a yoga instructor with 20 years of experience. The program is geared towards rejuvenation, stress reduction, weight loss, and body pampering Although the spa program is mostly tailored to the need of women, some men only weeks and family weeks are available. The entire facility and program can be reserved for a family, group of friends, or by a company (1-8 guests).

OREGON

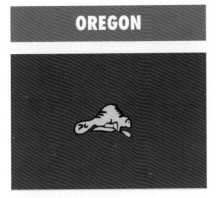

AREA: 97,073 sq. mi. (251,419 sq. km.)
POPULATION: 2,853,733
CAPITAL: Salem
TIME ZONE: Pacific Time

DETROIT
꜒ 503
✈ Salem Municipal Airport, 50 mi. / 80 km.

Breitenbush Hot Springs
♥♥♥

P.O. Box 578, Detroit, OR 97342. Tel: (503) 854-3314.

Fax: (503) 854-3819. TYPE: Rustic Hot-springs resort. LOCATION: In Oregon's Cascade Mountains. DESCRIPTION: Spa with hot spring baths, organic vegetarian cuisine, massage, yoga, guided meditations and hikes. 42 cabins, 10 tents.

WARM SPRINGS
꜒ 541
✈ Redmond Municipal Airport
34 mi. / 54 km.

Kah-Nee-Ta Resort
♥♥♥♥

PO Box K, Warm Springs, OR 97761. Tel: (541) 553-1112. Fax: (541) 553-1071. TYPE: First Class resort owned by the Confederated Tribes of Warm Springs. LOCATION: 11 mi. / 18 km. from Warm Springs, 1 hour from Redmond Airport. DESCRIPTION: First class resort owned by the Confederated Tribes of Warm Springs. Spa with mineral baths, gym, sauna, massage. 138 rooms, 11 suites, 20 tepees, nonsmoker rooms, wheelchair access. Restaurants (2), coffee shop, lounge, casino, meeting facilities, pools (2), 18-hole golf course, tennis courts (2). Hotel rates: from $95.

PENNSYLVANIA

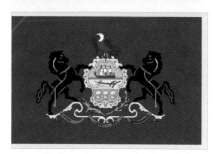

AREA: 45,308 sq. mi. (117,348 sq. km.)
POPULATION: 11,924,000
CAPITAL: Harrisburg
TIME ZONE: Eastern Time

EAST STROUDSBURG

⟩ 717

✈ Allentown/Bethlehem AP (ABE) 30 mi. / 48 km.

East Stroudsburg, population 8,000, is a year round resort in the Pocono Mountains of northeastern Pennsylvania. The Pocono Mountains is a scenic country with pine forests, blue lakes, deep canyons, and pure mountain air. East Stroudsburg can be reached from Philadelphia via SR 611 north. From New York City, take I-80 west to Stroudsburg.

Deerfield Manor
♥♥

🚶 ⊙

RD #1, (Rte. 402), E. Stroudsburg, PA 18301. Tel: (717) 223-0160. TYPE: Health Spa Retreat. MANAGER: Frieda Eisenkraft, Dir. LOCATION: In the Pocono Mountains. CLIENTELE: Women and men. SPECIAL RESTRICTIONS: Over 18 years. Pets not permitted on Spa grounds.

* Rooms: 22 w/private bath
* Airport: Allentown (PA) 1 hour drive, limo, bus
* Reservations: deposit required
* Credit Cards: MC/VISA/AMEX
* Open: April 20 - November 4

* Rates: from $795/week; TAC: 10%
* Spa on premises
* **Spa Facilities**: Heated outdoor swimming pool, gymnasium, Swedish Sauna, Massage Room
* **Spa Programs**: Weight loss & control. supervised diet plans; short period water fast, juice fast (350 calories/day), and low calorie diet (750 - 900 calories)
* **Spa Treatments**: diets, massage (Swedish, Shiatsu), aerobics, water exercises, body toning, walks, yoga, reflexology
* **Spa Packages**: Weekly, mini-week, and weekends

DESCRIPTION: Located in the scenic Pocono Mountains on 12 acres of landscaped woodland, Deerfield Manor specializes in a regimented weight reduction through water or juice only fasting, or a modified diet based on low calorie intake. It offers a stress free environment and provides the basics for weight loss and general fitness.

FARMINGTON

⟩ 724

✈ Pittsburgh Int'l Airport (PIT) 80 mi. / 130 km.

Farmington is a small town in the Laurel Mountains of PA, 13 mi. / 20 km. southeast of Uniontown on US 40. The region is known for its historic sites, national parks, antique shopping, factory outlets and year round retreats and resorts. **Fort Necessity National Battlefield** is a reconstructed fort near Farmington. The park offers picnic areas, and cross-country skiing trails for all class of skiers. Frank Lloyd Wright's Fallingwater, 10 mi. / 16 km. north of Farmington on RD 1.

Nemacolin Woodlands
♥♥♥

🚶 🎿

Route 40, Farmington, PA 15437. Tel: (724) 329-8555. Toll Free: (800) 422-2736. TYPE: Resort & Spa. LOCATION: In the Laurel Mountains (PA). SPA CLIENTELE: Women and men. SPECIAL RESTRICTIONS: No one admitted under 18.

* Rooms: 96 w/priv. bath. Suites: 20; Apartments: 58

* Airport: Pittsburgh, 80 mi. / 130 km.
  on location runway for small planes
* Transportation from Airport: bus
* Reservations: required
* Credit Cards: MC/VISA/AMEX
* Open: Year round
* Hotel Rates: from $119
* Spa on premises
* **Spa Facilities**: sauna, steam room, whirlpool,
  lap pool, weight, aerobic & massage rooms
* **Spa Programs**: Behavior modification, stress
  management, stop smoking
* **Spa Treatments**: fitness, beauty, pampering
* **Spa Packages**: 1, 3 and 6 day packages

DESCRIPTION: Historic resort with elegant rooms and condominium units with wood burning fireplace and fully
equipped kitchen. The Spa consists of a three story 20,000
sq.ft. / 1,818 sq.m. facility. For your dining needs there
are several restaurants including Allures serving low calorie
spa cuisine. Recreation: tennis, horseback riding, winter
skating, cross country skiing, and golf.

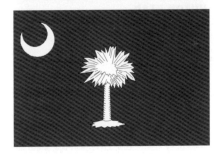

SOUTH CAROLINA

AREA: 31,113 sq. mi. (80,583 sq. km.)
POPULATION: 3,505,700
CAPITAL: Columbia
TIME ZONE: Eastern Time

CHARLESTON
☎ 843
✈ Charleston Int'l Airport (CHS) 13 mi. / 21 km.

Charles Harbor Hilton Resort
♥♥♥♥

20 Patriot's Point Rd, Mt. Pleasant, SC 29464. Tel: (843)
856-0028. Fax: (843) 856-0028. TYPE: Hotel & Spa.
LOCATION: On Charleston Harbor across from downtown
Charleston. DESCRIPTION: New classic southern-style resort
hotel with full service spa and exercise room. 125 rooms,
6 suites, restaurant, bar & lounge, entertainment, meeting
facilities, business services, 18-hole golf course, beach,
pool. Hotel rates: from $109.

Woodlands Resort Inn
♥♥♥♥

125 Parsons Road, Summerville, SC 29483. Tel: (843)
875-2600. Fax: (843) 875-2603. TYPE: Hotel & Spa.
LOCATION: In Summerville, 15 mi. / 24 km. to Charleston
Int'l Airport, 28 mi. / 45 km. to downtown Charleston.
DESCRIPTION: Superior first class stately manor house and
spa with massage therapy, body treatments & nail care. 20

rooms, nonsmoking policy, restaurant, bar, meeting rooms, outdoor pool, 2 tennis courts. Hotel rates: from $225.

HILTON HEAD
✈ 843

✈ Municipal Airport (HHH)
Savannah Int'l Airport, GA (SAV) 35 mi. / 56 km.

Hilton Head, population 18,000, is a year round resort island, known for its fine beaches, unpolluted marine inlet, and a pleasant climate. The island is located just off the southern coast of South Carolina. Although, the island was inhabited by Indians some 3,800 years ago, it was not until the mid 1950's that the island went through a rapid development. Today, it is a popular resort with beautiful marinas, manicured gardens, luxury condominiums, retirement villas, fine restaurants, & shops. Sports and recreation: golf, tennis, biking, horseback riding, deep sea fishing. Nature lovers can enjoy a walk through nature preserves at the Sea Pine Plantation. Hilton Head Island is accessible via US 278.

Hilton Head Health Institute
❤❤❤❤

14 Valencia Road, Hilton Head Island, SC 29928. Tel: (843) 785-7292. Toll Free (800) 292-2440. Fax: (843) 686-5659. TYPE: Health & Fitness Institute. LOCATION: A resort island off southeast corner of South Carolina, about 1 hour drive north of Savannah (GA). SPA CLIENTELE: Women and men. SPECIAL RESTRICTIONS: Minimum age 18 to participate in the programs.

* Rooms: 45 w/private bath in 20 cottages w/cooking facilities
* Airport: Hilton Head, 6 mi. (10 km.)
* Airport Transportation: taxi, limo
* Reservations: deposit required
* Credit Cards: MC/VISA
* Open: Year round
* Rates: from $2,300 (6 nts); rates Include: room,

food, medical screening, health seminars, exercise, and treatments
* TAC: 10%
* Spa on premises
* **Spa Facilities**: Indoor & outdoor facilities
* **Spa Programs**: Health & weight control (12 or 26 days)
* **Spa Treatments**: Nutritional planning, low calorie meals, exercises, low impact aerobics, calisthenics, aqua exercises,health education, stress management, decrease dependency on medications, smoking & drinking.
* **Indications**: obesity, health promotion, behavior modification, cholesterol reduction, lower blood pressure
* **Contraindications**: none
* Medical Supervision: 1 MD, 1 RN

DESCRIPTION: The Hilton Head Health Institute is geared toward long-term education rather than temporary changes in weight, appearance and behavior. It is directed by Peter M. Miller Ph. D. an expert in habit control and self-management. The Institute is located at The Cottages in Shipyard Plantation. Clients participating in the program can choose between an informal campus-like setting accommodations or luxuriously appointed villas. The programs are medically supervised and tailored to the needs of each individual.

Hyatt Regency Hilton Head Resort
❤❤❤❤❤

1 Hyatt Circle, PO Box 6167, Palmetto Dunes, SC 29938. Tel: (843) 785-1234. Fax: (843) 842-4695. TYPE: Deluxe golf & tennis resort. LOCATION: On the Atlantic oceanfront. DESCRIPTION: Golf & tennis resort with complete spa & fitness center, jogging, bicycling. 448 rooms, 26 Regency rooms, 31 suites, nonsmoker rooms, wheelchair access. Restaurants (5), lounges, bars, meeting facilities, pools, tennis center, 90-holes of golf, beach, deep sea fishing. Hotel rates: from $125.

TENNESSEE

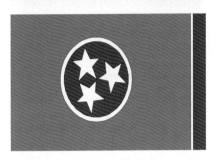

AREA: 42,144 sq. mi. (109,153 sq. km.)
POPULATION: 4,896,640
CAPITAL: Memphis
TIME ZONE: Eastern/Central Time

WAYNESBORO
ↄ 931

✈ Memphis Int'l Airport (MEM)

Waynesboro is in south central Tennessee east of Memphis and southwest of Nashville, near the Natchez Trace Parkway.

Tennessee Fitness Spa
❤❤❤

299 Natural Bridge Park Road, Waynesboro, TN 38485. Tel: (931) 722-5589. Toll Free: (800) 235-8365, Fax: (931) 722-9113. TYPE: Fitness spa. DESCRIPTION: Spa specializes in weight loss and fitness, Low fat nutrition program, massage, herbal wraps, beauty shop, cardiovascular & circuit training equipment. 30 rooms, heated indoor pool.

TEXAS

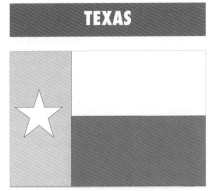

AREA: 266,807 sq. mi. (691,030 sq. km.)
POPULATION: 17,059,805
CAPITAL: Austin
TIME ZONE: Central Time

ARLINGTON
ↄ 817

✈ Dallas/Ft. Worth Int'l Airport (DFW) 20 mi.
(32 km.) NE or Arlington

Arlington, population 160,000, is located between two major cities: Dallas and Fort Worth. This particular location makes it an ideal base to explore the elegant shopping centers and historical sites of both cities. Arlington is mostly known for its huge entertainment center - Six Flags Over Texas, featuring historic themes of Texas under flags of Spain, France, Mexico, the Republic of Texas.

The Greenhouse
❤❤❤❤❤

P.O. Box 1144, Arlington, TX 76010. Tel: (817) 640-4000. Fax: (817) 649-0422. TYPE: Luxury Spa. LOCATION: On beautifully landscaped property. SPA CLIENTELE: Women only. SPECIAL RESTRICTIONS: No alcohol.

* Rooms: 37 w/priv. bath. Suites: 2
* Phone, CTV, A/C
* Dining Room
* Airport: DFW Airport, 20 mi. (32 km.)

* Airport Transportation: Free Pick Up
* Reservations: $500 deposit Required
* Credit Cards: MC/VISA/AMEX/NEIMAN MARCUS
* Open: Year round (closed 2 wks. in summer and 2 wks. in winter)
* Rates: from $3,225 week (Sun-Sun), rates include accommodations, meals, programs, treatments and use of Spa facilities; TAC: 10%
* **Spa Facilities**: Indoor swimming & exercise pool, solarium, sauna, whirlpool, beauty department
* **Spa Programs**: Health, beauty, weight loss
* **Spa Treatments**: exercises, aerobics, facials, massages, sauna & whirlpool baths, loofah baths, beauty care, basic skin care, daily facial massage, hair treatments, diet meals
* Medical Supervision: 1 MD, 2 RN
* Number of Customers per Doctor: 40
* Treatments Approved by Medical/Professional Assoc.

DESCRIPTION: Luxurious Spa retreat for women only. Deluxe accommodations are stylishly designed and deco-rated to provide total comfort, quiet and relaxation. Public spaces are tastefully and lavishly decorated with objets d'art, classic design and a lush array of tropical greenery. The Spa program emphasizes fitness, exercises, beauty care and pampering. Women who wish to loose weight can enjoy the specially prepared low calorie gourmet meals.

AUSTIN

⟩ 512

✈ Robert Mueller Municipal AP (AUS) 4 mi. / 6 km.

Austin, population 350,000, is the capital of Texas and an important education, research and governmental center. It is a fast moving, fun-loving city with a flare for health and sports. Its location is in the heart of Texas, on the Highland Lakes chain with the beautiful Lake Austin and Town Lake quietly flowing through the town.

Barton Creek Conference Resort
♥♥♥♥♥

🏃 🦌

8212 Barton Club Drive, Austin, TX 78735. Tel: (512) 329-4000, Fax: (512) 329-4597. TYPE: Spa Hotel &

Conference center. LOCATION: In Texas Hill Country, 15 minutes to downtown. DESCRIPTION: Stylish spa hotel with spa center and health & beauty treatments. 143 rooms, 4 suites, nonsmoker rooms, wheelchair access. Restaurants (6), lounge meeting facilities, business center 54-holes of golf. 12 tennis courts. pro shop, indoor/outdoor pools.

Lake Austin Resort
♥♥♥♥

1705 S. Quinlan Park Road, Austin, TX 78732. Tel: (512)266-2444. Toll Free (800) 847-5637. Fax: (512) 266-4386. TYPE: Health & Fitness Resort. LOCATION: On the shore of Lake Austin off F.M. 620. SPA CLIENTELE: Women and men. SPECIAL RESTRICTIONS: Age limit 14 years or older.

* Rooms: 40 w/private bath
* Phone, CTV, A/C, hair dryer
* Airport: Robert Mueller AIRPORT, 18 mi. / 29 km.
* Airport Transportation: courtesy transportation
* Reservations: deposit required
* Credit Cards: AMEX/VISA/MC
* Open: January 1 - December 24
* Hotel Rates: from $250; TAC: 10%
* Spa on premises
* **Spa Facilities**: Indoor and outdoor pools, jacuzzi, weight room, sports field, paddleboats, granite walking/jogging trail
* **Spa Programs**: Improvement in fitness, nutrition & self image.
* **Spa Treatments**: full range of movement & exercise, water toning & water aerobics, nutrition counselling, complex carbohydrate menus (900 - 1,200 calories), complete beauty services, European facials, skin analysis, massages
* Medical Supervision: 1 RN, 1 LUN, MD on call

DESCRIPTION: Wellness oriented health resort with accom-modations ranging from standard to deluxe rooms. Pro-grams are designed to meet the needs of the fitness and nutrition minded individuals. The fitness program offers 16 physical fitness classes daily. The nutrition program is sup-plemented with low fat cooking classes featuring guest chefs. Daily lifestyle enrichment programs include subjects ranging from behavior modification to fine arts.

DALLAS
ꓕ 214 / 972

✈ Dallas/Ft. Worth Int'l AP (DFW) 13 mi. / 20 km. Love Field Airport (DAL) 6 mi. / 10 km.

Dallas, population one million plus, is one of the country's most artistically and cuturally inclined cities, The Opera and Symphony Orchestra are the finest in the USA. The city has a striking furtistic style with many tall blue-tinted glass covered office buildings and hotels. The Galleria mall with over 200 shops offers fine luxury shopping.

The Spa at The Cooper Aerobics Center
❤❤❤

12100 Preston Rd., Dallas, TX 75230. Tel: (972) 392-7729. Toll Free (888) 964-8875. Fax: (972) 788-2056. TYPE: Day Spa and Fitness Center. LOCATION: North Dallas, on Preston Road, between LBJ Freeway (635) and Forest Lane. SPA DIRECTOR: Anne Witte. SPA CLIENTELE: Men, women, children 13 and over.

* The Guest Lodge: 50 rooms, 12 suites, on premises
* Phone, CTV, A/C, C/H
* Two Restaurants, Meeting Facilities
* Airport: Love Field and Dallas/Ft. Worth Int'l
* Reservations: Required
* Credit Cards: AMEX/VISA/MC/DIS
* Season: Year round
* Spa Rates: Based on individual needs, for rates and Cooper Wellness video Tel: (800) 444-5192
* Spa on premises
* **Spa Facilities:** Eight treatment rooms and salon; sauna, steam room and whirlpool in both men and womens locker rooms; indoor and outdoor track, two heated outdoor pools; group exercise classes (yoga, tai chi, pilates), cardiovascular and elliptical equipment, Cybex strength training equipment and free weights; Personal trainers, boxing, tennis, basketball, martial arts and nutrition counseling

* **Spa Packages:** Earth and Sea Sensation, Rain Forest Rejuvenator, Mediterranean Meditation, or Individualized Package. Gift certificates available
* **Spa Treatments:** Skin care facials, waxing, massage therapy, body cleansing and exfoliation, body wraps, cool gel masque, seaweed masque, Italian fango, Dead Sea fango, manicure, pedicure, acrylics and wraps, paraffin treatments
* **Spa Programs:** The Cooper Wellness Program developed by Dr. Kenneth H. Cooper for serious rejuvenation, fitness and good heath, or tailored programs for permanent, life-enhancing changes

DESCRIPTION: The spa is located on the 30-acre Cooper Aerobics Center campus in North Dallas known worldwide for its fitness center, preventive medicine and research. The Mediterranean style spa provides spacious accommodations in two levels. The spa details present a first class elegant environment for men and women.

Wyndham Anatole Hotel
❤❤❤❤❤

2201 Stemmons Freeway, Dallas, TX 75207. Tel: (214) 748-1200. Fax: (214) 761-7520. TYPE: Hotel & Spa. LOCATION: 5 minutes to the business district, 20 minutes to DFW Airport. DESCRIPTION: Moderate deluxe hotel featuring spa with complete services and Sports center with 8 racquetball, 6 tennis, 2 squash courts, indoor & outdoor pools, gym, sauna, jogging track. 1,475 rooms, 145 suites, nonsmoker rooms, wheelchair access. Restaurants (5), coffee shop, nightclub, meeting facilities, business center. Hotel rates: from $229.

Four Seasons Resort & Club
❤❤❤❤❤

4150 N. MacArthur Blvd., Irving, TX 75038. Tel: (972) 717-0700. Toll Free (800) 332-3442. Fax: (972) 717-2486. TYPE: Deluxe Resort Hotel & Spa. LOCATION: 8 mi. / 13 km. to DFW Airport. DESCRIPTION: Impressive resort hotel in the Dallas International airport area with full service European spa and emphasis on fitness. 362 rooms, 13 suites, 2 executive villas, nonsmoker rooms, wheelchair access. Restaurants (3), cafe bar, meeting facilities, business center, 18-hole golf course, tennis courts (12), pools (4). Hotel rates: from $275.

HOUSTON
⌐ 713
✈ G. B. Intercontinental AP (IAH) 20 mi. / 32 km.
Hobby Airport (HOU) 10 mi. / 16 km.

Houston, population 1,500,000, is a fast growing metropolis and major shipping port on the Buffalo Bayou, a part of a man-made waterway leading to the Gulf of Mexico. It is an important cultural center for the performing arts with fine theatrical productions, thriving night life and elegant shopping centers.

The Spa at The Houstonian
❤❤❤❤❤

111 North Post Oak Lane, Houston, TX 77024. Tel: (713) 685-6718. Fax: (713) 680-0626. TYPE: Health Spa. LOCATION: On the grounds of the Houstonian Hotel Club, within 5 mi. (8 km.) of The Galleria; 10 mi. (16 km.) of downtown, museum & art districts; 25 mi. (40 km.) from Johnson Space Center and Medical Center. SPA CLIENTELE: Women only. (1st wk of each month open for couples).

* Rooms: 15 w/private bath
* Phone, CTV, A/C, hair dryer
* Airport: Houston Int'l / Hobby AP, 20 mi. (32 km.)
* Airport Transportation: free pick-up, limo
* Reservations: $1,000 deposit required
* Credit Cards: AMEX/VISA/MC/DC
* Open: Year round
* Rates: $2100-$2500; TAC: 10%
* Spa on premises: Day Spa
* **Spa Facilities**: exercise studios, weight equipment, gym, olympic heated pool, whirlpool, sauna, steam and swedish shower, 8 racquetball, 5 tennis courts,
* **Spa Programs**: The Ultimate Week, six exercise classes, 1,000 calorie/day gourmet meals, body massages, beauty treatments; Fitness Week Plus - exercise, meals, massage & beauty treatments, yoga, tai-chi and relaxation classes

* Medical Supervision: complete medical services available (not included in program); nutritionists, G.P., Psychiatrists, Plastic and Orthopedic Surgeons; Eating Disorder Specialist.

DESCRIPTION: A small mansion converted into Spa on 22 wooded acres right in the heart of Houston. The Spa maintains the quality of its services by limiting the number of participating guests to 15 per week. As a part of the Houstonian Medical Center - a respected health and fitness center, it offers individual treatment programs combining diet, exercise, behavior modification and physical examination.

The Woodlands Executive Conference Center & Resort
❤❤❤❤

2301 N. Millbend Drive, Woodlands, TX 77380, Tel: (713) 367-1100 Fax: (713) 364-6338. TYPE: Superior first class Rustic Lodge & Conference Center. LOCATION: On 25,000 forested acres, 18 miles to Houston Intercontinental Airport. DESCRIPTION: Superior first class rustic lodge & conference center with complete spa facilities; Roman & Japanese baths. 191 room, 77 suites, nonsmoker rooms, wheelchair access. Restaurants (5), bars (5), meeting facilities, business center, outdoor pool, 36 holes of golf, 24 tennis courts.

SAN ANTONIO
⌐ 210
✈ San Antonio Int'l Airport (SAT) 8.5 mi. / 13.6 km.

Alamo Plaza Spa, The Menger Hotel
❤❤❤❤

204 Alamo Plaza, San Antonio, TX 78205. Tel: (210) 223-5772. Fax: (210) 228-0022. TYPE: Hotel & Spa. LOCATION In Alamo Plaza Park adjacent to Rivercenter Mall & River Walk. DESCRIPTION: 19th century style first class historic hotel with full service spa for relaxation, reflection and revitalization. 300 rooms, 20 suites, nonsmoker rooms, wheelchair access, restaurant, lounge bar, meeting facilities, outdoor pool, jacuzzi. Hotel rates: from $129.

UTAH

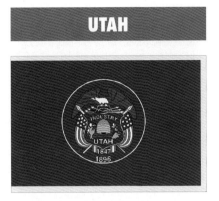

AREA: 56,345 sq. mi. (145,934 sq. km.)
POPULATION: 11,466,682
CAPITAL: Chicago
TIME ZONE: Central Time

HURRICANE
) **435**
✈ Municipal Airport (SGU)

Pah Tempe Hot Springs Resort
♥♥

825 North 800 East, Hurricane, UT 84737. Tel: (435) 635-2879. Toll Free: (888) 726-8367. Fax: (435) 635-2353. TYPE: Bed & Breakfast & Hot Springs. LOCATION: On the Virgin River. Description: 3 natural cliff side soaking pools, swimming pool, private massage and jacuzzi rooms.

IVINS
) **435**
✈ Municipal Airport (SGU)

Red Mountain Spa
♥♥♥

202 N. Snow Canyon Rd., Box 380938, Ivins, UT 84738. Tel: (435) 673-4905. Toll Free: (800)407-3002. Fax: (435) 673- 1363. TYPE: Fitness Resort. LOCATION: Base

of Snow Canyon 10 mi. / 16 km. north of St. George, and about 2 hours drive northeast of Las Vegas (NV). SPA CLIENTELE: Women and men. SPECIAL RESTRICTIONS: Guests must be 18 or older. No wheelchair access facilities available.

* Rooms: 52; 48 w/private bath
* Phone, CTV, A/C, C/H
* Airport: St. George (UT) 9 mi. / 14 km.
* Airport Transportation: free Shuttle van
* Reservations: deposit required
* Credit Cards: MC/VISA
* Open: Year round
* Length of Stay: Monday-Sunday (one week)
* Rates: from $794/week
* TAC: 10%
* Spa on premises
* Year Established: 1974
* **Spa Facilities**: Racquetball court, tennis court, aerobic dance floor/gymnasium, indoor heated pool, weight training equipment
* **Spa Programs**: Fitness, weight loss, low fat cooking, lectures on health, stress reduction
* **Spa Treatments**: aerobics, step aerobics, body toning, stretch, yoga, aquacize, vigorous walking, jogging, bicycling, weight training, low-fat high fiber diet, swedish massages, European facials, aromatherapy; full service beauty salon
* **Indications**: obesity, stress, physical fitness, stabilize blood sugar, lower cholesterol, lower blood pressure
* Medical Supervision: 4 RN
* Documentation from Physician: not required, but suggested for those who may be limited from fitness activities
* Maximum number of guest: 145

DESCRIPTION: Fitness and health education resort built in futuristic design emphasizing life-style changes with a low-fat nutrition program and a variety of supervised physical activities. The average stay at the Spa is 4.5 weeks. The expected average weight loss is a pound per day for men, and about 1/2 pound a day for women. (Formerly Franklin Quest Institute of Fitness and Formerly National Institute of Fitness).

ST. GEORGE
꒭ 435
✈ Municipal Airport (SGU), 1 mi. / 0.6 km. West

St. George, population 13,200, lies in the southwestern rugged desert corner of Utah at an elevation of 2,800 ft. (850 m.). This corner of southern Utah is blessed with scenic beauty and attracts tourism from the US and overseas. The climate is mild and pleasant year round, though summers can be hot. St. George is located 120 mi. / 192 km. northeast of Las Vegas (NV), and 300 mi. / 480 km. southwest of Salt Lake City.

Green Valley Spa
Tennis & Fitness Resort
❤❤❤❤

1515 W. Canyon View Dr., St. George, UT 84770. Tel: (801) 628-8060. Toll Free (800) 237-1068. Fax: (801) 673-4084. TYPE: Resort & Spa. LOCATION: In the Green Valley area of St. George. SPA CLIENTELE: Women and men, family oriented. SPECIAL RESTRICTIONS: Must be 18 years or older to use the spa.

* Suites: 50 1-to-3 bedroom condos
* Phone, CTV, A/C, kitchen, balcony
* Spa dining room
* Airport: St. George Municipal, 6 mi. / 10 km.
* Airport Transportation: free pick up
* Reservations: deposit required
* Credit Cards: MC/VISA
* Open: Year round
* Hotel rates: from $110
* Spa Rates: from $1,795 (7 days)
* TAC: 10%
* Spa on premises
* **Spa Facilities**: Fitness, stress control, and weight loss clinic, Olympic-style pool, lap pool, jacuzzi, exercise studio, aerobic room, yoga room, spa & beauty center based on herbal and natural products.
* **Spa Programs**: Weight loss, fitness - exercise, beauty/pampering, cellulite reduction
* **Spa Treatments**: aerobics, brisk walks in the red rock canyons, aquacise, yoga, meditation, stretch and

tone, one on one training in the weight room, lap swimming, diet counseling, cooking classes, stress management classes, exercise counselling and body fat evaluation, massages, head and shoulder facial, foot reflexology, aroma water therapy, pear body rubs, herbal wraps
* **Indication**: exercise, diet, and stress control
* Medical Supervision: 2 RN, and 1 exercise physiologist

DESCRIPTION: Nestled among the red rocks of southern Utah, Green Valley is a desert resort and health center. The Spa accepts 20 guests per week to insure personalized attention and quality service. The spa offers a "no-diet" program for weight loss that teaches how to control your set point with exercise, correct nutrition and addiction control. Another program 'Adventure Bound' is offered for the very fit who prefer outdoor workout.

PARK CITY
꒭ 435
✈ Salt Lake City Airport (SLC), 35 mi. / 56 km.

Park City, population 3,000, is an historic silver mining village which was founded in the late 19th century. Park City is experiencing a new revival as a 'Four Season' resort thanks to the sophisticated, world class ski area in Deer Valley about 10 minutes drive from Park City. Deer Valley offers first class skiing facilities, luxurious resort accommodations and gourmet dining and it a favorite resort for many celebrities and jet setters.Deer Valley is located near Park City and is accessible by car from Salt Lake City, driving time is about 45 minutes.

Stein Eriksen Lodge
❤❤❤❤❤

P.O. Box 3779, Park City, UT 84060. Tel: (435) 649-3700. Toll Free (800) 453-1302. Fax: (435) 649-5825. TYPE: Ski Resort & Spa. LOCATION: Heart of the Deer Valley Resort, in Park City (UT). SPA CLIENTELE: Women and men, mostly corporate executives and their wives.

* Rooms: 120 w/priv. bath. Suites: 50
* Restaurants, games & recreation lounge

* Airport: Salt Lake City 30 mi. / 48 km., taxi
* Reservations: 1 day deposit req'd
* Credit Cards: AMEX/VISA/MC/CB/DC
* Open: Year round
* Hotel Rates: from $175
* TAC: 10%
* Spa on premises
* **Spa Facilities**: Outdoor heated pool; Indoor pool, hot tub, jacuzzi, sauna, well equipped exercise and weight room, gym, massage rooms, sun terrace
* **Spa Programs**: 7 day program of diet, exercise & beauty in the Summer.
* **Spa Treatments**: sauna, jacuzzi, hot tubs, exercise, weights, massages

DESCRIPTION: Rustic ski lodge with Scandinavian ambiance. All the units are beautifully appointed with designer furnishings. During the summer the hotel caters mainly to corporate executives and conventions. Exercise instructors are available for workout in the Health Spa which specializes in fitness and sports. Recreation: skiing, golf and tennis.

SNOWBIRD
ꀯ 435

✈ Salt Lake City Int'l Airport (SLC) 30 mi. (48 km.)

Snowbird is a year round mountain resort and a major ski area in Little Cottonwood Canyon. The resort lies in high altitude of 7,900 - 11,000 ft. (2,408 - 3,352 m.) and offers excellent amenities for skiing. Salt Lake City is only 25 mi. / 40 km. northwest.

The Cliff Lodge & Spa
❤❤❤❤

P.O. Box 92900 Snowbird, UT 84092. Tel: (801) 933-2225 ext: 5900 Fax: (801) 933-2283. TYPE: Spa & Fitness Resort. SPA DIRECTOR: Paul Wright. LOCATION: 25 mi. (40 km.) southeast of Salt Lake City on UT 210 in Little Cottonwood Canyon at an altitude of 7,900 - 11,000 ft. (2,400 - 3,350 m.) SPA CLIENTELE: Women and men.

* Accommodations: The Cliff Lodge, 532 rooms Tel: (800) 895-9090 or (801) 742-2222.
* Reservations: 50% deposit
* Credit Cards: AMEX/VISA/MC/DISC
* Open: Year round
* Rates: $88 -$380/day (room only)
* SPA Program rates: Single Day packages $160 - $ 285; Multi-Day Packages $878 - $2,003 (including accommodations and treatments)
* TAC: 10%
* **Spa Facilities**: heated pool; steam room, beauty salon, sauna, solarium, aerobic room, weight & stretching room, whirlpool, café serving healthful fare
* **Spa Programs**: Exercise, Stretch "Met" Program (Movement Energy Therapy), Yoga, Massage, Beauty & Skin Care, Personal Training
* **Spa Treatments**: therapeutic massages, hydro massage, herbal wraps, mud baths, balneotherapy, salt glows, skin nail & hair care
* **Contraindications**: Persons with heart, respiratory or hypertension conditions should take precautions due to the high altitude.
* **Special Restrictions**: Smoking is not permitted, children under 18 are not permitted in the Spa.
* E-Mail: pwright@snowbird.com
* Web: http://www.snowbird.com

DESCRIPTION: The Cliff Spa offers a unique resort spa experience in a pristine alpine setting. Spa programs emphasize Health, Fitness & Beauty. Guests may make a single a la carte choice or enroll in half-day, full-day, or several day packaged programs. Spa Plans include all Spa services plus 3 Spa meals a day featuring low fat, low cholesterol dishes, and a personal fitness consultation. Recreation: skiing, golfing, tennis, summer dance festival, concerts and Octoberfest. Supervised children's camp is available for kids five and up.

VERMONT

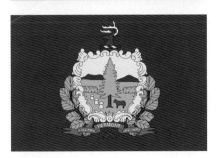

AREA: 9,614 sq. mi. (24,900 sq. km.)
POPULATION: 564,964
CAPITAL: Montpelier
TIME ZONE: Eastern Time

KILLINGTON SKI AREA
↷ 802

 Rutland Airport (RUT) 17 mi. / 27 km.

The Killington ski area offers year round recreational opportunities including downhill or cross country skiing, hiking, biking, tennis, swimming, golf and boating. The surrounding villages have a wide array of antique shops, collectibles, flea markets and weekly auctions.

Killington at the Woods
♥♥♥♥

RR 1, Killington Rd, PO Box 2151, Killington, VT 05751. Tel: (802) 773-9924. Fax: (802) 773-9928. TYPE: Resort & Spa. LOCATION: 12 mi. / 19 km. to Rutland, DESCRIPTION: First class condominium resort with spa. The emphasis is on fitness with cardiovascular fitness room, indoor pool, gym, sauna, steam room, jacuzzi. 75 condo units 1 to 3 bedroom, restaurant, 3 tennis courts. Hotel rates: from $100.

New Life Hiking Spa
♥♥♥

PO Box 395, Killington, VT 05751. Tel: (802) 422-4302. Toll Free: (800) 228-4676. Fax: (802) 422-3690. DESCRIPTION: Spa features stress-reduction, physical activity & relaxation with exhilarating hikes, low-fat cuisine, massages, facials, and fitness classes. 25 rooms.

Green Mountain at Fox Run
♥♥♥

P.O. Box 164, Fox Lane, Ludlow, VT 05149. Tel: (802) 228-8885. Toll Free: (800) 448-8106. Fax: (802) 228-8887. TYPE: Health & Fitness Resort. MANAGER: Dr. Alan H. Wayler, Thelma J. Wayler, MS, RD. LOCATION: Green Mountain National Forest. SPA CLIENTELE: Women only.

* Rooms: 13 w/priv. bath
* Airport: Lebanon (NH) 33 mi. / 52 km.
* Airport Transportation: free pick-up
* Reservations: $500 deposit required
* Credit Cards: VISA/MC
* Open: Year round
* Rates: from $900/week; TAC: 10%
* Spa on premises
* **Spa Facilities:** swimming pool, walk/jog track, exercise/dance rooms, fitness trails, sauna
* **Spa Programs:** Health Management Program (7, 14, and 28 day programs); Special Mother-Daughter Program, Executive Women
* **Spa Treatments:** nutrition classes, personalized exercise, behavior modification
* **Indications:** weight control, aging, healthy lifestyle changes
* **Contraindications:** cardiovascular disorders are handled on a case by case basis
* Medical Supervision: 1 MD, plus dietitians, exercise physiologist, nutritional biochemist, physical education specialists, psychologists
* Treatments Approved by: American Dietetic Association, American Nurses Association

DESCRIPTION: One of the country's oldest and well respected residential weight and health management center for women only. It offers an "anti-diet" approach which allows women to take home with them a more livable attitude towards a long-term weight and health management. Professional staff is equipped to handle women with cardiovascular, orthopedic, and metabolic special needs.

MANCHESTER VILLAGE
☽ 802

✈ Rutland Airport (RUT) 32 mi. / 51 km.

Manchester Village is a year round resort in the Green Mountains of Vermont. This historic New England town is a show case of Greek revival style homes, wide tree-lined streets mostly sugar-maple that burst into a rainbow of colors each fall, and majestic mountains including Mount Equinox with its popular ski-slopes. For shopping visit the Equinox Junior complex or some of the fashionable brand name clothing factory outlets along route 7. Manchester Village is accessible by car from Boston via Route 2 to Greenfield, then follow I-91 to Brattleboro. From Brattleboro drive northwest on Route 30 to Manchester Center. Travel time is approximately 3-1/2 hours.

The Equinox Hotel Resort & Spa
❤❤❤❤

Rte 7A, Manchester Village, VT 05254. Tel: (802) 362-4747, Toll Free: (800) 362-4747. Fax: (802) 362-4861. TYPE: Resort Complex & Spa. SPA MANAGER: Susan Thorne-Thomsen. LOCATION: At the foot of Mt. Equinox in southern Vermont. SPA CLIENTELE: Mixed.

* Rooms: 176 bedrooms w/private bath
* Suites: 16; 10 w/cooking facilities
* Dining room, tavern
* Airport: Albany AP 65 mi. / 104 km.
* Airport Transportation: taxi, limo (special arrangement with the hotel)
* Reservations: 50% deposit required
* Credit Cards: MC/VISA/AMEX
* Open: Year round
* Hotel Rates: from $159
* TAC: 10% (on room only)
* Spa on premises
* **Spa Facilities**: heated pools, Nautilus weight equipment room, steam rooms, sauna, whirlpools

* **Spa Programs**: Fitness, beauty & pampering
* **Spa Treatments**: thalassotherapy, exercise, skin care, massages, herbal wraps, aerobics, low-calorie, fat free spa meals, aquamotion
* **Contraindications**: thalassotherapy should be avoided if allergic to iodine and seaweed; herbal wrap/thalassotherapy should be avoided by pregnant women

DESCRIPTION: Elegant resort in a charming New England town. Accommodations are spacious and furnished in great style and comfort. Some have views of the town and mountains. Daily spa package includes beauty and pampering treatments with or without accommodations. Weight watchers can enjoy gourmet low-calorie, fat free meals. Recreation: golf, fly-fishing, Alpine skiing at Stratton or Bromley Mountains, and cross-country skiing at the Robert Todd Lincoln's Estate.

STOWE
☽ 802

✈ Burlington Int'l Airport (BTV) 34 mi. / 54 km.

Stowe is a romantic New England village in a scenic mountain setting. Known as the home of Mt. Mansfield, it offers excellent ski conditions in the winter. During the summer, the area burst in a fantastic showcase of colors with wild flower blossoms covering the mountains and valleys. Recreation: hot air balloon riding, flying and gliding, horseback riding, fishing and canoeing.

Golden Eagle Resort
❤❤❤

P.O. Box 1090, Mountain Rd., Stowe VT 05672. Tel: (802) 253-4811. Toll Free (800) 626-1010. TYPE: Resort Motor Inn. LOCATION: In the Green Mountains. SPA CLIENTELE: Women & men. DESCRIPTION: The Golden Eagle Resort is an inn in a scenic mountain setting. All 95 rooms w/ private bath, oversized beds, balconies, refrigerators, some with own jacuzzi & fireplace. The Health Club (exercise and massage) is mainly for recreation and does not feature any planned programs or treatments. Restaurant, coffee shop, lounges. Hotel Rates: from $79.

Stowflake Resort & Spa
♥♥♥♥

🏃 🚶

1746 Mountain Rd., P.O. Box 369, Stowe VT 05672. Tel: (802) 253-7355. Toll Free: (800) 253-2232. Fax: (802) 253-6858. TYPE: Resort & Spa. LOCATION: Between the village and the ski area. SPA DIRECTOR: Emile Willett. SPA CLIENTELE: Men, women, children age 16 and older.

* Rooms: 91, Suites: 7, Condos: 24
* Phone, CTV, A/C, C/H
* Restaurant, Bar, Jacuzzi
* Airport: Burlington Int'l, 35 minutes, taxi
* Reservation: Required
* Credit Cards: MC/VISA/AMEX
* Open: Year round
* Hotel rates: from $110
* Spa Treatment Rates: from $45
* Spa on premises: **Stoweflake Spa & Sports Club**
* **Spa Facilities**: treatment rooms, whirlpool, steam room, sauna, showers, lockers, exercise room and equipment, indoor pool, seasonal outdoor pool, squash/racquetball courst, tennis courts
* **Spa Programs**: Massage, fitness classes, sports activities, bike rentals, hiking
* **Spa Treatments**: Salt loofa, herbal wrap, spirulina wrap, clay body masque, paraffin dip; Swedish, shiatsu, combo, aromatherapy, sports, deep tissue, Thai, and prenatal massages; reflexolgy, craniosacral, Reiki; body toning, aqua-fit, yoga, tai chi, wally ball, cardio boxing, stretch body & mind classes; adult and kid's tennis clinic; personal training exercise prescription, comprehensive fitness evaluation
* Medical Supervision: none
* Stoweflk @ sover.net
* Web: www.stoweflake.com

DESCRIPTION: Contemporary style resort with ski house and spa & sports club "Where fitness & relaxation go hand in hand..."

Topnotch at Stowe Resort & Spa
♥♥♥♥♥

🐵 🏃 🚶

4000 Mountain Rd, Stowe, VT 05672. Tel: (802) 253-8585. Toll Free: (800) 451-8686. Fax: (802) 253-9263. TYPE: Resort & Spa. LOCATION: In the heart of Vermont's Green Mountains. SPA CLIENTELE: Women and men, family oriented.

* Rooms: 86 w/priv. bath. Suites: 4
* Condos: 18. Townhouses: 6
* Restaurants (2), wine cellar, fireplace lounge
* Airport: Burlington Int'l, 36 mi. (57 km.)
* Airport Transportation: limo
* Reservation: 1 day deposit
* Credit Cards: MC/VISA/AMEX/DC/CB/DIS
* Open: Year round
* Hotel Rates: from $130
* Spa on premises
* **Spa Facilities**: 3 exercise studios with resistance weight training equipment, large exercise pool, jacuzzi and waterfalls for hydromassage, 10 massage rooms, luxurious locker rooms, beauty salon
* **Spa Programs**: Fitness, nutrition, stress management
* **Spa Treatments**: European hydrotherapy, herbal wraps, salt-glo loofah, facials, relaxation techniques
* Medical Supervision: 1 MD on call, 2 RN 1 licensed therapist

DESCRIPTION: Elegant resort with a 22,000 sq.ft. Spa that is fitness and exercise oriented. Beauty and pampering services are available for both men and women. Recreation: tennis, skiing, Equestrian center, water sports, and mountain hikes. The Spa features a gourmet Spa cuisine prepared by a master chef.

STRATTON MOUNTAIN
🤙 **802**

✈ Albany County AP (NY)

Stratton Mountain is a popular year round resort area some 15 mi. / 24 km. east of Manchester. The area is noted for its beautiful scenery, quaint New England villages, and year round recreational activities: golf, tennis, sailing, swimming, and fly-fishing. Cross-country skiing is available between mid November and April. There is also an annual

Arts Festival that takes place during the fall season at the Stratton Mountain Base Lodge. Stratton Mountain is accessible by car from Manchester off SR 30.

New Life Spa
❤❤❤

c/o Liftline Lodge, P.O. Box 144, Stratton Mt., VT 05155. Tel: (802) 422-4302. Toll Free (800) 545-9407. TYPE: Resort Spa. MANAGER: Jimmy LeSage. LOCATION: In the heart of Southern Vermont's Green Mountain National Forest. 3-1/2 hours drive northwest of Boston (MA) and 4-1/2 hrs. drive north of New York City (NY). SPA CLIENTELE: Men, Women (no children).

* Rooms: 24 w/private bath
* Airport: Albany (NY) 70 mi. / 112 km.
* Airport Transportation: bus
* Reservations: $150 deposit required
* Credit Cards: VISA/MC
* Open: May - October
* Rates: from $1,295
* TAC: 10%
* Spa on premises
* **Spa Facilities**: swimming pool, outdoor & indoor tennis court, hot tub, sauna, massage, facial & exercise rooms, indoor lap pool
* **Spa Program**: fitness plan - balancing cardiovascular fitness with stretching and strengthening; Diet - 800 calories per day based on high complex carbohydrate, moderate protein, low-fat diet; intensive spa week - accelerated fitness program.
* **Spa Treatments**: massage, facials, aerobics, body conditioning, yoga, aquaerobics

DESCRIPTION: Austrian chalet type accommodations at the base of Stratton Mountain. The New Life Spa, operating during the summer only, offers complete fitness program designed to heighten cardiovascular endurance, strengthen muscles and help build a positive self-image. The spa cuisine is high in fiber, complex carbohydrate and is especially prepared to help eliminate toxins and lose weight. Recreation: tennis, racquetball, hikes and excursions in the Vermont countryside.

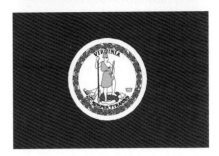

VIRGINIA

AREA: 40,767 sq. mi. (105,587 sq. km.)
POPULATION: 6,216,568
CAPITAL: Richmond
TIME ZONE: Eastern Time

HOT SPRINGS
⌐ 540
✈ Ingalls Field Airport, 17 mi. / 27 km.

Hot Springs, population 700, is in the George Washington National Forest of western Virginia. The forest offers clean mountain air and recreation opportunities. The mineral springs at the Homestead are naturally heated water, high in sulfur and magnesium ontent, at a constant temperature of 104°F (40°c). The hot springs are excellent for a hydrotherapy. The Homestead Ski area offers good winter skiing facilities and an Olympic-size ice-skating rink. Hot Springs can be reached by car from Washington D.C., New York, Pittsburgh and other major Eastern Cities.

The Homestead
❤❤❤❤❤

US 220 N., Hot Springs, VA 24445. Tel: (540) 839-1766. Toll Free (800) 336-5771. Fax: (540) 839-7656. Spa Toll Free (800) 838-1766. TYPE: Mountain Resort. LOCATION: In the Allegheny Mountains. SPA CLIENTELE: Women and men. SPECIAL RESTRICTIONS: Spa guests must be at least 16 years.

* Rooms: 521 w/priv. bath; 75 parlor suites
* Dinning room, buffet & tavern
* Airport: Ingalls Field AP 17 mi. / 28 km.
* Airport Transportation: taxi, limo
* Open: Year round
* Credit Cards: MC/VISA/AMEX
* Hotel Rates: from $297
* TAC: 10%
* Spa on premises
* **SPA Facilities**: thermal baths, gym, indoor pool with mineral and well water, outdoor pools (2), locker room amenities, beauty salon, spa shops, fitness center, aerobic room, relaxation lounges
* **Spa Programs**: Hydrotherapies, fitness, beauty, pampering, anti-stress
* **Spa Treatments**: hydrotherapy, swedish massage, aromatherapy, Dr. Goode's spout bath, clay body wrap, seaweed body wrap, raspberry relaxer, herbal wrap, karisoftness nourisher, golfer's glow, body polish, facials, european facials, alpha-lifting, oxygenating treatment, spa manicure, hand fitness
* **Spa Packages**: The Cascades, The Tradition, The rejuvenator, The Cure

DESCRIPTION: Deluxe resort and conference hotel filled with charming old world decor. Guest rooms feature sophisticated amenities and twice-daily maid service. The Spa offers a European style hydrotherapy for recreation and relaxation. Beauty and fitness services are available on à la carte basis. Recreation: golf, tennis, racquetball, fishing, horseback rides, cross country skiing in the winter, pop and rock concerts and dancing.

WILLIAMSBURG

✆ **757**

✈ Newport News / Williamsburg Int'l Airport (PHF) 15 mi. / 24 km. SE

Spa at Kingsmill Resort
♥♥♥♥

1010 Kingsmill Road, Williamsburg, VA 23185. Tel: (757) 253-1703. Toll free (800) 832-5665. Fax: (757) 253-8237. TYPE: Resort & Spa. LOCATION: on the James River a few minutes from Williamsburg. DESCRIPTION: Superior first class condominium resort & conference center. Classic pampering spa with a wide selection of services and facilities including skin, body, massage, salon services, and fitness, nautilus equipment, racquetball, whirlpool. 250 rooms, 160 condos 1 to 3 bedroom, nonsmoker rooms, wheelchair access. 3 restaurants, lounge, entertainment, meeting rooms, 4 pools, 15 tennis courts, 3 golf courses. Hotel rates: from $125.

WASHINGTON

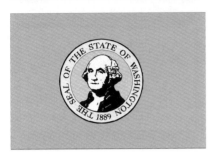

AREA: 68,139 sq. mi. (176,480 sq. km.)
POPULATION: 4,887,940
CAPITAL: Olympia
TIME ZONE: Pacific Time

BELLLEVUE
) 360

✈ Sea-Tac Int'l Airport (SEA) 28 mi. (45 km.) SE

The Spa at Bellevue Club Hotel
♥♥♥♥

11200 Se 6th St., Bellevue, WA 98004. Tel: (425) 454-
-4424, Fax: (425) 688-3101. TYPE: Hotel & Spa. LOCA-
TION: 15 minutes west of Seattle. DESCRIPTION: First class
hotel with a full service spa and athletic facilities including
swimming pool, gym, weight rooms (2), aerobic studio,
racquetball courts (4), squash courts (4), tennis courts
(11). 64 rooms, 3 suites, 2 restaurants, meeting facilities.
Hotel rates: from $190.

ORCAS ISLAND
) 360

✈ East Sound Airport, 5 mi. / 8 km.

San Juan Islands are a cluster of 172 picturesque islands in
the Pacific Northwest, the largest of which are: Orcas
Island, San Juan Island, Lopez Island and Fidalgo Island.
San Juan shores abound in shellfish and various species of
salmon and white fish. The abundance of shellfish and

seafood contributed to the excellence and nutritional value
of the local cuisine. The islands offer hidden coves and
rugged coastlines; their isolated location provides an ideal
escape from the stress of the mainland. How to get there:
By car - Washington State Ferry Service to Orcas Island is
provided from Anacortes, WA, and Sidney B.C. (on Vancouver Island). By Air - San Juan Airlines serves Eastsound
Airport direct from Seattle - Tacoma Int'l Airport. By Seaplane - fly from downtown Seattle to Rosario with Lake
Union Air.

Rosario Resort & Spa
♥♥♥

One Rosario Way, Eastsound, WA 98245. Tel: (360) 376-
2222. Fax: (360) 376-3680. TYPE: Resort & Spa. LOCA-
TION: On 55 sq.mi. private island in Puget Sound. SPA
CLIENTELE: Women and men. SPECIAL RESTRICTION: Non
smoking policy.

* Rooms: 130 w/priv. bath; 45 suites
* Phone, CTV, coffee maker, balcony
* Restaurants & Cafe
* Airport: Seattle/Tacoma Int'l, 90 mi. / 144 km.
* Airport Transportation: air, car, boat
* Reservation: deposit required
* Credit Cards: MC/VISA/AMEX/DC
* Open: Year round
* Hotel Rates: from $120
* TAC: 10%
* Spa on premises
* **Spa Facilities:** Fitness,exercise rooms, beauty
  salon, whirlpool, sauna, indoor pool
* **Spa Programs:** Diet, fitness, beauty
* **Spa Packages:** 3 night/4 day
* **Spa Treatments:** Ocean body wraps, massages,
  salt glow, pampering, exercise and fitness

DESCRIPTION: Victorian mansion built in the early 1900's
and listed on the National Historic Register. The hotel-condo
complex features an elegant blend of antique and modern.
The historic Moran Mansion offers a complete spa facility
for fitness and pampering. For weight maintenance a well
balanced gourmet spa meal provides between 1400 -

1900 calories. Recreation: water skiing, boating, lawn games, dancing and entertainment.

SNOQUALMIE
 425

✈ Sea-Tac Int'l Airport (SEA) 43 mi. (69 km.) SW

The Salish Lodge & Spa
❤❤❤❤

6501 Railroad Ave. SE, PO Box 1109, Snoqualmie, WA 98065-1109. Tel: (425) 888-2556. Fax: (425) 888-9634. TYPE: County Inn & Spa. LOCATION: Top of Snoqualmie Fall, 40 minutes to Sea-Tac Int'l Airport. DESCRIPTION: Moderate deluxe county inn with a full service health spa, rooftop hot tub. 87 rooms, 4 suites, nonsmoker rooms, wheelchair access, dining room, lounge, library. Hotel rates: from $195.

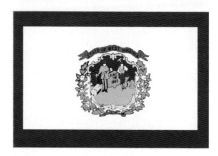

WEST VIRGINIA

AREA: 24,231 sq. mi. (62,758 sq. km.)
POPULATION: 1,801,625
CAPITAL: Charleston
TIME ZONE: Eastern Time

BERKELEY SPRINGS
〉 **304**

✈ Winchester Regional AP (VA), 33 mi. / 53 km.

Berkeley Springs, population 1,000, is a small old-fashioned spa resort in the Eastern Panhandle of West Virginia. From pre-colonial times, the warm mineral springs attracted many visitors for health and recreation. Berkeley Springs is only 2 hrs. from Washington and Baltimore, and 3 hrs. from Pittsburgh.

Coolfont Resort
❤❤

Cold Run Valley Road, Berkeley Springs, WV 25411. Tel: (304) 258-4500. Fax: (304) 258-5499. TYPE: Resort & Spa. LOCATION: In a hidden valley between Cacapon Mountain and Warm Springs near Berkeley Springs. SPA CLIENTELE: Women and men.

* Rooms: 227 w/priv. bath. Chalets: 30
* Phone, CTV, A/C, kitchenette, fireplace, jacuzzi
* Restaurant, lounge, meeting facilities
* Train Station: Martinsburg WV, 35 mi. / 56 km.
* Reservations: deposit required

* Credit Cards: MC/VISA/AMEX/DC
* Open: Year round
* Hotel Rates: from $112
* TAC: 10%
* Spa on premises
* **Spa Facilities**: pool for lap and water aerobics, gym with resistance and cardiovascular training equipment
* **Spa Programs**: Weight loss, stop smoking, fitness, stress management
* **Spa Treatments**: non medical; exercise, massages, beauty, low calorie diets (1200 - 1500 calories per day, 900 calories diet available)
* **Contraindications**: insulin dependent diabetics, heart disease patients
* Medical Supervision: MD on call

DESCRIPTION: The Coolfont is a rustic Conference and Retreat center in a mountain setting. Accommodations are in a lodge (standard hotel/motel rooms), in the historic manor, or in chalets with a jacuzzi tub. The Spa offers weekly programs to stop smoking based on a group dynamics, and weight loss based on low fat, high carbohydrate meals of 1200 to 1500 calories per day and daily exercise. Some programs are available on a Weekend basis. Recreation: hiking, fishing, horseback riding, tennis, swimming, Ice skating and cross-country skiing in winter.

WHITE SULPHUR SPRINGS
304

Greenbrier Airport, 12 mi. / 20 km.

White Sulphur Springs, population 3,500, is an historic spa in the West Virginia Mountains. The hot springs were used by the colonials for curative purposes as early as 1772, and later became a meeting place for wealthy visitors. Recreation: fishing, swimming, camping, and lake water

sports. White Sulphur Springs is located 250 mi. / 400 km., southwest of Washington, D.C., and it is easily accessible by air, automobile and train from most major cities.

The Greenbrier

White Sulphur Springs, WV 24986. Tel: (304) 536-1110. Toll Free (800) 624-6070. Fax: (304) 536-7834. TYPE: Resort & Spa. LOCATION: On a secluded 6,500-acre estate in upland valley of the Alleghenies. SPA CLIENTELE: Women and men.

* Rooms: 674 w/priv. bath, Suites: 33, Cottages: 121
* Phone, CTV, A/C, fireplace, kitchenette, balcony
* Dinning Rooms, cafe, bar, pool lounge
* Airport: Greenbrier 12 mi / 20 km, taxi, limo
* Open: Year round
* Credit Cards: MC/VISA/AMEX
* Hotel Rates: from $198
* TAC: 10%
* Spa on premises
* **Spa Facilities**: Spa & mineral bath, Olympic-size pool, medical clinic
* **Spa Programs**: hydrotherapy, fitness, beauty
* **Spa Treatments**: hydrotherapy, aerobics, weight training, massages, mud and seaweed
* Medical Supervision: at the Medical Clinic

DESCRIPTION: Prestigious mountain resort with health spa. Accommodations vary from spacious hotel rooms to lavish suites and cottages. The Greenbrier Spa & Mineral Baths offers European hydrotherapy and American fitness programs. Recreation: golf, tennis, horseback riding, jogging and hiking trails, trap and skeet shooting, feature films and dancing.

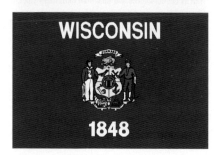

WISCONSIN
WISCONSIN
1848

AREA: 56,153 sq. mi. (145,436 sq. km.)
POPULATION: 4,906,745
CAPITAL: Madison
TIME ZONE: Central Time

LAKE GENEVA / FONTANA
✈ 414

Milwaukee's General Mitchell Airport (MKE) 45 mi. / 72 km. NE of Lake Geneva

Lake Geneva, population 5,600, is a year round resort and recreation center on the eastern shore of Lake Geneva. Activities include water sports in the lake and cross-country skiing, ice fishing and ice boating in the winter. Lake Geneva can be reached by car from Milwaukee (WI) 45 mi. / 72 km., or Chicago (IL) 65 mi. / 104 km.

Fontana Spa at The Abbey Resort
♥♥♥♥

269 Fontana Blvd. PO Box 50. Fontana, WI 53125. Tel: (414) 275-6811. Toll Free: (800) SPA-1000. Fax: (414) 275-5948. TYPE: Resort & Spa. LOCATION: On an inlet of Lake Geneva. DESCRIPTION: Rustic year round resort complex with a full service spa with 33 personal services and treatments. 317 rooms, 13 suites, 24 condos, nonsmoker rooms, wheelchair access, 3 dining rooms, cocktail lounge, entertainment, meeting rooms, pools (5), tennis courts (6), recreation center, shops, marina. Hotel rates: from $99.

Grand Geneva Resort & Spa
♥♥♥♥

7036 Grand Geneva Way, Lake Geneva, WI 53147. Tel: (414) 248-8811. Fax: (414) 248-3192. TYPE: Resort & Spa. LOCATION: On 1300 acres, 45 mi. / 72 km. from Milwaukee. DESCRIPTION: Superior first class resort conference center & spa. Spa & sports center & aerobics studio, cardiovascular workouts, body treatments, facials, massage. 318 room, 37 suites. Restaurants (3), meeting rooms, 36 hole of golf, tennis courts (10), indoor & outdoor pools, riding stable. Hotel rates: from $115.

Interlaken Resort & Country Spa
♥♥♥♥

West 4240 State Road 50, Lake Geneva, WI 53147. Tel: (414) 248-9121. Toll Free: (800) 225 5558. Fax: (414) 245-5016. TYPE: Resort & Spa. LOCATION: On Lake Como. SPA CLIENTELE: Women and men.

* Rooms: 144 w/priv. bath. Villas: 286
* Apartment Villas: 30
* Dining room, nightly entertainment
* Airport: Milwaukee 45 mi. / 72 km.
* Airport Transportation: rent-a-car
* Credit Cards: MC/VISA/AMEX/DC/CB
* Rates: $95 - $195/day (room only); SPA packages available.
* TAC: 10%
* Spa on premises
* **Spa Facilities**: Fully equipped Country Spa - gym, 3 pools, Health Club
* **Spa Programs**: Country spa escape - fitness getaway, beauty care, weight loss
* **Spa Treatments**: Swedish massage, hand & foot treatments, herbal wraps, mineral baths, body sculpting, cardio-respiratory development, dance aerobics, aquacise & hydrotherapy, low calorie meals,skin care

DESCRIPTION: Country spa nestled in a wooded valley on the shores of Lake Como. Spa programs are designed to initiate an exercise program or expand current fitness routines. Diet and beauty treatments complete the spa package. Recreation: tennis, nearby golf, boating and skiing (in winter).

OSCEOLA
 715

✈ Minneapolis/St. Paul AP (MSP) 64 mi. / 102 km.

Osceloa is on east bank of the St Croix River, the border between Wisconsin and Minnesota, 45 mi. / 72 km. northwest of St. Paul, MN.

Aveda Spa Retreat
♥♥♥

1015 Cascade St., Osceola, WI 54020. Tel: (800) 283-3202, Fax: (715) 294-2196. TYPE: Operates as a day spa. LOCATION: Woodland setting. DESCRIPTION: Wellness programs, beauty, plant essences.15 rooms available separate from spa.

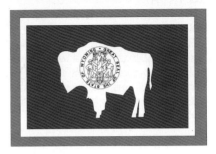

WYOMING

AREA: 97,809 sq. mi. (253,325 sq. km.)
POPULATION: 455,975
CAPITAL: Cheyenne
TIME ZONE: Mountain Time

JACKSON
307

✈ Jackson Hole Airport (JAC)
10 mi. / 16 km.

The Spa at Grand Targhee
Ski & Summer Resort
♥♥♥

Ski Hill Road., PO Box SKI, Alta, WY 83422. Tel: (307) 353-2300. Fax: (307) 353-8148. TYPE: First class year-round resort. LOCATION: At the Idaho border and Targee National Forest. DESCRIPTION: Full service spa with weekly & single day packages include aromatherapy, herbal & mud wraps, massage, sauna. 96 rooms., nonsmoker rooms, wheelchair access. Restaurants (5), bar, nightclub, meeting rooms, outdoor pool, hot tub, tennis court, horseback riding. Hotel rates: from $59.

THERMOPOLIS
(HOT SPRINGS STATE PARK)
307

✈ Cody Regional Airport (COD)
70 mi. / 112 km.

Holiday Inn of the Waters
♥♥♥

115 E. Pioneer St., PO Box 1323, Thermopolis, WY 82443. Tel: (307) 864-3131. Fax: (307) 864-3131 ext 299. TYPE: Spa Motel. LOCATION: Adjacent to Hot Spring State Park. DESCRIPTION: Spa motel with hot mineral pool, mineral baths, messages, hot tubs, exercise & therapy rooms, sauna. 80 rooms, nonsmoker rooms, wheelchair access, restaurant, coffee shop, lounge, bar, meeting facilities. Hotel rates: from $79.

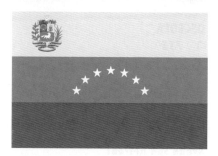

VENEZUELA

AREA: 352,143 sq. mi. (912,050 sq. km.)
POPULATION: 19,300,000
CAPITAL: Caracas
OFFICIAL LANGUAGES: Spanish
CURRENCY: Bolívar
EXCHANGE RATE: 1 US$ = Bolívars 574
COUNTRY TELEPHONE CODE: 58

CUMANAGOTO
ꙅ 93

Sofitel Cumanagoto
♥♥♥♥

Ave. Universidad Plya San Luis, Cumana, Sucre. Tel: (93) 32-16-24. Fax: (93) 32-16-24.TYPE: Hotel & Spa. LOCATION: Beachfront 15 min. from National Park. SPA CLIENTELE: Women and men. DESCRIPTION: Modern resort hotel with health spa, gym, Turkish bath. Hotel rates: from US$150.

MARGARITA ISLAND
ꙅ 95

✈ Gen. Santiago Marino AP (PMV) 9 mi. / 14 km.

Margarita island is located in the Caribbean off the Northern Coast of Venezuela. It is a Caribbean holiday destination with beautiful beaches, quaint villages, national parks and fascinating lagoons. Most of the resort hotels are located at **Porlamar**, about 11 km. / 7 mi. from the airport. The climate is pleasant and dry year round.

Isla Bonita Golf & Beach Hotel
♥♥♥♥♥

Playas de Puerto Viejo & Puerto Cruz, Pedro Gonzalez. Tel: (95) 657111. Fax: (95) 657211. TYPE: Hotel & Spa. LOCATION: Oceanfront overlooking the Caribbean and surrounded by park with lakes and everglades. SPA CLIENTELE: Women and men.

* Rooms: 312 w/priv. bath. Suites: 17
* Phone, CTV, minibar, safe deposit
* Restaurants, bars, cafeteria, beach club
* Airport: Internacional del Canbe AP, 25 min.
* Airport Transportation: free shuttle
* Reservations: deposit requested
* Open: Year round
* Rates: from $180 (room only)
* TAC: 10%
* Spa on premises
* **Spa Facilities**: European Spa, gyms, saunas turkish bath, scottish showers
* **Spa Programs**: Beauty and pampering
* **Spa Treatments**: massages, body wraps, facials, aromatherapy, body glo, hydrotherapy, aerobics, fitness training, weight loss

DESCRIPTION: Beautiful beach resort offering spacious rooms and suites. European health spa with medical services offers a variety of massages, facials, and hydrotherapy. Recreation: tennis , horseback riding, water, sports, 18-hole golf course, casinos nearby

La Samanna Hotel & Thalassotherapy Center
♥♥♥♥♥

Urb. Costa Azul, Av. FCO Esteban Gomez, Porlamar, Margarita Island. Tel: (95) 621267. Fax: (95) 620989.

TYPE: Resort Hotel & Spa. SPA MANAGER: Carolina Casanova. LOCATION: Beachfront in Porlamar. SPA CLIENTELE: Women and men. DESCRIPTION: Beach resort hotel with a full service health & beauty spa.

PUERTO LA CRUZ
ᒐ 81

✈ Barcelona Int'l Airport

Puerto La Cruz, population 220,000, is located east of Caracas on the north coast of Venezuela. Originally a small fishing village it is becoming an enormously popular holiday destination for North Americans and Venezuelans.

Golden Rainbow Maremares
♥♥♥♥

Avda. Americo Vespucio con Avda R-17. Tel: (81) 813028. Fax: (81) 813028. TYPE: Waterfront Resort & Spa. LOCATION: On the beach in the El Morro section near shopping & nightlife. SPA CLIENTELE: Women and men.

* Rooms: 500 w/priv. bath.
* Phone, CTV, minibar, safe deposit
* Restaurants, pool bar, cocktail lounge
* Airport: Barcelona Int'l AP, 20 min., free shuttle
* Reservations: deposit requested
* Open: Year round
* Hotel Rates: from $120 (room only)
* Spa Packages: from $675 (5-night) pp
* TAC: 10%
* **Spa Facilities**: Health Spa with aerobic rooms, steam room, sauna, facial rooms, massage rooms, beauty salon, swimming pool
* **Spa Programs**: Beauty & Pampering
* **Spa Treatments**: massages, aerobics,facials, mud baths, herbal wraps

DESCRIPTION: Low-rise resort hotel & Spa overlooking the golf course, waterway and marina. Recreation: water sports, scuba, golf and tennis. Recreation: tennis, horseback riding, water sports, 18-hole golf course, casinos nearby.

VIRGIN ISLANDS (US)

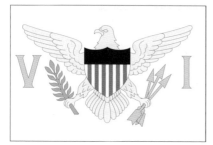

AREA: 146 sq. mi. (390 sq. km.)
POPULATION: 155,000
CAPITAL: Charlotte Amalie
OFFICIAL LANGUAGES: English
CURRENCY: US$
INTERNATIONAL PHONE CODE: 340

ℹ Virgin Islands Dept. of Tourism
PO Box 6400, St. Thomas, USVI 00804.
Tel: (340) 774-8784 Fax: (340) 774-4390

The U.S. Virgin Islands are among the most beautiful in the Caribbean. They have US territory status and are located 70 mi. / 112 km. east of Puerto Rico and 1,000 mi. / 1,600 km. south of the tip of Florida. The climate is tropical and stable year round at 76˚ F (25˚c) with cooling trade winds. The US Virgin islands are comprised of three major islands: St. Croix, St. John and St. Thomas and many smaller cays and islets. The islands offer great beaches, national parks, excellent scuba diving and duty free shopping.

ST. CROIX
✈ Alexander Hamilton AP (STX) 7.5 mi. / 12 km.

The Buccaneer
❤❤❤❤❤

Gallows Bay, PO Box 25200, St. Croix, USVI 00824-5200. Tel: 773-2100. Fax: 773-0010. TYPE: Hotel &

Spa. LOCATION: Beach resort on a landscaped peninsula 2 mi. / 3 km. from Christiansted. SPA CLIENTELE: Women and men. DESCRIPTION: Deluxe beach resort with health club, sauna, tennis and water sports.

ST. THOMAS
✈ Cyril E. King AP (STT) 2 mi. / 3 km.

Bolongo Bay Beach Club & Villas
❤❤❤❤

7150 Bolongo, St. Thomas, USVI 00802. Tel: 775-1800. Fax: 775-3208. TYPE: Resort Hotel & Spa. LOCATION: Oceanfront on palm lined beach, 8 mi. / 13 km. to airport. DESCRIPTION: Charming beach resort hotel with Spa and fitness center. 75 hotel units (rooms & efficiencies w/kitchen). Restaurants (2), bars (2), entertainment, pools (3), tennis courts (2), volleyball courts (2), water sports, scuba. Hotel rates: from $170.

Marriott Frenchman's Reef & Morningstar Resorts
❤❤❤❤❤

PO Box 7110 St. Thomas, USVI 00801. Tel: 776-8500, Fax: 776-3054. TYPE: Resort Complex & Spa. LOCATION: On an inlet surrounded by the Caribbean sea overlooking Charlotte Amalie harbor. SPA CLIENTELE: Women and men.

* Rooms: 504 w/priv. bath. Suites: 88
* Restaurants, bars and lounges
* Airport: Cyril E. King AP, 6 mi. / 10 km.
* Open: Year round
* Hotel Rates: from $240
* Spa on premises
* **Spa Facilities**: health club, gym, sauna, whirlpool, steam room, exercise equipment, beauty salon
* **Spa Treatments**: massages, body wraps, facials, aerobics, exercise training

DESCRIPTION: Large resort complex near Coral World, Atlantis Submarine and Bluebeards Castle with full service health, fitness & beauty spa.

SPAS AT SEA

If you need a spa vacation, and want to combine it with a cruise, telephone the following cruise lines for more details. (International Telephone Access Codes: Vary)

CARNIVAL CRUISE LINE
3655 NW 87th Ave., Miami, FL 33178-2428 USA. Tel: +1-305-599-2600. Fax: +1-305-406-8630.

Carnival Destiny - Health Spa; saunas, whirlpools, outdoor pool; special diets catered. **Sailing**: 7-day Caribbean, departing Miami, FL.

Carnival Triumph - Health Spa; 7 whirlpools, 4 pools; special diets catered. **Sailing**: 7-day Caribbean, from Miami, Fl.; 4- & 5-day Canada/New England, from New York, & 11-day millennium cruise.

MS Ecstasy - Health Spa, 2 saunas; 6 whirlpools, 3 pools, special diets catered. **Sailing**: 3- & 4-day to Bahamas, Key West and Cozumel, from Miami, FL.

Elation - Nautica Spa, exercise equipment, health and beauty treatments; 6 whirlpools, 3 pools, special diets catered. **Sailing**: 7-day to Mexican Riviera, departing Los Angeles, CA.

MS Fantasy - Health Spa; jogging track, 2 saunas, 6 whirlpools, 3 pools, special diets catered. **Sailing**: 3- & 4-day to Bahamas, departing, port Canaveral, FL; 7-day western Caribbean millennium cruise.

MS Fascination - Health Spa; 2 saunas, 6 whirlpools, 3 outdoor pools, special diets catered. **Sailing**: 7-day Southern Caribbean departing San Juan, PR; 11-day millennium cruise.

MS Imagination - Health Spa; 2 saunas, 6 whirlpools, 3 outdoor pools, special diets catered. **Sailing**: 4-, 5-, & 7-day Caribbean & Mexico, 9 day millennium cruise.

MS Inspiration - Health Spa; 2 saunas, 6 whirlpools, 3 outdoor pools, special diets catered. **Sailing**: 7-day Southern Caribbean.

Paradise - Health & Fitness Facilities, special diets catered. **Sailing**: 7-day Caribbean, from Miami, FL.

CELEBRITY CRUISES
1050 Caribbean Way, Miami, FL 333132 USA. Tel: +1-305-539-6000. Fax: +1-305-375-0711.

Century - 10,053 sq. ft. full service AquaSpa with hydrotherapy, thalassotherapy, and massages; fitness equipment, aerobics and exercise classes; whirlpools, 2 outdoor pools. **Sailing**: 5- to 15 night to Caribbean, Mediterranean and Scandinavia.

Galaxy - 10,053 sq. ft. full service AquaSpa with massages, hydrotherapy baths, and revitalization therapies; fitness equipment, aerobics and exercise classes; whirlpools, 5 pools. **Sailing**: 7- to 17-night Caribbean, Alaska and Panama Canal.

MV Horizon - AquaSpa program with massages, hydrotherapy baths, and revitalization therapies; sauna, 3 whirlpools, 2 outdoor pools; dietetic, low-calorie, low-salt and vegetarian menus. **Sailing**: 7- to 11-night Caribbean and Bermuda

Mercury - 10,053 sq. ft. full service AquaSpa featuring thalassotherapy, hydrotherapy baths, and massages; fitness equipment, aerobics and exercise classes; whirlpools, 5 pools. **Sailing**: 7- to 15-night Western Caribbean, Alaska and Panama Canal.

MS Zenith - AquaSpa program with massages, hydrotherapy baths, and revitalization therapies; sauna, whirlpool, aerobic and exercise classes, 2 outdoor pools; dietetic, low-calorie, kosher, low-salt and vegetarian menus. **Sailing**: 7- to 15 night Caribbean and Panama Canal, and to Bermuda, from New York, NY.

COSTA CRUISE LINES
World Trade Center, 80 SW 8th St., Miami, FL 33130-3097 USA. Tel: +1-305-358-7325. Fax: +1-305-375-0676.

MV CostaAllegra - Caracalla Spa on 2 levels; solarium, 3 whirlpools, pool; special diets catered. **Sailing**: 7- to 13-night North Cape, Fjords, the Baltics, Russia and Mediterranean.

MV CostaClassica - Health Spa; 4 whirlpools, sauna, 2 outdoor pools; special diets catered. **Sailing**: 5- to 7-night Mediterranean.

MV CostaMarina - Health Spa; 3 whirlpools, sauna, outdoor pool; special diets catered. **Sailing**: 7-night Scandinavian Fjords, Baltic Sea and Russia, departing Copenhagen, Denmark; 10-night Mediterranean cruise.

SS CostaRiviera - Health Spa, whirlpool, sauna, outdoor pool; special diets catered. **Sailing**: 10- to 11-night Mediterranean, departing from Savona.

MV CostaRomantica - Health Spa; exercise classes, 4 whirlpools, 2 outdoor pools, special menus available. **Sailing**: 5- to 7- night Caribbean and Mediterranean; 16-day east and west bound transatlantic cruises.

MV CostaVictoria - Full Service Spa, 6 whirlpools, 3 outdoor pools, 1 indoor pool. **Sailing**: 5- to 7-night Mediterranean, Caribbean, and transatlantic crossings.

CRYSTAL CRUISES

2049 Century Park East, Ste 1400, Los Angeles, CA 90067 USA. Tel: +1-310-785-9300. Fax: +1-310-785-0011.

Crystal Harmony - Crystal Spa & Salon; aerobics, exercise classes, exercise equipment, saunas, steam rooms, personal trainers, massage, 2 jacuzzi pools, indoor/outdoor pool; special diets catered. **Sailing**: 7- to 16-day Mexican Riviera, Hawaii, Mediterranean, Western Europe, Northern European Capitals, Black Sea, Transatlantic, South America and Panama Canal.

Crystal Symphony - Crystal Spa & Salon; aerobics, exercise classes, exercise equipment, saunas, steam rooms, personal trainers, massage, lap pool with jacuzzi, indoor/outdoor pool; special diets catered. **Sailing**: 7- to 99-day Panama Canal, Caribbean, Mexico, Alaska/Canada, US East Coast, New England/Canada,, Asia, Australia/New Zealand and South America.

CUNARD

6100 Blue Lagoon Drive, Suite 400, Miami, FL 33126 USA. Tel: +1-305-463-3000. Fax: +1-305-463-3010.

Queen Elizabeth 2 - Health Spa; 4 whirlpools, 2 saunas, indoor/outdoor pool; special diets catered. **Sailing**: 3- to 17-day Bermuda, Caribbean, New England, Canada, Scandinavia, Iceland and Mediterranean; 6-day transatlantic; and 105-day world cruise.

Sea Goddess I - Health Spa; aerobics, massage, sauna, whirlpool, outdoor pool. **Sailing**: 7- to 9-day Caribbean, Mediterranean and Africa.

Sea Goddess II - Health Spa; aerobics, massage, sauna, whirlpool, outdoor pool. **Sailing**: 7- to 14-day Southeast Asia, Indian Ocean, Middle East, Mediterranean, Canary Islands, Caribbean and Australia.

Vistaafjord - Health Spa; sauna, 2 whirlpools, gym, indoor and outdoor pools. **Sailing**: 7- to 21-day Panama Canal, Mediterranean, Middle East.

DISNEY CRUISE LINE

210 Celebration Place, Ste. 400, Celebration, Fl 34747-4600 USA. Tel: +1-407-566-3500. Fax: +1-407-566-3751.

Disney Magic - Ocean View Spa & Salon; aerobics, exercise equipment, saunas, steam rooms, jogging, 3 pools. **Sailing**: 3- or 4-day to the Bahamas plus 3- or 4-day Walt Disney World Land Package.

Disney Wonder - Ocean View Spa & Salon; aerobics, exercise equipment, saunas, steam rooms, jogging, 3 pools. **Sailing**: 3- or 4-day to the Bahamas plus 3- or 4-day Walt Disney World Land Package.

FIRST EUROPEAN CRUISES

95 Madison Ave., Suite 1203, New York, NY 10016 USA. Tel: +1-212-779-7168. Fax: +1-212-779-0948.

MV The Azur - Spa - sauna, massage, exercise classes, gym, 2 outdoor pools. **Sailing**: 4- to 13 day Mediterranean and Canary Islands.

Mistral - Fitness Center with Thalassotherapy Spa; sauna, massage, 2 outdoor pools; special diets catered. **Sailing**: Mediterranean & Caribbean cruises starting July, 1999.

FRED OLSEN CRUISE LINES

Fred Olsen House, White House Rd., Ipswich, Suffolk IP1 5LL England. Tel: +44-(0)1472-292200. Fax: +44-(0)1473-2923345.

MS Black Prince - Health Spa; exercise classes, sauna, weight room, gym, outdoor pool; diabetic, low calorie, low-cholesterol, low-salt and vegetarian meals available. **Sailing**: 8- to 36-day Canary Islands, British Isles, Mediterranean, Scandinavia, South America and Caribbean.

HOLLAND AMERICAN LINE

300 Elliott Ave. W., Seattle, WA 98119 USA, Tel: +1-206-281-35356, Fax: +1-206-281-7110.

Maasdam - Ocean Spa & Passport to Fitness Program; aerobics, massage, beauty salon, sun deck, pools, special diets catered. **Sailing**: 10- to 12-day Panama Canal, Caribbean, Mediterranean, Europe & Transatlantic.

Nieuw Amsterdam - Ocean Spa & Passport to Fitness Program; 2 saunas, whirlpool, jogging track, 2 outdoor pools; special diets catered. **Sailing**:5- to 17-day Caribbean, Panama Canal, Alaska, Transpacific, Asia, Australia, New Zealand and Indonesia.

Noordam - Ocean Spa & Passport to Fitness Program; sauna, whirlpool, jogging, outdoor pool; special diets catered. Sailing: 7-day Alaska; 10- to 14-day Caribbean; 10 to 19-day Panama Canal; and 16-day South America.

Rotterdam VI - Ocean Spa & Passport to Fitness Program; saunas, steam rooms, Swedish massage, exercise room, beauty salon, sun deck, two outdoor pools. **Sailing**: 7- to 14-day Caribbean; 14- day Panama Canal; 10- to 12-day Mediterranean, Black Sea, Western Europe, Norwegian Fjords, Scandinavia, Russia, transatlantic; 97-day World cruise.

Ryndam - Ocean Spa & Passport to Fitness Program; gym,sauna, massage, 2 pools; special diets catered. **Sailing**: 7-day Alaska; 7- to 10-day Caribbean; and 19- to 20 day Panama Canal.

Statendam - Ocean Spa & Passport to Fitness Program; deck sports, jogging track, 2 outdoor pools; special diets catered. **Sailing**: 7-day Alaska; 10-day Southern Caribbean; 10-day Mexico; 10- to 16- day Hawaii; 16- day Panama Canal.

Veendam - Ocean Spa & Passport to Fitness Program; deck sports, sauna, 2 whirlpools, indoor & outdoor pools; special diets catered. Sailing: 7-day Alaska; 7-day Eastern and Western Caribbean; 18- to 19-day Panama Canal cruises.

LEISURE CRUISES SA

Neue Jonastrasse 91. PO Box 1312, Rapperswil, SG CH 8640 Switzerland. Tel: +41-55-220-8400. Fax: +41-55-220-8484.

MS Switzerland - Aqua Vitalis Wellness Center & Health Club; sauna, 2 whirlpools, outdoor pool. **Sailing**: 4- to 9-day Mediterranean and Canary Islands.

NORWEGIAN CRUISE LINE

7665 Corporate Center Drive, miami, FL 33126 USA. Tel: +1-305-436-4000. Fax: +1-305-436-4106.

MS Leeward - Fitness Center and Spa; exercise equipment, jogging track, outdoor pool, jacuzzi, beauty salon, light cuisine available. **Sailing**: 3- to 4-night Bahamas, Key West and Mexico, from Miami, FL.

SS Norway - Full European Spa; gym, massage, 2 saunas, indoor pool, 2 outdoor pools; special diets catered. **Sailing**: 3- to 4-day Caribbean & Mediterranean.

Norwegian Dream - Health Spa; massage, aerobic and exercise classes, gym, weight room, sauna, whirlpool, jacuzzi, 2 outdoor pools, special diets catered (dietetic, kosher, low-calorie, low-cholesterol, low-salt, and vegetarian). **Sailing**: 7-day Caribbean; 12- to 14-day to Europe.

Norwegian Dynasty - Olympic Spa, massage, sauna, aerobics, fitness equipment, 3 whirlpools, outdoor pool, special diets catered. **Sailing**: Panama Canal and Mexican Rivera from January to March; Hawaii in April; Alaska from May to August.

MS Norwegian Majesty - Fitness Center & Spa, aerobic, exercise equipment, whirlpool, pool. Norwegian Sky - Full Service Spa; aerobics, gym, beauty salon, 6 jacuzzis, 2 outdoor pools. **Sailing**: 7-day to Bermuda, from Boston; 10- to 11-day Caribbean and Panama Canal.

Norwegian Sky - Full Service Spa; aerobics, exercise gym, 6 jacuzzis, 2 outdoor pools, beauty salon. **Sailing**: 7- to 15-day Europe, New England/ Canada, Caribbean and transatlantic.

Norwegian Star - Fitness Center & Spa; exercise equipment, aerobics, massage, walking track, outdoor pool, 3 whirlpools, beauty salon, light cuisine available. **Sailing**: South Pacific from Australia.

Norwegian Wind - Health Spa, aerobics and exercise classes, 2 outdoor pools, sauna, whirlpool, jacuzzi; special diets catered. **Sailing**: 7-day Southern Caribbean from March to April; 7- day Alaska May to September; Hawaii cruises September to November.

P & O CRUISES

77 New Oxford St., London, WC1A 1PP England, Tel: +44-(0)171-800-2345, Fax: +44-(0)171-831-1410.

Oriana - Health Spa; jacuzzi, sauna, massage, 3 outdoor pools. **Sailing:** 4- to 24-day Canary Islands, Mediterranean, Scandinavia, and Caribbean; 92-day World cruise.

PAQUET FRENCH CRUISES

5 Blvd. Malesherbes, Paris, 75008 France. Tel: +33-1-4924-8319. Fax: +33-1-4924-4201.

MS Mermoz - Hydrotherapy Spa; weight room, sauna, whirlpools, 2 outdoor pools; special diets catered. **Sailing:** vary.

PRINCESS CRUISES

10100 Santa Monica Blvd., Ste. 1800, Los Angeles, CA 90067-4189. Tel: +1-310-553-6330. Fax: +1-310-277-6175.

Dawn Princess - Health Spa; gym, weight room, aerobic and exercise classes, massage, sauna, 3 pools; special diets catered. **Sailing:** 3-day US West Coast; 7-day Caribbean and Alaska; 11- to 21-day Panama Canal repositioning cruises.

Grand Princess - Full Service Spa; sauna, whirlpool, 4 pools; special diets catered. Sailing: 7-day Caribbean; 12-day Mediterranean and Transatlantic cruises.

Sun Princess - Spa & Health Center; aerobics, sauna, massage, gym, 2 whirlpools, pool; special diets catered. **Sailing:** 4- to 21-day Alaska, Mexico, Caribbean and Panama Canal.

RADISSON SEVEN SEAS CRUISES

600 Corporate Dr., Ste. 410, Fort Lauderdale, FL 33334 USA. Tel: +1-954-776-6123. Fax: +1-954-772-3763.

Paul Gauguin - Spa & Fitness Center; aromatherapy, thalassotherapy, massages, facials, steam room, exercise equipment, beauty salon, water sports marina, scuba diving program. **Sailing:** 7-night South Pacific, from Tahiti.

SSC Radisson Diamond - Complete Health Spa, European style sauna, massages, exercise classes, jogging track, pool; special diets catered. **Sailing:** 5- to 21-day Caribbean, Panama Canal and Costa Rica; Transatlantic; Mediterranean and Europe.

Seven Seas Navigator - Full Service Spa & Fitness Center; aromatherapy, massages, facials,

manicure, pedicures, steam room, exercise equipment, fitness track, 2 whirlpools, outdoor pool. Sailing: 8- to 17-day Mediterranean and Caribbean, beginning August, 1999.

RENAISSANCE CRUISES

1800 Eller Dr., Suite 300. PO Box 350307, Fort Lauderdale, FL 33335-0307 USA. Tel: +1-954-463-0982. Fax: +1-954-463-9216.

R1/R2/R3/R4 - Spa & Fitness Center; hydrotherapy bath, thalassotherapy whirlpool, fog shower, massage, aerobics, fitness track. **Sailing:** 10-day Eastern Mediterranean and South Pacific.

ROYAL CARIBBEAN INTERNATIONAL

1050 Caribbean Way, Miami, FL 33132 USA. Tel: +1-305-539-6000. Fax: +1-305-374-7354.

Enchantment of The Seas - Indian Themed Solarium Spa; 2-story spa, work-out are, fitness classes, fitness machines, jogging track, massage, sauna, 6 whirlpools, swimming pools. **Sailing:** 7-night alternating Eastern/Western Caribbean, from Miami.

Grandeur of the Seas - Moorish Themed Solarium Spa & ShipShape Fitness Center, massage, sauna, jogging, 6 whirlpools, 2 swimming pools. **Sailing:** 7-night Eastern Caribbean, from Miami.

Rhapsody of The Sea - Egyptian Themed Solarium Spa; gym, jogging, massage, exercise classes, indoor/outdoor swimming pools. **Sailing:** 7-night Alaska, Southern Caribbean, Mexico; 11- to 13-night Hawaii and Panama Canal cruises.

Vision of the Seas - Full Service Spa & ShipShape Fitness Center; jogging track, 6 whirlpools, indoor/outdoor pool, outdoor pool. **Sailing:** 7-night Alaska; 11- to 12-night Hawaii; 10-, 11-, and 14-night Panama Canal cruises.

ROYAL OLYMPIC CRUISES

Akti Miaouli 87, Piraeus, 18538 Greece. Tel: +30-1-429-1000. Fax: +30-1-429-0946.

Olympic Countess - Health Spa; sauna, whirlpool, outdoor pool; special diets catered. **Sailing:** 7-day summer Greek Isles and Turkey; 10- to 11-day winter Caribbean and Venezuela Rainforest.

SEABOURN CRUISE LINE

55 Francisco St., Suite 710, San Francisco, CA 94133 USA. Tel: +1-415-391-7444. Fax: +1-415-391-8518.

Seabourn Legend - Health Spa; herbal body wrap, massage, sauna, steam room, gym, 2 whirlpools, outdoor pool; special diets available. **Sailing**: 5- to 21-day Caribbean, Mediterranean and Panama Canal.

Seabourn Pride - Health Spa; 2 saunas, 3 whirlpools, outdoor pool; special diets available. **Sailing**: 6- to 23-day Panama Canal, South America, Caribbean, British Isles, Scandinavia, New England, and Canada.

Seabourn Spirit - Health Spa; 2 saunas, 3 whirlpools, outdoor pool; special diets available. **Sailing**: 6- to 14-day Asia, Middle East, Mediterranean and Indian Ocean.

SILVERSEA CRUISES

110 E. Broward Blvd., Fort Lauderdale, FL 33301 USA. Tel: +1-954-522-4477. Fax: +1-954-522-4499.

Silver Cloud - Health Spa & Fitness Center; sauna, massage, jogging track, 2 whirlpools, outdoor pool. **Sailing**: 8- to 16-day South Pacific, Australia, Asia, Indian Ocean, Middle East, Mediterranean, Europe, Scandinavia, Transatlantic, New England, Canada, Caribbean, South America, Panama Canal, Mexico, and Hawaii.

Silver Wind - Health Spa & Fitness Center; sauna, massage, jogging track, 2 whirlpools, outdoor pool.

Sailing: 3- to 16-day Southeast Asia, Australia, South Pacific, Hawaii, California, Mexico, Panama Canal, Caribbean, Transatlantic, and Mediterranean.

STAR CRUISES

391 Orchard Road., 21-01 Tower B, Singapore, 238874 Singapore. Tel: +65-733-9766, Fax: +65-733-3622.

MV Superstar Gemini - Health Spa; whirlpools, jogging deck, outdoor pool; special diets catered. **Sailing**: 7-day Malaysia and Thailand, from Singapore.

SUN CRUISES SINGAPORE

304 Orchard Rd., #05-02, Lucky Plaza, 238863 Singapore. Tel: +65-733-8866. Fax: +65-835-2222.

Sun Vista - Health Spa; 2 saunas, 4 whirlpools, indoor and outdoor pools; special diets catered. **Sailing**: 7-night Southeast Asia, from Singapore.

WINDSTAR CRUISES

300 Elliott Ave. W. Seattle, WA 98119 USA. Tel: +1-206-281-3535, Fax: +1-206-286-3229.

Wind Surf - WindSpa: body wraps, massage, facials, stress management, aerobics, fitness center, sauna, 2 hot tubs, 2 outdoor pools, watersports launching platform; special health and vegetarian menu selections. **Sailing**: 7- to 15-day Mediterranean featuring Venice, Rome, French & Italian Rivieras; Transatlantic; Caribbean; Repositioning cruises.

INTERNATIONAL DAY SPAS

If you need pampering, but only have a few hours, call the nearest day spa and find out what they offer! (International Telephone Country Access Codes: Vary)

CANADA

Fayez Beauty Spa
2224 Wharncliff Road South, London, ON N6P 1L1.
Tel: +1 (519) 652-2780.

Wheels Country Spa
615 Richmond St., Chatham ON N0P 1M0.
Tel: +1 (519) 436-5505.

In Touch Massage Therapy
4816 - 50th Avenue, Camrose, Alberta T4V 0R9
Tel: +1 (403) 672-0700.

Institut de Beaute Carol St. Piere Day Spa
33 Wharf Road, Hudson, Quebec J0P 1H0.
Tel: +1 (514) 458-5607.

Aqua Cite
666 Sherbrooke Street West, 16th Fl., Montreal, Quebec H3A 1E7, Tel: +1 (514) 845-8455.

Civello Salon Spa
887 Yonge St., Toronto, ON M4W 2H2, Canada,
Tel: +1 (416) 924-9244.

Estee Lauder Spa
Hlt Renfrew, 50 Bloor St. West, Toronto, ON M4M 1A1.
Tel: +1 (416) 960-2909.

HealthWinds The Health & Wellness Spa
2401 Yonge St.,, Suite LLo1, Toronto, ON M4P 2E7.
Tel: +1 (416) 488-9545.

Mira Linder Spa
108 Avenue Rd., Toronto, ON M5R 2K6
Tel: +1 (416) 961-6900.

Spa at the Century
Century Plaza Hotel, 1015 Burrard St., Lobby Level, Vancouver, BC V6Z 1Y5., Tel: +1 (800) 663-1818.

Versailles Spa Ltd.
1838 West First Ave., Vancouver, BC V6J 1G5.
Tel: +1 (604) 732-7865, Fax: +1 (604) 732-1863.

Estetica Beauty Institute
2407 Dougall Avenue, Windsor, ON N8X1T3
Tel: +1 (519) 969-8848.

ENGLAND

Elizabeth Arden Red Door Hair & Beauty Spa
29 Davies St., London, England W1Y 1FN.
Tel: +44 (0)1716-294488.

HONG KONG

Renewal Day Spa
Ground Floor, Printing House, 6 Duddell St., Hong Kong,
Tel: +852 (297) 36669.

MALAYSIA

Renewal Day Spa
JW Marriott Hotel. 183 Jalan Bukit, Bintang 55100 Luala Lumpur, Tel: +60 (3) 245-1889

PORTUGAL

Thalgo Portela
Urbanization Da Portela 197, Portela LRS, P-2685.
Tel: +351 (1) 94301470, Fax: +351 (1) 943-6690.

SINGAPORE

Alexandra Wellness Spa
356D Alexandra Roa, Singapore 159949.
Tel: +65-476-8211.

Renewal Day Spa
#07-02 Tong Bldg., 302 Orchard Rd., Singapore 238862.
Tel: +65-738-0988.

SWEDEN

Sturebadet
Styregallerian 36, 11446 Stockholm.
Tel: +46 (468) 5450-1500.

U.S.A. DAY SPAS

If you need pampering, but only have a few hours, call the nearest day spa and find out what they offer! (International Telephone Access Code: +1)

ALABAMA

Deborah Stone A Day Spa & Salon
3439 Colonnade Parkway, Birmingham, AL 35243.
Tel: (205) 967-1170.

ALASKA

Opulence Grand Salon and Day Spa
450 E. Tudor Rd., Anchorage, AK 99503
Tel: (907) 562-2060.

ARKANSAS

Quy's Color Salon & Day Spa,
3101-C Maumelle Club Manor, Maumelle, AK 72113
Tel: (501) 851-3641, Fax: (501) 851-1168.

ARIZONA

The Perfect Day
5000 E. Via Esrancia Miraval, Catalina, AZ 85739
Tel: (520) 825-5105, Fax: (520) 825-5199.

DMB Racquet Clubs
4444 East Camelback Road, Phoenix, AZ 85018
Tel: (602) 840-6412.

Candela Skin Care Center
6939 East Main Street, Scottsdale, AZ 85251
Tel: (602) 949-0100, Fax: (602) 949-0143.

Spa Du Soleil
7040 East Third Avenue, Scottsdale, AZ 85251
Tel: (602) 994-5400.

Gadabout Hair, Skin, Nails & Day Spa
3325 N. Dodge, Tucson, AZ 85716
Tel: (520) 322-9434.

Gadabout Day Spa - East Tucson
6393 E. Grant Road, Tucson, AZ 85715
Tel: (520) 885-0000.

Gadabout Day Spa - St. Philip's Plaza
1990 E. River Road, Tucson, AZ 85718
Tel: (520) 577-2000.

The Personal Services Center
3660 East Sunrise Drive, Tucson, AZ 85718
Tel: (520) 742-7866, Fax: (520) 722-2292.

CALIFORNIA

Estee Lauder Spa
Neiman Marcus Beverly Hills, 9700 Wilshire Blvd.,
Beverly Hills, CA 90212. Tel: 310-550-2056.

Georgette Klinger
131 South Rodeo Drive, Beverly Hills, CA 90212.
Tel: (310) 274-6347.

Spa Thira
417 N. Canon Drive, Beverly Hills, CA 90210.
Tel: (800) 708-4472 or (310) 274-3207

Lavender Hill
1015 Foothill Blvd., Calistoga, CA 94515.
Tel: (707) 942-4495.

E.D.C.'s Isis Oasis
7th and San Carlos (Hampton Court), PO Box 222771,
Carmel, CA 93922. Tel: 408-626-2722.

Glen Ivy Hot Springs Spa
25000 Glen Ivy Road, Corona, CA 91719.
Tel: 888-CLUB-MUD or 909-277-3529.

Georgette Klinger
South Coast Plaza, 2nd Level, 3333 Bristol St., Costa
Mesa, CA 92626. Tel: (714) 850-1212.

The Spa at South Coast Plaza
695 Town Center Drive, Suite 180, Costa Mesa, CA
92626. Tel: (714) 850-0050, Fax: (714) 850-0825.

Bellissima Day Spa at the Paladion
122 East Grand Avenue, Escondido, CA 92025.
Tel: (619) 480-9072, Fax: (619) 480-9851.

The Skin Spa
17401 Ventura Blvd., Encino, CA 91316.
Tel: (818) 907-9888.

Spa off The Plaza
706 Headsburg Ave., Healdsburg, CA 95448.
Tel: (707) 431-7938.

Gaia Day Spa
1299 Prospect St., Suite 105, La Jolla, CA 92037.
Tel: (619) 456-8797, Fax: (619) 456-9396.

The Chopra Center for Well-Being
7630 Fay Ave., La Jolla, CA 92037.
Tel: (619) 551-7788, Fax: (619) 551-7825.

Spa Thira
7917 Ivanhoe Ave., La Jolla, CA 92037.
Tel: (619) 551-6700, Fax: (619) 551-6707.

The Body Clinic
8820 S., Sepulveda Blvd., Suite 104, Los Angeles, CA
90045. Tel: (310) 568-0303.

The Massage Therapy Center
2130 S. Sawtelle Blvd., Suite 207, Los Angeles, CA
90025. Tel: (310) 444-8989.

Tea Gardens Springs
38 Miller Ave., Mill Valley, CA 94941.
Tel: (415) 389-7123.

Skin Care Institute / Day Spa
250 Coast Village Rd., Montecito, CA 93108
Tel: (805) 969-6454.

Spat Thira
401 Newport Center Drive #216, Newport Beach, CA
92660. Tel: (714) 644-4677, Fax: (714) 64-6614.

Body Essentials
111 S. Signal St., Ojai, CA 93023.
Tel: (805) 646-0906.

La Belle Day Spa
36 Standford Shopping Center, Palo Alto, CA 94304.
Tel: (650) 326-8522.

La Belle Day Spa
95 Town & Country Village, Palo Alto, CA 94301.
Tel: (650) 327-6964.

The Huntington Spa and Salon
1401 S. Oak Knoll Ave., Pasadena, CA 91104.
Tel: (626) 585-6414.

A New Beginning Salon Spa
138 N. Lake Ave., Pasadena, CA 91101.
Tel: (626) 449-1231, Fax: (626) 449-1235.

The Pleasanton Spa
3059-K Hoyard Rd., Pleasanton, CA 94588.
Tel: (510) 846-0544.

International Skin & Body Care
325 Cajon Street, Redlands, CA 92373
Tel: (909) 793-9080.

Yamaguchi Salon & Coastal Day Spa
3260 Telegraph Rd., San Bueanventura, CA 93003.
Tel: (800) 572-5661 or (805) 658-7909.

Anatomy Day Spa
1205 University Ave., San Diego, CA 92103.
Tel: (619) 296-6224.

Beauty Kliniek Aromatheraphy Day Spa
3268 Governor Drive, San Diego, CA 92122.
Tel: (619) 457-0191.

World Spa
10397 Friars Rd., San Diego, CA 92120.
Tel: (619) 624-0506.

La Belle Day Spa
233 Grant Ave., The Penthouse, San Francisco, CA
94108. Tel: (415) 433-7644.

Mister Lee, Beauty, Hair & Health Spa
834 Jones St., San Francisco, CA 94109
Tel: (415) 474-6002 or (800) 693-2977.

Harmonie European Day Spa
14501 Big Basin Way, Saratoga, CA 95070.
Tel: (408)-741-4997 or (800) 391-3300.

Preston Wynne Spa
14567 Big Basin Way, Saratoga, CA 95070.
Tel: (408) 741-5525, Fax: (408) 741-4903.

Osmosis Enzyme Bath & Massage
209 Bohemian Hwy, Sebastopol, CA 95472.
Tel: (707) 823-8231.

Complexions Day Spa & Wellness Center
1350 Pacific Coast Hwy, Seal Beach, CA 90740.
Tel: (562) 493-2442.

Gauthier Total Image Spa
14449 Ventura Blvd., Sherman Oaks, CA 91423
Tel: (817) 501-4423.

Skytop Fitness Retreat, Inc.
23883 Broken Bit Rd., Sonora, CA 95370
Tel: 209-586-7777.

Yamaguchi Salon & Coastal Day Spa
3260 Telegraph Road, Ventura, CA 93003.
Tel: (800) 572-5661 or (310) 658-7909.

COLORADO

Aspen Club Day Spa
1450 Crystal Lake Road, Aspen CO 81611.
Tel: (970) 925-8900, Fax: (970) 925-9548

Total Beauty Centre at Hyatt Regency
50 E. Thomas Place, Beaver Creek, CO 81629,
Tel: (970) 845-2816.

Essentiels Spa
2660 Canyon Blvd. Boulder, CO 80302
Tel: (303) 440-0711 or (888) 889-4SPA.

John Douillard's Life Spa
3065 Center Green Dr., Suite 110, Boulder, CO 80301.
Tel: (303) 442-1164.

A+ European Body & Health
3879 East 120th Ave., Suite 141, Denver, CO 80233.
Tel: (303) 553-2194.

Skin Care Institute / Day Spa
3150 East 3rd Ave., Denver, CO 80206.
Tel: (303) 377-7676.

Spa Thira
242 Milwaukee St.,Denver, CO 80206.
Tel: (303) 388-3800, Fax: (303) 388-8807.

Ambiance Day Spa
1895 Youngfield St., Golden, CO 80401.
Tel: (303) 238-9611.

CONNECTICUT

Hands on Massage
28 Lafayette Place, Greenwich, CT 06830.
Tel: (203) 531-7829.

Spa Thira
44-48 W. Putnam Ave., Pickwick Commons, Greenwich,
CT 06830. Tel: (203) 622-0300, Fax: (203) 622-8377.

Adam Broderick Image Group
89 Danbury Road, Richfield, CT 06877.
Tel: (203) 431-3994, Fax: (203) 431-4156.

Noelle Spa for Beauty & Wellness
1100 High Ridge Road, Stamford, CT 06905.
Tel: (203) 322-3445, Fax: (203) 321-1477.

Derma Clinic European Day Spa
299 Post Road East, Westport, CT 06881
Tel: (800) 752-4993 or (203) 227-0771.

DISTRICT OF COLUMBIA

Elizabeth Arden Red Door Salon & Spa
5225 Wisconsin Ave., N.W., Washington, DC 20015
Tel: (202) 362-9890.

Georgette Klinger
Chevy Chase Pavilion, 5345 Wisconsin Ave., N.W.,
Washington, DC 20015. Tel: (202) 686-8880.

FLORIDA

Spa Thira
459 Plaza Real, Mizner Park, Boca Raton, FL 33432.
Tel: (561) 416-4044, Fax: (561) 416-4049.

La Bella Spa
3505 North Courtenay Parkway, Merritt Island, FL 32953.
Tel: (407) 453-1510.

Cleopatra's Secrets - Advanced Beauty Care
Center, 2554 NE Miami Gardens Dr., North Miami Beach,
Fl 33180, Tel: (305) 933-2722.

Spa Thira
634 Collins Ave., Miami Beach, FL 33139
Tel: (305) 531-0881, Fax: (305) 531-4788.

The Veranda Pampering Salon
40 North Beach St., Ormond Beach, FL 32174.
Tel: (904) 676-7622.

The Babor Institut
303 Royal Poinciana Plaza, Palm Beach, FL 33480.
Tel: (561) 802-6160 or (888) 222-6891.

Georgette Klinger
Espanade, 150 Worth Ave., Palm Beach, FL 33480.
Tel: (561) 659-1522.

Spa Thira
230 Worth Avenue, Palm Beach, FL 33480.
Tel: (561) 833-0353, Fax: (561) 833-9518.

M Spa at Mettlers
35 South Blvd, of Presidents, Sarasota, FL 34236.
Tel: (941) 388-1772.

GEORGIA

Don & Sylvoas Shaw Salon (DASS)
4505 Ashford Dunwoody Road, Atlanta, GA 30346.
Tel: (770) 393-8303, Fax: (770) 395-1091.

Key Lime Pie Salon & Day Spa
806 N Highlands Avenue, Atlanta, GA 30306.
Tel: (404) 873-6512, Fax: (404) 873-0386.

Natural Body Day Spa
1402-1 N. Highland Ave., Atlanta, GA 30306.
Tel: (404) 872-1039.

HAWAII

Paul Brown Salon and Day Spa
1200 Alamona Blvd., Honolulu, HI 96814.
Tel: (808) 591-1881, Fax: (808) 596-0755

Lei Spa
505 Front St., Lahaina, HI 96761.
Tel: (808) 661-1178, Fax: (808) 667-7727.

ILLINOIS

Bettye O. Day Spa
5200 South Harper Ave., Chicago, IL 60615.
Tel: (773) 752-3600 or (800) 262-6104.

Elizabeth Arden Red Door Salon & Spa
919 N. Michigan Ave., Chicago, IL 60611.
Tel: (312) 988-9191.

Georgette Klinger
Water Tower Place, Level 3, 835 N. Michigan Ave.,
Chicago, IL 60611, Tel: (312) 787-4300

Michael Anthony Salon & Day Spa
1001 West North Ave., Chicago, IL 60622.
Tel: (312) 649-0707, Fax: (312) 649-0623.

Rodica European Skin & Body Care Centers
Water Tower Place, 845 No. Michigan Ave., Suite 944E,
Chicago, IL 60611. Tel: (312) 527-1459.

Spa Thira
840 North Michigan Ave., Chicago, IL 60611.
Tel: (312) 867-5720, Fax: (312) 867-4550.

Annabella Salon & Day Spa
1115 Randal Court, Geneva, IL 60134.
Tel: (630) 262-1556.

Weis Morris DaySpa Salon
4108 Morsay Dr., Rockford, IL 61107.
Tel: (815) 398-4000.

Estee Lauder Spa
Marshall Field's, Old Orchard Rd. Skokie, IL 60077.
Tel: (847) 329-2SPA, Fax: (847) 329-2602.

Day Escape, The Ultimate Spa
150 East Ogden Ave., 2nd floor, Westmont, IL 60559.
Tel: (630) 455-0660, Fax: (630) 455-0669.

INDIANA
European Skin Care by Zizi-Day Spa
3901 Hogan Street, Suite A, Bloomington, IN 47401.
Tel: (812) 339-6704.

Escape Day Spa
9747 Fall Creek Rd., Indianapolis, IN 46256.
Tel: (317) 595-0404.

House Of Bianco Beauty Concepts & Day Spa
1000 E. 80th Place, Merrillville, IN 46410.
Tel: (219) 769-1010

Nob City Salon & Day Spa
216 Lakeview Dr., Noblesville, IN 46060.
Tel: (317) 773-8636.

Emerald Cut Salon & Day Spa
6331 University Commons, South Bend, IN 46635.
Tel: (219) 272-1225.

LOUISIANA
Rigsby Frederick Salon Gallery Spa
7520 Perkins, Rd., Baton Rouge, LA 70808.
Tel: (504) 769-7903.

H2O Salon & Spa
441 Metairie Road, Metairie, LA 70005.
Tel: (504) 835-4377, Fax: (504) 828-8532.

Belladonna Day Spa
2900 Magazine Street (at Sixth Street), New Orleans, LA
70115. Tel: (504) 891-4393, Fax: (504) 891-1004.

MAINE
Cythia's Day Spa & Salon
24 First South St., Bal Harbor, ME 04609.
Tel: (207) 288-3426.

MARYLAND
About Faces Day Spa
894 Kenilworth Drive, Baltimore, MD 21204.
Tel: (410) 828-8666, Fax: (410) 828-6438.

Robert Andrew Day Spa Salon
11 51 Route 3 North, Gambrills, MD 21054.
Tel: (301) 261-3844, Fax: (301) 261-6889.

A Perfect Face European Day Spa
82nd St. and Coastal Hwy, Ocean City, MD 21842.
Tel: (800) 476-5524 or (410) 524-2390.

MASSACHUSETTS
Moodz Day Spa & Salon
556 Massachusetts Ave., Acton, MA 01720.
Tel: (978) 263-3017, Fax: (978) 263-0203

4 C's Health Spa
19 Putnam St., Beverly, MA 01915.
Tel: (978) 922-5524.

Daryl Christopher Spa & Salon
37 Newbury St., Boston, MA 02116.
Tel: (617) 424-0250.

Guiliano The Spa for Beauty & Wellness
338 Newbury St., Boston, MA 02115
Tel: (617) 262-2220, Fax: (617) 262-5861.

Backstage Salon & Day Spa
225 Turnpike Road, Route1, Rowley, MA 01969.
Tel: (508) 948-7772, Fax: (508) 948-7476.

MICHIGAN
Heidi Christine's Salon Day Spa
500 Ada Drive, Ada, MI 49301.
Tel: (616) 676-3304.

Jeffrey Michael Powers Beauty Spa
206 South Fifth Street, Ann Arbor, MI 48104.
Tel: (313) 996-5585, Fax: (313) 996-1511.

Emile Salon & Spa
31409 Southfield Rd., Beverly Hills, MI 48025.
Tel: (248) 642-3315.

Margot's Euro Spa
280 North Old Woodward Ave., Birmingham, MI 48009.
Tel: (248) 642-3770, Fax: (248) 642-3739.

Capelli Spa
1939 South Telegraph Road, Bloomfield, MI 48302.
Tel: (248) 332-3434, Fax: (248) 332-8921.

Kitty Wagner Facial Salon & Spa
6895 Orchard Lake Rd., East Bloomfield, MI 48322.
Tel: (248)626-1231.

Mira Linder Spa in the City
29935 Northwestern Hwy, Southfield, MI 48034.
Tel: (248) 356-5810.

Hudson's Somerset Collection
2752 Big Beaver Rd., Troy, MI 48084.
Tel: (810) 816-4255.

Spa Nordstrom
2850 West Big Beaver Rd., Troy, MI 48084.
Tel: (248) 816-7502 or (248) 816-7595.

Spa Thira
2800 Big Beaver Rd., Troy, MI 48084.
Tel: (810) 614-8952, Fax: (810) 614-8972.

MINNESOTA

Simonson's Salon & Day Spa
646 East River Road, Anoka, MN 55303.
Tel: (612) 427-0761.

Estee Lauder Spa
100 South Dale Center, Edina, MN 55435.
Tel: (612) 924-6638, Fax: (612) 924-4750.

The Day Spa
7575 France Ave. S., Edina, MN 55435.
Tel: (612) 830-0100.

Spa Thira
3680 Galleria, Edina, MN 55435.
Tel: (612) 915-1234, Fax: (612) 915-9491.

Simonson's Salon & Day Spa
13744 83rd Way, Maple Grove, MN 55369.
Tel: (612) 494-4863.

Healing Touch Therapeutic Massage Center
Mayo Clinic, Rochester, MN.
Tel: (800) 305-6162.

Rodico Facial Salon
681 E. Lake Street, Suite 257, Wayzata, MN 55391.
Tel: (612) 475-3111.

MISSOURI

The Day Spa Salon, Inc.
13359 Olive St. Rd. Chesterfield, MO 63017.
Tel: (314) 576-4704.

Persona
408 West 74th Terrace, Kansas City, MO 64113.
Tel: (816) 822-0600.

MONTANA

Alpenglow Massage & Spa
Shoshone Lodge, PO Box 160218, Big Sky, MT 59716.
Tel: (800) 851-1561 or (406) 995-4663.

Montana Body Care & Day Spa
16 N. Grand Ave., Bozeman MT 59715.
Tel: (406) 585-3006, Fax: (406) 585-3047.

NEBRASKA

Healthy Lifestyles Retreat Center
6001 South 58th Street, Bldg. D, Lincoln, NE 68516.
Tel: (402) 421-7410.

NEVADA

Natural Nouveaux Nontoxic Salon & Spa
2231 E. Desert Inn Rd., Las Vegas, NV 89109.
Tel: (702) 222-1919.

Forever Slender
475 S. Arlington Ave., #1A, Reno, NV 89501.
Tel: (775) 322-9966.

NEW HAMPSHIRE

River Valley Club
33 Morgan Dr., Lebanon, NH 03766.
Tel: (603) 643-7720.

Jaimie European Day Spa
46C Nashua Road, Londonderry, NH 03053.
Tel: (603) 421-0700.

NEW JERSEY

The Day Spa of Le Salon Classique
1465 Rte. 31 South, Annadale, NJ 08801.
Tel: (908) 730-6288, Fax: (908) 730-6867.

Beauty Spa of Englewood
363 Grand Avenue, Englewood, NJ 07631.
Tel: (201) 567-6020.

The Botanical - A day Spa
302 Broadway, Hillsdale, NJ 07642.
Tel: (201) 666-4300.

Spa at Rizzieri
6001 West Lincoln Dr., Marlton, NJ 08053.
Tel: (609) 985-0554, Fax: (609) 983-1680.

The Spa at DePasquale
Rt. 10 East Powder Mill Plaza, Morris Plains, NJ 07950.
Tel: (201) 538-3811, Fax: (201) 359-8940.

Balneo-Esthetic
218 Franklin Ave, Nutley, NJ 07110.
Tel: (973) 661-1818, Fax: (973) 2840170.

The Fountain European Day Spa
1100 Rt. 17, Ramsay NJ 07446.
Tel: (201) 327-5155, Fax: (201) 327-4243.

Estee Lauder Spa
Bloomingdales, Short Hills Mall, JFK Parkway, Rte. 24 West, Short Hills, NJ 07078. Tel: (973) 376-1722.

Skin Dynamics
154 Mt. Bethel Road, Warren, NJ 07059.
Tel: (908) 647-720.

NEW MEXICO

Face Place
2501, E. 20th St., Farmington, NM 87401.
Tel: (505) 325-6266.

Sante Fe Massage
100 E. San Francisco Street, Sante Fe, NM 87501
Tel: (505) 986-8466.

Ten Thousand Waves Japanese Health Spa
PO Box 10200, Sante Fe, NM 87504.
Tel: (505) 982-9304, Fax: (505) 989-5077.

The Sterling Silver Institute de Beauty
402 Don GasPar Ave., Sante Fe, NM 87501.
Tel: (505) 984-3223, Fax: (505) 984-3223.

NEW YORK

Complexions Spa for Beauty & Wellness
Wolf Road Shoppers Park, 6 Metro Park Rd., Albany, NY 12205. Tel: (518) 489-5231.

Natural Beauty Spa
10 Main Street, East Hampton, NY 1937.
Tel: (516) 329-0006.

DeFranco Spangnolo Salon & Day Spa
200 Middle Neck Road, Great Neck, NY 11021.
Tel: (516) 466-6752, Fax: (516) 466-2618.

RiverSpa
50 South Buckhout St., Suite 202, Irvington on Hudson, NY 10533. Tel: (914) 591-5757.

David Michaels - The Day Spa
510 Old Louden Rd. Latham. NY 12210.
Tel: (518) 783-6342.

Kimberley's A Day Spa Ltd.
637 New Loudon Road, Latham, NY 12110.
Tel: (518) 785-5868.

4-Ever Beautiful Salon & Day Spa
1704 Rockaway Ave., Lynbrook, NY 11563.
Tel: (516) 887-4440.

Estee Lauder Spa
The American at Manhasset, 2100S Northern Blvd., Manhasset, NY 11030, Tel: (516) 869-9100.

Spa Thira
1950 Northern Blvd., A2 Manhasset, NY 11030-3527, Tel: (516) 869-0100, Fax: (516) 869-0177.

Advance Skin Care Day Spa
532 Madison Ave., 3rd Floor, New York, NY 10022.
Tel: (212) 644-5500.

Allure Day Spa & Hair Design
139 East 55th Street, 3rd Floor, New York, NY 10022.
Tel: (212) 644-5500.

Anushka
241 East 60th Street, New York, NY 10022.
Tel: (212) 355-6404.

Carapan Urban Spa & Store
5 W. 16th Street, Garden Level, New York, NY 10011.
Tel: (212) 633-6220.

Diane Higgins Beauty Basics
1166 Lexington Ave. (at 80th St.)
Tel: (212) 288-7781.

Dorit Baxter Skin Care
47 W 57th Street, New York, NY 10019.
Tel: (212) 371-4542, Fax: (212) 371-4549.

Elizabeth Arden Red Door Salon & Spa
691 Fifth Avenue, 7 th Floor, New York, NY10022.
Tel: (212) 546-0200, Fax: (212) 546-0304.

The Spa at Eqinox
140 E. 63rd, New York, NY 10021.
Tel: (212) 750-4900, Fax: (212) 750-2858.

Equinox Urban Spa
205 E 85th Street, New York NY 10028.
Tel: (212) 439-8500, Fax: (212) 717-0230.

Estee Lauder Spa
Bloomingdales New York, 1000 Third Ave., Loge Level,
New York, NY 10022. Tel: (212) 705-2318.

Ettia
239 West 72nd Street, New York, NY 10023.
Tel: (212) 362-7109.

Feline Salon Spa
60 West 75th Street, New York, NY 10023.
Tel: (212) 496-7415.

Gazelle Beauty Center & Day Spa
509 Madison Ave., 14th Floor, New York, NY 10022.
Tel: (212) 751-5144, Fax: (212) 751-5144.

Georgette Klinger
501 Madison Ave., New York, NY 10022.
Tel: (212) 838-3200.

Georgette Klinger
978 Madison Ave., New York, NY 10021.
Tel: (212) 744-6900.

La Casa Day Spa
41 E. 20th St., New York, NY 10003.
Tel: (212) 673-2272.

Lia Schoor Skin Care
686 Lexington, Ave., New York, NY 10022.
Tel: (212) 334-5550.

Millefleurs Day Spa
130 Franklin St., New York, NY 10013.
Tel: (212) 966-3656.

New York Health & Racquet Club Spa
115 E. 57th St., New York, NY 10022
Tel: (212) 826-9640.

Origins Feel-Good Spa
The Sports Center Chelsea Piers/Pier 60, 23rd St. & Hudson
River, New York, NY 10011, Tel: (212) 336-6780.

Park Avenue Spa & Fitness
Swissotel, 440 Park Ave., at 56th St., New York, NY
10022, Tel: (212) 756-3968.

Paul La Brecque Salon & Spa
160 Columbus Ave., New York, NY 10023.
Tel: (212) 595-0099, Fax: (212) 362-3434.

Peninsula Spa
700 Fifth Ave., 21st Floor, New York, NY 10019
Tel: (212) 903-3910, Fax: (212) 903-3958.

Scott J. Salon & Spa
257 Columbus Ave., New York, NY 10023.
Tel: (212)769-0107.

SoHo Sanctuary
119 Mercer Street, New York, NY 10012.
Tel: (212) 334-5550.

Susan Ciminelli Day Spa
754 Fifth Ave., 9th floor, New York, NY 10019.
Tel: (212) 872-2650.

Terme Di Saturnia at Studio 57
57 W. 57th Street, Suite 710, New York, NY 10019.
Tel: (212) 758-6383.

Gabriella Day Spa
355 S. Oyster Bay Rd., Plainview, NY 11801.
Tel: (516) 932-8374.

Scott Miller Salon & Spa
3340 Monroe Ave., Rochester, NY 14618.
Tel: (716) 264-9940.

Pure Maximus Spa & Salon
The Source, 1504 Old Country Rd, Suite 226, Westbury,
NY 11590, Tel: (516)222-8880, Fax: (516) 222-5175.

Capellini Salon & Day Spa
964 Broadway, Woodmere, NY 11598.
Tel: (516) 374-1060.

NORTH CAROLINA
Charles Grayson European SpaSaloon
6401 Morrison Blvd., Suite 4B, Charlotte, NC 28211.
Tel: (704) 364-2944, Fax: (704) 364-8662.

ABBA Herbal Touch Day Spa
6164 B Falls Neuse Road, Raleigh, NC 27609
Tel: (919) 850-0785, Fax: (919) 850-9372.

Platinum Studios Salon & Day Spa
205 South Stratford Rd., Winston-Salem, NC 27103.
Tel: (910) 724-4940, Fax: (910) 777-1696.

OHIO
Vickie Lynn's Skin Care & Salon
205 South Main, Akron, OH 44308.
Tel: (330) 374-6950.

The Spa at Glenmoor
4191 Glenmoor Road Road NW, Canton, OH 44718.
Tel: (330) 966-3524 or (888) 456-6667.

Mitchell's Salon & Day Spa
8118 Montgomery Rd. Cincinnati, OH 45236.
Tel: (513) 793-0900.

Phyllis at the Madison
2324 Madison Rd., Cincinnati, OH 45208.
Tel: (513) 321-1300.

OKLAHOMA

Face Beautiful Euro - Clinical Day Spa
7108 North Western, Suite D2, Oklahoma City, OK
73116. Tel: (405) 840-3223.

OREGON

Atrium Center for Body Therapies
51 Water St., Suite 111, Ashland, OR 97520.
Tel: (541) 488-8775, Fax: (541) 488-8692.

The Phoenix
2425 Siskiyou Blvd., Ashland, OR 97520.
Tel: (541) 488-1281.

Joie De Vie Spa Salon
715 SW Morrison, Suite 905, Portland, OR 97205.
Tel: (800) 322-5643 or (503) 224-8636.

Paradise Day Spa & Salon
2905 NE Broadway, Portland, OR 97232.
Tel: (503) 287-7977.

Sylvie Day Spa
1706 NW Gliason St., Portland, OR 97209.
Tel: (503) 222-5054, Fax: (503) 274-8267.

PENNSYLVANIA

Currie Hair-Skin-Nails
567 Wilmington, Rte. 202, Glen Mills, PA 19342
Tel: (610) 558-4247.

The Spa at Felicita
2201 Fishing Creek Valley Rd., Harrisburg, PA 18938,
Tel: (717) 599-7550.

Spa Bi Ba
261 Old York Rd., Jenkintown, PA 19046.
Tel: (215) 576-7000, Fax: (215) 576-6988.

Soothing Touch Day Spa
2938 Columbia Ave., Suite 202, Lancaster, PA 17603.
Tel: (717) 399-0190.

Pierre & Carlo European Spa
Bellvue Hotel, 200 S. Broad St., Philadelphia, PA 19102.
Tel: (215) 790-0902, Fax: (215) 790-9158.

Adolf Biecker Spa & Salon
Rittenhouse, 210 W. Rittenhouse Sq., 3rd Floor,
Philadelphia, PA 19103. Tel: (215) 735-6404.

L'Avantage Day Spa
441 N. York Rd., New Hope, PA 18938.
Tel: (215) 862-3456.

Toppers Spa Salons
745 W. Lancaster Ave., Suite 200, Wayne, PA 19087.
Tel: (610) 225-0480,   Fax: (610) 225-0485.

European Body Concepts
1013 Brookside Rd., Wescoville, PA 18106
Tel: (610) 398-7556.

RHODE ISLAND

Judy's Hair Company & Day Spa
1037 Aquidneck Ave., Middletown, RI 02842.
Tel: (401) 846-4444, Fax: (401) 846-7713.

SOUTH CAROLINA

Earthling Day Spa
334 East Bay Street, Suite K, Charleston, SC 29401.
Tel: (803) 722-4737, Fax: (803) 722-1459.

Spa Adagio
387 King Street, Charleston, SC 29403.
Tel: (803) 577-2444, Fax: (803) 577-2445.

The European Spa
115 The Executive Center, Hilton Head, SC 29928.
Tel: (803) 842-9355, Fax: (803) 842-2456.

TENNESSEE

Illusions Spa
5 115 Harding Road, Nashville, TN 37205.
Tel: (615) 352-4464, Fax: (615) 352-4395.

Tiba de Nuhad Khoury
2126 Abbott Martin Rd., Suite 132, Nashville, TN
37215. Tel: (615) 269-5121, Fax: (615) 297-1193.

TEXAS

Citiview B & B and Spa
1405 East Riverside Dr., Austin, TX 78741.
Tel: (512) 441-2606, Fax: (512) 441-2949.

Day Break Salon & Spa
11930 Preston Rd., Suite 108, Dallas, TX 75230.
Tel: (972) 387-4247.

Georgette Klinger
1265 Galleria, Dallas, TX 75240.
Tel: (973) 385-9393.

Estee Lauder Spa, Neiman Marcus NorthPark
400 NorthPark Center, Dallas, TX 75225.
Tel: (214) 891-1280.

Renee Rouleau Skin Spa
19009 Preston Road, Suite 206, Dallas, TX 75252.
Tel: (972) 248-6131, Fax: (972) 248-5826.

Spa Thira
5560 West Lovers Lane, Dallas, TX 7520.
Tel: (214) 654-9800, Fax: (214) 654-9807.

The Spa at the Crescent
400 Crescent Court, Suite 100, Dallas, TX 75201.
Tel: (214) 871-3232, Fax: (214) 871-3281.

Ash Britt Je'Ne Personal Enhancement Spa
206A South Cedar Ridge, Ducanville, TX 78205.
Tel: (210) 223-5772.

Spa Thira
2535 Kirby Drive, Houston, TX 77019-6320.
Tel: (713) 529-2444, Fax: (713) 529-4557.

Tovas Hair Studio & Day Spa
1409 South Post Oak Lane, Houston, TX 77015.
Tel: (713) 439-1414.

Alamo Plaza Spa
204 Alamo Plaza, San Antonio, TX 78205.
Tel: (210) 223-5772, Fax: (210) 228-0022.

UTAH

Silver Mountain Spa
2080 Dust Lane, Park City, UT 84060.
Tel: (435) 655-8484.

Sanctuary Day Spa
36 S. State St., Suite 115, Slat Lake City, UT 84111.
Tel: (801) 533-2720.

Skin Care World
3350 S. Highland Dr., Salt Lake City, UT 87106
Tel: (801) 484-0574, Fax: (801) 487-2870.

VIRGINIA

Bazzak Day Spa
617 King St., 2nd Floor, Alexandria, VA 22134.
Tel: (703) 548-9873.

Circe Day Spa & Wellness Center
116 Commerce St., Alexandria, VA 22314.
Tel: (703) 519-8528.

Petra's Skin Spa
3915 Old Lee Hwy, Suite 21A, Fairfax, VA 22030
Tel: (703) 385-6800, Fax: (703) 385-3675.

Eden Spa
1700 Tysons Blvd., McLean, VA 22102.
Tel: (703) 506-8412.

Estee Lauder Spa
Bloomingdale's, Tyson Corner, 1961 Chain Bridge Rd.,
McLean, VA 22101. Tel: (703) 556-4651.

Elizabeth Arden Red Door Salon
8075 Leesburg Pike, Suite 110, Vienna, VA 22182.
Tel: (703) 448-8388, Fax: (703) 848-0729.

WASHINGTON

Gene Juarez Salon & Spa
Redmond Town Center, 7730 Leary Way Ne, Suite E
155, Redmond, WA 98052, Tel: (425) 882-9000.

Gene Juarez Salon & Spa
601 Pine St., 4th Floor, Seattle, WA 98101.
Tel: (206) 326-6000.

Ummelina Int'l Day Spa
1525 Fourth Ave., Seattle, WA 98052.
Tel: (206) 624-1370.

Gene Juarez Salon & Spa
1139 Tacoma Mall, Tacoma, WA 98409.
Tel: (253) 472-9999.

WISCONSIN

Sports Core Salon and Day Spa
100 Willow Creek Dr., Kohler, WI 53044.
Tel: (920) 457-4444, Fax: (920) 457-0290.

The Watermark Day Spa
319 8th Street South, Wisconsin Rapids, WI
54494. Tel: (715) 423-8808, Fax: (715) 424-2848.

WYOMING

The Body Sage, at the Rusty Parrot Lodge
175 N. Jackson St., Jackson Hole, WY 83001.
Tel: (307) 733-2000.

MARKET PLACE

AROMATHERAPY

The Essential Oil Company
1719 SE Umatilla St., Portland OR 97202
Toll Free (800) 729-5912
Email: catalog@essentialoil.com

Rainbow Meadow
pure essential oils
Toll Free (800) 207-4047
Web: www.rainbowmeadow.com

Young Living Essential Oils
Toll Free (800) 683-1802

ASSOCIATIONS

American Polarity Therapy Association
2888 Bluff St., Ste #149
Boulder CO 80301
Tel: (303) 545-2080. Fax: (303) 545-2161
Toll Free (800) 359-5620
Web: www.PolarityTherapy.org

International Herb Association
PO Box 317, Mundelein IL 60060
Tel: (847) 949-4372. Fax: (847) 949-5896

International Yoga Association
3000 Connecticut Ave., NW Suite 308
Washington DC 20008
Tel: (202) 387-6555. Fax: (202) 332-0531
Web: www.imagroup.com

Relais Santé
Canadian Spa Association. C.P. 971 / PO Box 971, Oka QC
JON 1E0, Canada. Tel: (450) 479-1690. Toll Free (800)
788-7594. Fax: (450) 479-1662. Ms. Jocelyna Dubuc,
president. Email: relais.sante@videotron.ca

HEALTH & BEAUTY AIDS

Aubrey Organics
Natural hair and skin care products. Tel: (800) 282-7394.

Healing Garden
unique line of holistic fragrances for mind, body and spirit.
Tel: (800) 400-1114.

HERBS

Ayurveda Resources
natural herbal health products
Tel: (888) 880-8088

BioForce
The fresh herb company
Tel: (800) 641-7555

Flora
Liquid herbal formulas
Toll Free (800) 446-2110
Web: www.florainc.com

Herbs & More
Tel: (402) 330-4372
Web: www.herbs-more.com

Kneipp
herbal products wellness for daily living
Toll Free (800) 937-4372

Nature's Herbs
Time released herbal supplements. Tel: (800) 437-HERB

Nature's Way
Natural herbs and botanical medicines. Tel: (800)
9NATURE.

Maharishi Ayur-Veda Products
Holistic health care products. Tel: (800) 255-8332.

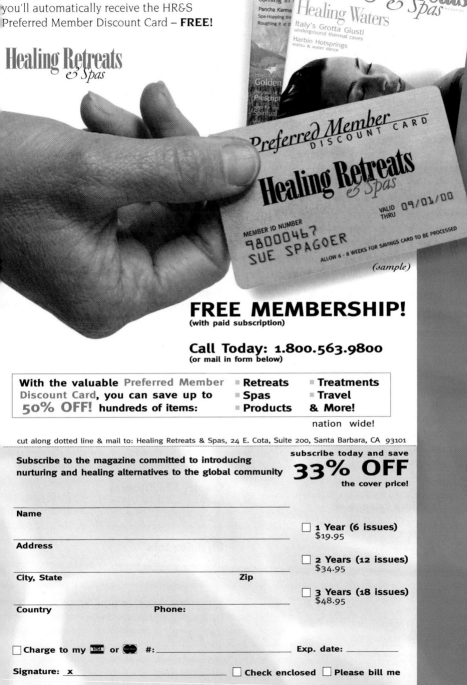

MAGAZINES

Alternative Medicine
21 1/2Main St., Tilburn CA 94920. Tel: (415) 789-8700. Fax: (415) 789-9138.
Web: www.alternativemedicine.com

Cooking Light
The magazine of food and fitness
PO Box 1748, Birmingham AL 35201.
Tel: (205) 877-6000. Fax: (205) 877-6600
Email: letters@cookinglight.com

Eating Well
The magazine of food and health, published by Telemedia Communications, PO Box 1001, Charlotte VT 05445-1001. Tel: (800) 678-0541. Email: EWellEdit@aol.com

Healing Retreats & Spas
Nurturing and healing alternatives for the global community, 24 E. Cota, Suite 101, Santa Barbara CA 93101. Tel: (805) 962-7107. Fax: (805) 962-1337.
Email: walters@grayphics.com

Healthy Living
Magazine for natural remedies, spirituality, stress reduction, diet and exercise. Published by Hearst Communications, 959 Eighth Ave., New York NY 10019. Tel: (212) 649-3220. Fax: (212) 977-4153.

The Herb Companion
PO Box 7714, Red Oak IA 51591-0714
Tel: (800) 456-5835
Web: www.Interweave.com

Men's Fitness
21100 Erwin St., Woodland Hills CA 91367.
Tel: (818) 884-6800. Fax: (818) 716-5626
Web: www.menfitness.com

Natural Health
70 Lincoln St., 5th Fl., Boston MA 02111.
Tel: (617) 753-8900. Fax: (617) 457-0966.

Self
Women's lifestyle magazine, published by The Condé Nast Publications Inc., 350 Madison Ave., New York NY 10017.

Spa
Travel, well being and renewal magazine, 5305 Shilshole Ave. NW, Suite 200 Seattle WA 98107. Tel: (206) 789-6506. Fax: (206) 789-9193.

Spa Vacations
Destinations spas in the USA. Magazine published annually by The Destination Spa Group, 1871 West Canyon View Drive, St. George UT 84770. Tel: (801) 628-8060.

Yoga Journal
PO Box 12008, Berkeley CA 94712-3008.
Tel: (510) 841-9200. Fax: (510) 644-3101
Web: www.yogajournal.com

NUTRITIONAL SUPPLEMENTS

Bodyonics
Longevity age erasers nutritional supplements. Tel: (888) 588-9898.

Country Life Vitamins
Our product line includes an effective combination of herbs, minerals, and vitamins. (888) 476-8647.

Olympian Labs
nutritional supplements. Tel: (800) 473-5883.

Solgar Vitamin and Herb Company
500 Willow Tree Road, Leonia NJ 07605.
Web: www.solgar.com

REJUVENATION CLINICS

Bio Pulse
Toll Free (888) 552-2855
Web: www.biopulse.com

SKIN CARE

Alba Botanica
PO Box 40339, Santa Barbara CA 93140
Web: www.albabotanica.com

Jasön
Natural cosmetics
8468 Warner Drive, Culver City CA 90232-2484.
Tel: (310) 838-7543. Fax: (310) 838-9274
Web: www.jason-natural.com

Reborn
Holistic skin care
248 Todt Hill Rd., Staten Island NY 10314
Tel: (888) 732-6768. Fax: (718) 982-8003
Web: awabi.com/reborn

Zia Natural Skin Care
Tel: (800) 334-7546
Web: www.ziacosmetics.com

TOUR OPERATORS

Custom Spa Vacations
1318 Beacon St., Suite 20, Brookline, MA 02446, Tel: (617) 566-5144. Fax: (617) 731-0599. Toll Free: (800) 443- SPAS (7727). Manager: Naomi Wagman, president. Individual and group services worldwide. Health, stress and fitness holidays in Europe, the USA, the Caribbean, Mexico, Asia and elsewhere. Customized itineraries and programs for weight loss, anti-cellulite, therapies, arthritic diseases, psoriasis and revitalization.
Email: csv@tiac.net Web: www.spatours.com

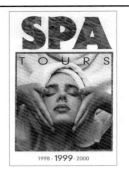
Spa Tours
6033 West Century Blvd., Suite 830, Los Angeles CA 90045. Tel: (310) 417-8726. Toll Free (800) 429-8762. Fax: (310) 417-8369. Health spa vacations and fine tours to 40 spas in 18 countries. Free 48 page SpaTours brochure. Contact: Daniel Zbyvatel.
Email: spatours@aol.com

Spa Traveler
15246 NW Greenbrier Parkway, Beaverton, OR 97006. Manager: Lynn Nicholson. We specialize in the Spas of Mexico, the Caribbean, Central & South America. Call for our free brochure. Tel: (503) 690-8003, Toll Free (800) 300-1565.Fax: (503) 645-7088.
Email: info@spatraveler.com
Web: www. spatraveler.com

Spa World Travel
101 S. Coast Hwy #104, Encinitas CA 92024. Tel: (760) 635-1297. Toll Free (888) 772-9675. Fax: (760) 635-1299.

GLOSSARY

Acupuncture: the insertion of needles into parts of the body, discovered and developed more than three thousand years ago in the Far East.

Affusion Shower: stretched out on a table, the curist receives warm seawater jets over the entire body surface. This technique is in fact a whole-body alternative massotherapy.

Aerobics: rhythmic set of exercises and movements supported by oxygen delivered to the working muscles. Aerobics stimulate the blood circulation, the capacity of the heart and lungs and help burning fat.

Algotherapy: The skin is covered with sea algae and mud, then wrapped in a thalassotherapeutic warming blanket. The progressive heat soothe the muscles.

Anaerobics: exercise and muscular work that is not supported by blood circulation and delivery of oxygen to the working muscles. Weight lifting and body building are examples of anaerobic exercise.

Anthrotherapy: treatments in humid caves where the atmosphere is very vaporous (between 30°c-°42c / 86°F - 107°F); in dry caves the atmosphere takes the heat from the spring (between 50°c-70°c / 122°F - 158°F).

Aqua-aerobics: exercise in a swimming pool utilizing the water resistance to strengthen the body and tone the muscles. This activity is also commonly known as aquacize.

Aquaciser: Equipment that helps you choose the level of activity desired without stressing any joints, muscles or ligaments. It is an ideal introduction to exercise.

Aromatherapy: a full-body massage with fragrant oils in Shiatsu style using flower lavender, jasmine, lemon grass) or other essences with different oils used for different therapeutic benefits (lymph drainage, relaxing, or energizing).

Aslan Therapy: the use of either Gerovital H3 or Aslavital

drugs, both developed by Dr. Ana Aslan of Romania. Both are used for their regenerative effect in fighting the aging process.

Aslavital: a biotrophic drug developed by Dr. Aslan of Romania whose anti atheroscleroyic and neurotrophic effects recommend it especially in the treatment of aging process of the cardio-vascular apparatus and central nervous system.

Athletic Massage: a very deep penetrating massage for the active person that concentrates on all muscle groups, but particularly on the muscles primarily used in the persons sports activities.

Ayurvedic reflexology: a therapeutic treatment that incorporates an ancient healing art from India.

Behavior Modification: elimination of harmful habits such as bad eating patterns, smoking and other substance abuse.

Balneotherapy: generic term for mineral water treatments.

Basic cell regeneration (Dr. P. Niehans method): the renowned professor Paul Niehans is the creator of cell therapy. Live cell therapy is especially efficient in cases where the organs have begun to very slowly weaken and the signs of aging begin to appear. For this reason the treatment should be applied at the first signs of aging as its preventive effect is greater than its curative properties.

Biofeedback: the attempt to give conscious minds the same control over body functions that hypnosis can give in an unconscious state. It offers a greater degree of control over a variety of physiologic events. Many people who suffer from headaches, chronic pains and migraines can use feedback technics to reduce their dependency on drugs.

Body Composition: the relative percentage of each component that make up the total body weight such as fat, lean body mass, and body water.

Boicil Forte: a drug used to treat rheumatic diseases developed by Dr. Vasile Boici of Romania.

Brush and Tone: cleansing the skin with dry brushing to remove the layer of dead skin and increase circulation. Following dry brushing a lotion which nourishes and tones the skin is applied.

Calorie: the amount of heat needed to increase the temperature of 1 kg (2.2 lbs) of water by 1 degree centigrade, from 15°c-16°c. It is most commonly used to express the energy content of food.

Carnial Sacral Work: Carnial work promotes well-being by balancing the autonomic nervous system.

Cellular Therapy: also known as live cell therapy or fresh cell therapy, consists of the injection by an intramuscular route, of fresh embryonic animal cells, typically from sheep or cows, suspended in a physiological serum, or frozen, freeze-dried (lyophilized) cells from ampoules. Used for total body revitalization, to maintain or return the body to its state of healthy equilibrium and prevent premature aging. Developed in the early 1930s by Paul Niehan MD, a Swiss physician, it became popular with wealthy individuals and celebrities as a means of reversing the aging process. Wolfram Kuhnau MD, a colleague of Dr. Niehans introduced the treatment in Tijuana (Mexico) in the late 70s as a cancer treatment. It is also claimed to help build the immune system. In 1985 the FDA banned importation into the USA of all cellular powders and extracts intended for injection. In 1987 the Health Office of Germany suspended the product licenses of live-cell preparations.

Cellulite Treatment: treatments designed to reduce cellulite from the hips, thighs, and lovehandles (in men).

Cenegenics Therapies: Hormone replacement therapy supplementing those hormones as deficiencies are identified. These may include: human growth hormone (hGH); sex hormones (estrogen, progesterone, and testosterone); thyroid, DHEA and others.

Chelation Therapy: Intravenous administration of a synthetic amino acid called ethylenediamine tetracetic acid (EDTA), along with vitamins and other substances, to combat atherosclerosis as an alternative to the conventional coronary bypass surgery.

Chinese "Herbology" Polish: herbal mix containing high concentrates of Alpha-Hydroxy acids for exfoliation to encourage, assist, and enhance the body's own natural processes.

Cleopatra Soaks: hydrotherapy massages with mineral care unique minerals.

Collagen renewal treatment: restore the collagen lost from sun exposure and natural aging with the B2 actigen collagen treatment series. This application triggers your own natural collagen and enhances cellular regeneration.

Combined serum therapy: a general biological treatment for the regeneration of the entire organism.

Crenotherapy: every type of treatment carried out with mineral water, mud and vapor.

Cupping: The antique method of applying heated vacuum to painful areas to treat frozen shoulders, painful knees, and other small injuries.

Deep-cleansing facial: use of sophisticated machines to open pores, extract blackheads by hand, purify skin, close pores, and revitalizes skin.

DHEA: The biological accelerator for aging. It balances the human growth hormone, the sexual hormones, and the thyroid. It is extremely useful to fight a long list of chronic conditions from cancer, obesity to cardiovascular disease.

Douche Affusion (Shower): Soothing and relaxing gushing seawater shower while you lie in comfort and serenity.

Drinking Cures: drinking of mineral waters of various mineral content medically prescribed by amount and frequency by medical staff of spa for treatment of specific medical disorders.

Dulse scrub: a vigorous scrubbing of the entire body with a mixture of powdered dulse seaweed and oil or water to remove dead skin and provide a mineral and vitamin treatment to the skin; a gentle treatment for sensitive skin which leaves the skin incredibly smooth.

Electro-acupuncture: use of an electrical pencil-like instrument which is place on the same acupuncture points which generates current through the tip of the wand without penetration. It is highly sensitive to body heat and thus can pick up trouble spots, immediately.

Electromagnetic Field Therapy: this therapy identifies unbalanced electrical charges that have built up in the tissues and organs - creating the foundation for disease - and corrects them.

Electrotherapy: generic term for the treatment of disease by means of electricity (e.g. nemectron, galvanionization, ultrashort waves, infrared rays, ultraviolet rays, illumination - partial and total baths, diadynamic currents, ultrasound).

Essential Oils: aromatic liquid substances which are extracted from certain species of flowers, grasses, fruit, leaves, roots and trees which are used in the medicine, food and cosmetic industries. The positive effect of essential oils on blood circulation is due to bringing oxygen and nutrients t the tissues while assisting in the disposal of carbon dioxide and other waste products that are produced by the cell metabolism.

European Facial: A custom facial with a complete skin analysis features the benefits of deep pore cleaning which gently removes surface impurities.

Exothermic mud: very rich in magnesium and trace elements, during application the mud releases progressive heat that allows a better penetration of active products. Can be used locally and soothes arthritic pain.

Fango therapy or Fango pack: dehydrated highly mineralized mud is mixed with water or wax (paraffin) and applied as a heat pack to soothe muscles, increase blood flow and sweat out toxins.

Fat: Organic nutrient that provides the most concentrated source of calories . Each gram of fat = 9 calories. Saturated fat is usually of animal origin and can be found in products such as lard, butter and exotic oils. It is known to increase the levels of bad cholesterol in the body; Monosaturated fat is mostly of vegetarian origin such as olive oil, canola oil and avocados. Saturated fat may reduce blood cholesterol levels in the body.Polyunsaturated Fat of plant or fish origin may reduce the cholesterol levels in the body.

Feng Shui: a term from traditional Chinese culture to indicate the proper way to arrange furniture, rooms, houses, offices, churches, tombs, and other humanmade structures with respect to maximizing the favorable energies of location, shape, size, color, weather and other subtle influences.

Finnish Sauna: A simple form of traditional bathing that aims at cleansing the body through perspiration. A pile of stones covering the stove is heated by wood, preferably birch, spruce or pine until it turns red hot. Water is than thrown over the heated stones to generate steam; leafy birch twigs are used to stimulate the circulation by beating the body.

Fresh Cell Therapy: see Cellular Therapy

Gastein Cure: radon treatments taken at the spas of the Gastein Valley in Austria. Radon is a radioactive inert gas which is absorbed into the body, stimulates organic functions and promotes glandular secretion without radiation damage.

Golden Needles: the use of acupuncture applied to the face as an anti-wrinkle program at Clinic La Prairie. The insertion of golden needles restimulates blood circulation, re-intensify the strength of relaxed muscles, and tightens up the face again. A natural alternative to a surgical face lift.

Herbal wrap: linen strips soaked in herbal preparations are wrapped tightly around the body, then the client lies relaxed in a quiet place for a period of time covered by a sheet; opens pores and induces temporary, but not permanent weight loss.

Herbalism: use of plants and plant essence in their natural form to cure instead of synthetic drugs. Herbalism is common to all types of traditional folk medicine and has its roots in Judeo-Christianity based upon the Biblical tree of life.

Herod Wrap: Herod mud wraps with low-sodium Dead Sea mud enriched with Aloe-Vera.

Holistic Medicine: general term for various forms of alternative medicine that include: homeopathy, chelation therapy, clinical ecology, acupuncture, stress reduction, nutritional therapy and other alternative medicine methods.

Holistic Spa: spas focusing on alternative healing methods and nutrition, mainly vegetarian or microbiotic. holistic healing seeks "high level of wellness" integrating body and mind in a higher consciousness.

Homeopathics: Homeopathy alters the basic environment so that infections or degeneration cannot prosper. It is effective in all areas of illness (excepting the mechanical - such as broken bones) reversing situations without need for antibiotics or surgery.

Human Growth Hormone (hGH): After age 25. levels of this hormone decrease sharply. An adequate level of hGH keeps muscle mass firm, stimulates the absorption of calcium and other minerals and allows the body to metabolize nutrients better. The course of treatment 5 shots (1 ampule) every two weeks for 6 months can be repeated every year.

Hydrotherapy: generic term for water therapies using jets, underwater massage and mineral baths (e.g. scotch hose, swiss shower, Vichy treatment, thermal pools).

Immunotherapy: a biological therapy for revitalization and improvement of the immune system that consist of cell therapy, enzymes, placenta and/or vitamins. Some trade names are Omnigen and Transvital.

Inhalation therapy: inhaling steam from hot mineral water, often enhanced with medication or natural herbal substance for treatment of respiratory, pulmonary and sinus problems.

Iridology: The art of reading the iris of the eye as a minia-

ture map of the body's organs.

Japanese Enzyme Bath: a three part treatment that lasts about an hour. First you are served hot enzyme tea, then you submerge in large wooden tubs filled with fragrant blend of cedar fibers and plant enzymes imported from Japan. The enzyme bath stimulates circulation and metabolism.

Kinesitherapy: physical active or passive movement of various areas of the body. Known more generally as physiotherapy.

Kniepp System: highly regarded European therapies using special mineral and herbal treatments. Named after Pastor Sebastian Kneipp (1821-1897). Popular in Austria, Switzerland and West Germany. Kneipp combined the practice of physical exercise with healthy diet and hydrotherapy to achieve physical and emotional well being.

LaStone Therapy: a powerful massage technique combining the healing power of heat and the energies of stones. This patented therapy was developed in Arizona using stones from "the heart of the volcano".

Live Cell Therapy: see Cellular Therapy

Lomi Lomi massage: Hawaiian style traditional massage. Lomi Lomi means "touch with loving hands." Massage strokes are more vigorous, rhythmical, and faster than Swedish massage.

Loofah scrub: full body massage with loofah sponge for exfoliation of skin and renewed circulation. Deep but soft massage of skin and subcutaneous tissues of specific body sites located around lymph nodes. Used extensively for neck, head and shoulders in facial massage.

Magnetotherapy: following an acupuncture treatment a small magnet is taped over the treatment point and left for a period of approximately one week. This provides for a continuos treatment rather than intermittent and thus more efficacious.

Massage therapies: include Athletic Lymph Drainage,

Polarity, Reflexology, Rolfing, Shiatsu, Sports, Swedish, or Trager Body Work.

Massercise: a thermal mask applied to the lower body combined with massage to break up cellulite.

Maternity massage: designed to give relief to the special needs of the mother-to-be.

Medicinal Water: mineral water, which has curative effects that have been confirmed by medical observation and experiments. Medicinal water can be cold or hot, but their curative effect and composition is essential. Most medicinal waters are thermal waters.

Meditation Therapy: A full body massage treatment designed around a meditation session that allows your body to relax and your mind to unwind to the sounds of ocean waves.

Metabolism: the chemical and physical processes continuously going on in living organisms and cells, comprising those by which assimilated food is built up (Anabolism) into protoplasm and those by which protoplasm is used and broken down (catabolism) into simpler substances or waste matter, with the release of energy for all vital processes.

Mineral Water: water from springs and wells, which contain a minimum of 1,000 mgr/l solid components of rare, biologically active elements or compounds, more than a definite value. Mineral waters can be cold or hot, but their composition is essential.

Naturopathy: natural medicine based on the healing power of nature. The term was coined in 1895 by Dr. John Scheel from New York to describe his methods of health care. Naturopaths believe that virtually all diseases are within the scope of their practice. Current methods include: fasting, "natural food" diets, vitamins, herbs, homeopathy, tissue minerals, cell salts, manipulation, massage, exercise, colonic enemas, acupuncture, "Chinese Medicine", natural childbirth, minor surgery, and applications of water, heat, cold, air, sunlight and electricity. Radiation may be used for diagnosis but not for treatments.

Neural Therapy: mini injections of procaine to relief pain

from sport injuries, surgeries, neuralgia, migraines toothaches and tension headaches.

Onsen: Japanese natural mineral hot springs.

Osteopatic Treatment: treatment for recent or chronicle vertebral and articular pains, traumatism consequences, stiffness and muscular strains.

Oxygen treatment facial: scientific method of delivering 87 different vitamins, live enzymes, amino acids and minerals to the skin to treat and prevent environmental damage and to stimulate the production of collagen and elastin.

Pedi-Luve and Manu-Luve: Alternating seawater baths that have a bubbling effect on the hands, arms and feet. Activate circulation in the extremities; help combat venous insufficiency in the lower limbs and help resorb oedemas.

Pell-Amar: a sapropelic mud extract devised by Dr. Ionescu-Calinesti of Romania used in drug or cosmetic form a variety of diseases (e.g. rheumatism, gynecological and skin diseases).

Physiochineitherapy: a therapeutic method that uses heat, light, electricity, mechanical means and movement.

Phytotherapy: use of natural herbs, essences or oils of plants or flora in mud packs, baths massage or inhalation to enhance specific treatments and therapeutic benefits (i.e. eliminate body toxins).

Placenta implants: implantation of a tiny piece of live placenta, generally in a small incision around the waist area, used for the revitalization of the entire system. Placenta regenerates new cells and renews organs and glands retarding aging and helps overcome illness.

Polarity Massage: gentle massage created by the Austrian born Dr. Randolph Stone, designed to release energy blocks and balance the body energetic system.

Polarity Therapy: concept created by the Austrian born Dr. Randolpf Stone, based on principles of energy and a philosophy based primarily on the East Indian Ayurvedic principles. It provides understanding of energy moving through body, mind and spirit. Polarity is designed to balance the body's subtle or electromagnetic energy through touch, stretching exercises, diet and mental-emotional balanced attitude. Polarity seeks to balance the flow of life force through a free flowing exchange between the giver and receiver of a polarity session.

Pressotherapy: Inflatable boots with intermittent and alternating compression that improve circulation by promoting venous and lymphatic factors. Pressotherapy reduces and controls limb oedema by reducing the excess interstitial liquid that causes swelling.

Pritikin Therapy: strict program with a 'military like' attitude toward health, especially the health of the heart. Pritikin insists that one must cut all fat from the diet except for small amounts found in whole grains and vegetables. Use of any kind of animal or dairy products are limited. Use of carbohydrates such as sugar, syrup, molasses, and honey is forbidden, also forbidden are alcohol, salt, soda pop, coffee and black tea. According to the Pritikin Program you can eat - unrefined, complex carbohydrate foods, whole grains, potatoes, vegetables and fruit. Avocados and soybeans are not allowed in the diet. The Pritikin Program does not allow for any vitamins or nutritional supplements and limit the daily fat intake to 10% fat.

Procain (H3) therapy: a therapy based on the revitalization substance H7, a further development of H3 (Aslan therapy). This therapy normalizes and regulates metabolic processes and improves the oxygen supply to cells and tissue.

Reflexology massage: hand, foot or ear massage using pressure points to release blockages and help re-establish energy flows to treat a variety of other sites on the body similar to acupressure.

Reflexology: American concept based on ancient Oriental wisdom. This is a bodywork technic of stroking or applying pressure to one part of the body in order to effect changes in another part of the body, relax muscles, and stimulate the body's own natural ability to heal itself. Reflexology uses foot massage or other parts of the body to effect phys-

iological changes which may trigger psychoemotional benefits. Reflexology is recommended for chronic conditions such as asthma, headaches and migraines.

Reiki with Chakra balancing: *Reiki* means universal life energy. Reiki is a key that opens the door to your heart and helps heal your life. At the inner core of each one of us spin seven wheel-like energy centers called *chakras*. Each chakra reflects and aspect of consciousness essential to our lives.

Rejuvenate: use of therapy to make an organism younger or youthful again; bring back to youthful strength, appearance, etc.

Revitalization: the stimulation of fatigued or ageing organism. The use of therapy to assist an organism in defending itself and resisting the wear and tear of time, ageing.

Repechage massage or facial: combination of masks including herbal or aloe, moisturizing, seaweed and finally clay or mud to create a hardened mask for deepest cleansing and moisturizing.

Rolfing massage: deep, powerful and sometimes painful structural massage technique designed to realign the body skeletal system as used by chiropractors and osteopaths.

Roman bath: heated sea water jacuzzi with jets, equipped with benches for seated bathing.

Salt glo/glow rub: the entire body is massaged with coarse salt and fragrant oils for removal of dead skin and renewed circulation.

Sauna: use of dry heat, less than 10% humidity, to open pores, sweat out impurities and let the body take higher temperatures. After a sauna, a cool to cold shower closes the pores & brings down body temperature.

Seaweed wrap: similar to herbal wraps, using seaweed liquids rich in minerals combined with heat packs to eliminate toxins, remineralize skin and restore skin elasticity.

Scotch hose: standing body massage delivered by therapist with high pressure hoses using hot and cold sea or fresh water within seconds, intermittently, for circulation.

Shiatsu massage: "finger pressure", a cross between acupuncture and massage developed in Japan by Tokujiro Namikoshi in the 40's. Shiatsu is used to treat a variety of illnesses. It can be used to overcome sexual problems and enhance the enjoyment of sexual relations.

Solomon's Coat: hot mud treatments with a unique blend of Dead Sea mud and Donuliella seaweeds and Ylang-Ylang oil.

Sports massage: athletic massage using Swedish massage techniques for deep treatment of specific muscle groups.

Structured Spa: Spas with a strict set of rules whose entire facility is geared towards the achievement of a particular goal such as weight loss, or fitness.

Swan Waterfall: Concentrated warm seawater used to give a potent facial massage as well as localized neck massage.

Swedish massage: manipulation techniques of the body set down by Per Henrik Ling in 1812 using five different movements (long gliding strokes; kneading of individual muscles; percussive, tapping movement; rolling of the figures; and vibration) and oils beneficial to the skin.

Swiss showers: standing full body massage under powerful needlelike jets usually administered by a therapist using hose.

Thalassotherapy: individual baths of sea water equipped with powerful underwater jets for deep massage; or therapist applies manual massage to body with hoses.

Thermal Water: the temperature of water is steadily higher than 35°c (95°F).

Thermotherapy: heat treatment involving the use of various forms of heat for therapeutic purposes.

Thymus therapy: treatments based on the stimulative effect that T lymphocytes or the substances produced by the thymus gland have on the defense system. This therapy restores the immune defense system.

Trager Body Work massage: gentle rhythmic movements developed by Dr. Milton Trager for releasing tension and realigning the body structure.

Underwater Shower: underwater hydromassage with a manually controlled spray to help remove accumulated fat and cellulitis and to soothe tension spots. This treatment is vigorous but not painful.

Ulcosilvanil: a drug devised by Dr. Ioan Puscas of Romania effective in the treatment of ulcerous diseases.

Vichy therapy: combination of Swiss shower treatment and salt glo scrub or loofah scrub.

Waxing: removal of facial, bikini, leg or arm hair by paraffin application and removal.